13th Edition

CHAMBERLAIN'S

SYMPTOMS AND SIGNS IN CLINICAL MEDICINE

An Introduction to Medical Diagnosis

13th Edition

CHAMBERLAIN'S

SYMPTOMS AND SIGNS IN CLINICAL MEDICINE

An Introduction to Medical Diagnosis

Edited by

Andrew R Houghton MA(Oxon) DM FRCP(Lond) FRCP(Glasg)
Consultant Physician and Cardiologist, Grantham and District
Hospital, Grantham, and Visiting Fellow, University of Lincoln,
Lincoln, UK

David Gray DM MPH BMedSci BM BS FRCP(Lond) FRSPH
Reader in Medicine and Honorary Consultant Physician,
Department of Cardiovascular Medicine, Nottingham University
Hospitals NHS Trust, Queen's Medical Centre, Nottingham, UK

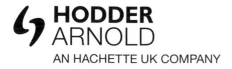

HODDER
ARNOLD

AN HACHETTE UK COMPANY

First published in Great Britain in 1936
Second edition 1938
Third edition 1943
Fourth edition 1947
Fifth edition 1952
Sixth edition 1957
Seventh edition 1961
Eighth edition 1967
Ninth edition 1974
Tenth edition 1980
Eleventh edition 1987
Twelfth edition 1997
This thirteenth edition published in 2010 by
Hodder Arnold, an imprint of Hodder Education, an Hachette Livre UK Company,
338 Euston Road, London NW1 3BH

http://www.hodderarnold.com

© 2010 Edward Arnold (Publishers) Ltd

Whilst the advice and information in this book are believed to be true and accurate at the date of going to press, neither the editors nor the publisher can accept any legal responsibility or liability for any errors or omissions that may be made. In particular (but without limiting the generality of the preceding disclaimer) every effort has been made to check drug dosages; however it is still possible that errors have been missed. Furthermore, dosage schedules are constantly being revised and new side-effects recognized. For these reasons the reader is strongly urged to consult the drug companies' printed instructions before administering any of the drugs recommended in this book.

British Library Cataloguing in Publication Data
A catalogue record for this book is available from the British Library

Library of Congress Cataloging-in-Publication Data
A catalog record for this book is available from the Library of Congress

ISBN-13   978 0 340 974 254

1 2 3 4 5 6 7 8 9 10

Commissioning Editor:	Joanna Koster
Production Editor:	Jane Tod
Production Controller:	Kate Harris
Cover Designer:	Amina Dudhia
Indexer:	Linda Antoniw

Typeset in 10 pt Minion by Phoenix Photosetting, Chatham, Kent
Printed and bound in India

What do you think about this book? Or any other Hodder Arnold title?
Please visit our website: www.hodderarnold.com

Contents

INSTRUCTIONS FOR COMPANION WEBSITE

This book has a companion website available at:

http://www.hodderplus.com/chamberlainssymptomsandsigns

To access the image library and multiple choice questions included on the website, please register on the website using the following access details:

Serial number: kwlt294ndpxm

Once you have registered, you will not need the serial number but can log in using the username and password you will create during registration.

Preface

The student of medicine has to learn both the 'bottom up' approach of constructing a differential diagnosis from individual clinical findings, and the 'top down' approach of learning the key features pertaining to a particular diagnosis. In this textbook we have integrated both approaches into a coherent working framework that will assist the reader in preparing for academic and professional examinations, and in everyday practice. In so doing, we have remained true to the original intention of E Noble Chamberlain who, in 1936, wrote the following in the preface to the first edition of his textbook:

> As the title implies, an account has been given of the common symptoms and physical signs of disease, but since his student days the author has felt that these are often wrongly described divorced from diagnosis. An attempt has been made, therefore, to take the student a stage further to the visualisation of symptoms and signs as forming a clinical picture of some pathological process. In each chapter some of the commoner or more important diseases have been included to illustrate how symptoms and signs are pieced together in the jig-saw puzzle of diagnosis.
>
> E Noble Chamberlain
> *Symptoms and Signs in Clinical Medicine,*
> 1st edition (1936)

We have split this textbook into three sections. The first section introduces the basic skills underpinning much of what follows – how to take a history and perform an examination, how to devise a differential diagnosis and select appropriate investigations, and how to record your findings in the case notes and present cases on ward rounds.

The second section takes a systems-based approach to history taking and examining patients, and also includes information on relevant diagnostic tests and common diagnoses for each system. Each chapter begins with the individual 'building blocks' of the history and examination, and ends by drawing these elements together into relevant diagnoses. A selection of self-assessment questions pertaining to each chapter is also available on the companion website so you can test what you have learnt.

The third and final section of the book covers 'special situations', including the assessment of the newborn, infants and children, the acutely ill patient, the patient with impaired consciousness, the older patient and death and the dying patient.

We are grateful to all of our contributors for sharing their expertise in the chapters they have written. We hope that today's reader finds the 13th edition of *Chamberlain's Symptoms and Signs in Clinical Medicine* to be as useful and informative as previous generations have done since 1936.

Andrew R Houghton
David Gray
2010

List of contributors

Guruprasad P Aithal MD PhD FRCP
Consultant Hepatobiliary Physician, Nottingham Digestive Disease Centre; NIHR Biomedical Research Unit, Nottingham University Hospitals NHS Trust, Queen's Medical Centre Campus, Nottingham, UK

David Baldwin MD FRCP
Consultant Respiratory Physician, Respiratory Medicine Unit, David Evans Centre, Nottingham University Hospitals NHS Trust, City Campus, Nottingham, UK

Christine A Bowman MA FRCP
Consultant Physician in Genitourinary Medicine, Sheffield Teaching Hospitals NHS Foundation Trust, Sheffield, UK

Stuart N Cohen BMedSci (Hons) MMedSci (Clin Ed) MRCP
Consultant Dermatologist, Department of Dermatology, Nottingham University Hospitals NHS Trust, Queen's Medical Centre Campus, Nottingham, UK

Declan Costello MA MBBS FRCS(ORL-HNS)
Specialist Registrar in Otolaryngology, Ear, Nose and Throat Department, John Radcliffe Hospital, Oxford, UK

Robert N Davidson MD FRCP DTM&H
Consultant Physician in Infection and Tropical Medicine, Department of Infection and Tropical Medicine, Lister Unit, Northwick Park Hospital, Harrow, Middlesex, UK

Alastair K Denniston PhD MA MRCP MRCOphth
Clinical Lecturer and Honorary Specialist Registrar in Ophthalmology, Academic Unit of Ophthalmology, University of Birmingham, Birmingham and Midland Eye Centre, City Hospital, Birmingham, UK

Chris Dewhurst MbChB MRCPCH PgCTLCP
Specialist Registrar in Neonatology, Liverpool Women's Hospital, Liverpool, UK

John S C English FRCP
Consultant Dermatologist, Department of Dermatology, Nottingham University Hospitals NHS Trust, Queen's Medical Centre Campus, Nottingham, UK

Jennifer Eremin MBBS DMRT FRCR
Senior Medical Researcher and Former Consultant Clinical Oncologist, United Lincolnshire Hospitals NHS Trust, Lincoln, UK

Oleg Eremin MB ChB MD FRACS FRCSEd FRCST(Hon) FMedSci DSc (Hon)
Consultant Breast Surgeon and Lead Clinician for Breast Services, United Lincolnshire Hospitals NHS Trust, Lincoln, UK

David Gray DM MPH BMedSci BM BS FRCP(Lond) FRSPH
Reader in Medicine and Honorary Consultant Physician, Department of Cardiovascular Medicine, Nottingham University Hospitals NHS Trust, Queen's Medical Centre Campus, Nottingham, UK

Alan J Hakim MA FRCP
Consultant Physician and Rheumatologist, Associate Director for Emergency Medicine and Director of Strategy and Business Improvement, Whipps Cross University Hospital NHS Trust, London, UK

Rowan H Harwood MA MSc MD FRCP
Consultant Physician in General, Geriatric and Stroke Medicine, Nottingham University Hospitals NHS Trust, Queen's Medical Centre Campus, Nottingham, UK

Andrew R Houghton MA(Oxon) DM FRCP(Lond) FRCP(Glasg)
Consultant Physician and Cardiologist, Grantham and District Hospital, Grantham, and Visiting Fellow, University of Lincoln, Lincoln, UK

Martin R Howard MD FRCP FRCPath
Consultant Haematologist York Hospital, and Clinical Senior Lecturer, Hull, York Medical School, Department of Haematology, York Hospital, York, UK

Prathap Kumar Kanagala MBBS MRCP
Specialist Registrar in Cardiology, Department of
Medicine, Grantham and District Hospital,
Grantham, UK

Peter Mansell DM FRCP
Associate Professor and Honorary Consultant
Physician, Department of Diabetes and
Endocrinology, Nottingham University Hospitals
NHS Trust, Queen's Medical Centre Campus,
Nottingham, UK

Philip I Murray PhD FRCP FRCS FRCOphth
Professor of Ophthalmology, Academic Unit
of Ophthalmology, University of Birmingham,
Birmingham and Midland Eye Centre, City Hospital,
Birmingham, UK

Leena Patel MD FRCPCH MHPE MD
Senior Lecturer in Child Health and Honorary
Consultant Paediatrician, University of Manchester,
Royal Manchester Children's Hospital, Central
Manchester University Hospitals Foundation Trust,
Manchester, UK

Hina Pattani BSc MBBS MRCP
Specialist Registrar in Intensive Care and
Respiratory Medicine, Nottingham University
Hospitals NHS Trust, Queen's Medical Centre
Campus, Nottingham

**Basant K Puri MA PhD MB BChir BSc(Hons)MathSci
MRCPsych DipStat PGCertMaths MMath**
Professor and Honorary Consultant in Imaging and
Psychiatry, Hammersmith Hospital and Imperial
College London, London, UK

Venkataraman Subramanian DM MD MRCP
Walport Lecturer, Nottingham Digestive Disease
Centre: NIHR Biomedical Research Unit, Nottingham
University Hospitals NHS Trust, Queen's Medical
Centre Campus, Nottingham, UK

Peter Topham MD FRCP
Senior Lecturer in Nephrology, John Walls Renal Unit,
University Hospitals of Leicester, Leicester, UK

Ian H Treasaden MB BS LRCP MRCS FRCPsych LLM
Honorary Clinical Senior Lecturer in Psychiatry,
Imperial College London, London, and Consultant
Forensic Psychiatrist Three Bridges Medium Secure
Unit, West London Mental Health NHS Trust,
Middlesex, UK

Adrian Wills BSc(Hons) MMedSci MD FRCP
Consultant Neurologist, Department of Neurosciences,
Nottingham University Hospitals NHS Trust, Queen's
Medical Centre Campus, Nottingham

Bob Winter DM FRCP FRCA
Consultant in Intensive Care Medicine, Nottingham
University Hospitals NHS Trust, Queen's Medical
Centre Campus, Nottingham, UK

Chamberlain and his textbook of symptoms and signs

The first edition of *Symptoms and Signs in Clinical Medicine: An Introduction to Medical Diagnosis* was published in 1936 by John Wright & Sons (Bristol). It was written by Ernest Noble ('Joey') Chamberlain and included a chapter on 'The Examination of Sick Children' by Norman B Capon.

At the time his textbook was published, Chamberlain was working at the Liverpool Royal Infirmary as a lecturer in medicine and as assistant physician to the cardiologist Henry Wallace Jones. Prior to this he had served in the Royal Naval Air Service and also as a ship's surgeon, before becoming a physician to outpatients and to the new cardiology department at the Royal Southern Hospital, Liverpool, where he studied for an MSc, his thesis being on *Studies in the Chemical Physiology of Cholesterol* (Munk's Roll, vol. VI, p. 97 © Royal College of Physicians of London).

Chamberlain's textbook was advertised in the *Quarterly Journal of Medicine* (Fig. 1), at a cost of 25 shillings (the equivalent of over £60 today!), and a favourable review appeared in the *Journal of the American Medical Association* (*JAMA*):

> *The text is well written and there are numerous splendid illustrations. The chapters on diseases of the heart and vessels and the digestive system are complete and deserve special commendation.*
> Journal of the American Medical Association
> 1936, **107**: 1997.
> © 1936 American Medical Association.
> All rights reserved.

The textbook rapidly became popular, requiring a reprint within the same year, and a second edition was soon published in 1938. Further editions followed, including special Commonwealth and Japanese editions, and by the time of the eighth edition Chamberlain's textbook had expanded to over 500 pages and was attracting great praise from a reviewer in the *Archives of Internal Medicine*:

> *It is a remarkable course in diagnosis with the eyes; if well studied, it would almost convert a recent medical school graduate into a good diagnostician. The reviewer has never seen anything to equal it.*
> Archives of Internal Medicine
> 1969, **123**: 106–107. © 1969 American Medical Association.
> All rights reserved.

Chamberlain retired from his post as senior physician at the Royal Southern Hospital, Liverpool, in 1964. He died on 9 February 1974, aged 75, the day after he had completed the proofreading of the ninth edition of his textbook. His obituary in the *British Medical Journal* described him as:

> *a consultant physician of the old school. A man of great kindliness and courtesy, he dedicated most of his time to medicine, and equally he lived a full and gracious professional life. We have yet to feel the full impact of losing men of his type.*
> British Medical Journal 1974, **i**: 464, with permission from BMJ Publishing Group.

When the ninth edition (co-authored by Colin Ogilvie) was published, it brought the total number of copies sold to over 100 000. Further editions, still bearing Chamberlain's name, have continued to be published at regular intervals up to the present day.

Recently Published.   Large 8vo.   436 pp., with 282 Illustrations, of which 17 are in colour.
25s. *net, postage* 6d.

SYMPTOMS AND SIGNS IN CLINICAL MEDICINE
An Introduction to Medical Diagnosis.

By E. NOBLE CHAMBERLAIN, M.D., M.Sc., M.R.C.P., Lecturer in Medicine, University of Liverpool; Assistant Physician, Royal Infirmary, Liverpool; Visiting Physician, Smithdown Road Hospital, Liverpool.

With a Chapter on the Examination of Sick Children.

By NORMAN B. CAPON, M.D., F.R.C.P., Lecturer in Diseases of Children, University of Liverpool.

The aim of this book is to help the student and young practitioner to master the technique of medical examination and to apply it to the problems of diagnosis and practice.

'The volume must be counted a fine achievement. . . . The illustrations are well chosen and, together with the rest of the volume, excellently produced.'—*The Practitioner.*

Acknowledgements

We would like to thank everyone who provided suggestions and constructive criticism while we prepared *Chamberlain's Symptoms and Signs in Clinical Medicine*, 13th edition. We are particularly indebted to the following:

- The Health Informatics Unit of the Royal College of Physicians for permission to reproduce their guidance on standards for medical record keeping in Chapter 5.
- The General Medical Council for permission to reproduce extracts from Good Medical Practice (2006).
- The UK Foundation Programme Office for permission to use extracts from the Foundation Programme Curriculum (2007).
- The United Lincolnshire Hospitals NHS Trust for permission to reproduce their 'fast track' breast cancer referral guidelines in Chapter 16.
- The American Journal of Clinical Oncology and the Eastern Cooperative Oncology Group (Robert Comis MD, Group Chair) for permission to use the Eastern Cooperative Oncology Group (ECOG) performance status scale in Chapter 17.
- Miss Hope-Ross, Mr Kumar, Mr Kinshuck and the photographers of the Birmingham and Midland Eye Centre for providing additional photographs in Chapter 19.
- The Child Growth Foundation for permission to use the growth charts in Chapter 22.
- The Society of Critical Care Medicine for permission to reproduce their Guidelines for Management of Severe Sepsis and Septic Shock (2008) in Chapter 23.
- The Academy of Medical Royal Colleges for permission to reproduce extracts from their guideline *A code of practice for the diagnosis and confirmation of death* (2008) in Chapter 26.
- The editors, authors, contributors and publishers of the following textbooks for permission to reproduce photographs and illustrations:
  - Gray D, Toghill P (eds). 2001. *An introduction to the symptoms and signs of clinical medicine*. London: Hodder Arnold.
  - Kinirons M, Ellis H (eds). 2005. *French's index of differential diagnosis*, 14th edn). London: Hodder Arnold.
  - Marks R. 2003. *Roxburgh's common skin diseases*, 17th edn. London: Hodder Arnold.
  - Ogilvie C, Evans CC (eds). 1997. *Chamberlain's symptoms and signs in clinical medicine*, 12th edn. London: Hodder Arnold.
  - Puri BK, Laking PJ, Treasaden IH. 2003. *Textbook of psychiatry*, 2nd edn. Edinburgh: Churchill Livingstone.
  - Puri BK, Treasaden IH. 2008. *Emergencies in psychiatry*. Oxford: Oxford University Press.
  - Ryan S, Gregg J, Patel L. 2003. *Core paediatrics*. London: Hodder Arnold.
- The following organizations for permission to reproduce material:
  - American Medical Association
  - BMJ Publishing Group
  - Cambridge University Press
  - Elsevier
  - Macmillan Publishers
  - Nature Publishing Group
  - Oxford University Press
  - Royal College of Physicians of London
  - Wiley-Liss, a subsidiary of John Wiley & Sons

We are of course grateful to all of our contributors who have given us their valuable time and expertise in preparing their chapters. We would also like to express our gratitude to those patients who have kindly consented to be photographed for educational purposes.

We would like to thank our wives, Kathryn Ann Houghton and Caroline Gray, for their support and patience during the preparation of this book.

Finally, we would like to thank Dr Joanna Koster (Head of Health Science Textbooks), Jane Tod (Senior Project Editor), Lotika Singha (Freelance Editorial Consultant) and the rest of the team at Hodder Arnold for their encouragement, guidance and support throughout this project.

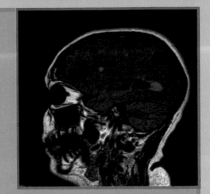

A THE BASICS

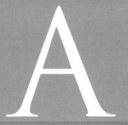

1 TAKING A HISTORY

Prathap Kumar Kanagala

INTRODUCTION

To this day, history taking forms the basis of medical practice worldwide. After all, in the majority of cases, the correct diagnosis can be made from the history alone. Viewed simplistically, the medical history is an exercise in data gathering. This dataset can not only help formulate diagnoses but also ascertain possible causes, assess the impact of illness on patients and guide more focused examination, investigation and subsequent management.

Current practice (see Box 1.1), however, dictates that we adopt a different approach to the history compared with traditional models. We now require a greater volume and quality of information than ever before in order to manage our patients more holistically. Moreover, healthcare professionals are dealing with more demanding and knowledgeable patients with access to masses of information via the internet and other media outlets. Healthcare professionals, in turn, are under different pressures to obtain data. As examples, consider the busy hospital on-call doctor and 10-minute general practitioner (GP) consultations, not to mention medical exams!

This chapter deals with the art of deriving these data effectively through good communication and the concept of set, dialogue, closure.

BOX 1.1 GENERAL MEDICAL COUNCIL – *GOOD MEDICAL PRACTICE* (2006)

Good clinical care must include:
- adequately assessing the patient's conditions, taking account of the history (including the symptoms, and psychological and social factors), the patient's views, and where necessary examining the patient
- providing or arranging advice, investigations or treatment where necessary
- referring a patient to another practitioner, when this is in the patient's best interests.

On the topic of history taking, the Foundation Programme Curriculum (2007) states that the following knowledge is required of foundation doctors:

- symptom patterns
- incidence patterns in primary care
- alarm symptoms
- the appropriate use of open/closed questions.

The Curriculum goes on to say that foundation doctors must develop the following attitudes/behaviours. Foundation doctors must consider the impact of:

- physical problems on psychological and social well-being
- physical illness presenting with psychiatric symptoms
- psychiatric illness presenting with physical symptoms
- psychological/social distress on physical symptoms (somatization)
- family dynamics
- poor nutrition.

Foundation doctors must be able to show empathy with patients when:

- English is not the patient's first language
- the patient is confused
- they have impaired hearing
- they are using complementary/alternative medicines
- they have psychiatric/psychological problems where there are doubts over the informant's reliability
- they have learning disabilities
- the doctor asks appropriate questions on sexual behaviour and orientation
- the patient is a child and the informant is the child and/or carer
- there is a possible vulnerable child/elder protection issue.

The core competencies and skills listed in the Curriculum are listed below.

F1 level:

- demonstrates accomplished, concise and focused (targeted) history taking and communication, including in difficult circumstances
- includes the importance of clinical, psychological, social, cultural and nutritional factors, particularly those relating to ethnicity, race, cultural or religious beliefs and preferences, sexual orientation, gender and disability
- takes a focused family history, and constructs and interprets a family tree where relevant
- incorporates the patient's concerns, expectations and understanding
- takes a history from patients with learning disabilities and those for whom English is not their main language.

F2 level:

- encourages and teaches the above
- checks on patients' understanding, concerns and expectations
- begins to develop skills to manage three-way consultations, for example with children and their family/carers.

COMMUNICATION SKILLS

Most patients are only too willing to volunteer information. After all, many patients think that the more they talk, the more you will be able to help. The key is getting the relevant information through effective communication.

Language

Keep it simple and talk clearly. Study the patient's speech and body language. Matching these can help build rapport quickly. Avoid medical jargon. If it is obvious the patient doesn't understand you, try rephrasing the question, preferably using lay terms.

Active listening

Don't just listen; show the patient you are interested in what they have to say! Adopt an attentive posture, maintain good eye contact, gesture with your hands or nod your head accordingly. Avoid unnecessary interruptions. Summarizing salient points not only suggests you have been listening but can quite often evoke further points that may otherwise have been missed.

Questioning

Begin with a series of 'open' questions, those that are likely to provide a long response:

- 'Why have you come to hospital today?'
- 'Tell me more about these chest pains.'

As the interview proceeds use more 'closed' questions, those that are likely to provide a shorter response:

- 'Any difficulty breathing?'
- 'Any problems with your waterworks?'

Control

Manage the pace and direction of the interview. Patients prefer a doctor who is slightly authoritative. Appearing too laid back or aloof rarely instils confidence.

Signposting

This is the process of telling patients where the interview might go next. As a doctor, use it to steer the patient towards the questions that you want answered. 'Mrs X, that was very useful, thank you. But moving on, could you tell me if you are on any regular medications?' This also ensures a smooth dialogue without any awkward pauses.

Cues

Cues can be verbal or non-verbal and are a way in which patients signpost their real concerns unintentionally and should be explored further.

- 'I'm not going to get admitted am I doctor? I cannot afford to be off work' says Mr Y, constantly looking at his watch
- 'Could it be cancer doctor?' asks Mrs Z, whose mother recently died of colonic carcinoma.

SET, DIALOGUE, CLOSURE

In simple terms, this means knowing what to do before, during and after a consultation. This approach provides a clear structure to the interview, acts as an *aide memoire* for reference, maximizes information and ensures salient points are not overlooked. In fact, the format can be applied to almost any communication skills exercise in medical practice, be it teaching, breaking bad news or even practical procedures!

SET: setting the scene

As stated in the introduction, history taking is ultimately a data-gathering exercise. Even before engaging the patient in medical dialogue, it pays to be well prepared and organized. A few simple steps can get the patient on your side and maximize this information.

Ensure privacy – draw the curtains and make the surroundings as quiet as possible. Read accompanying correspondence (GP/clinic letters), and look through old notes. This provides valuable objective and subjective information from other healthcare professionals. Dress appropriately and in line with local infection control policy.

Introduce yourself and ask the patient how they would prefer to be addressed. Explain your aims, seek consent to proceed and reiterate that all information provided will be handled with confidentiality. These assurances should quickly establish rapport and instil confidence. Patients are more likely to provide intimate personal details if they know your specific role in their care. Note the GP's details in case certain points need to be clarified later (e.g. drug history).

A few moments spent observing the patient and establishing ethnicity, occupation and the spoken language can be extremely useful. Remember, many diseases have associations with particular ethnic groups and occupations (for example: Middle Eastern background – thalassaemia; Caucasian – cystic fibrosis; publicans – alcoholic liver disease; shipbuilders – asbestosis). Would you need a translator? General inspection can provide insight into the patient's functional status. Are they on oxygen, or in a wheelchair?

DIALOGUE: the actual content of the medical history

PC – presenting complaint(s)

The presenting complaint(s) are the main symptom(s), in the patient's own words, that have brought him/her forwards for medical attention. The patient presents with 'passing black motion' not 'melaena'. Simple 'open' questions such as 'What has brought you to hospital today?' or 'What has been troubling you recently?' are often all that is needed to generate this information.

Many patients see this opening gambit as a cue to express all of their symptoms and concerns in a seemingly illogical and disconnected manner. The key is not to fear and not to interrupt! Instead, be attentive and formulate a list of the patient's chief concerns. Contrary to popular belief, this may actually save you time.

HPC – history of presenting complaint(s)

Symptoms are a consequence of dysfunction of an organ system. In most cases, the organ involved gives rise to a classic cluster of symptoms, e.g. pneumonia can cause breathlessness, cough and purulent sputum. The extent of dysfunction largely determines the breadth and severity of the symptoms. At the same time, we know that disease can involve more than one system, similar symptoms can arise from different organs (chest pain – cardiac versus respiratory versus musculoskeletal), and patients can present with multiple diseases. It is the evaluation of these symptoms, through careful questioning, that is dealt with here.

The combination of history of presenting complaints and systems enquiry (dealt with later) should answer the following questions:

- Which system do the symptoms come from?
- How severe are the symptoms?
- How many systems are involved?

As a general guide, explore the following.

- The patient's interpretation of that symptom:
  - 'Exactly what do you mean by palpitations?'
- Duration and onset:
  - 'When and how did it start?'
  - 'Was it sudden or gradual?'
  - 'What were you doing at the time?'
- Severity and functional status:
  - 'What sort of things can you not do now compared with when you were last well?'
- Precipitating, exacerbating and alleviating factors:
  - 'What seems to bring it on?'
  - 'What makes it worse?'
  - 'What makes it better?'
- Previous similar episodes and if so, find out the outcome:
  - 'What was the diagnosis?'
  - 'What investigations and treatments were carried out?'
- Associated symptoms from that system:
  - If the patient has dysuria, ask about polyuria, nocturia and haematuria.
- In addition, if the presenting complaint is pain, determine the:
  - site
  - character (stabbing, squeezing, crushing, etc.)
  - severity (no pain = 0, worst ever =10)
  - radiation
  - temporal relationship (worse at certain times, continuous or intermittent?).

CLINICAL PEARL

A useful mnemonic when taking a pain history is SOCRATES:

- Site
- Onset (sudden or gradual)
- Character
- Radiation
- Associations (other symptoms or signs)
- Time course
- Exacerbating and relieving factors
- Severity

IMPORTANT *i*

'Red flag symptoms' – these are alarm symptoms which, by their very presence, pattern of behaviour or association with other elements in the history, indicate potentially serious underlying medical conditions such as carcinoma. These symptoms warrant prompt assessment and management. Examples include:

- Haemoptysis alone (?carcinoma, tuberculosis, pulmonary embolism)
- Back pain that is getting worse, lasts longer than 6 weeks, is associated with neurological symptoms such as sphincter disturbance, loss of perianal sensation or progressive motor weakness (?cauda equina syndrome)
- Tight central chest pain lasting longer than 15 minutes, with no relief following glyceryl trinitrate spray, in a patient who has diabetes, hypertension and a history of previous percutaneous coronary intervention (?acute coronary syndrome).

PMH/PSH – past medical and surgical history

In chronological order, for each condition specifically enquire about:

- diagnosis – when, where and how?
- complications
- treatment details
- any active problems
- follow-up arrangements (hospital, GP).

CLINICAL PEARL

A useful mnemonic for reviewing the PMH/PSH for commonly occurring and serious conditions is 'MJ THREADS':

- Myocardial infarction
- Jaundice
- Tuberculosis
- Hypertension
- Rheumatic fever
- Epilepsy
- Asthma and chronic obstructive pulmonary disease
- Diabetes
- Stroke

DH – drug history

The reasons for conducting a detailed drug history are numerous and include:

- assessment of the patient's treatment response to date
- the patient's symptoms may be related to drug side effects or interactions
- a medication list can provide valuable clues about the medical history that the patient may have forgotten to mention.

Enquire about current and past treatments. Details should include:

- indications (what was the medical reason?)
- response to treatment
- monitoring (e.g. warfarin and international normalized ratio (INR) checks)
- dosage and frequency (and any recent changes)
- side effects
- compliance:
  - does the patient know the doses and have they ever missed any?
  - do they get any help taking their medications?
  - district nurse administered medications or dosette boxes?
- do they take any over-the-counter preparations (e.g. aspirin) or herbal remedies?
- any illicit drug usage (for recreational or medicinal purposes)?

Allergies and adverse reactions – drugs, chemicals, food

Document any previous allergies and adverse reactions, severity (mild, moderate, severe or life-threatening) and management. This reduces future risk from prescribing errors. Try to ascertain if what the patient had was a true allergy, simple intolerance or troublesome side effects.

SH – social history

Exploring the social welfare of patients is perhaps the least well-practised section (and often the most relevant to the patient) in the traditional history-taking model. Yet, a detailed enquiry can provide the most useful insight(s) into the patient's problems. Often, failure of social well-being and support networks can contribute to illness. Conversely, physical ailments can have detrimental effects on the quality of day-to-day life. Pay particular attention to:

- family and friends (including marital status):
  - their health and relationship well-being
  - frequency of visits.
- accommodation:
  - flat or house
  - nursing or residential home
  - flights of stairs or chair lift
  - toilet location – upstairs versus downstairs
  - modification to appliances – bathroom rails, door handles.

Help
- Who?
  - Family, friends, neighbours
  - Social services, district nurses
  - Meals on wheels
  - Carers
- What with?
  - Cooking, cleaning, dressing, shopping
  - Mobility – any walking aids?
- How often?
  - Once a day, twice a day, etc.

Occupation
- Nature of work – is the illness due to the patient's occupation (e.g. asthma)?
- Consider the effects of illness on work (e.g. any absences)?

Leisure

- Hobbies (e.g. pet birds – psittacosis)
- Smoker? If so, what, and current or previous? Calculate the number of pack-years (see Box 1.2).
- Alcohol? Calculate the average units per week (current recommended weekly allowance is 21 units for men and 14 units for women).

BOX 1.2 SMOKING PACK-YEAR CALCULATION

Assumption: 1 pack contains 20 cigarettes

Pack-years = packs smoked per day × years of smoking

So, 40 cigarettes smoked per day for 15 years = 2 packs per day × 15 years = 30 pack-year smoking history.

FH – family history

The FH provides valuable insight into whether the patient's symptoms are related to a familial condition. Enquiries should be 'open' questions and serve as a screen.

- 'Is the family well?'
- 'Are there any illnesses that run in the family?'

If the answers are positive, construct a detailed family tree (see Fig. 22.2, p. 393). In particular, find out who is affected, the age, health and the cause of death, if known. Remember to be empathetic when discussing these potentially sensitive matters.

SE – systems enquiry

The systems enquiry is sometimes called the systems review, functional enquiry or review of systems. This is a brief review of symptoms from other systems and therefore a screen for illness elsewhere. Ask about:

- general:
  - weight
  - appetite
  - lethargy
  - fever
  - mood
- cardiovascular:
  - chest pain
  - exercise tolerance
  - breathlessness
  - paroxysmal nocturnal dyspnoea
  - orthopnoea
  - ankle swelling
  - palpitations
- respiratory:
  - cough
  - sputum
  - breathlessness
  - haemoptysis
  - wheeze
  - chest pain
- gastrointestinal:
  - abdominal pain
  - indigestion
  - dysphagia
  - nausea
  - vomiting
  - bowel habit
- neurological:
  - fits
  - faints
  - 'funny turns'
  - headaches
  - weakness
  - altered sensation
  - speech problems
  - blackouts
  - sphincter disturbance
- genitourinary:
  - urinary frequency
  - dysuria
  - polyuria
  - nocturia
  - haematuria
  - impotence
  - menstruation
- musculoskeletal:
  - aches and pains
  - joint stiffness
  - swelling.

If any of the answers are positive, explore them in further detail.

Patient's concerns, expectations and wishes

As you take the history, explore how the patient perceives their symptoms and the treatment they

Table 1.1 Example of history taking in a patient with jaundice

	Data	Possible implications
Set		
Inspection	Yellow discoloration Unkempt Tattoos	Jaundice Not coping Hepatitis B and C
Language	Confused, slurred speech	Encephalopathy
Age	Young Elderly	Hepatitis more likely Malignancy
Occupation	Farm worker	Weil's disease
Dialogue		
Presenting complaint	'I've been turning yellow doctor'	
History of presenting complaint(s)	Longstanding symptoms Travel abroad Pale stools, dark urine Blood transfusions Previous similar episodes	Chronic liver disease Shellfish, hepatitis A Obstructive jaundice Hepatitis C Haemolysis, Gilbert's syndrome
Past medical and surgical history	Liver disease Gallstones Diabetes mellitus Recent abdominal surgery	Decompensation of chronic disease Common bile duct stone Haemochromatosis Injury to biliary tract
Drug history	Intravenous drug use Contraceptive pill General anaesthetic	Hepatitis C, human immunodeficiency virus (HIV) Hepatocellular Hepatocellular
Allergies	Any new medications	
Social history	Relationship problems, unemployment Smoking	Alcohol excess Malignancy
Family history	Autosomal recessive	Haemochromatosis, Wilson's disease
Systems enquiry	Cardiac – breathlessness Respiratory – dry cough Gastrointestinal – pale stools Neurology – confused, psychiatric Genitourinary – dark urine Genitourinary – unprotected sex Musculoskeletal – arthralgia	Haemochromatosis (cardiomyopathy) Primary biliary cirrhosis (lung fibrosis) Obstructive jaundice Wilson's disease, encephalopathy Obstructive jaundice Hepatitis, HIV Haemochromatosis
Closure	30-year-old man with jaundice	Problem – hepatitis Cause – viral Examination focus – tattoos etc. Investigations – hepatitis screen etc.

anticipate. Ascertain their health-related goals. This is also a suitable point at which to enquire whether they are happy for information about their illness to be shared with family or friends.

CLOSURE: concluding

Use this opportunity to summarize the main points from the history. Ask about any outstanding issues. Then thank the patient by name. Create a mental list of the patient's problems and the possible causes. Use closure to plan the next few steps: confirming or refuting diagnoses and tackling these problems through focused examination, investigation and treatment.

DIFFICULT SCENARIOS

Despite the best efforts of this chapter, history taking is not always plain sailing! Occasionally, you will face patients from whom data gathering is difficult. This does not mean that the patients themselves are difficult. Do not be prejudiced or judgemental. Their conduct during the consultation could in itself be explained by their underlying problems.

- Are they having difficulties at home, e.g. financial, relationships?
- Is the problem with the hospital itself, e.g. long waiting times, perceived poor previous experience?
- Are there any medical problems, e.g. psychiatric illness, alcohol or drug misuse?

The key to dealing with these scenarios is prompt recognition so that appropriate action can be taken.

The angry patient

Remember that, despite the best intentions or approach, anger can quickly turn to hostility or a physical threat. Be prepared. Inform staff early and position yourself near an exit for that quick getaway!

Key points

- Recognition of anger is usually obvious. Body language can reveal intimidating or aggressive posturing, clenched fists, finger pointing. The spoken language could include shouting, swearing or repeating themselves.
- Pause, be attentive and let the patient vent their anger.

- Acknowledge the situation. Empathize, and apologize if appropriate. ('That is a long time to wait to see a doctor. It must be frustrating. I can understand why it would be frustrating.')
- Attempt to resolve the situation. ('I'll try to find out what caused the delay. It may be avoidable in future.')
- Re-direct back to the interview ('Now that we have resolved the issue, tell me, what brings you to hospital?')

Avoid:

- being defensive
- being confrontational
- criticism of colleagues ('Sounds like Dr X got it wrong')
- taking it to heart.

The reserved patient

Key points

- Remain patient.
- Use 'open' questions. ('Headaches? Tell me more.')
- Actively encourage the patient. Show an interest; gesture approvingly, smile, echo what is being said 'Okay, right, yes'.
- Take control. ('I can't help you as much, without your help.')

Avoid:

- Rushing the patient. Remember – only they know their symptoms.

The 'rambling' patient

Key points

- Use 'closed' questions.
- Summarize.
- Interrupt politely.
- Signpost (re-direct) questions ('I am sorry to interrupt you. I can see you feel strongly about that and I shall try to come back to that later, but for the moment I would like to move on and ask you about your bowels').
- Ask the patient to prioritize symptoms.
- Make them aware of time constraints.

Avoid:

- showing frustration or anger.

The elderly patient

Key points

- The social history is of vital importance in this vulnerable population. Are they at risk from neglect or confusion? Are they coping?
- Visual and hearing loss is common. Ensure adequate lighting is present and hearing aids are working. (If not, move closer.) Speak clearly and perhaps at a slower pace. Write down questions if needed.
- Polypharmacy is frequently encountered with resultant issues of compliance and side effects.
- Dementia may present problems with confusion and memory recall. Look for other sources to corroborate the history (relatives, carers, GP, etc.) and document this.

Avoid:

- making prejudicial statements or judgements. Not all elderly patients are the same!
- patronizing language such as 'dear'.

SUMMARY

Use the principles of:

- set
- dialogue
- closure

to structure your medical history-taking.
Cover the following aspects in taking the medical history:

- PC – presenting complaint(s)
- HPC – history of presenting complaint(s)
- PMH/PSH – past medical/surgical history
- DH – drug history
- Allergies and adverse reactions
- SH – social history
- FH – family history
- SE – systems enquiry
- Patient's concerns, expectations and wishes.

FURTHER READING

Fishman J, Fishman L, Grossman A (eds). 2005. *History taking in medicine and surgery*. Knutsford: PasTest.

Goldberg C, Thompson J. 2004. *A practical guide to clinical medicine*. University of California, San Diego. Available at: http://meded.ucsd.edu/clinicalmed/introduction.htm (accessed 1 November 2009).

General Medical Council. 2006. *Good medical practice*. London: General Medical Council. Available at: www.gmc-uk.org/guidance/good_medical_practice/index.asp (accessed 1 November 2009).

The Foundation Programme Curriculum, 2007. Available at: www.foundationprogramme.nhs.uk (accessed 1 November 2009).

2 AN APPROACH TO THE PHYSICAL EXAMINATION

David Gray

INTRODUCTION

Why carry out a physical examination when twenty-first century imaging using ultrasound, computed tomography (CT) and magnetic resonance imaging (MRI) provide non-invasive, almost 'anatomical' pictures and are readily available in most hospitals in the developed world? These investigations can make clinical examination seem redundant and even 'antiquated'.

However, there are many reasons why physical examination skills will always be important.

- The appropriate *selection* of a test depends upon your differential diagnosis, which in turn is based on your clinical findings. Physical examination can avoid the need for unnecessary tests, thereby:
  - saving time
  - avoiding potential risk and discomfort for the patient
  - saving resources.
- The appropriate *interpretation* of a test result depends on the pre-test probability (see Table 4.2, p. 26) of disease being present, which in turn is determined by the clinical context as judged by your initial clinical assessment.
- You might not have *immediate access* to imaging technology, for instance when:
  - assessing a patient in the community
  - the scanner is not working
  - demand exceeds availability.
- Assessment of *physical examination skills* remains one of the most important components of undergraduate and postgraduate medical examinations.
- There is a great deal of *professional satisfaction* to be gained from the ability to make diagnoses simply by taking a history and examining a patient.

Performing a physical examination should be an active and adaptable process – it is all too easy to get into a 'routine' of examining particular systems in isolation, but it is more useful (and more efficient) to adapt your 'routine' according to the findings you make as you go along.

You should begin with the preliminary differential diagnosis that you have compiled from the patient's history, and then use the physical examination to 'test' the different possible diagnoses in turn, looking for evidence that might support or refute each diagnosis. This 'focused' approach helps to avoid overlooking potentially useful information that might not otherwise be part of a 'standard' systems-based examination (e.g. on finding aortic regurgitation during a 'cardiovascular' system examination, a skilled doctor will go on to look for potential causes in other systems – such as evidence of Marfan's syndrome or ankylosing spondylitis). It also shows where you can safely 'cut corners', so that you do not needlessly perform parts of the examination which are not going to contribute to the diagnostic process.

It takes time, and experience, to accumulate the knowledge and skills to be able to do this well. This is why careful study and plenty of hands-on experience are crucial, and why continuing professional development is so important. Doctors never stop learning.

On the topic of clinical examination, the Foundation Programme Curriculum (2007) states that foundation doctors should demonstrate a knowledge of patterns of clinical signs including mental state. Foundation doctors should:

- be willing to share expertise with other (less experienced) foundation doctors
- consider patient dignity and the need for a chaperone.

The core competencies and skills listed in the Curriculum are given below.

F1 level:

- explains the examination procedure, gains appropriate consent for the examination and minimizes patient discomfort

- elicits individual clinical signs and adopts a coordinated approach to target detailed examination as suggested from the patient's symptoms, with attention to patient dignity
- performs a mental state assessment.

F2 level:

- demonstrates and teaches examination techniques to others
- demonstrates an awareness of safeguarding children and vulnerable adults.

STRUCTURING THE EXAMINATION

First things first

Before you start the examination, make sure that you:

- introduce yourself – a handshake is appropriate in many cultures, but not in all, so if your handshake is declined, offer a smile instead
- gain appropriate consent for the examination
- check the patient knows what you intend to do – intermittent comments such as 'I'm just going to examine your heart' or 'I just want to feel your abdomen' may help your patient to relax
- have available all the equipment you need to complete the examination – sphygmomanometer, stethoscope, ophthalmoscope and otoscope, tongue depressor, gloves (if an internal examination is appropriate), patella hammer, disposable pins for testing sensation
- are standing on the patient's right side
- have adjusted the bed to the appropriate height for your comfort – if the bed cannot be elevated, kneel down if necessary
- have ensured the room or cubicle is well lit, and curtains or screens are adequate to allow privacy
- have checked that the patient is comfortable, and is suitably undressed ready to be examined
- only expose those parts of the body being examined – preserve a patient's modesty at all times, but not to the point where important signs may be missed
- keep a female patient's breasts covered, unless they are the focus of the examination

- always keep the groin covered (in both males and females) to maintain modesty
- ask a nurse to chaperone if you are examining a member of the opposite sex
- avoid causing the patient discomfort at all times.

Although there can be no 'set routine' for clinical examination, the physical examination usually follows a predetermined sequence of:

- inspection
- palpation
- percussion
- auscultation
- when necessary, functional assessment.

In time you will develop your own sequence of doing things. In emergency situations, following the 'A B C D E' principle will serve you well (see Chapter 23); in less acute situations, the history may suggest which system takes priority for clinical examination, and more detailed examination of specific systems may be necessary (Box 2.1).

BOX 2.1 WHEN YOU MAY NEED TO 'CUT CORNERS'...

- Patient A gives a 2-month history of abdominal discomfort. Stools have been darker than normal. His wife had called the ambulance when he collapsed after having passed fresh blood rectally. On admission, he looked pale and was breathless and could not sit up without feeling dizzy. His abdomen is soft but tender. You diagnose a bleeding gastric ulcer. You take an urgent blood sample, request 4 units of whole blood and start intravenous fluids for presumed severe symptomatic anaemia and fluid loss. Once fluid resuscitation has been started, you carry on with the remainder of the examination.
- Patient B has a history of myocardial infarction followed by coronary bypass surgery. He woke up suddenly in the night with acute breathlessness. He arrives in the hospital very breathless, despite the paramedics having given him oxygen therapy on arrival, but he is not in pain. He is drenched in sweat and he says he thought he was going to die. You decide he needs immediate help so you check his blood pressure (120/88 mmHg).

On auscultation, you cannot hear any murmurs, but find fine inspiratory crepitations at the lung bases. You give him an intravenous opiate and furosemide for pulmonary oedema and request an immediate electrocardiogram (ECG). You plan to review him and then complete the examination as soon as the ECG is available.

- Patient C is a young man who is normally fit and active but has been increasingly breathless over the previous 2 days. He has been coughing up bloody sputum and it hurts to breathe deeply. The ambulance crew have given him 28 per cent oxygen. He has a temperature of 38.4 °C, is reluctant to breathe deeply and you hear localized crepitations over the right mid-zone. Suspecting acute lobar pneumonia, you make arrangements for an urgent chest X-ray, full blood count and blood gases and then continue with the remainder of the examination.

Initial impression

Your first impression is important. Start by looking at the patient from the end of the bed. The most important thing to decide is: *does the patient look ill or healthy?* The critically ill patient will usually be lying horizontally and still or slouched, breathing may be intermittent and laboured or rattling *in extremis*. If the patient is ill, start by assessing the system you suspect to be at fault based on the history; this will get easier as you gain experience. By contrast, the patient who is sitting up in bed talking to relatives may have an illness but is unlikely to need your urgent attention.

Some easily obtainable clinical signs convey important physiological information – pulse, blood pressure, temperature and respiratory rate are usually checked by nursing staff as part of their ward routine. Even so, get in the habit of checking these yourself as they may well influence your management.

Some **smells** are characteristic:

- cigarette smoke can linger on clothing long after a person stops smoking
- alcohol on the breath of a patient in a morning clinic

- the sweet smell of ketones (just like pear drops) in diabetic ketoacidosis or extreme vomiting
- the offensive smell of suppurating breast carcinoma or gangrenous ulceration
- the strong smell of melaena
- stale urine in urinary incontinence
- fishy smell of abnormal vaginal discharge.

Patient **colour** can be informative:

- pallor may indicate:
  - *shock* – a reduction in cardiac output, usually accompanied by low blood pressure, tachycardia and clammy skin
  - *anaemia* – a low haemoglobin
  - a natural variant
- cyanosis, a blue discoloration of skin and mucous membranes, which may be:
  - *central* – seen best in the tongue
  - *peripheral* – seen best in the hands and fingernails (prolonged exposure to cold is a common cause)
- yellow tinge – this occurs in *jaundice* – as the serum level of bilirubin increases, it is deposited in the skin (often traversed by scratch marks) and sclera. In haemolytic anaemia, the colour is lemon-yellow
- blue/grey discoloration – may occur in patients taking long-term amiodarone.

The patient's **facial appearance** ('facies') may carry clues to their illness:

- round 'moon face' cushingoid appearance due to endogenous or iatrogenic steroids
- dull, lifeless expression of an underactive thyroid (myxoedema)
- open mouth, epicanthic folds and upward slant of the eyes in Down's syndrome
- expressionless face of Parkinson's disease
- slack jaw and drooping eyes of myotonic dystrophy.

The hands

Nails

- *Clubbing* is sometimes a marker of cardiovascular, respiratory or gastrointestinal disease; occasionally it is inherited.
- *Leuconychia* or pallor and opacification of the nail bed – from chronic liver disease or hypoalbuminaemia.

- *Yellow* – from yellow nail syndrome.
- *Splinter haemorrhages* – seen in vasculitis and endocarditis.
- *Spoon-shaped* – in iron deficiency anaemia.
- *Onycholysis* – or separation of the nail from the nail bed from psoriasis.
- *Transverse lines (Beau's lines)* – in malnutrition and cachexia.
- *Capillary refill* – if you press then release the nail, colour should return in about a second if the circulation is normal.

Palms

- Palmar erythema – reddened thenar and hypothenar eminences, seen in chronic liver disease, pregnancy, thyrotoxicosis, polycythaemia or rheumatoid disease.
- Pale creases – seen in anaemia, haemolysis, or malabsorption of folate or vitamin B12.
- Dupuytren's contracture – thickening and contracture of the palmar fascia causing permanent flexion of the ring or little finger.

Joint deformity

See Chapter 14.

The arterial pulse

Check the radial pulse for rate (time over 10 seconds), rhythm (sinus rhythm is regular, ectopic beats interrupt an otherwise regular rhythm, while in atrial fibrillation the pulse is irregularly irregular), character (the wave form is slow rising in aortic stenosis and falls away rapidly in aortic regurgitation) and volume (normal or low). The left radial pulse should be equally palpable, and there should be no radial–radial or radio-femoral delay (see Chapter 7). Aortic regurgitation may cause the pulse to have a collapsing quality – but ask about pain in shoulder before lifting it up.

The face

- Perform a general inspection of facial appearance as outlined earlier in this chapter.
- The eyes may show an arcus (a white line around the iris suggestive of familial hypercholesterolaemia, but common in old age) and the sclerae should be white.

- Mucous membranes should be pink.
  - Check the mouth for central cyanosis, for dental hygiene and for mouth ulcers, which are occasionally seen in Crohn's disease and coeliac disease.
  - Fungal infection in the mouth causes white spots (candidiasis), often seen after treatment with steroids, chemotherapy or broad spectrum antibiotics, which changes the natural flora.
- The tongue may be:
  - *coated*, especially in smokers, but this is rarely associated with disease
  - smooth (*glossitis*) due to atrophied papillae, seen in iron, folate and vitamin B12 deficiency and in alcoholics
  - enlarged (*macroglossia*) in Down's syndrome or when infiltrated with tumour.

The neck

- Look at the neck for the jugular venous pressure (JVP) – this is an indirect measure of pressure in the right side of the heart, the pulsations reflecting changes in the right atrium (see Chapter 7).
- Palpate the carotid arteries for pulse volume and character.
- Examine the neck for lymph nodes and move behind the patient to check the thyroid – it is normal for it to rise on swallowing.

The praecordium

Inspect the praecordium for signs of deformity and for surgical scars. Then, use palpation to assess the position of the apex beat, the most lateral and downward point at which the tip of the heart can be felt, and also its character (Chapter 7). In thin people, pulsation of the apex may be visible.

Next, feel for a *parasternal heave* with the heel of your hand – if the right ventricle has to work hard (right ventricular hypertrophy) to eject blood (e.g. pulmonary hypertension), you will be able to feel its impulse easily. Place your hand over the upper chest and then the lower chest to feel for vibrations or valvular *thrills* (not often felt, but when present they are indicative of a significant valve lesion).

Auscultate the heart and simultaneously palpate the arterial pulse so that you know when systole occurs (a murmur coinciding with a palpable pulse means the murmur must be systolic; if murmur and pulse alternate, the murmur is diastolic). Use the bell of the stethoscope at the apex, the best place to hear mitral stenosis – if you hear a loud first heart sound (the easiest sound to hear) then listen carefully for a diastolic murmur characteristic of mitral stenosis (on a busy noisy ward you might not hear the murmur, but you should still hear the loud first heart sound). Using the diaphragm, listen in the same area for the first and second sounds and any murmurs. Listen in the axilla for radiation of a pansystolic murmur of mitral regurgitation.

Move the stethoscope in stages to the lower left sternal edge, then up towards the upper right sternal edge. An ejection systolic murmur here is likely to be aortic stenosis – it should be heard over the carotids (easier to hear if the patient stops breathing for a few seconds to eliminate breath sounds). Sit the patient forward – this makes aortic regurgitation easier to hear and gives you an opportunity to check for sacral oedema.

CLINICAL PEARL

Making sense of murmurs

Try to put all the pieces together as you examine the cardiovascular system. Make things simple by:

- palpating a large pulse (brachial or carotid artery) so that you can time the murmur – if the pulse and murmur coincide, the murmur must be systolic; if they alternate, then it must be diastolic. In clinical practice, systolic murmurs are more common
- asking the patient to breathe *in* deeply if you are unsure whether a murmur might be from the right side of the heart or the left: increased venous return on inspiration enhances *right*-sided murmurs; left-sided murmurs get louder if the patient breathes *out*, as the insulating effect of air in the lungs is removed
- tricuspid regurgitation is *the murmur you see rather than hear* (large 'v' waves in the JVP in time with the pulse), as it can be quiet
- position the patient to optimize sound from any murmur – for mitral regurgitation, roll the patient well onto their left side; for aortic valve disease, sit the patient up.

The lungs

Now watch the patient breathe – the lungs should expand symmetrically; disease may prevent one side moving as much as the other (Chapter 8). Ask the patient to take a deep breath if there is any doubt. Check the position of the trachea, it should be central but may be pushed or pulled to one side by disease. Now percuss the lungs – mentally divide the lungs into upper, middle and lower zones, put your left hand firmly on the left chest wall upper zone and tap the left middle finger with the right. A normal percussion note is resonant, dullness may indicate an effusion or infection and hyper-resonance an over-inflated chest. Repeat over the right upper zone so you can compare the left and right sides. Repeat over the middle and lower zones on the front of the chest. Check for transmission of breath sounds through the chest wall with the edge of the hand:

- *tactile vocal fremitus* – ask the patient to say '99' and you can 'feel' the vibration

or

- *vocal resonance* – ask the patient to say '99' and listen with the scope.

If the sounds are louder than normal, this indicates a disease process.

Now listen with the stethoscope in the same areas that you percussed – breath sounds are normally heard during all of inspiration and the first part of expiration ('vesicular'). Reduced sounds occur with airways obstruction as in asthma (a 'silent chest' is an ominous sign) and emphysema. Sit the patient forward, observe respiratory movements again and repeat percussion and auscultation on the back of the chest.

You may hear additional sounds – a musical wheeze can occur in asthma and bronchitis, fine crackles in heart failure and fibrosis.

The abdomen

Expose the patient's abdomen for examination. The patient should be lying flat on the bed. Observe the abdomen moving with respiration. In thin people you may see pulsation of the abdominal aorta, peristalsis and the edge of an enlarged liver. The abdomen is normally slightly concave; any swelling due to fluid (ascites) tends to gravitate to the flanks, but with massive ascites the umbilicus becomes everted and venous drainage may be altered by portal hypertension. The skin may have striae, especially after pregnancy or weight loss. In Cushing's syndrome, striae may appear purple. The location of surgical scars is usually a clue to the type of operation performed.

Next, make sure your hands are warm ready to palpate the abdomen. Ask if any area is painful or tender. Using the palmar surface of your right hand, gently press your hand into each of the abdomen's nine segments in turn. You may elicit pain as you do, so watch the patient's face. After one 'circuit', perform a second circuit, this time using firmer pressure and visualizing the anatomy of abdominal organs (Table 2.1). It takes considerable practice to learn what is normal, but you may feel the liver, spleen, kidneys and colon easily in thin people.

Table 2.1 Which organ is it?

Organ	How to identify it
Liver	Expands below costal margin on right
Spleen	Emerges from left costal margin Cannot get hand between costal margin and spleen Enlarges towards right iliac fossa in line of ninth rib Dull to percussion – anterior to bowel gas May be notched More easily felt with patient lying on right side
Kidneys	Move downwards on inspiration Resonant to percussion – posterior to bowel gas Can get hand between costal margin and kidney

Liver

If you ask the patient to take a deep breath, you will feel the liver being pushed down towards your hand placed just below the costal margin – use the edge of your hand rather than your fingertips (Fig. 2.1a). The edge should be smooth, firm, non-tender and

CLINICAL PEARL

Sometimes a normal liver may appear to be enlarged – a Riedel's lobe, a projection of the right lobe of the liver towards the right iliac fossa, can be deceiving.

The gallbladder is occasionally felt just below the liver as a rounded mass that moves downwards on inspiration. Even a grossly enlarged gallbladder may be impalpable.

The spleen enlarges to emerge from the left costal margin towards the right iliac fossa; in inspiration, the spleen moves this way too, in the line of the ninth rib. It is best felt using a two-hand technique (Fig. 2.2). Place the left hand over the left lower ribs and the right hand on the abdomen, starting below the umbilicus. If you start too near the costal margin, you may miss a large spleen. As the patient breathes in, you may feel the spleen move downwards; if not, move your right hand closer to the costal margin. If no spleen is felt, roll the patient onto the right side and try again; a spleen has to be about twice its normal size to be palpable. The spleen may be notched when swollen.

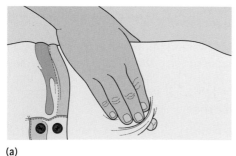
(a)

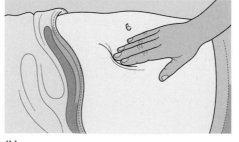
(b)

Figure 2.1 (a) Start palpation of the liver with the index finger parallel to the lower border of the liver; this will enable you to assess the general size of the liver. (b) Define the edge more accurately with the fingers parallel to the long axis of the body. From: Gray D, Toghill P. (eds), *An introduction to the symptoms and signs of clinical medicine*, with permission. © 2001 London: Hodder Arnold.

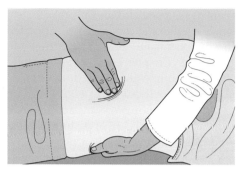

Figure 2.2 Palpation of the spleen. From: Gray D, Toghill P. (eds), *An introduction to the symptoms and signs of clinical medicine*, with permission. © 2001 London: Hodder Arnold.

well defined – use your fingertips to define the liver edge more accurately (Fig. 2.1b). The surface in disease may be hard, tender and irregular and occasionally pulsatile in tricuspid regurgitation.

Kidneys

The kidneys move down on inspiration; the left is more easily felt than the right. The kidneys also require a bimanual technique (Fig. 2.3). Start with the right kidney – place your left hand underneath the patient's right loin and your right hand over their right upper abdominal quadrant. Gently bring the hands together to feel the kidney between your fingers. You should try to bounce the kidney upwards with your left hand towards the right. Reverse the hands to feel the left kidney. The kidneys have a dull percussion note contrasting with resonant bowel gas.

Organ size

Having palpated the major organs, you need to percuss these in turn to confirm organ size. The upper limit of the liver is normally level with the sixth rib in the mid-clavicular line. This can be defined by percussing down from the mid-chest until the percussion note changes from resonant (over lung) to dull (over liver). The lower limit of the liver is very variable and normally is protected by the ribs. The maximum size of the normal liver is about 13 cm, but clinical examination may underestimate by up to 5 cm. In disease, it usually enlarges downwards, though in emphysema it may be pushed down due to hyperinflation. Start percussing in the right iliac

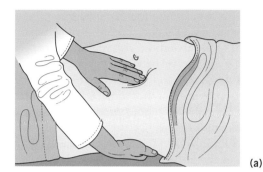

(a)

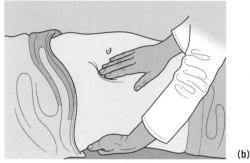

(b)

Figure 2.3 Palpation of (**a**) the left and (**b**) the right kidney. From: Gray D, Toghill P. (eds), *An introduction to the symptoms and signs of clinical medicine*, with permission. © 2001 London: Hodder Arnold.

fossa and gradually work your way upwards; when you reach the lower edge, the note will change from resonant (due to bowel gas) to dull (over the liver's solid tissue).

Spleen

To percuss the spleen, start again in the right iliac fossa, this time percussing towards the left costal margin; you may need to percuss over the lower ribs. When you reach the spleen, the note will change from resonant to dull.

Bladder

You can recognize the bladder as an area of suprapubic dullness.

Ascites

Large amounts of fluid (about 2 L) in the abdomen (ascites) can collect in the flanks under the influence of gravity, lifting up the gas-containing bowel; this can be detected using percussion. Start percussing in the midline and map out the areas of dullness (fluid) and resonance (gas). Keeping the flat of your hand on the left side of the abdomen, with your middle finger demarcating the border between dullness and resonance, ask the patient to roll over towards you. Wait about 15 seconds to allow the fluid to redistribute due to gravity. The percussion note under your hand will change – the dull area will become resonant if there is ascites. Another way to detect ascites, particularly if massive, is to ask the patient to put the medial edge of their hand firmly on the middle of their abdomen; a flick of the abdomen on one side will be transmitted to the other, easily palpable by your hand.

Rectum

Finally, carry out a rectal examination. Place the patient in the left lateral position with the knees drawn up. Check for piles, skin tags (seen with piles or Crohn's disease), rectal prolapse or fistula. Ask the patient to strain and bear down; note any incontinence, leakage or prolapse. Now, with the patient relaxed, insert a gloved and lubricated finger gently into the anus; the sphincter will relax if the patient breathes quietly. Palpate the anterior rectal wall for:

- the prostate in men – this is normally rubbery with a central furrow, obliterated in prostatic hypertrophy or hard and nodular in prostatic cancer
- the cervix in women.

The finger is advanced as far as possible and withdrawn; check the glove for blood.

The legs

Check the major pulses in both legs – femoral, popliteal, dorsalis pedis and posterior tibial. Then check for peripheral oedema by gently pressing over the medial side of the tibia for a few seconds. When you remove your finger, the presence of a dimple that gradually fills in confirms pitting oedema.

The nervous system

Now it is time to examine the nervous system. You may well have formed some opinion about the integrity of the nervous system already from the patient's speech and understanding during the history and from the patient's movements during the clinical examination. Start with the cranial nerves, and then examine the peripheral nervous system; these are described in detail in Chapter 12.

The above is an outline of a basic clinical examination which will suffice for most patients. There are many other signs that you might come across, some eponymous, many of which are of historical value only. In appropriate circumstances, you may need to conduct a detailed examination of the genitourinary (Chapter 11), musculoskeletal (Chapter 14), endocrine (Chapter 15) or haematological systems (Chapter 17).

SUMMARY

The physical examination usually follows a predetermined sequence of:

- inspection
- palpation
- percussion
- auscultation
- when necessary, functional assessment.

A 'standard' physical examination includes an assessment of:

- initial impression:
  - does the patient look ill or healthy?
  - pulse, blood pressure, temperature and respiratory rate
  - characteristic smells
  - patient colour can be informative: pallor; cyanosis; jaundice; blue/grey discoloration (amiodarone)
  - facial appearance ('facies')
- hands:
  - nails
  - palms
  - joint deformity
- arterial pulses
- head
- neck
  - jugular venous pressure (JVP)
  - carotid arteries
  - lymph nodes
  - thyroid

- praecordium:
  - inspect for deformity and surgical scars
  - apex beat
  - heaves and thrills
  - auscultate the heart
- lungs:
  - observe while the patient breathes
  - check the position of the trachea
  - percuss the lungs
  - check tactile vocal fremitus and vocal resonance
  - auscultate with the stethoscope
- abdomen:
  - inspect the abdomen
  - palpate the abdomen
  - liver
  - spleen
  - kidneys
  - ascites
  - rectal examination
- legs
- nervous system:
  - cranial nerves
  - peripheral nervous system.

In appropriate circumstances, you may need to conduct a detailed examination of the genitourinary (Chapter 11), musculoskeletal (Chapter 14), endocrine (Chapter 15) or haematological systems (Chapter 17).

FURTHER READING

Douglas G, Nicol F, Robertson C. 2009. *Macleod's clinical examination*, 12th edn. Edinburgh: Churchill Livingstone.

Epstein O, Perkin GD, Cookson J, *et al.* 2008. *Clinical examination*, 4th edn. London: Mosby.

Talley NJ, O'Connor S. 2005. *Clinical examination: a systematic guide to physical diagnosis*, 5th edn. Edinburgh: Churchill Livingstone.

The Foundation Programme Curriculum, 2007. Available at www.foundationprogramme.nhs.uk (accessed 1 November 2009).

3 DEVISING A DIFFERENTIAL DIAGNOSIS

David Gray

INTRODUCTION

After taking a history, completing an examination, and writing up your findings, you will need to give some thought as to the cause of your patient's symptoms. A diagnosis is the most rational explanation for the symptoms and signs that your patient has. It may be immediately obvious – the thunderclap headache of a subarachnoid haemorrhage, the facial droop and unilateral weakness of a stroke, or a knife still sticking out of the chest wall.

Many diseases present with 'classic' symptoms and signs, and to make a diagnosis all you have to do is recognize the pattern. For example, an undergraduate student presents complaining of feeling unwell for a couple of days, a severe headache, fever, photophobia and a stiff neck. On examination, the temperature is 38 °C; the patient cannot voluntarily flex the cervical spine, and when you try to flex it, there is obvious resistance. You cannot examine the fundi, because 'the bright light is too painful'. There is a petechial rash. You decide that the constellation of symptoms and signs is characteristic of meningococcal meningitis.

But what if the diagnosis is not so obvious and you remain unsure as to the cause of the presenting symptoms? Usually, the history provides the key. In a study of diagnoses made in the outpatient department, 83 per cent of cases were diagnosed on the basis of the referral letter and history alone (Hampton et al., 1975). So the first thing you should do in this setting is to review the history, asking more questions of the patient, relatives and if necessary the general practitioner. Try to establish a clear timeline of events:

- When was the patient last completely well?
- What was the first clue that things weren't quite right?
- What happened next?

On the topic of diagnosis and clinical decision-making, the Foundation Programme Curriculum (2007) states that foundation doctors should demonstrate knowledge of the principles of clinical reasoning in medicine. Foundation doctors should understand the impact on differential diagnosis of the different clinical settings of primary and secondary care.

The core competencies and skills listed in the Curriculum are given below.

F1 level:

- establishes a differential diagnosis/problem list in the order of likelihood/importance on the basis of information available. This should include a principal or working diagnosis and diagnoses which (though less likely) are too important to be missed
- constructs a management plan including investigations, treatments and requests/instructions to other healthcare professionals (taking account of ethnicity and the patient's cultural or religious beliefs and preferences as well as wishes)
- pursues further history, examination and investigation in the light of the differential diagnosis
- makes a judgement about prioritizing actions on the basis of the differential diagnosis and clinical setting.

F2 level:

- describes the different epidemiology of patient presentations in primary and secondary care
- takes account of probabilities in ranking differential diagnoses
- helps other foundation doctors prioritize their actions.

THE DIFFERENTIAL AND WORKING DIAGNOSES

You may find that there are several possibilities for an illness. Start by listing all the diseases that *might* explain the problem facing you. There should be sufficient information for you to at least decide which body system is likely to be at fault. Medical problems may of course affect more than one body system, but this in itself reduces the range of likely diseases – connective tissue and autoimmune disorders commonly wander through body systems. Examples include:

- rheumatoid disease, which classically affects peripheral joints but systemic features such as fever, weight loss and malaise may be prominent and body secretions can dry up, causing dry eyes or dry mouth (Sjögren's syndrome)
- vasculitis causing gut ischaemia, stroke, peripheral gangrene or destructive changes in the nerves leading to a mononeuritis multiplex.

If you 'get stuck', systematically go through the information you have and make a short list of all possible diagnoses that spring to mind – you will probably end up with three or more illnesses to consider. These may all be within a single body system. For example, you may think that the cause of a person's breathlessness, cough and blood-stained sputum is entirely due to some form of disease process within the respiratory system, but are not sure *which* disease, your differential diagnosis being lobar pneumonia, carcinoma bronchus and bronchiectasis. You can now consider which investigations are the most appropriate to eliminate two of these so that you end up with a firm diagnosis.

The cause of a patient's breathlessness may lie outside the respiratory system and there may be features in the history and examination that make you consider:

- a cardiovascular cause (history of ischaemic heart disease, sudden onset of symptoms, bi-basal crepitations)
- a metabolic disorder (patient has 'air hunger', you can smell ketones as you enter the treatment area)
- a haematological problem (deathly pale appearance, petechial haemorrhages appear under the blood pressure cuff).

So the best advice is to:

- think broadly
- remember that 'common things occur commonly' and rare things really are 'rare'.

When devising your list, you should put the most likely diagnosis first – this is the *working diagnosis*, the one that will shape your treatment plan, at least until you have more information to add more certainty to your diagnosis.

By listing the possible diagnoses in rank order, you will have devised a *differential diagnosis*. This allows anyone reading the notes to appreciate:

- what *you* made of the presenting features when *you* saw the patient
- what other diagnoses were not considered at the time (but may be considered later when the clinical picture may have developed).

The differential diagnosis will allow you to:

- decide whether your patient may have a life-threatening disease
- arrange appropriate investigations to confirm or refute the various diagnoses
- plan treatment based on the most likely cause, the number one in your differential diagnosis, the *working diagnosis*.

Think about it...

Your basic clinical knowledge can help you eliminate a lot of potential diagnoses, even if you don't know a great deal about them. Take the example of a 55-year-old man who has just come in to your ward; an hour previously, he suddenly found it difficult to breathe. There are several things to consider:

- What is a common cause of breathlessness? Rather than think of *individual* disease processes, think first in *systems,* then specific diseases within each system. Cardiac and respiratory causes are the most common, but if nothing in the history or examination points towards these, think of less common problems as the underlying cause:
  - neurological problems (phrenic nerve lesion, Guillain–Barré syndrome)
  - haematological problems (anaemia)
  - metabolic problems (diabetic ketoacidosis)
- What is common in your area? Clearly, diseases that a man living in the middle of a city in the UK might have would be different from those that a man living in the middle of Kenya might have.

- Which diseases might cause breathlessness of *sudden* onset?
  - Pulmonary embolism would be high up the list if he had recently undergone surgery or undertaken a long-haul flight.
  - Myocardial infarction - if he had 'tight' central chest pain.
- Which diseases might a *middle-aged man* have?
- What associated features might help distinguish one cause from another?

What if you are really stuck?

Some presenting complaints are fairly non-specific and so the differential diagnosis can be very wide – a headache may be due to:

- extracranial disease – including stress, fever associated with an upper respiratory tract infection, a mechanical problem such as cervical spondylosis, heat stroke, trauma, herpes zoster, dental disease, cluster headache
- a serious intracranial event – such as subarachnoid haemorrhage or cerebral tumour
- miscellaneous conditions such as drug side effects, carbon monoxide inhalation or poisoning with lead.

The list seems endless. In these circumstances, attention to detail in the history and examination may pay dividends. You are going to need advice from a more senior colleague.

Outside assistance

You can also get some help from books such as *French's index of differential diagnosis*. Your hospital may have constructed some diagnostic algorithms, a step-by-step method of solving a problem or making a decision (e.g. http://med.oxfordradcliffe.net/guidelines/PE). Computer-based diagnostic decision support software can help with diagnosis. Because medical diagnosis is inherently probabilistic, decision support systems or artificial intelligence can be harnessed to assist in diagnosis in a range of illnesses (e.g. acute abdominal pain). Such systems may have been approved for use in your hospital.

SUMMARY

- Take a thorough history – the better the history, the more likely you will be to make a diagnosis.
- If you are faced with a complex problem, be prepared to think widely and then devise a short list or differential diagnosis.
- If you are having problems, you may need to go back to the patient and ask more searching questions, or obtain some collateral history from the patient's relatives or general practitioner.
- Do not be afraid to discuss cases with your more senior colleagues.
- As you become more experienced, your diagnostic abilities will improve.
- Until then, read widely and follow any locally available diagnostic algorithms.

FURTHER READING

Ellis H, Kinirons M (eds). 2005. *French's index of differential diagnosis: an A–Z.* London: Hodder Arnold.

Hampton JR, Harrison MJ, Mitchell JRA, *et al.* 1975. Relative contributions of history-taking, physical examination and laboratory investigation to diagnosis and management of medical outpatients. *British Medical Journal* **2**: 486–489.

Hopcroft K, Forte V. 2007. *Symptom sorter*, 3rd edn. Oxford: Radcliffe Publishing.

Raftery AT, Lim E. 2005. *Churchill's pocketbook of differential diagnosis*, 2nd edn. Edinburgh: Churchill Livingstone.

The Foundation Programme Curriculum, 2007. Available at: www.foundationprogramme.nhs.uk (accessed 1 November 2009).

4 ORDERING BASIC INVESTIGATIONS

David Gray

INTRODUCTION

Having taken a history, performed a clinical examination and constructed a differential diagnosis, your next step is to consider what investigations are needed to:

- confirm that the most likely diagnosis, the *working diagnosis*, is correct
- exclude other potential diagnoses.

On the topic of investigations, the Foundation Programme Curriculum (2007) states that for each of the investigations listed in Table 4.1, foundation doctors should be able to:

- explain the investigation to patients
- explain why it is needed
- explain the implications of possible and actual results
- gain informed consent.

For all investigations it is vital that foundation doctors are able to recognize abnormalities that need immediate action. They should also be able to:

- recognize the need for an investigation result to impact on management
- avoid unnecessary investigations
- recognize that investigation reports often require the opinion of another professional who will need relevant information on the request form
- recognize that reports may need reviewing as circumstances change
- act on the results in a timely and appropriate fashion
- prioritize the importance of results and ask for help appropriately
- chase results when they have not arrived in a timely fashion.

The core competencies and skills listed in the Curriculum are given below.

F1 level:

- requests common investigations appropriate for patients' needs
- discusses, to the patient's level of expertise, the risks, possible outcomes and (when available) the results
- recognizes normal and abnormal results in adults
- prioritizes importance of results and asks for appropriate help
- ensures results are available and timely.

F2 level:

- supports F1 doctors or students in requesting, interpreting and acting on the results of common investigations
- understands local systems and asks for appropriate help.

Confirming and excluding diagnoses

Imagine a patient presenting with chest pain and breathlessness, where your differential diagnosis is:

- acute myocardial infarction
- pulmonary embolus
- reflux oesophagitis
- musculoskeletal chest pain.
  You would order investigations to:
- confirm the clinical impression you formed after taking a history and examination – for example, an electrocardiogram (ECG) that shows ST segment elevation in chest leads V2–V6 confirms your most likely diagnosis of an acute myocardial infarction (in this case an acute *anterior* myocardial infarction); this test also helps to rule out other pathologies as the cause of the symptoms
- refute other conditions as the cause of symptoms – for instance, a computed tomography (CT) pulmonary angiogram, or a lung ventilation–perfusion scan, to exclude a pulmonary embolus

Table 4.1 Frequently used investigations that foundation doctors should be able to select, appropriately request and accurately interpret reports for[1]

Investigation	Knowledge	Skills
Full blood count	Circumstances requiring urgent results	Use results reporting system
Urea and electrolytes	Significance of major abnormalities and general irrelevance of minor variations from 'normal' values	Record and tabulate where appropriate
Blood glucose	When to initiate pregnancy testing	Interpret results and know when to request further specialist advice
Cardiac markers	Where to look up age-related reference ranges for children	
Liver function tests		
Amylase		
Calcium and phosphate		
Coagulation studies		
Arterial blood gases		
Inflammatory markers		
12-lead ECG	Normal ECG patterns	Use of ECG machines, including how to connect limb and chest leads
	Patterns for common abnormalities in adult patients	Recognize: common abnormalities, normal variants, abnormally connected leads, when to repeat
Peak flow, spirometry	Normal patterns	Use of ECG machines, including how to connect limb and chest leads
	Patterns of common abnormality	Recognize: common abnormalities, normal variants, abnormally connected leads, when to repeat
12-lead ECG	Normal ECG patterns	Use of peak flow and spirometer devices
	Patterns for common abnormalities in adult patients	Recognize common abnormalities
		Give instructions to patients and colleagues about when to call for help
Chest X-ray	Circumstances requiring: urgent requests, particular views	Communicate well with radiologists, radiographers and other staff
Abdominal X-ray	Normal findings of chest and abdominal X-ray	Identify the need for radiological advice
Trauma radiography	Imaging appearances of common abnormalities on chest and abdominal X-rays	Recognize common abnormalities
Ultrasound, CT and MRI	Recognition of the risks of radiation, including risks in pregnancy	Identify when ultrasound, CT or MRI might be required
Microbiological samples	Type of samples and collection method required	Interpret results

[1]From: The Foundation Programme Curriculum (2007). Available at: www.foundationprogramme.nhs.uk.
ECG, electrocardiogram; CT, computed tomography; MRI, magnetic resonance imaging.

- establish a physiological baseline of measurements prior to starting treatment – for example, an angiotensin-converting enzyme inhibitor, recommended for secondary prevention, can adversely affect renal function, so urea and electrolytes are measured on admission
- allow you to monitor the effectiveness of treatment – for instance, an ECG must be performed 90 minutes after the start of coronary reperfusion therapy with a thrombolytic drug. If this has restored perfusion of the blocked coronary artery, the height of the pretreatment ST segment elevation is reduced by at least 50 per cent
- provide an indication of disease severity – for example, a myocardial infarction may impair cardiac function; echocardiography will show whether left ventricular function has been adversely affected.

To take a different example, in suspected overdose blood tests may confirm:

- an excess of a prescribed drug such as digoxin – the level detected being outside the therapeutic range
- a suspected overdose of a drug such as paracetamol – blood levels at least 4 hours after ingestion can confirm the ingestion of paracetamol, give an indication of whether the patient is at high risk and help to guide appropriate treatment.

CHOOSING AN APPROPRIATE TEST

You might think that the more investigations you request, the quicker you will arrive at the correct diagnosis. Unfortunately this is not so. A single test swings the odds in favour of a disease but is rarely 'diagnostic' and can sometimes be completely wrong; about 5 per cent of patients with chest pain seen in an emergency department who are sent home on the basis of a single 'normal' ECG turn out to have had a myocardial infarction.

A perfect test would distinguish those patients who genuinely have a particular disease from those who genuinely do not – that is, the test would have 100 per cent sensitivity and 100 per cent specificity (Table 4.2).

So you may request:

- a test with a 95 per cent sensitivity – this means that 5 per cent of patients will be given the 'all clear', incorrectly, when they really do have an illness; these test results are 'false negatives'
- a test with 95 per cent specificity – this means that 5 per cent of patients will be told, incorrectly, that they had a particular illness; these test results are 'false positives'.

What does a normal test result mean? All biological variables have a gaussian or normal bell-shaped distribution, with 95 per cent of the population falling within two standard deviations from the median value. Medical tests such as blood tests are no different – 95 per cent of people will have a blood test result within two standard deviations of the median (the 'normal range'). What is 'normal' may, however, vary with such factors as age, gender, race and pregnancy.

A test result that is *just outside* this normal range does not automatically indicate 'disease' as 5 per cent of normal people will be, by definition, outside the normal range. Generally, the more abnormal the test result, the more likely it is to indicate disease. Sometimes tests may be affected by:

- diet – the anticoagulant effect of warfarin can be antagonized by food containing vitamin K, such as spinach
- drugs – diuretics, selective serotonin reuptake inhibitors and antiepileptic drugs may cause hyponatraemia
- other diseases – cardiac failure may cause hepatic congestion and abnormal liver function test results.

When ordering 'uncommon' tests, it is wise to contact your local laboratory to ensure that there are no specific requirements. For example:

- cryoglobulins precipitate on cooling, so must be collected, transported and handled at 37 °C
- urine for a catecholamine assay must be collected in an acid medium.

Which tests should you order? Tests may be carried out:

- to help with diagnosis – for example, full blood count, erythrocyte sedimentation rate (ESR) and blood cultures in an intravenous drug user presenting with a fever

Table 4.2 Some useful terminology

True positive	A test result that is positive when the person tested does have the condition in question
True negative	A test result that is negative when the person tested does not have the condition in question
False positive	A test result that is positive even though the person tested does not have the condition in question
False negative	A test result that is negative even though the person tested does have the condition in question
Sensitivity	The proportion of people with a condition who will be correctly identified by a test for that condition – a test with a sensitivity of 85 per cent will be positive in 85 per cent of individuals who have the condition, but will produce a false negative result in 15 per cent $$Sensitivity = \frac{number\ of\ true\ positives}{number\ of\ true\ positives + number\ of\ false\ negatives}$$
Specificity	The proportion of people without a condition who will be correctly identified as not having that condition – a test with a specificity of 98 per cent will be negative in 98 per cent of normal individuals, but will produce a false positive result in 2 per cent $$Specificity = \frac{number\ of\ true\ negatives}{number\ of\ true\ negatives + number\ of\ false\ positives}$$
Positive predictive value (PPV)	The proportion of individuals with a positive test result who have been correctly identified $$PPV = \frac{number\ of\ true\ positives}{number\ of\ true\ positives + number\ of\ false\ positives}$$
Negative predictive value (NPV)	The proportion of individuals with a negative test result who have been correctly identified $$NPV = \frac{number\ of\ true\ negatives}{number\ of\ true\ negatives + number\ of\ false\ negatives}$$
Pre-test probability	The likelihood that an individual has a particular condition before a test for that condition is performed. This estimate may be based on clinical experience, a knowledge of disease prevalence, a risk prediction tool, or a combination of all three

- to assess the severity of disease – monitoring a patient's creatinine and estimated glomerular filtration rate (eGFR) will help determine at what point renal replacement therapy (dialysis) may be needed
- to monitor the effect of treatment – in sepsis, you would expect markers of infection and inflammation, ESR and C-reactive protein (CRP), to be high at the time of diagnosis and to gradually return to normal with intensive antibiotic treatment
- to 'screen' – some hospitals carry out an automated 'battery' or 'panel' of common tests including urea and electrolytes, liver function, troponin, full blood count and thyroid function.

Tests that are invasive usually involve an element of risk for a patient. For instance, there is a 1:1000 risk of death, myocardial infarction, stroke or vascular damage during cardiac catheterization – which needs to be explained to a patient before seeking consent to proceed, preferably by the person carrying out the test. In choosing the test to perform, you need to balance the usefulness of the test against the potential risks. You should only:

- request investigations that are likely to affect the patient's management
- interpret results of investigations in the appropriate clinical context.

Tests that are within the normal range may be thought of as 'negative'. 'Negative' results can be as informative as 'positive' results, as the former can 'rule out' an illness that can be just as important as a positive result 'ruling in' a disease. For example, D-dimer (a fibrinogen degradation product) is often requested when a patient has suspected deep vein thrombosis – a negative result practically rules out thrombosis, while a positive result *may* indicate thrombosis (but does not rule out other possible causes).

Some tests are time-dependent. For example, it may:

- take up to 12 hours before the troponin level is elevated in an acute coronary syndrome
- be days before viral titres are raised after the onset of symptoms
- take several months before human immunodeficiency virus (HIV) infection can be confirmed.

At some point, you may come across conflicting results, or results that just do not fit the clinical picture. Discuss these with the appropriate department – a sample may have been incorrectly collected, the laboratory may have made a mistake, or the reports have been filed in the wrong patient's notes.

DOCUMENTING TESTS (AND RESULTS)

Everyone involved in a patient's care needs to know what tests have been requested and what the results have shown – the best place to do this is in the patient's notes. Remember that other doctors will be providing care 'out of hours' and so a clear and up-to-date record of tests and results is essential.

Listing each test requested on a separate line makes it easier to see what has been done (and what has not). Writing the result alongside will also make it easier to see what results are still outstanding. Where tests are being repeated on a regular basis, tabulating them in the form of a flow chart makes trends much easier to spot (Table. 4.3).

Before writing results or filing paper reports in the notes, always check the patient's identification details on each one to ensure that you are putting them in the correct notes.

DISCUSSING TEST RESULTS WITH PATIENTS

You will need to keep the patient informed about test results as you get them. Of special interest to them will be the invasive tests, which are generally landmarks in their investigation history. If a test has involved a biopsy, explain that results will take several days. Be prepared to answer questions to explain the significance of test results and what is likely to happen next – have a more senior colleague with you until you have more experience. And do not be afraid to admit it when you do not know the answer, but reassure the patient that you will arrange for them to speak to someone who can answer their questions.

SUMMARY

Investigations are undertaken to:

- confirm that the most likely diagnosis, the *working diagnosis*, is correct
- exclude other potential diagnoses.

For the investigations you need to undertake, you must be able to:

- select tests appropriately
- request tests appropriately
- interpret test reports accurately
- recognize abnormalities needing immediate action.

You must be able to explain tests to patients, including the implications of possible and actual results, and thereby gain informed consent.

Table 4.3 Tabulating test results makes trends easier to spot. This table shows urea and electrolyte results for a patient who developed renal impairment with an angiotensin-converting enzyme inhibitor (ACE-I)

	ACE-I started ↓			ACE-I stopped ↓				
	Day 1	Day 2	Day 3	Day 4	Day 5	Day 6	Day 7	Day 8
Sodium (mmol/L)	140	138	139	138	137	138	139	138
Potassium (mmol/L)	4.3	4.2	4.4	4.7	4.9	5.4	5.2	4.9
Urea (mmol/L)	5.8	6.1	7.2	9.8	11.1	13.7	13.4	11.0
Creatinine (µmol/L)	112	117	130	168	188	205	192	178

FURTHER READING

Higgins C. 2007. *Understanding laboratory investigations: for nurses and health professionals*, 2nd edn. Chichester, UK: Wiley-Blackwell.

Provan D (ed). *Oxford handbook of clinical and laboratory investigation*, 2nd edn. Oxford: Oxford University Press, 2005.

Royal College of Radiologists. *Making the best use of clinical radiology services: referral guidelines*, 6th edn. London: Royal College of Radiologists, 2007.

The Foundation Programme Curriculum, 2007. Available at: www.foundationprogramme.nhs.uk (accessed 1 November 2009).

5 MEDICAL RECORDS

Andrew R Houghton

INTRODUCTION

Medical records are a means of recording details about a patient's care and communicating that information between healthcare professionals. The information contained within the medical records can also be used to monitor service activity, and for audit and research purposes. It is therefore essential that records are clear, accurate and legible, and that they are made contemporaneously (see Box 5.1).

BOX 5.1 GENERAL MEDICAL COUNCIL – GOOD MEDICAL PRACTICE (2006)

In providing [good clinical] care you must:
- keep clear, accurate and legible records, reporting:
  - the relevant clinical findings
  - the decisions made
  - the information given to patients
  - any drugs prescribed
  - any other investigation or treatment
- make records at the same time as the events you are recording or as soon as possible afterwards.

On the topic of medical record-keeping, the Foundation Programme Curriculum (2007) states that the following knowledge is required of foundation doctors.

- Structure of:
  - medical notes
  - discharge letters
  - discharge summaries
  - outpatient letters
  - prescriptions.
- Role of medical records in generation of central data returns and audit.
- Importance of good medical records as a sound basis for any subsequent legal action.
- An understanding that all notes may be read by the patient.

The Curriculum goes on to say that foundation doctors must develop the following attitudes/behaviours:

- strive to ensure that notes are accessible to all members of the team and to patients when requested
- consider the importance of:
  - timely recording of communications
  - effective use of the team and National Health Service (NHS) resources
  - time
  - prompt and accurate communication between primary and secondary care
- understand the importance of clear definition of diagnosis and procedures for coding for central returns
- willing to keep records of own experience in order to facilitate learning by reflection.

The core competencies and skills listed in the Curriculum are given below.

F1 level:

- routinely records accurate, logical, comprehensive and pertinent accounts of history, examination, investigations, management plans and clinical decisions that are timed, dated and clearly attributable (name written in capitals with your General Medical Council (GMC) reference number) with the understanding that they may be read by the patient
- routinely records patients' progress, including diagnoses, decision paths and evolving management plans, with details of input from other healthcare professionals
- routinely records information given to patients, details of discussion with patients, and patients' views on investigative and therapeutic options
- maintains personal knowledge of outcomes for the patients he/she has cared for
- effectively uses both written and computer-based information systems

- adapts style of record-keeping to multidiscipli-nary case record where appropriate
- updates clinical records appropriately.

F2 level:

- structures letters clearly to communicate findings and outcome of episodes so that they can be read and understood by patients
- ensures that letters and discharge summaries are written and sent out in a timely and efficient manner

- conveys the medico-legal importance of good record keeping to other foundation doctors
- demonstrates record keeping and intra/internet access skills to F1 doctors or students.

RECORD KEEPING STANDARDS

Generic standards

Generic standards are those that apply to all forms of medical record keeping. In 2007 the Health

Table 5.1 Generic standards for medical record keeping[1]

Standard	Description
1	The patient's complete medical record should be available at all times during their stay in hospital
2	Every page in the medical record should include the patient's name, identification number (NHS number[2]) and location in the hospital
3	The contents of the medical record should have a standardized structure and layout
4	Documentation within the medical record should reflect the continuum of patient care and should be viewable in chronological order
5	Data recorded or communicated on admission, handover and discharge should be recorded using a standardized proforma[3]
6	Every entry in the medical record should be dated, timed (24 hour clock), legible and signed by the person making the entry. The name and designation of the person making the entry should be legibly printed against their signature. Deletions and alterations should be countersigned, dated and timed
7	Entries to the medical record should be made as soon as possible after the event to be documented (e.g. change in clinical state, ward round, investigation) and before the relevant staff member goes off duty. If there is a delay, the time of the event and the delay should be recorded
8	Every entry in the medical record should identify the most senior healthcare professional present (who is responsible for decision making) at the time the entry is made
9	On each occasion the consultant responsible for the patient's care changes, the name of the new responsible consultant and the date and time of the agreed transfer of care should be recorded
10	An entry should be made in the medical record whenever a patient is seen by a doctor. When there is no entry in the hospital record for more than four (4) days for acute medical care or seven (7) days for long-stay continuing care, the next entry should explain why[4]
11	The discharge record/discharge summary should be commenced at the time a patient is admitted to hospital
12	Advance Decisions to Refuse Treatment, Consent, Cardio-Pulmonary Resuscitation decisions must be clearly recorded in the medical record. In circumstances where the patient is not the decision maker, that person should be identified e.g. Lasting Power of Attorney.

[1]Reproduced with permission from the Health Informatics Unit, Royal College of Physicians, London.
[2]In the UK the NHS number is being introduced as the required patient identifier.
[3]This standard is not intended to mean that a handover proforma should be used for every handover of every patient, rather that any patient handover information should have a standardized structure.
[4]The maximum interval between entries in the record would in normal circumstances be one day or less. The maximum interval that would cover a public holiday weekend, however, should be four days.

Informatics Unit of the Royal College of Physicians (RCP), London, published 12 standards (Table 5.1).

Standards for structure and content

A recent consultation process has shown that over 90 per cent of doctors think that there should be structured documentation across the NHS. In a project funded by NHS Connecting for Health, the Royal College of Physicians (RCP) Health Informatics Unit has developed profession-wide standards for the structure and content of hospital patient records, and these have been approved by the Academy of Medical Royal Colleges. Standards have been developed for the following types of patient record:

- hospital admission record
- handover document
- discharge summary.

Hospital admission record

Box 5.2 summarizes the headings that should be included in a hospital admission record. The doctor completing the record should note down their name, grade and contact details, and also (in the UK) their GMC number (which acts as a unique identifier). A detailed description

---

BOX 5.2 HOSPITAL ADMISSION RECORD – HEADINGS (REPRODUCED WITH PERMISSION FROM THE HEALTH INFORMATICS UNIT, RCP, LONDON)

- Responsible consultant
- Clerking doctor
- Source of referral
- Time and date patient seen
- Time and date of clerking
- Patient's location
- Reason for admission and presenting complaints
- History of each presenting complaint
- Past medical, surgical and mental health history
- Medication record
  - Current medications
  - Relevant previous medications
- Relevant legal information
  - Mental capacity
  - Advance decisions to refuse treatment
  - Lasting power of attorney or deputy
  - Organ donation
- Allergies and adverse reactions
- Risks and warnings
- Social history
  - Lifestyle
  - Social and personal circumstances
  - Services and carers
- Family history
- Systems enquiry
- Patient's concerns, expectations and wishes

- Observations and findings
  - General appearance
  - Structured scales
  - Vital signs
  - Mental state
  - Cardiovascular system
  - Respiratory system
  - Abdomen
  - Genitourinary
  - Nervous system
  - Musculoskeletal system
  - Skin
- Problem list and/or differential diagnosis
- Relevant risk factors
- Discharge planning
- Management plan
  - Summary and interpretation of findings
  - Next steps
  - Special monitoring required
  - Resuscitation status
- Information given to the patient and/or authorized representative
- Investigations and initial procedures
- Person completing clerking
  - Doctor's name
  - Grade
  - Doctor's signature
- Specialist registrar/senior review
- Post-take ward round

BOX 5.3 HANDOVER DOCUMENTS – HEADINGS (REPRODUCED WITH PERMISSION FROM THE HEALTH INFORMATICS UNIT, RCP, LONDON)

- Date
- Time
- Patient details
  - Patient surname, forename
  - Date of birth
  - NHS number
  - Gender
  - Current location
  - Intended location
- Clinical details
  - Date of admission
  - Expected date of discharge
  - Responsible consultant
  - New responsible consultant
  - Diagnosis/problem list/differential diagnosis
  - Mental capacity
  - Advance decisions to refuse treatment and resuscitation status
  - Mental state
  - Patient at high risk
  - Allergies
  - Risks and warnings
- Reason for handover

- Management plan
  - Clinical narrative (consultant to consultant team handover only)
  - Current treatment/investigations
  - Aims and limitations of treatment and special instructions
  - Escalation plan
  - Agreed with patient or legitimate patient representative (Y/N)
- Outstanding issues
  - Tasks which must be done
  - Tasks to be done if possible
  - Information given to patient and/or authorized representatives
- Doctor handing over
  - Name
  - Grade
  - Specialty
  - Bleep number/contact details
- Doctor receiving handover
  - Name
  - Grade
  - Specialty
- Senior clinical contact

of the type of information that applies under each heading, together with a downloadable sample pro forma, is available on the Health Informatics Unit website (see Further reading) for the hospital admission record and for the other documents described below.

Handover document

Patient handovers occur when a patient's care is transferred between different consultants or between on-call teams (e.g. at weekends or at night). The handover process is often poorly done, with little or no documentation as part of the process. To maintain good patient care, safety and communication, it is important to ensure that key information is handed over between teams and that a written record of this information is available. Box 5.3 summarizes the headings that can be included in a handover document.

Discharge summary

Box 5.4 summarizes the suggested headings for inclusion in a discharge summary. It is important that discharge summaries include the information that general practitioners (GPs) want and need. As well as details pertaining to the patient's admission, the discharge summary must include details of future plans with clear and specific information about any future actions that may be required by the hospital, GP and allied health professionals.

USE OF ABBREVIATIONS IN NOTES

Avoid the use of abbreviations in medical records – even abbreviations that appear well known can prove

---

BOX 5.4 DISCHARGE SUMMARY – HEADINGS (REPRODUCED WITH PERMISSION FROM THE HEALTH INFORMATICS UNIT, RCP, LONDON)

- GP details
  - GP name
  - GP practice address
  - GP practice code
- Patient details
  - Patient surname, forename
  - Name known as
  - Date of birth
  - Gender
  - NHS number
  - Patient address
  - Patient telephone number(s)
- Admission details
  - Method of admission
  - Source of admission
  - Hospital site
  - Responsible trust
  - Date of admission
  - Time of admission
- Discharge details
  - Date of discharge
  - Time of discharge
  - Discharge method
  - Discharge destination
    - Type of destination
    - Destination address
    - Living alone
  - Discharging consultant
  - Discharging specialty/department
- Clinical information
  - Diagnosis at discharge
  - Operations and procedures

- Reason for admission and presenting complaints
- Mental capacity
- Advance decisions to refuse treatment and resuscitation status
- Allergies
- Risks and warnings
- Clinical narrative
- Relevant investigations and results
- Relevant treatments and changes made to treatments
- Measures of physical ability and cognitive function
- Medication changes
- Discharge medications
- Medication recommendations
- Advice, recommendations and future plan
  - Hospital (actions required/planned)
  - GP (actions required)
  - Community and specialist services (actions requested/planned/agreed)
- Information given to patient and/or authorized representative
- Patient's concerns, expectations and wishes
- Results awaited
- Person completing summary
  - Doctor's name
  - Grade
  - Specialty
  - Doctor's signature
  - Date of completion of discharge record
- Distribution list

---

misleading. For instance, does 'MS' refer to 'multiple sclerosis' or 'mitral stenosis'? Does 'PID' refer to 'pelvic inflammatory disease' or a 'prolapsed intervertebral disc'? Abbreviations such as 'L' and 'R' for 'left' and 'right' must also be avoided to minimize the risk of confusion. Do not abbreviate drug names or dosage instructions – for instance, 'IU' ('International Unit') can easily be mistaken for 'IV' ('intravenous'). A 2007 study reported that 4.7 per cent of medication errors could be attributed to the use of abbreviations. The *British National Formulary* recommends that 'in general, titles of drugs and preparations should be written in full. Unofficial abbreviations should not be used as they may be misinterpreted'.

SUMMARY

Medical records must be:

- clear
- accurate
- legible
- contemporaneous.

All medical records should meet the 12 generic standards listed in Table 5.1. There are published standards for the structure and content of the:

- hospital admission record (Box 5.2)
- handover document (Box 5.3)
- discharge summary (Box 5.4).

FURTHER READING

General Medical Council. *Good medical practice*. London: General Medical Council, 2006. Available at: www.gmc-uk.org/guidance/good_medical_practice/index.asp (accessed 1 November 2009).

Royal College of Physicians. Medical record keeping standards, 2008. Available at: www.rcplondon.ac.uk/clinical-standards/hiu/medical-records (accessed 1 November 2009).

The Foundation Programme Curriculum, 2007. Available at; www.foundationprogramme.nhs.uk (accessed 1 November 2009).

6 PRESENTING CASES

Andrew R Houghton

INTRODUCTION

Once you have taken the history, carried out a clinical examination and documented your findings, your job is not yet over – you will also need to communicate your assessment of the patient to others. In many situations, you will be expected to present your findings orally:

- presenting a new case on a ward round following admission
- updating your team on a patient's progress during an inpatient ward round
- performing a patient handover between shifts
- obtaining telephone advice from a senior colleague
- making a formal case presentation at a grand round meeting.

The key to an effective case presentation is to be clear and concise, including all the important findings (key positives and negatives) while leaving out superfluous information. Learning what to include and what to omit is a skill that comes with practice and experience – the more cases you present (and the more constructive feedback you seek), the better you will become.

Begin with an arresting sentence; close with a strong summary; in between speak simply, clearly, and always to the point; and above all be brief.
William J Mayo,
co-founder of the Mayo Clinic

THE OPENING STATEMENT

An effective case presentation begins with a clear one-sentence summary of the case:

Mr Jones is a 54-year-old man who presented this morning with an acute inferior ST-elevation myocardial infarction.

The opening statement has the same role as a newspaper headline – it should give your 'audience' a clear idea of what is going to follow. This makes it much easier for listeners to focus on the key elements of the story. Imagine that you are listening to a case presentation – as soon as you hear an opening statement like the one above, the key points you would expect to hear in the rest of the history include:

- the precise nature of the chest pain (site, radiation, duration, etc.)
- associated symptoms (e.g. breathlessness, nausea, sweating)
- relevant past history (e.g. previous angina, coronary revascularization procedures)
- drug history (e.g. prior use of antianginal drugs)
- social history (e.g. smoking history)
- family history (e.g. first degree relatives with a history of cardiovascular events)
- cardiovascular risk factors.

You will also expect to hear about relevant examination findings:

- pulse and blood pressure
- jugular venous pressure
- heart sounds
- chest auscultation
- peripheral pulses.

And also relevant investigations:

- electrocardiogram
- cardiac markers (troponins, creatine kinase)
- lipid profile.

The key point is that it is much easier for your audience to pick out the relevant details from your presentation if they know where it is heading from the outset. On many occasions, a presenting doctor or medical student will 'dive in at the deep end' with a long list of symptoms and examination findings that they have elicited but without any clear sense of direction until the diagnosis is revealed like a punchline at the very end – at which point the audience has to think back over everything they've heard and pick out the relevant bits in retrospect (if they can recall them). When you are on a long post-take ward round, this can make things very tiring for everyone.

Starting your presentation with a 'headline' diagnosis is also a good way to give *yourself* focus, and to reassess for yourself whether your findings really do support that diagnosis. For instance, it is not uncommon to hear that an elderly patient has a 'chest infection' when they present with confusion or a fall, and yet on closer examination the diagnosis does not have a lot to support it – they may be pyrexial with raised inflammatory markers, but there is no cough or sputum, no chest signs, and the chest X-ray is entirely clear. If you are planning to present such a case, think to yourself – what elements of my story actually support the diagnosis that I am about to state? And if, on reflection, there is indeed very little supporting evidence, this may be an indicator that you need to revise your diagnosis – for instance, have you checked the patient's urine, and discovered whether their confusion and pyrexia is actually due to a urinary tract infection, or cellulitis, or some other source of sepsis?

So, beginning with a headline diagnosis is an effective way to engage your audience and also for you to self-assess whether your diagnosis is likely to be correct. But what if you have not made a diagnosis? If the diagnosis remains unclear, you should still begin your presentation with a 'headline', but this time it should be a summary of the key findings or a problem list, or a list of possible diagnoses (differential diagnosis) where appropriate:

Mrs Smith is a 43-year-old woman who presented yesterday with sudden onset headache but a normal CT brain scan and lumbar puncture.

PRESENTING THE CASE

After the opening statement, present your findings in a structured and logical order – generally, this should follow an order similar to that you would use to assess the patient and record your findings:

- history
  - presenting complaint(s)
  - history of presenting complaint(s)
  - past medical/surgical history

- drug history
- allergies and adverse reactions
- social history
- family history
- systems enquiry
- physical examination
  - general appearance
  - vital signs
  - system-by-system findings
- investigations
  - which tests have been requested
  - key results (when available)
- problem list
- differential diagnosis
- plan for further investigation and management.

As you present the case, speak clearly – there may be several team members on the round, and all will need to hear your presentation, not just your seniors. At the same time, be alert to the need to protect the patient's privacy and confidentiality – do not present the case so loudly that every other patient and relative in the ward can overhear what is being said.

CLINICAL PEARL

As you gain experience, you will learn how to 'trim' your presentation to the key positive and negative findings. It takes time to acquire this skill, and your senior colleagues will be able to guide you on honing your presentation technique. Be sure to seek constructive feedback and endeavour to act on the advice you are given.

THE CLOSING SUMMARY

As with the opening statement, the closing summary should be short and to the point, and needs to condense all the key findings of the case you have presented into a final paragraph:

In summary, Mrs Brown is a 67-year-old woman who presented yesterday with a 4-day history of breathlessness and cough productive of green sputum. On examination she was febrile and had chest signs consistent with consolidation in the right middle lobe, confirmed on chest X-ray.

Her inflammatory markers are elevated and she has a CURB-65 risk score of 2. She is responding well to antibiotics.

As well as using the closing summary to end a full case presentation, a variant of it can also be used on subsequent ward rounds to remind the team of the key points of each case and the progress so far. As you arrive at each patient's bedside, give the team a short summary to bring everyone 'up to speed':

Mr Green is an 88-year-old man who presented 8 days ago with congestive cardiac failure. He has responded well to intravenous furosemide and is now on oral diuretics, and his electrolytes and renal function remain stable. We anticipate that he will shortly be medically fit for discharge, but he and his family have expressed concerns about returning back home and so we are planning a case conference this afternoon to discuss discharge arrangements.

A short case summary prepared for each ward round will not only ensure the smooth and efficient running of the round, but will also help you to remain focused on the key issues and plans for each patient.

SUMMARY

William J Mayo summarized it best. When presenting a case:

- begin with an arresting sentence
- close with a strong summary
- in between, speak:
  - simply
  - clearly
  - always to the point
- and above all be brief.

FURTHER READING

Parrott T, Crook G. In press. *Effective communication skills for hospital doctors*. Nottingham: DevelopMedica.

Rawlins K. 1999. *Presentation and communication skills: a handbook for practitioners*. London: EMAP Healthcare.

B

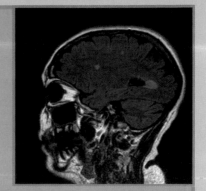

INDIVIDUAL SYSTEMS

7 THE CARDIOVASCULAR SYSTEM

Andrew R Houghton and David Gray

INTRODUCTION

There is a just small number of presenting symptoms of cardiovascular disease, namely chest discomfort, breathlessness, palpitation, dizziness and syncope, and peripheral oedema. There are, however, a multitude of physical signs, but these are relatively straightforward to interpret as long as you bear in mind the underlying cardiovascular physiology and pathophysiology.

CLINICAL HISTORY

Presenting complaint

Chest discomfort

Patients with angina often say that the symptom they experience in the chest is not a *pain* but a feeling of *discomfort*. It's important to recognize this – if you only ask the direct question 'Do you get chest pain?', and the patient answers 'No', you might move on and miss a vital part of the patient's history.

 IMPORTANT
If you must ask a leading question, enquire about chest discomfort rather than chest pain.

There are many different causes of chest discomfort, each of which has its own key characteristics (Table 7.1). Enquire about the following features:

- location and radiation:
    - central (retrosternal), radiating to the arms, neck and jaw in angina and myocardial infarction
    - retrosternal in gastro-oesophageal reflux and oesophageal spasm
    - between the shoulder blades (interscapular) in aortic dissection
    - tends to be localized with musculoskeletal

or pleuritic pain, although the pain of massive pulmonary embolism can mimic that of angina
- character:
    - tight, heavy, crushing in angina or myocardial infarction
    - 'tearing' in aortic dissection
    - sharp/stabbing with pleuritic pain (e.g. pulmonary embolism)
    - sharp or 'raw' with pericarditis
    - sharp/stabbing or dull with musculoskeletal pain
- severity:
    - graded by the patient on a scale of 0–10, where 10 represents the worst pain ever
- duration and onset:
    - angina – onset with exertion/emotional stress and usually lasting less than 10 minutes
    - myocardial infarction – onset often at rest, lasting more than 10 minutes
    - pulmonary embolism – pleuritic chest pain of sudden onset
    - aortic dissection – sudden onset
    - musculoskeletal – may be of sudden onset (e.g. with movement) and lasts a few seconds, or be more gradual and chronic (e.g. costochondritis)
- precipitating, exacerbating and alleviating factors:
    - angina – brought on by exertion/emotional stress, particularly in cold windy weather and/or after a heavy meal, and rapidly relieved by rest or sublingual glyceryl trinitrate (GTN)
    - myocardial infarction – pain continues despite resting or using GTN
    - pericarditis – exacerbated by lying flat and respiration, relieved by sitting upright and leaning forwards
    - pleuritic pain – worsened by inspiration and coughing
    - musculoskeletal – worsened by movement

Table 7.1 Common causes of chest discomfort and their characteristic features

System	Cause	Characteristic features
Cardiovascular	Angina	Tight or heavy central chest discomfort, radiating to left and/or right arm, neck and jaw, worsened by exertion or stress and relieved with glyceryl trinitrate. Associated with breathlessness
	Myocardial infarction	Similar in character to angina but usually more severe and not relieved with glyceryl trinitrate. Often occurs at rest. Associated with breathlessness, sweating, nausea and vomiting
	Pericarditis	Chest pain may be sharp or 'raw'. Exacerbated by lying flat and respiration. Eased by leaning forwards. May be associated with breathlessness and fever
	Aortic dissection	Severe 'tearing' interscapular pain. May be associated with ischaemia in other regions if the blood supply is compromised, e.g. stroke (cerebrovascular ischaemia), abdominal pain (mesenteric ischaemia), paraplegia (spinal cord ischaemia)
Respiratory	Pleuritic pain (e.g. pulmonary embolism)	Sharp/stabbing pain, exacerbated by inspiration. Associations depend upon underlying cause (e.g. breathlessness and haemoptysis in pulmonary embolism, productive cough and fever in pneumonia)
Gastrointestinal	Gastro-oesophageal reflux	A burning discomfort rising from the stomach or lower chest up towards the neck. Exacerbated by bending over, straining or lying down, especially after a meal. Associated with waterbrash
	Oesophageal spasm	Central chest discomfort that can mimic angina, even being relieved by glyceryl trinitrate (although usually taking longer than 5 minutes). Unlike angina, it is unrelated to exertion and often occurs at rest
Musculoskeletal	E.g. costochondritis (Tietze's syndrome), rib fracture, malignant chest wall involvement	Localized chest discomfort which may be of sudden onset (e.g. with movement) and lasts a few seconds, or be more gradual and chronic (e.g. costochondritis). Usually exacerbated by movement
Dermatological	Shingles (herpes zoster)	Usually unilateral in a nerve root distribution and with a blistering rash

- associated symptoms
  - angina – breathlessness (which may be more of a feature than chest discomfort)
  - myocardial infarction – breathlessness, sweating, nausea and vomiting
  - pericarditis – breathlessness, fever
  - pulmonary embolism – breathlessness, haemoptysis
  - pneumonia – breathlessness, productive cough, fever
  - gastro-oesophageal reflux – waterbrash.

The characteristic features of the common causes of chest discomfort are discussed in more detail under the individual sections for angina (p. 65), acute coronary syndromes (p. 66), pericarditis (p. 76), aortic dissection (p. 67), pulmonary embolism (p. 106), pneumothorax (p. 106) and dyspepsia (p. 109).

Breathlessness

A degree of breathlessness (dyspnoea) is normal on heavy exertion, but breathlessness becomes *abnormal* when it is disproportionate to the level of activity undertaken. As with chest pain, you should ask about:

- severity (heart failure symptoms can be graded using the New York Heart Association (NYHA) functional classification, see Table 7.2)
- duration and onset
- precipitating, exacerbating and alleviating factors
- associated symptoms (e.g. chest discomfort).

Table 7.2 The New York Heart Association (NYHA) functional classification of heart failure symptoms

NYHA class	Description
Class I	No limitation of physical activity. Ordinary physical activity does not cause undue fatigue, palpitation, or dyspnoea
Class II	Slight limitation of physical activity. Comfortable at rest, but ordinary physical activity results in fatigue, palpitation, or dyspnoea
Class III	Marked limitation of physical activity. Comfortable at rest, but less than ordinary activity causes fatigue, palpitation or dyspnoea
Class IV	Unable to carry out any physical activity without discomfort. Symptoms of cardiac insufficiency at rest. If any physical activity is undertaken, discomfort is increased

From: The Criteria Committee of the New York Heart Association. 1994. *Nomenclature and criteria for diagnosis of diseases of the heart and great vessels*, 9th edn. Boston, MA: Little, Brown & Co, 253–256.

Left ventricular dysfunction (p. 67) is a common cardiac cause of breathlessness and can result from systolic dysfunction (a 'weak' ventricle with impaired contractility and a low ejection fraction), diastolic dysfunction (a 'stiff' ventricle with impaired relaxation and filling), or a combination of the two. This leads to an elevation in filling pressures (end-diastolic pressure) which in turns raises left atrial pressure and pulmonary venous pressure. Pulmonary venous congestion occurs, 'stiffening' the lungs and exacerbating the sensation of breathlessness, and can ultimately progress to frank pulmonary oedema.

Orthopnoea is the sensation of breathlessness on lying flat. Orthopnoea occurs because of increased venous return and a redistribution of interstitial oedema throughout the lungs. Patients who are prone to orthopnoea may report using several pillows (ask how many) to prop themselves upright in bed, or may even resort to sleeping in a chair.

Paroxysmal nocturnal dyspnoea (**PND**) is the development of breathlessness while the patient is lying down asleep, waking the patient and usually forcing them to sit upright or even lean out of an open window to regain their breath. It results from the development of orthopnoea while the patient is sleeping. Patients often find PND an alarming symptom.

Breathlessness is also a feature of myocardial ischaemia, and indeed breathlessness may be the predominant (or even only) symptom. The respiratory causes of breathlessness are discussed in Chapter 8.

Palpitation

Palpitation is an awareness of the heartbeat, but patients use the term in a variety of ways, so it is important to obtain a detailed description of what they are experiencing. It is particularly important to determine whether the palpitations are:

- fast or slow
- regular or irregular.

Ask the patient to 'tap out' the rhythm by clapping their hands – this will usually make it clearer whether the rhythm is regular or irregular. If it is irregular, determine whether it is 'regularly irregular' (e.g. bigeminy) or 'irregularly irregular' (e.g. atrial fibrillation).

The patient's description can give a strong clue as to the nature of the palpitation – intermittent 'skipped beats' are commonly ectopic beats, a rapid regular palpitation with gradual onset and termination and occurring with stress is commonly sinus tachycardia, whilst a rapid irregularly irregular palpitation is likely to be atrial fibrillation (which can occur in self-limiting episodes – 'paroxysmal atrial fibrillation' – as well as being persistent). In general, palpitations which have an *abrupt* onset and termination are more likely to be due to a 'significant' arrhythmia than palpitations which start gradually and later on fade away.

CLINICAL PEARL

Sometimes the patient is aware of just a fleeting sensation, perceived as a 'missed beat' or 'extra beat', which is typically due to an ectopic beat – this is often described as the heart having 'jumped', 'lurched' or 'skipped a beat'.

Palpitations are usually episodic, and so you should ask the following questions.

- How often do the episodes occur?
- Do they occur at rest, during exercise or both?
- How does each episode begin:
  - sudden or gradual onset
  - any apparent triggers (e.g. alcohol, caffeine)?
- How long does each episode last?
- How does each episode terminate:
  - sudden or gradual termination
  - does anything terminate an episode (e.g. Valsalva manoeuvre)?
- Have they been prescribed any medication (e.g. β-blocker), and does it help?

Table 7.3 lists many of the commoner causes of palpitation and their key features. To make a definitive diagnosis, it is necessary to capture the heart rhythm on an electrocardiogram (ECG) during a typical episode (see *Ambulatory ECG*, p. 62).

Ask the patient whether they have any additional symptoms during an episode of palpitation, such as dizziness or syncope (see below), chest pain or breathlessness, as this will indicate how troublesome the episodes are and therefore guide the urgency of treatment . Some patients notice a need to pass urine just after an episode of supraventricular tachycardia.

Pre-syncope and syncope

Syncope refers to a transient loss of consciousness resulting from transient global cerebral hypoperfusion (in contrast to other causes of loss of consciousness, such as epilepsy (p. 205)). The cerebral hypoperfusion is a consequence of a fall in cardiac output and/or a fall in peripheral vascular resistance. Syncope is characterized by:

- a rapid onset
- a short duration
- a full recovery.

Patients with syncope may experience a prodrome (**pre-syncope**) in which they have a feeling of lightheadedness, ringing in the ears, visual disturbance, nausea and sweating. These prodromal symptoms last just a few seconds before the syncopal event occurs – if the patient is able to lie down (to improve cerebral perfusion) during that time, they might avoid a syncopal event altogether. Ask the patient about:

- frequency of pre-syncopal and syncopal episodes
- any prodromal symptoms (pre-syncope)
- specific triggers (e.g. pain, micturition, sudden standing, head-turning, exertion)
- speed of onset of symptoms
- any associated symptoms (e.g. palpitations, chest pain, fits, tongue biting, incontinence)

Table 7.3 Characteristic features of common arrhythmias

Arrhythmia	Regularity	Fast or slow	Other features
Ectopic beats (atrial or ventricular)	Usually isolated 'missed beats'	Neither	If occurring in a predictable pattern (e.g. bigeminy, trigeminy), can feel 'regularly irregular'
Atrial fibrillation	Irregularly irregular	Usually fast, but rate can be normal depending upon degree of atrioventricular block	Often associated with breathlessness and fatigue
Atrial flutter	Regular (unless variable atrioventricular block)	Usually fast, but rate can be normal depending upon degree of atrioventricular block	Classically (but not always) presents with a ventricular rate of 150 bpm
Supraventricular tachycardia	Regular	Fast	Usually abrupt onset and termination
Ventricular tachycardia	Regular	Fast	Usually symptomatic (breathlessness, dizziness, syncope)

- duration of event
- rapidity of recovery
- any residual symptoms after the event.

> **CLINICAL PEARL**
>
> In a patient with syncope, make every effort to obtain a detailed description of the syncopal events from a witness. Patients typically recall little or nothing about the syncopal events themselves, so information from a witness can prove invaluable in making a diagnosis.

The cardiovascular causes of syncope can be classified as:

- reflex (neurally mediated) syncope
- syncope secondary to orthostatic hypotension
- cardiac syncope.

Reflex (neurally mediated) syncope can be predominantly vasodepressor (i.e. fall in blood pressure), predominantly cardio-inhibitory (i.e. fall in heart rate), or a mixed vasodepressor/cardio-inhibitory type. Examples include:

- vasovagal syncope, which can occur with pain or emotional stress, or in specific situations such as during micturition or coughing
- carotid sinus hypersensitivity, where pressure over the carotid sinus (e.g. tight collar, head turning) triggers syncope.

Syncope secondary to orthostatic hypotension (often called 'postural hypotension', p. 50) is typically seen with hypovolaemia (e.g. haemorrhage or dehydration), autonomic failure or secondary to certain drugs (e.g. vasodilators such as angiotensin-converting enzyme inhibitors or α-receptor blockers). Patients with orthostatic hypotension report pre-syncopal symptoms and/or syncope occurring after suddenly standing.

Cardiac syncope is seen with some arrhythmias (e.g. bradycardia, such as complete heart block or sick sinus syndrome, and tachycardia, such as ventricular tachycardia) and also with structural heart disease where there is an obstruction to blood flow (e.g. aortic stenosis, hypertrophic obstructive cardiomyopathy, atrial myxoma). With obstruction to left ventricular outflow (aortic stenosis and hypertrophic obstructive cardiomyopathy) the pre-syncope/syncope typically occurs on exertion; with atrial myxoma it can occur at any time if the myxoma transiently obstructs flow through the mitral or tricuspid valve.

> **CLINICAL PEARL**
>
> Dizziness is a vague term that can be used to refer to a feeling of vertigo, light-headedness, pre-syncope or unsteadiness ('disequilibrium'). It is important to obtain as much detail as possible about the symptoms, and how and when they occur, to characterize the patient's complaint more fully. Dizziness can be cardiovascular in origin, but can also result from inner ear pathology (p. 351) or a neurological disorder (p. 187). Ask about associated symptoms such as vertigo (do the surroundings 'spin round'?), hearing disturbance, muscle weakness and falls.

Peripheral oedema

Peripheral oedema is both a *symptom* and a *sign*, because it is a physical abnormality which is visible to the patient. It is typically noticed as ankle swelling, often worse in the evening, but can extend all the way up the legs and involve the abdomen (and, in recumbent patients, the sacrum). Peripheral oedema is most commonly associated with heart failure, but there are a number of other causes. Oedema is described as pitting (where finger pressure leaves an indentation) or non-pitting. The causes of pitting oedema are listed in Table 7.4. Non-pitting oedema is seen in hypothyroidism (pre-tibial myxoedema) and in lymphoedema.

The rest of the history

Past medical/surgical history

Enquire about:

- a known diagnosis of angina or myocardial infarction
  - how certain was the diagnosis?

Table 7.4 Causes of pitting oedema

System	Causes
Cardiac	Congestive cardiac failure Constrictive pericarditis
Vascular	Deep vein thrombosis (usually unilateral) Chronic venous insufficiency (uni- or bilateral) Venous compression by pelvic or abdominal mass (uni- or bilateral) Inferior vena cava obstruction
Gastrointestinal	Hypoalbuminaemia secondary to malabsorption, protein-losing enteropathy, cirrhosis of the liver
Renal	Hypoalbuminaemia secondary to nephrotic syndrome
Pharmacological	Calcium channel blockers Fludrocortisone
Metabolic	Thiamine deficiency (wet beri-beri)
General	Immobility ('dependent oedema')

- previous investigations, such as coronary angiograms
- previous cardiac operations or procedures:
  - coronary revascularization (coronary artery bypass grafting or percutaneous coronary intervention)
  - valve surgery (valvotomy, repair or replacement)
  - permanent pacemaker implant
  - implantable cardioverter-defibrillator implant
- known congenital heart disease, and any corrective surgery
- rheumatic fever in childhood
- other known cardiovascular conditions, such as heart failure, arrhythmias, murmurs or palpitations.

Cardiovascular risk factors

These can be divided into modifiable and non-modifiable risk factors.

- Modifiable risk factors are:
  - hypertension
  - diabetes mellitus
  - hyperlipidaemia
  - tobacco smoking.

- Non-modifiable risk factors are:
  - age
  - gender
  - family history (see below).

Drug history

Note down the drugs currently being taken by the patient. Also enquire about drugs taken previously, together with any adverse effects they might have had.

Allergies and adverse reactions

Document details of any known allergies and adverse reactions. Examples with particular relevance to cardiology include:

- aspirin allergy
- aspirin intolerance (e.g. excessive bleeding, gastrointestinal upset, worsening asthma)
- β-blocker intolerance (e.g. bronchospasm)
- angio-oedema, intolerable cough or renal impairment with angiotensin-converting enzyme inhibitors
- rhabdomyolysis with statins
- allergy to iodine-based contrast agents (e.g. during coronary angiography).

Social history

Smoking

- Smoking is strongly associated with the development of cardiovascular disease.
- Record whether the patient is a current or ex-smoker, or has never smoked.
- For cigarette smokers, calculate the lifetime consumption in terms of 'pack-years' (see Box 1.2, p. 7). Thus 40 cigarettes (2 packs) per day for 15 years is a 30 pack-year smoking history.

Alcohol

- Excessive alcohol consumption can be a causative factor in hypertension, atrial fibrillation and dilated cardiomyopathy
- Record alcohol consumption in terms of units per week, but also describe the pattern of drinking (e.g. 14 units per week could equal 2 units every day or 'binge' drinking of 14 units all in 1 day).

Caffeine

Caffeine consumption can be a factor in palpitations, so document the patient's consumption of caffeine-containing drinks (e.g. coffee, cola drinks)

Recreational drug use

- Cocaine can cause coronary artery spasm, which further causes myocardial ischaemia and infarction.
- Volatile substance (e.g. butane gas) misuse can cause arrhythmias.
- Infective endocarditis affecting the right heart can occur in intravenous drug users.

Occupation

Ask about the patient's occupation. A diagnosis of cardiovascular disease can have serious career implications (e.g. pilots, military personnel, 'occupational' drivers). Where appropriate, patients should seek advice from their occupational health department.

Driving

- Ask whether the patient drives a vehicle, and the type of driver's licence that they hold (e.g. 'standard' licence, heavy goods or public service vehicle licence).
- Rules vary according to the nature of the driving (e.g. there are special rules for 'occupational' driving) and the underlying cardiovascular condition.
- In the UK, detailed guidance is available from the Driver and Vehicle Licensing Agency (DVLA) in its regularly updated 'At a Glance' document on Medical Standards of Fitness to Drive (see www.dft.gov.uk/dvla/medical.aspx)

Effects of the cardiovascular condition on home and family life

- Impaired mobility due to chest pain or breathlessness.
- Psychological effects (e.g. fear of dying).
- Sexual function (e.g. impotence due to use of β-blockers).

Family history

Enquire about any family history of sudden cardiac death, which may indicate a familial disorder that predisposes to arrhythmias (e.g. long QT syndrome, Brugada syndrome).

Other cardiovascular conditions with a genetic basis include:

- Marfan's syndrome
- hypertrophic cardiomyopathy
- familial hypercholesterolaemia (see www.nice.org.uk/CG71).

> **CLINICAL PEARL**
>
> A family history of coronary artery disease increases an individual's risk by half, but only where it affects a first-degree relative at a 'premature' age (younger than 55 years for male relatives and 65 years for female relatives). If more than one first-degree relative is affected, the patient's risk is doubled.

PHYSICAL EXAMINATION

General examination

Begin the cardiovascular examination by ensuring that the patient is reclining comfortably on a couch at an angle of 45°. Take a step back, and inspect the patient's general appearance. Do they appear:

- comfortable at rest
- breathless
- sweaty or clammy ('diaphoretic')
- cachectic (e.g. as a result of longstanding heart failure – cardiac cachexia)?

Be alert to the features of specific genetic and endocrine diseases that can be associated with cardiac problems:

- Marfan's syndrome
  - tall stature, high-arched palate, lens dislocation
  - mitral valve prolapse, aortic dilatation, aortic dissection
- Ehlers–Danlos syndrome
  - joint hypermobility, elastic skin, easy bruising
  - mitral valve prolapse, aortic (and other arterial) aneurysms
- Down's syndrome
  - microgenia, macroglossia, epicanthic folds, single transverse palmar crease
  - complete atrioventricular septal defects

- Turner's syndrome˙
  - short stature, broad chest, webbed neck
  - bicuspid aortic valve, coarctation of the aorta
- thyrotoxicosis
  - heat intolerance, weight loss, tremor
  - tachycardia
- hypothyroidism
  - cold intolerance, fatigue, weight gain, depression
  - bradycardia
- acromegaly
  - enlargement of hands and feet, prominent brow
  - cardiomyopathy.

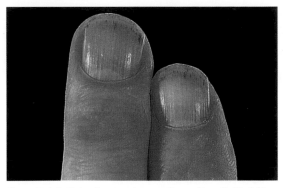

Figure 7.1 Splinter haemorrhages. From: Gray D, Toghill P. (eds), *An introduction to the symptoms and signs of clinical medicine*, with permission. © 2001 London: Hodder Arnold

The hands

Look for signs of:

- cyanosis (e.g. right-to-left intracardiac shunt)
- clubbing (p. 88) – causes are listed in Table 7.5
- splinter haemorrhages (Fig. 7.1) – narrow red/brown lines beneath the nails, aligned in the direction of nail growth, most commonly due to trauma but also found in infective endocarditis
- Osler's nodes – an uncommon manifestation of infective endocarditis, these are tender, red lesions that occur on the fingertips, palms and soles

Table 7.5 Causes of clubbing

Cardiovascular	Cyanotic congenital heart disease Infective endocarditis Atrial myxoma Axillary artery aneurysm (unilateral clubbing)
Respiratory	Lung cancer Mesothelioma Fibrosing alveolitis Bronchiectasis Cystic fibrosis Empyema
Gastrointestinal	Malabsorption (e.g. coeliac disease) Crohn's disease Ulcerative colitis Cirrhosis
Endocrine	Thyroid acropachy
Familial	'Pseudoclubbing'

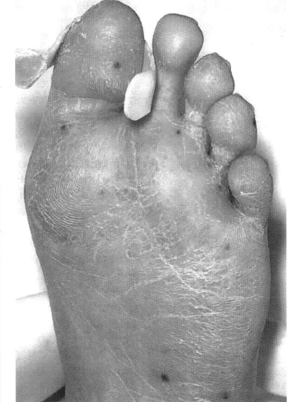

Figure 7.2 Multiple Janeway lesions on the sole of the foot and toes in S*taphylococcus aureus* endocarditis. Reproduced from *Heart*, Davies MK, **74**: 540 © 1995 with permission from BMJ Publishing Group Ltd.

- Janeway lesions (Fig. 7.2) – also seen in infective endocarditis (infrequently), these are maculo-papular lesions that occur on the palms and soles but, unlike Osler's nodes, are non-tender
- tendon xanthoma – yellowish cholesterol deposits in the tendons, often in the hands or at the elbow/knee, seen in hyperlipidaemia
- staining of the fingers as a consequence of cigarette consumption.

Arterial pulses

During or after your examination of the hands, check the patient's radial pulse at the wrist using the tips of your forefinger and middle finger. Assess:

- pulse rate
- pulse rhythm.

Rate and rhythm can also be assessed at the brachial pulse in the antecubital fossa, medial to the biceps tendon.

Pulse rate

Count the number of pulsations over a period of 30 seconds, and then double this figure to obtain the pulse rate in beats per minute (bpm). A normal pulse rate is between 60 and 100 bpm. A rate <60 bpm is termed bradycardia, and >100 bpm is called tachycardia.

Bradycardia

Bradycardia may result from slowing of the heart's sinoatrial node ('sinus bradycardia'), which may be due to a normal physiological cause (as seen in athletes, or during sleep), a problem within the node itself (e.g. sick sinus syndrome) or an external factor (e.g. hypothyroidism, hypothermia). Several drugs slow the sinoatrial node, including β-blockers, verapamil, diltiazem and digoxin. Alternatively, the sinoatrial node itself may be working normally but not all its impulses are reaching the ventricles (e.g. in second- or third-degree atrioventricular block). Abnormal rhythms such as atrial fibrillation or flutter may also be associated with bradycardia if there is a high degree of atrioventricular block.

Bradycardia may also be an 'apparent' bradycardia rather than a 'true' bradycardia. This can occur when the patient is experiencing ventricular ectopic beats – these are 'weaker' than normal beats, and so palpation of the radial pulse may fail to detect them, leading to an underestimation of the true heart rate.

Tachycardia

Tachycardia may result from a high sinoatrial rate ('sinus tachycardia'), which may be due to a normal physiological cause (as seen with pregnancy, anxiety, or pain), a problem with the node itself (e.g. 'inappropriate sinus tachycardia') or an external factor (e.g. thyrotoxicosis, blood loss). Several drugs increase the sinoatrial rate, including atropine, dobutamine and salbutamol. Abnormal rhythms such as supraventricular tachycardia or ventricular tachycardia cause a fast heart rate, as do (usually) atrial fibrillation or flutter.

Pulse rhythm

The pulse rhythm can be described as:

- regular
- irregular:
  - 'regularly irregular'
  - 'irregularly irregular'.

Sinus rhythm is usually regular, although in younger patients there can be a noticeable variation in heart rate with respiration (sinus arrhythmia) – this is normal. Several abnormal rhythms can be regular too, including supraventricular tachycardia (atrioventricular re-entry tachycardia and atrioventricular nodal re-entry tachycardia (AVNRT)), atrial tachycardia, atrial flutter (with regular block), and ventricular tachycardia.

A 'regularly irregular' rhythm is one in which there is a predictable change in rhythm – this can be seen in second-degree Mobitz I heart block (Wenckebach's phenomenon), where a beat is 'dropped' on a regular basis, or with regular ventricular ectopic beats (e.g. ventricular bigeminy, trigeminy, etc.). An 'irregularly irregular' rhythm is one in which the occurrence of each beat is chaotic and unpredictable, and is usually the result of atrial fibrillation.

Pulse character and volume

With the exception of a collapsing pulse, pulse character and volume are not easily assessed at the radial pulse because it is so far from the heart (so the pulse has become quite 'damped'). In most cases it is easier and better to assess pulse character and pulse volume using the brachial pulse or, even better, the carotid pulse.

Several types of abnormal pulse character are recognized.

- Slow-rising pulse ('pulsus parvus et tardus') – with a gradual 'upslope' which peaks in late systole, this pulse is also weak and is characteristic of severe aortic stenosis.
- Collapsing pulse – assessed by raising the patient's arm above their head while palpating the radial pulse (Fig. 7.3 – ask the patient if they have any shoulder pain first!), this pulse has an early peak followed by a sharp descent and indicates aortic regurgitation. It is also known as a 'water hammer' pulse.
- Biphasic pulse ('pulsus bisferiens') – this describes a 'double peak' pulse and is classically found in mixed aortic stenosis and regurgitation, and also in hypertrophic obstructive cardiomyopathy.
- Alternating pulse ('pulsus alternans') – this describes alternate strong and weak beats, and is found in severe left ventricular systolic dysfunction.
- Pulsus paradoxus – this refers to an exaggeration of the normal variation in pulse volume with respiration (which decreases on inspiration and increases on expiration). It is seen in cardiac tamponade, and also in severe asthma and chronic obstructive pulmonary disease.

A large volume pulse is seen with increased cardiac output (e.g. pregnancy, anaemia, thyrotoxicosis, sepsis) and in aortic regurgitation. A small volume pulse is seen with reduced cardiac output (e.g. severe left ventricular failure, severe aortic stenosis) and/or reduced circulating volume (e.g. haemorrhage, dehydration).

Finally, check for radio-femoral delay by palpating the radial and femoral pulses simultaneously. Normally the two pulses occur together, but the femoral pulse is delayed relative to the radial

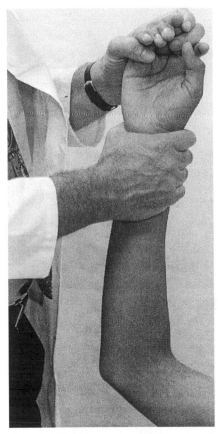

Figure 7.3 Checking for a collapsing pulse. From: Ogilvie C, Evans CC (eds), *Chamberlain's symptoms and signs in clinical medicine* (12th edition), with permission. © 1997 London: Hodder Arnold.

pulse in the presence of coarctation of the aorta (p. 75).

Blood pressure

Before taking a patient's blood pressure (BP), explain what you are about to do and try to ensure that the patient is as relaxed as possible. Standard BP measurements are made in a warm environment, with the patient sitting and the arm supported at the level of the heart. Patients should be seated for 5 minutes before the measurement is taken. Which arm is used is unimportant, but it is a good idea to check BP in *both* arms on a patient's first visit.

BOX 7.1 BRITISH HYPERTENSION SOCIETY (WWW. BHSOC.ORG) CUFF SIZE RECOMMENDATIONS
- A standard cuff (bladder 12 × 26 cm) for most adults.
- A large cuff (bladder 12 × 40 cm) for obese arms.
- A small cuff (bladder 12 × 18 cm) for lean adult arms and children.

Locate the position of the brachial artery in the antecubital fossa and position the BP cuff 2–3 cm above the antecubital fossa with the centre of the cuff's bladder over the line of the artery. Using a cuff that is too small leads to an overestimation of blood pressure, and vice versa (see Box 7.1).

Before using the stethoscope, estimate the systolic pressure by palpating the brachial artery and inflating the cuff until the brachial pulse disappears – this is the systolic pressure estimated by palpation.

Next, place your stethoscope over the brachial artery (without applying excessive pressure) and reinflate the cuff to 30 mmHg above the systolic pressure estimated by palpation. Gradually reduce the pressure at 2–3 mmHg per second and listen carefully for the point at which repetitive, clear tapping sounds first appear for two or more consecutive beats – this marks the *systolic blood pressure* (Korotkoff phase 1, Table 7.6). Continue to deflate

Table 7.6 Korotkoff phases

Korotkoff phase	Description
1	A repetitive, clear tapping sound which marks the systolic pressure
2	A brief period when there is a 'swishing' quality to the sounds, which may be followed by a period of silence ('auscultatory gap')
3	The return of crisper tapping sounds, similar to phase 1
4	An abrupt muffling of the sounds. Taken as the diastolic pressure if phase 5 cannot be clearly discerned (e.g. in pregnancy)
5	Silence, marking the diastolic pressure in most individuals

the cuff, and the point where the sounds finally disappear marks the *diastolic blood pressure* (Korotkoff phase 5). Both measurements should be taken to the nearest 2 mmHg.

In pregnancy, determining diastolic pressure is trickier as the sounds often continue all the way to zero. In this case, take the diastolic pressure as the point at which the sounds become muffled (Korotkoff phase 4).

Orthostatic hypotension

Normally on standing there is a modest drop in systolic BP and a modest rise in diastolic BP, keeping mean arterial pressure constant. Orthostatic hypotension refers to a fall in blood pressure on standing, and can occur in volume depletion (e.g. as a result of haemorrhage) and be a cause of syncope. However, testing for orthostatic hypotension is often performed incorrectly. When checking for a 'postural drop', it is important to check the pulse as well as the BP – a rise in pulse rate of ≥30 bpm or an inability to complete the test due to postural dizziness is a sensitive indicator of hypovolaemia (Brostoff, 2009). A drop in systolic BP of ≥20 mmHg or diastolic BP ≥10 mmHg is also often taken as an indicator of a 'significant' postural drop, but such a measurement must be taken after *at least* 1 minute of standing.

Face and eyes

Inspect the patient's face for signs of a malar flush – a reddish colour over the cheeks, seen in mitral stenosis with pulmonary hypertension. Next, take a closer look at the patient's eyes. Look for:

- xanthelasma (Fig. 7.4) – raised yellow deposits of cholesterol beneath the skin around the eyes
- anaemia – which can exacerbate angina and breathlessness
- jaundice (yellow sclerae) – which in the context of cardiovascular disease may indicate hepatic congestion (in congestive cardiac failure)
- corneal arcus – a white/yellow ring around the circumference of the cornea, which is seen in hyperlipidaemia (particularly when present in those aged <40 years) or in normal ageing ('senile arcus').

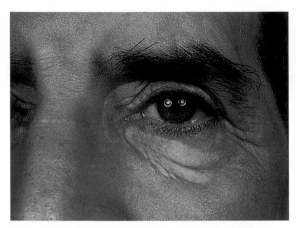

Figure 7.4 Xanthelasma. From: Gray D, Toghill P. (eds), *An introduction to the symptoms and signs of clinical medicine*, with permission. © 2001 London: Hodder Arnold.

Using an ophthalmoscope, carefully inspect the fundi, looking for:

- Roth spots – retinal haemorrhages with a pale centre, seen in infective endocarditis (but also in several other disorders, including leukaemia, anaemia and vascular diseases)
- hypertensive retinopathy (Table 7.7, Fig. 7.5).

Ask the patient to open their mouth. Look for:

- central cyanosis (blue tongue)
- poor dentition – which may pose a risk of bacteraemia and infective endocarditis
- high arched palate – a feature of Marfan's syndrome.

Table 7.7 Grades of hypertensive retinopathy

Grade	Findings
1	'Silver wiring' – mild narrowing and greater reflectivity of the retinal arteries
2	As grade 1, plus 'arteriovenous (AV) nipping' – focal indentation of the retinal veins where they are crossed by the arteries
3	As grade 2, plus the presence of flame-shaped retinal haemorrhages, soft exudates (cotton-wool spots) and hard exudates
4	As grade 3, plus papilloedema – accelerated (malignant) hypertensive retinopathy

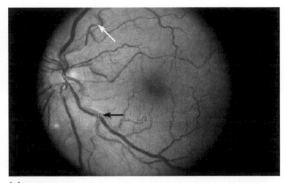

(a)

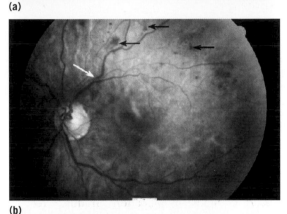

(b)

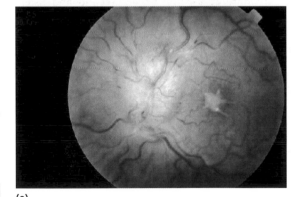

(c)

Figure 7.5 (a) Mild hypertensive retinopathy: AV nicking (black arrow) and focal narrowing (white arrow). (b) Moderate hypertensive retinopathy: retinal haemorrhages (black arrows), AV nicking (white arrow) and generalized retinal arteriolar narrowing. (c) Accelerated (malignant) retinopathy: swelling of optic disc, retinal haemorrhages and cotton-wool spots. Reproduced from Wong TY, McIntosh R. Hypertensive retinopathy signs as risk indicators of cardiovascular morbidity and mortality, *British Medical Bulletin*, 2005; **73-74**: 1, 57–70, by permission of Oxford University Press on behalf of The British Council.

Table 7.8 Distinguishing characteristics of venous and arterial neck pulsation

Internal jugular vein	Carotid artery
Two pulsations per cardiac cycle (if in sinus rhythm)	One pulsation per cardiac cycle
Prominent inward movement	Prominent outward movement
Varies with respiration	No variation with respiration
Varies with patient position	No variation with patient position
Palpable pulsation	Impalpable pulsation
Easily occluded by light pressure	Not easily occluded by light pressure

Jugular venous pressure

Examination of the jugular venous pressure (JVP) tells you about the pressure within the right atrium (judged from the 'height' of the JVP) and about right heart function (judged from the JVP waveform). With the patient reclining at an angle of 45° and with the neck muscles relaxed (use a pillow), inspect the right side of the neck to assess venous pulsation in the right internal jugular vein. This runs from the angle of the jaw, down the neck (passing deep to the sternocleidomastoid muscle), to the sternoclavicular joint. Avoid using the left internal jugular vein (which provides a less accurate guide to the JVP) or the external jugular veins (which are more superficial, and therefore more easily visible, but are more likely to 'kink').

Sometimes it can be tricky to distinguish between pulsation in the internal jugular vein and the carotid artery. Table 7.8 lists some helpful pointers.

Height of the JVP

> **IMPORTANT**
>
> Normal mean right atrial pressure is ≤9cm H₂O (which equates to ≤7 mmHg), so the height of the normal JVP is no more than 4cm above the sternal angle.

As there are no valves between the right atrium and the internal jugular veins, there is effectively a column of blood which acts as a manometer, the height of which reflects right atrial pressure. With the patient reclining at 45°, measure the height of the JVP (taken as the maximum height of pulsation in

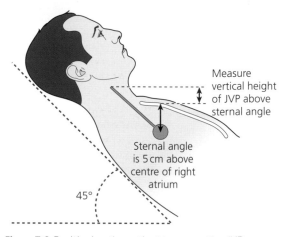

Measure vertical height of JVP above sternal angle

Sternal angle is 5 cm above centre of right atrium

45°

Figure 7.6 Positioning the patient to assess the JVP.

the right internal jugular vein) *vertically* in relation to the angle of the sternum, which itself lies approximately 5 cm above the centre of the right atrium (Fig. 7.6). Thus a JVP which lies exactly at the level of the sternal angle (0 cm) equates to a right atrial pressure of 5 cm H₂O.

You can state the height of the JVP either in relation to the sternal angle ('The JVP lies 2 cm above the sternal angle') or in terms of right atrial pressure (in cm H₂O) by adding 5 cm H₂O to your measurement ('The right atrial pressure is 7 cm H₂O', i.e. 2 + 5). Whichever way you choose to express the JVP, be clear and consistent with your terminology – simply writing 'JVP + 5' in the case notes does not make it clear whether the JVP is 5 cm above the sternal angle (abnormally elevated) or the right atrial pressure is 5 cm H₂O (normal). Box 7.2 lists the causes of raised JVP.

- Heart failure
- Fluid overload
- Superior vena cava obstruction
- Pulmonary embolism
- Constrictive pericarditis
- Cardiac tamponade

An additional manoeuvre that can be performed is the 'abdomino-jugular test', widely known as 'hepato-jugular reflux' (see Box 7.3). This tests the ability of the right heart to deal with an increase in venous return, and is positive if the right heart fails to do so, as in right ventricular failure, pericardial constriction, cardiac tamponade and tricuspid valve disease. The test is performed by applying firm pressure with your right hand over the patient's peri-umbilical area for 30 seconds while observing the height of the JVP. A *sustained* elevation of ≥4 cm in the JVP throughout the test represents a positive (abnormal) result.

Character of the JVP

The character or waveform of the JVP can be challenging to assess. The normal waveform has three peaks (a, c, v) and two descents (x, y), as shown in Figure 7.7.

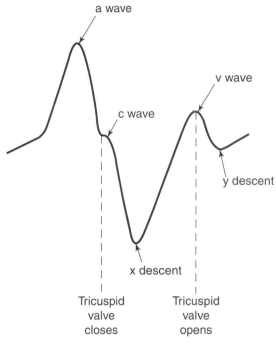

Figure 7.7 The normal JVP waveform.

BOX 7.3 'HEPATO-JUGULAR REFLUX'
The term 'hepato-jugular reflux' is widely used but rather misleading. First, pressure should be applied over the peri-umbilical area, not specifically the liver, to cause splanchnic (not hepatic) blood to return to the circulation. Second, the physiological mechanism is still not fully understood, so to call it 'reflux' may not be correct. Third, some textbooks refer to it as the 'hepato-jugular *reflex*', which is definitely incorrect. The best term may be 'abdomino-jugular test'. For an excellent discussion of this, and other topics, see Brostoff JM. Re-examining examination: misconceptions in clinical medicine. *Journal of the Royal Society of Medicine* 2009; **102**: 11–15.

- 'a' wave – represents right atrial contraction:
  - 'a' waves are prominent when right atrial pressure is raised (e.g. pulmonary hypertension, tricuspid stenosis)
  - giant 'a' waves ('cannon waves') are seen when atrial systole occurs against a closed tricuspid valve (e.g. complete heart block, ventricular tachycardia with retrograde atrial depolarization)
  - 'a' waves are absent in atrial fibrillation (no atrial systole).
- 'x' descent – represents atrial relaxation:
  - 'x' descent is prominent in cardiac tamponade and constrictive pericarditis.
- 'c' wave – interrupts the 'x' descent and represents a transmitted pulsation from the carotid artery; it also happens to mark the moment of tricuspid valve closure at the onset of ventricular systole.
- 'v' wave – represents atrial filling while the tricuspid valve is closed (during ventricular systole)
  - 'v' waves are prominent in tricuspid regurgitation due to regurgitation of blood from the right ventricle back into the right atrium.

- 'y' descent – represents rapid ventricular filling after the tricuspid valve opens:
  - 'y' descent is slow in tricuspid stenosis
  - 'y' descent is prominent in tricuspid regurgitation and constrictive pericarditis.

CLINICAL PEARL

Normally the height of the JVP falls on inspiration. However, if right ventricular filling is impaired (e.g. right ventricular infarction, constrictive pericarditis, cardiac tamponade) the opposite can happen – the JVP *rises* on inspiration. This is called Kussmaul's sign.

Inspection of the precordium

Carefully inspect the chest wall, looking for:

- chest wall deformities:
  - pigeon chest deformity (pectus carinatum)
  - funnel chest deformity (pectus excavatum)
- operation scars:
  - midline sternotomy (e.g. coronary artery bypass and/or valve surgery)
  - left lateral thoracotomy (mitral valvotomy)
- devices:
  - permanent pacemaker
  - implantable cardioverter-defibrillator (ICD)
  - implantable loop recorder
- visible pulsation:
  - apex beat.

Palpation of the praecordium

Using the flat of your hand and with your fingers outstretched, palpate the praecordium to:

- locate and characterize the apex beat
- check for a left parasternal heave
- check for thrills (apex, pulmonary and aortic areas).

The apex beat

The apex beat refers to the most lateral and inferior position in which the cardiac impulse can be palpated – usually the fifth left intercostal space in the left mid-clavicular line. Locate the apex with the index finger of your right hand and then, with your left hand, 'count down' the rib spaces until you reach the space in which the apex beat lies. You may need to ask the patient to roll to their left (the 'left lateral position') to make the apex beat more easily palpable.

Having located the apex beat (see Box 7.4), determine its *character* with your fingertips. Normally the pulsation of the apex beat is relatively gentle. However, a number of abnormalities are recognized. It is easy to tie yourself in knots over the terminology used to describe apex beat character, but essentially there are five distinct abnormalities you need to recognize.

- *Pressure-loaded apex* – a localized, heaving and sustained apex beat, which is found in pressure overload (e.g. left ventricular hypertrophy due to aortic stenosis or hypertension).
- *Volume-loaded apex* – a diffuse, thrusting and non-sustained apex beat, which is found in volume overload (e.g. mitral regurgitation).
- *Tapping apex* – a palpable loud first heart sound, found in mitral stenosis.
- *Double impulse apex* – two beats are felt during each systole. This is found in hypertrophic cardiomyopathy.
- *Dyskinetic apex* – an uncoordinated and diffuse apex beat, usually due to myocardial infarction.

BOX 7.4 CAUSES OF AN IMPALPABLE OR DISPLACED APEX BEAT

An impalpable apex beat may be a consequence of:

- overweight
- hyperinflated lungs (e.g. chronic obstructive pulmonary disease)
- pericardial effusion
- dextrocardia (in which case the apex beat is palpable on the *right* side of the chest).

Displacement of the apex beat (laterally and/or inferiorly) can result from:

- left and/or right ventricular enlargement
- mediastinal shift (so check tracheal position too)
  - tension pneumothorax
  - large pleural effusion
  - lung collapse
- funnel chest deformity (pectus excavatum).

Left parasternal heave

Use the heel of your right hand to check for a heave just to the left of the sternum ('left parasternal heave') which lifts your hand during systole. The presence of a left parasternal heave indicates right ventricular hypertrophy or dilatation.

Thrills

Finally, place the heel of your right hand in the aortic area with your fingers lying across the pulmonary area, and feel for a *thrill* (a vibrating sensation) in both areas. A thrill is caused by turbulent blood flow and represents a palpable murmur. Thrills may also be felt at the apex and left sternal edge (so be alert to them while palpating in these areas too). Apical thrills are more easily felt with the patient in the left lateral position; aortic and pulmonary area thrills are best felt with the patient leaning forwards and in end-expiration. Determine whether the thrill is systolic or diastolic by simultaneously palpating the right internal carotid artery with your left hand.

Auscultation

Auscultation of the heart begins by using the bell in the mitral area (apex, Fig. 7.8), pressing lightly so as not to make the underlying skin taut. The bell is good for low-pitched sounds such as the diastolic murmur of mitral stenosis (see below). Having listened with the bell, now listen again in the same area with the diaphragm of your stethoscope to pick up higher pitched sounds.

Sticking with the diaphragm, move on to the tricuspid area (lower left sternal edge), pulmonary area (second left intercostal space) and aortic area (second right intercostal space) in turn. As you auscultate in each area, palpate the carotid pulse to time the heart sounds with the cardiac cycle.

Auscultate also in the axilla (particularly to detect the radiation of a mitral regurgitation murmur) and over both carotid arteries (for the radiation of an aortic stenosis murmur, and for carotid bruits).

Next ask the patient to roll into the left lateral position and auscultate again with the bell in the mitral area, checking for mitral stenosis. Then ask the patient to sit upright and to lean forwards, and auscultate (during end-expiration: ask the patient to 'Take a breath in – And out – And stop there' – auscultate – 'Now breathe normally') with the diaphragm in the aortic area and lower left sternal edge for the early diastolic murmur of aortic regurgitation.

Heart sounds

First heart sound

Strictly speaking, the first heart sound (S_1) has two components (mitral and tricuspid) and is best heard at the apex. Mitral closure occurs a fraction earlier than tricuspid closure, but for all practical purposes the two occur so closely together that they are heard as a single sound.

A *loud S_1* is heard in:

- mitral stenosis (mitral leaflets are still widely open at the onset of systole)
- short PR interval (mitral leaflets are still widely open at the onset of systole)
- hyperdynamic circulation.

A *soft S_1* is heard in:

- mitral regurgitation (mitral valve leaflets fail to close properly)
- long PR interval (mitral leaflets already partly closed at the onset of systole)
- low cardiac output.

A *variable-intensity S_1* is heard in:

- atrial fibrillation
- ectopic beats
- complete heart block.

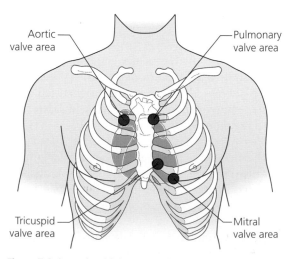

Aortic valve area

Pulmonary valve area

Tricuspid valve area

Mitral valve area

Figure 7.8 Areas in which to auscultate the heart.

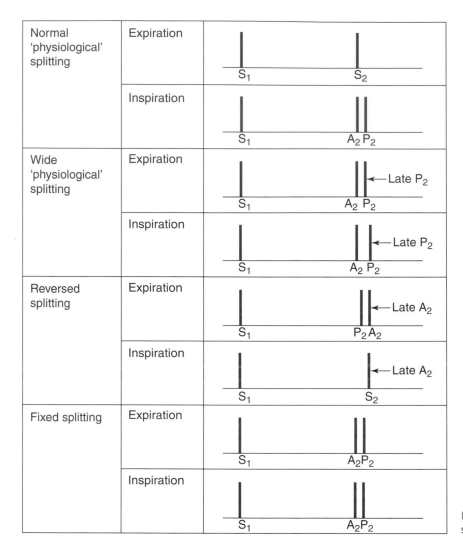

Figure 7.9 Splitting of the second heart sound.

Second heart sound

The second heart sound (S_2) is made up of two separate sounds that result from aortic valve (A_2) and pulmonary valve (P_2) closure. In expiration A_2 and P_2 are almost indistinguishable in adults and so are heard as a virtually single sound (S_2), but in inspiration P_2 is delayed (by an increase in venous return to the right heart) and so S_2 becomes split, with P_2 occurring about 50 ms after A_2 (Fig. 7.9). Splitting is easiest to hear when auscultating over the pulmonary area.

This normal or 'physiological' splitting of S_2 becomes wider if P_2 occurs later (due to delayed or prolonged right ventricular emptying caused by right bundle branch block or pulmonary stenosis), or if A_2 occurs earlier (due to shortened left ventricular emptying due to ventricular septal defect or mitral regurgitation).

Reversed splitting of S_2 (A_2 occurring *after* P_2) is heard in delayed or prolonged left ventricular emptying caused by left bundle branch block or aortic stenosis, and in this situation the splitting is best heard in *expiration* (as P_2 occurs, as normal, later during inspiration and therefore moves closer to the late A_2).

Fixed splitting occurs when there is no variation with respiration and is a characteristic feature of

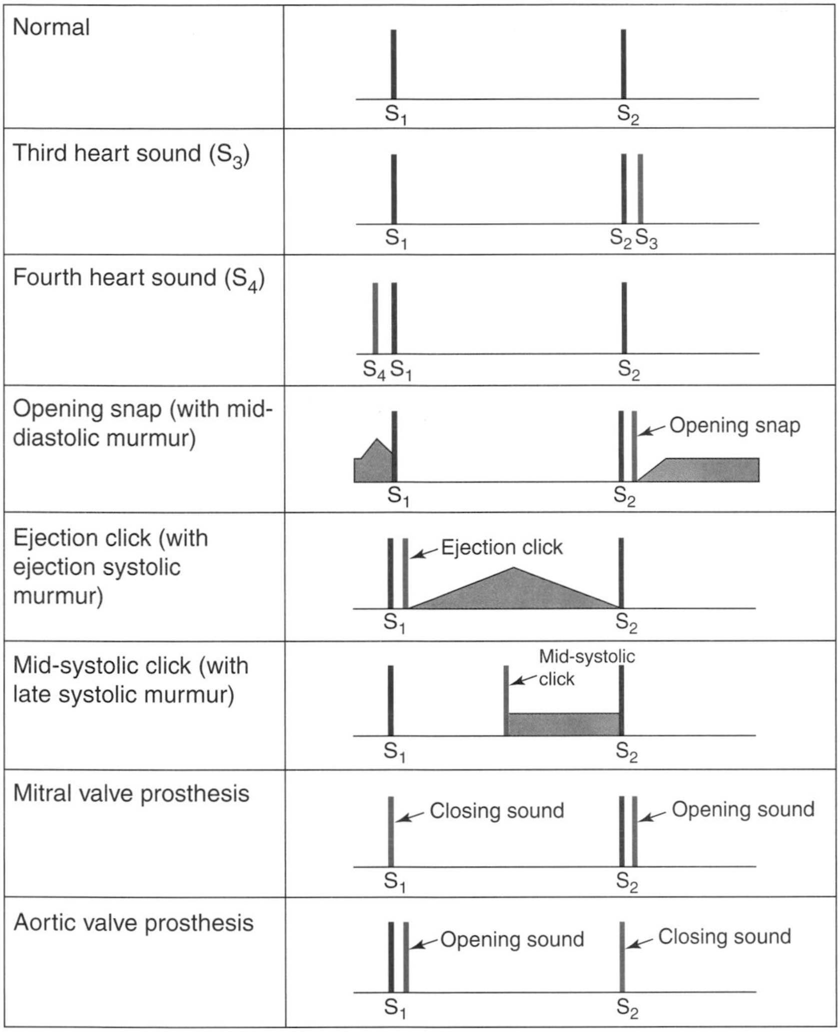
Normal
S1
S2
Third heart sound (S3)
S1
S2 S3
Fourth heart sound (S4)
S4 S1
S2
Opening snap (with mid-diastolic murmur)
Opening snap
S1
S2
Ejection click (with ejection systolic murmur)
Ejection click
S1
S2
Mid-systolic click (with late systolic murmur)
Mid-systolic click
S1
S2
Mitral valve prosthesis
Closing sound
Opening sound
S1
S2
Aortic valve prosthesis
Opening sound
Closing sound
S1
S2

Figure 7.10 Additional heart sounds.

atrial septal defect. The communication between right and left atria means that pressure changes with respiration affect both right and left heart equally.

A *loud* A_2 is heard in:

- systemic hypertension (forceful aortic valve closure).

A *soft* A_2 is heard in:

- calcific aortic stenosis (reduced cusp mobility)
- aortic regurgitation (failure of cusp coaptation).

A *loud* P_2 is heard in:

- pulmonary hypertension (forceful pulmonary valve closure).

Third heart sound

The third heart sound (S_3) is low-pitched and occurs in early diastole soon after S_2 (Fig. 7.10). It coincides with rapid ventricular filling and can be normal in younger patients, particularly athletes and in pregnancy, but in older patients it usually represents reduced left ventricular compliance as seen in heart failure and aortic or mitral regurgitation.

The combination of $S_1 + S_2 + S_3$ is like the cadence of the word 'Kentucky'. When the patient is tachycardic (as is usually the case when S_3 is pathological), this 'triple rhythm' is described as a 'gallop rhythm'. An S_3 arising from the left ventricle is best heard at the apex; from the right ventricle, an S_3 is best heard at the left sternal edge.

Fourth heart sound

The fourth heart sound (S_4) is also low-pitched and quite soft, occurring in late diastole just before S_1. It is caused by atrial contraction against a poorly compliant left ventricle and is therefore always pathological (e.g. left ventricular hypertrophy, ischaemic heart disease, hypertension, aortic stenosis). The combination of $S_4 + S_1 + S_2$ is like the cadence of the word 'Tennessee'. S_4 is best heard at the apex.

Additional heart sounds

Other heart sounds (Fig. 7.10) that may be heard include:

- **Opening snap** – a high-pitched sound best heard at the apex or left sternal edge just after the second heart sound. It occurs in mitral stenosis (and rarely tricuspid stenosis), due to sudden opening of the valve, and is followed by a mid-diastolic murmur.
- **Ejection click** – a high-pitched sound best heard in the aortic/pulmonary areas or left sternal edge just after the first heart sound. It occurs in aortic or pulmonary stenosis due to sudden opening of the valve (if the valve is still relatively mobile), and is followed by an ejection systolic murmur.
- **Mid-systolic click** – a high-pitched sound best heard at the apex in mid-systole. It occurs in mitral valve prolapse and is usually followed by a late systolic murmur.
- **Prosthetic mitral valve sounds** – a mechanical mitral valve will make a metallic opening sound (just after S_2) and closing sound (which coincides with S_1).
- **Prosthetic aortic valve sounds** – a mechanical aortic valve will make a metallic opening sound (just after S_1) and closing sound (which coincides with S_2).
- **Pericardial rub** – a 'scratchy' sound heard in both systole and diastole in pericarditis. Pericardial rubs can come and go quite rapidly, and are enhanced with the patient sitting upright and at end-expiration.

Heart murmurs

For any heart murmur, describe:

- timing – where it occurs in the cardiac cycle (Fig. 7.11); palpate the carotid pulse at the same time as auscultating the murmur to assess the timing

- duration – how long it lasts (e.g. ejection systolic, pansystolic, late systolic)
- character – high or low pitch, harsh, blowing
- loudness – graded on a scale of 1–6 (Table 7.9)
- location – the area of maximal intensity
- radiation – where else it can be heard beyond the area of maximal intensity.

Table 7.9 Grading of murmur intensity

Grade	Intensity
1	Very soft – often missed, and usually only heard by experts
2	Soft – but should not be missed under optimum conditions
3	Moderate intensity but no palpable thrill
4	Easy audible with a palpable thrill
5	Very loud with an easily palpable thrill
6	Extremely loud – can be heard even without the stethoscope touching the chest wall

CLINICAL PEARL
When assessing the intensity of a murmur, bear in mind that *intensity* is often a poor guide to the *severity* of the underlying valve lesion.

Systolic murmurs

There are three types of systolic murmur:

- ejection systolic
- pansystolic
- late systolic.

An *ejection systolic murmur* grows in loudness during early systole, peaks in mid-systole, and diminishes during late systole ('crescendo-decrescendo'). Ejection systolic murmurs result from:

- aortic stenosis
- pulmonary stenosis
- hypertrophic obstructive cardiomyopathy
- increased flow ('flow murmur')
  - pregnancy
  - anaemia
  - fever
  - atrial septal defect (left-to-right shunt).

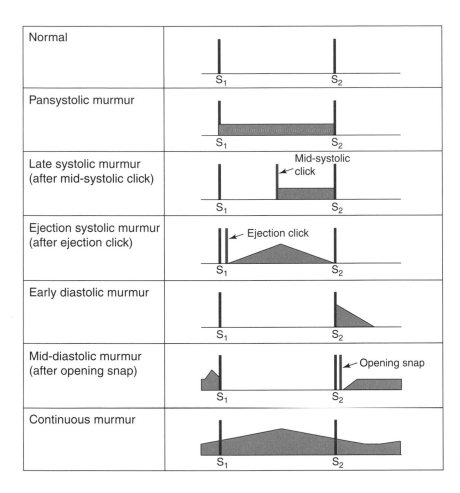

Normal	
Pansystolic murmur	
Late systolic murmur (after mid-systolic click)	
Ejection systolic murmur (after ejection click)	
Early diastolic murmur	
Mid-diastolic murmur (after opening snap)	
Continuous murmur	

Figure 7.11 Heart murmurs.

The ejection systolic murmur of aortic stenosis is usually best heard in the aortic area, and radiates to the carotid arteries. The murmur of pulmonary stenosis is best heard in the pulmonary area. In hypertrophic obstructive cardiomyopathy the murmur is usually loudest at the lower left sternal edge. Flow murmurs are generally best heard in the aortic area, except in the case of atrial septal defect in which case it is loudest in the pulmonary area.

A *pansystolic murmur* begins with S_1 and continues throughout systole to S_2. Pansystolic murmurs result from:

- mitral regurgitation
- tricuspid regurgitation
- ventricular septal defect.

The pansystolic murmur of mitral regurgitation is usually best heard at the apex and radiates to the axilla. The murmurs of tricuspid regurgitation and ventricular septal defect are best heard at the lower left sternal edge.

A *late systolic murmur* begins *after* S_1 and then continues throughout systole to S_2. Late systolic murmurs result from mitral regurgitation secondary to:

- mitral valve prolapse
- papillary muscle dysfunction.

Innocent murmurs

Innocent murmurs (also known as 'functional' or 'physiological' murmurs) are those which occur in the absence of any significant structural heart disease. They always occur in systole, are soft, and there are no other symptoms or signs of heart problems. Such murmurs are commonest in children.

Diastolic murmurs

There are two types of diastolic murmur:

- early diastolic
- mid-diastolic.

An *early diastolic murmur* peaks at the start of diastole and then gradually diminishes in loudness. Early diastolic murmurs result from:

- aortic regurgitation
- pulmonary regurgitation.

The early diastolic murmur of aortic regurgitation is usually best heard at the lower left sternal edge, and is enhanced with the patient sitting forward and in expiration. The murmur of pulmonary regurgitation is sometimes called a Graham Steell murmur and is generally found in the context of pulmonary hypertension.

A *mid-diastolic murmur* is a low-pitched 'rumbling' murmur which is loudest in the middle of diastole. Mid-diastolic murmurs result from:

- mitral stenosis
- tricuspid stenosis (rare).

The mid-diastolic murmur of mitral stenosis is best heard at the apex, and is enhanced with the patient rolled onto their left side. If the patient is in sinus rhythm, there may be an increase in the loudness of the murmur ('pre-systolic accentuation') at the end of diastole, coinciding with the 'kick' of atrial contraction which increases flow across the stenotic valve.

Continuous murmur

A continuous or 'machinery' murmur is heard during systole *and* diastole, and is most commonly due to a persistent (patent) ductus arteriosus (which connects the aorta to the pulmonary artery). The murmur is best heard at the upper left sternal edge and over the left scapula.

The chest and back

Ask the patient to lean forwards and perform a chest examination (Chapter 8). In particular, auscultate at the lung bases for the presence of inspiratory crackles, indicating the presence of pulmonary oedema (p. 67). As pulmonary oedema worsens,

> **CLINICAL PEARL**
>
> A number of bedside manoeuvres can affect the intensity of heart murmurs, and this can help in the diagnosis.
>
> - Inspiration makes right heart murmurs louder (due to an increase in venous return).
> - A Valsalva manoeuvre increases the loudness of the ejection systolic murmur of hypertrophic obstructive cardiomyopathy.
> - Rapid squatting from a standing position diminishes the murmur of hypertrophic obstructive cardiomyopathy. It also delays the mid-systolic click of mitral valve prolapse.
> - Sustained handgrip increases the intensity of the pansystolic murmur of mitral regurgitation and ventricular septal defect, but does not affect (or may diminish) the ejection systolic murmur of aortic stenosis.

the crackles may extend higher in the lung fields. A degree of bronchospasm may be evident causing an expiratory wheeze ('cardiac asthma'). Heart failure may also cause a pleural effusion, usually bilaterally but occasionally unilaterally.

While the patient is sitting forward, take this opportunity to check the sacral area for pitting oedema. Like ankle oedema, this is a sign of right heart/congestive cardiac failure, and is commonly found when such patients have been confined to bed.

The abdomen

Ask the patient to lie flat and perform an abdominal examination (Chapter 9). In particular, check for:

- hepatomegaly (as a sign of congestive cardiac failure)
- hepatic pulsatility (in tricuspid regurgitation or, rarely, aortic regurgitation)
- splenomegaly (in infective endocarditis)
- ascites (in congestive cardiac failure)
- abdominal aortic aneurysm (p. 77).

The lower limbs

Examine the lower limbs to assess:

- the arterial circulation (p. 77)

- the venous circulation (p. 79)
- peripheral oedema (p. 67).

Check for the presence of pitting peripheral oedema by applying finger pressure for 15 seconds:

- pitting is confirmed if a pit (indentation) remains after the finger is removed
- *be gentle* – pitting oedema can make the overlying skin very tender.

> **CLINICAL PEARL**
>
> If pitting oedema is present, assess how far up the leg it extends (it can sometimes involve the abdominal wall and scrotum). Remember to check for sacral oedema.

INVESTIGATIONS

Electrocardiogram

12-lead ECG

The 12-lead ECG is a relatively simple, safe and widely available tool that can reveal considerable amounts of information about the heart (Fig. 7.12). A detailed discussion of ECG interpretation is outside the scope of this chapter, but helpful textbooks are available (see Further reading, p. 81). In short, the 12-lead ECG uses information from 10 electrodes (four limb electrodes, one on each limb, and six chest electrodes) to generate 12 different 'leads' (or 'views') of the heart. Using this information, the ECG can provide information on:

- heart rate
- heart rhythm
- structural heart abnormalities (e.g. atrial enlargement, ventricular hypertrophy)
- myocardial ischaemia
- myocardial infarction
- electrolyte abnormalities
- drug effects on the heart
- miscellaneous abnormalities (e.g. hypothermia).

In reporting on a 12-lead ECG, always adopt a structured approach:

- check the patient's identification details
- check the date and time of the recording
- assess the heart rate
- assess the heart rhythm
- measure the cardiac axis (normally between −30° and +90°)
- inspect the P waves (= atrial depolarization, Fig. 7.13)
- measure the PR interval (normally between 120 and 200 ms)
- check for abnormal Q waves

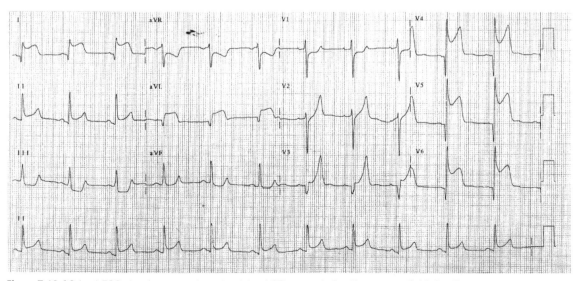

Figure 7.12 12-lead ECG showing an acute anterolateral ST-segment elevation myocardial infarction.

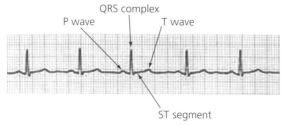

Figure 7.13 Components of the normal ECG.

- inspect the QRS complexes (= ventricular depolarization)
- assess the ST segments
- inspect the T waves
- measure the QT interval
- check for any additional features, e.g. J waves, U waves.

Ambulatory ECG

When investigating a patient who has episodic palpitations, there is no substitute for obtaining an ECG recording *during* an episode of palpitation. This usually requires some form of ambulatory ECG monitoring, with the patient wearing or carrying an ECG monitor for an extended period until a symptomatic event occurs. This can be achieved using one of the following methods:

- 24-hour ambulatory ECG recording
- event recorder
- implantable loop recorder.

The appropriate choice of method depends upon how frequently symptomatic episodes occur – there is little point in a 24-hour recording if the patient only experiences palpitations once every 3 months, for instance.

Exercise ECG

Exercise ECG testing can be useful in:

- diagnosing chest pain
- risk stratification in stable angina
- risk stratification after myocardial infarction
- assessing exercise-induced arrhythmias
- assessing the need for a permanent pacemaker
- assessing exercise tolerance
- assessing response to treatment.

Exercise ECG testing is usually performed using treadmill or bicycle exercise, with continuous 12-lead ECG and blood pressure monitoring. Any relevant symptoms (e.g. chest tightness and/or breathlessness) are noted, together with any ischaemic ECG changes (classically ST-segment depression, but sometimes T wave inversion), arrhythmias or abnormal blood pressure response.

Chest X-ray

The chest X-ray has many roles in cardiac assessment.

- *Assessing heart size* – the cardiothoracic ratio, which compares the transverse diameter of the heart to that of the thoracic cage, is normally <50 per cent. An increased cardiothoracic ratio indicates enlargement of the heart (cardiomegaly), e.g. due to dilated cardiomyopathy or pericardial effusion.
- *Assessing heart shape* – in certain conditions the cardiac silhouette may be abnormal (e.g. the 'boot-shaped' heart of tetralogy of Fallot, Fig. 7.14).
- Assessing lung fields:
  - left ventricular failure (upper lobe venous diversion, Kerley B lines, diffuse lung shadowing, pleural effusions)

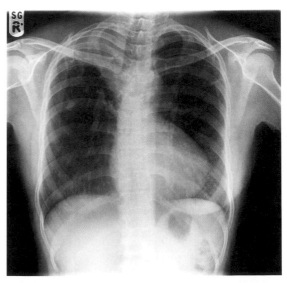

Figure 7.14 Chest X-ray showing the 'boot-shaped' heart of tetralogy of Fallot. This X-ray also shows right upper lobe collapse secondary to previous tuberculosis.

- enlarged pulmonary arteries (left-to-right shunts).
- Miscellaneous features:
  - rib notching in coarctation of the aorta
  - sternal sutures following cardiothoracic surgery
  - prosthetic heart valves.

Echocardiogram

Cardiac ultrasonography (echocardiography) is one of the most versatile of cardiac investigations, revealing detailed information about cardiac structure and function (Fig. 7.15). In transthoracic echo (TTE) an ultrasound probe is applied to the anterior chest wall to obtain 2-D (and, where available, 3-D) moving images of the heart, and also to assess blood flow using the Doppler principle. There are many indications for TTE, including the assessment of:

- breathlessness (e.g. left ventricular failure, pulmonary hypertension)
- heart murmurs
- infective endocarditis
- prosthetic valves
- cardiomyopathy
- pericardial disease (e.g. pericardial effusion)
- congenital heart disease.

TTE can be combined with stress (using exercise or a pharmacological stressor) to assess left ventricular function for signs of myocardial ischaemia or infarction ('stress echo').

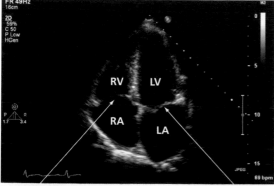

Tricuspid valve   Mitral valve

Figure 7.15 A normal echocardiogram ('apical 4-chamber view'). LA, left atrium; LV, left ventricle; RA, right atrium; RV, right ventricle.

Transoesophageal echo (TOE or TEE) uses the same principles as TTE, but the probe is passed into the patient's oesophagus. This provides clearer images, making TOE particularly useful when higher resolution imaging is necessary (such as the detection of small vegetations in suspected infective endocarditis). The commonest indications for a TOE study include assessment of:

- cardiac source of emboli
- suspected or proven infective endocarditis
- aortic diseases (e.g. aortic dissection/trauma)
- regurgitant heart valves, to judge suitability for surgical repair
- prosthetic valves (especially those in the mitral position)
- cardiac masses
- congenital heart disease and intracardiac shunts.

Nuclear cardiology

Myocardial perfusion imaging uses a radiopharmaceutical (e.g. thallium-201 or a technetium-99m-labelled radiopharmaceutical), administered intravenously, to assess myocardial blood flow, providing valuable information about coronary artery disease with a high degree of sensitivity and specificity (Fig. 7.16).

Radionuclide ventriculography assesses ventricular function using red blood cells labelled with technetium-99m. The count-rate of the radioactivity can be measured using a gamma camera at different stages of the cardiac cycle, and from this an accurate measure of ejection fraction can be derived.

Cardiac magnetic resonance imaging

Cardiac magnetic resonance imaging (MRI) is a highly versatile technique for cardiac imaging and provides both anatomical and functional information. Examples of its many uses include the assessment of:

- cardiac chamber dimensions and function
- valvular heart disease
- cardiomyopathies
- cardiac masses
- congenital heart disease
- pericardial disease
- aortic abnormalities.

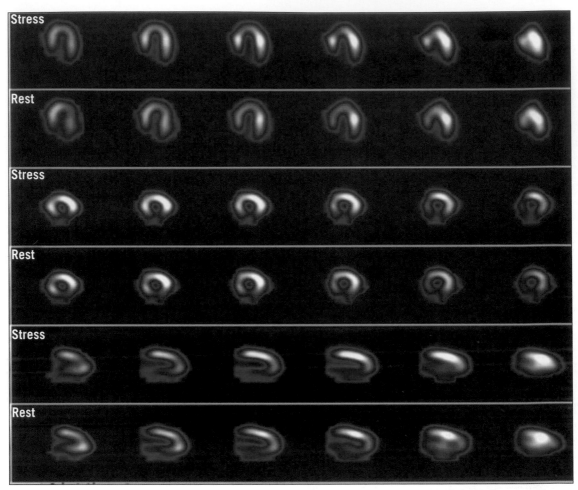

Figure 7.16 Myocardial perfusion imaging (showing inferior wall defect). From: Houghton AR. *Making sense of echocardiography*, with permission. © 2009 London: Hodder Arnold.

> ## *i* IMPORTANT
> Although cardiac MRI does not involve exposure to ionizing radiation, it does use a powerful magnetic field and is therefore contraindicated in patients with certain types of metallic implants (e.g. pacemakers, implantable defibrillators and cerebrovascular aneurysm clips).

Cardiac computed tomography

Multislice computed tomography (MSCT) is used to image the heart. MSCT scanners contain a gantry carrying an X-ray source that rotates around the patient, and multiple image 'slices' are obtained as the patient is moved through the gantry during the scan. The slices are then processed to generate images of the heart in any plane and from any angle, either as a three-dimensional volume rendered image (Fig. 7.17) or as cross-sectional slices.

Cardiac CT scanning is very fast (it takes just a few seconds to acquire the images) but processing and reporting the images usually takes 10–30 minutes.

The main use of cardiac CT is in assessment of the coronary arteries. A calcium score can be obtained (reflecting the amount of calcification present in the coronary arteries) and this correlates with the patient's risk of future cardiovascular events. With

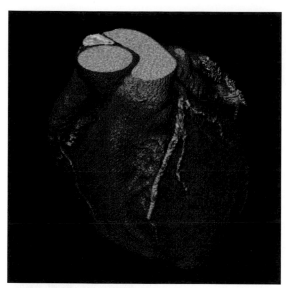

Figure 7.17 Cardiac computed tomography (CT) scan (volume rendered image). Reproduced from *Heart*, Roberts WT, Bax JJ, Davies LC, **94**: 781–92 © 2008 with permission from BMJ Publishing Group Ltd.

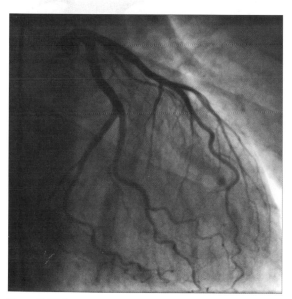

Figure 7.18 Coronary angiogram (showing a normal left coronary artery). From: Houghton AR. *Making sense of echocardiography*, with permission. © 2009 London: Hodder Arnold.

the injection of an intravenous contrast agent, the coronary arteries themselves can be imaged (CT coronary angiography).

Cardiac catheterization

Cardiac catheterization is an invasive technique, requiring a catheter to be passed to the heart via a peripheral vessel such as the radial or femoral artery. By injecting a contrast agent, the operator can image the coronary arteries (Fig. 7.18) and cardiac chambers. The catheter can also be used to measure intracardiac pressures and oxygen saturations.

COMMON DIAGNOSES

Angina

The discomfort of myocardial ischaemia (angina) is typically felt as a heavy, tight, squeezing or band-like sensation in the centre of the chest (retrosternal), and may radiate to the left and/or right arm, to the neck (causing a 'choking' discomfort) and to the jaw. When asked to indicate the location of the discomfort, patients with angina will often hold a clenched fist in front of the sternum (Levine's sign). Pain which is left sided and/or can be 'pointed to' with a finger is unlikely to be angina.

> **IMPORTANT** *i*
> Myocardial ischaemia can cause breathlessness as well as chest discomfort, and in many cases breathlessness is the *predominant* symptom (particularly in women). Be sure to ask about breathlessness in patients with suspected myocardial ischaemia, and similarly be sure to consider myocardial ischaemia in the differential diagnosis in patients presenting with breathlessness.

Angina is typically precipitated and/or exacerbated by physical exertion and is often reproducible, such that patients find that a certain amount of exertion under the same conditions predictably brings on their symptoms. However, some patients notice that their exercise tolerance improves for a while after an angina attack, a characteristic known as ischaemic preconditioning (or the 'warm-up phenomenon'). Conversely, angina is more easily provoked by exertion after a heavy meal, or by exercising in a cold environment. Many patients will say that their angina is at its worst when trying to walk into a cold headwind. The degree of functional limitation can be categorized as grade I to grade IV according to the Canadian Cardiovascular Society (CCS) angina grading scale (www.ccs.ca/download/position_statements/Grading%20of%20Angina.pdf).

Anginal symptoms are usually relieved quickly by rest or by the use of sublingual GTN – normally in less than 5 minutes. GTN will also relieve the symptoms of oesophageal spasm, but usually takes longer than 5 minutes to do so.

Chest pain is regarded as 'typical' of angina if it is retrosternal, brought on by stress, and relieved by rest or GTN. Pain which has just two of these characteristics is termed 'atypical', and pain with just one characteristic is termed 'non-specific'.

> **CLINICAL PEARL**
>
> A patient's response to GTN given as a 'test of treatment' can sometimes help with the diagnosis of angina. Angina usually improves rapidly with GTN. A response within 5 minutes has a sensitivity of around 60 per cent and a specificity of around 70 per cent for the diagnosis of angina. (Chun AA, McGee SR. Bedside diagnosis of coronary artery disease: a systematic review. *Am J Med* 2004; **117**: 334–43.)

Physical examination is usually unremarkable in stable angina, although there may be signs of associated risk factors such as hyperlipidaemia (tendon xanthoma, periorbital xanthelasma, corneal arcus) or hypertension. Look for evidence of vascular disease elsewhere (carotid artery bruits, diminished peripheral pulses). Auscultation of the heart *during* an angina attack may reveal evidence of ischaemic left ventricular dysfunction (third or fourth heart sound, ischaemic mitral regurgitation).

Angina usually occurs in the presence of coronary atheroma, but it can occur in the presence of normal coronary arteries if there is increased myocardial oxygen demand (e.g. hypertrophic cardiomyopathy) or reduced cardiac output (e.g. severe aortic stenosis). It can also result from coronary artery spasm ('Prinzmetal's angina') – the symptoms are similar in char-

acter to exertional angina, but typically occur at rest (particularly during the night) and are associated with transient ST segment elevation (rather than depression) on the ECG during episodes of pain. The occurrence of anginal symptoms and myocardial ischaemia in the absence of any anatomical obstruction to blood flow (e.g. coronary atheroma, aortic stenosis) or coronary artery spasm is termed syndrome X and is thought to result from microvascular dysfunction.

The investigation of angina can be *physiological* (stress testing with an exercise treadmill test, stress echocardiogram, stress cardiac MRI scan or nuclear myocardial perfusion scan) or *anatomical* (CT coronary angiogram or cardiac catheterization).

Acute coronary syndrome

The chest discomfort of an acute coronary syndrome (ACS) has similar characteristics to that of angina. However, the chest discomfort of ACS is typically:

- more severe ('crushing')
- longer lasting
- lacking an obvious precipitant (often occurring at rest)
- not relieved by GTN
- associated with sweating, nausea and vomiting.

Acute coronary syndrome is a medical emergency and you should advise patients to call the emergency medical services when they experience prolonged central chest pain that does not respond to GTN. ACS can be categorized as:

- unstable angina
- non-ST-segment elevation myocardial infarction (NSTEMI)
- ST-segment elevation myocardial infarction (STEMI).

The clinical features of all three types of ACS are the same, and the diagnosis is based initially on the ECG findings and subsequently on levels of cardiac markers in the blood (e.g. troponin I or T).

Physical examination in ACS will often reveal the patient to be unwell and obviously in pain, with sweating ('diaphoresis'), nausea and vomiting. The remainder of the examination should assess:

- heart rate:
  - bradycardic if parasympathetic overactivity/heart block

- tachycardiac if sympathetic overactivity/ tachyarrhythmias
- blood pressure:
  - low if parasympathetic overactivity/heart failure
  - high if pre-existing hypertension/sympathetic overactivity
- JVP – elevated JVP with right ventricular infarction
- heart sounds:
  - third or fourth heart sound in ischaemic left ventricular dysfunction
  - mid-late systolic murmur from ischaemic mitral regurgitation
  - pan-systolic murmur from papillary muscle rupture or acute ventricular septal defect
  - pericardial rub from pericarditis
- evidence of left ventricular failure.

Aortic dissection

Aortic dissection, a tear between the layers in the wall of the aorta, usually presents with pain that is:

- severe
- of sudden onset
- interscapular
- 'tearing' in character.

However, not all of these features will necessarily be present, and sometimes other features (such as those relating to compromised flow in vessels arising from the aorta, see below) may predominate. Such 'atypical' presentations mean that aortic dissection is a commonly overlooked diagnosis. You need to maintain a high index of suspicion so as not to miss the diagnosis.

Assess the patient for the presence of risk factors for aortic dissection:

- hypertension
- Marfan's syndrome
- Ehlers–Danlos syndrome
- chest trauma (e.g. blunt injury from a car accident)
- pregnancy
- bicuspid aortic valve
- aortic coarctation
- syphilitic aortitis.

A number of vessels arise from the aorta and these may be compromised by the dissection. Patients may therefore have features of:

- myocardial ischaemia/infarction (coronary artery involvement)
- neurological deficits (cerebral or spinal artery involvement)
- renal ischaemia
- mesenteric ischaemia.

The aortic dissection can involve the aortic root, causing aortic regurgitation, or rupture into the pericardium, leading to cardiac tamponade (p. 76). If the aortic dissection compromises flow down one or other subclavian artery, there may be a difference in blood pressure between the two arms – however, such a blood pressure deficit is found in less than a third of cases of dissection.

A chest X-ray may show a widened mediastinum. Investigations to image the aorta directly and confirm aortic dissection include MRI, CT angiography or transoesophageal echocardiography.

> **IMPORTANT** *i*
> Aortic dissection is a medical emergency, and must be distinguished from myocardial infarction – the use of a thrombolytic drug is *absolutely contraindicated* by the presence of an aortic dissection. Remember that the two conditions can occur at the same time, if the dissection involves the origin of one of the coronary arteries.

Heart failure and cardiomyopathy

Heart failure is common, affecting 1–2 per cent of the population (and is particularly common in the elderly, affecting over 10 per cent of those aged over 85 years). Heart failure is regarded as a clinical syndrome in which patients have the symptoms and signs of heart failure together with objective evidence of a structural or functional cardiac abnormality at rest. It can be classified as:

- left and/or right ventricular failure
- systolic and/or diastolic
- acute or chronic
- high output (e.g. thyrotoxicosis) or low output.

The functional status of patients with heart failure can be graded according to the NYHA scale (Table 7.2). When assessing the patient for symptoms and signs of heart failure, remember to look for evidence of the underlying cause (Box 7.5).

BOX 7.5 CAUSES OF SYSTOLIC HEART FAILURE
- Coronary artery disease
- Hypertension
- Valvular disease
- Viral myocarditis
- Cardiomyopathy
- Cardiotoxic drugs e.g. anthracyclines
- Alcohol.

Symptoms

Left ventricular failure may be asymptomatic or it may manifest as:

- exertional breathlessness
- orthopnoea
- paroxysmal nocturnal dyspnoea
- cough (sometimes with pink frothy sputum)
- fatigue.

Right ventricular failure:

- ankle swelling
- abdominal symptoms (due to hepatic congestion and/or ascites)
    - loss of appetite
    - abdominal discomfort
    - abdominal swelling.

Signs

Left ventricular failure:

- tachycardia
- alternating pulse ('pulsus alternans')
- hypotension with a narrow pulse pressure
- displaced, volume-loaded apex beat
- S3 and/or S4 (gallop rhythm)
- tachypnoea
- inspiratory crackles at lung bases
- pleural effusion (sometimes).

Right ventricular failure:

- elevated JVP

- ankle and/or sacral oedema
- hepatomegaly
- ascites.

In advanced heart failure patients may develop muscle wasting and weight loss ('cardiac cachexia'). Remember that the clinical features of left and right heart failure can co-exist.

Investigations

The cornerstone of investigating heart failure is an echocardiogram. Left ventricular size and function (commonly expressed in terms of 'ejection fraction') can be assessed, together with right ventricular size and function. Co-existent structural abnormalities (e.g. valvular heart disease), which may be causing or contributing to the heart failure, can be assessed at the same time. The chest X-ray may show an enlarged heart (cardiomegaly), pulmonary venous congestion, pulmonary oedema or pleural effusions.

Hypertrophic cardiomyopathy

Hypertrophic cardiomyopathy (HCM) is an autosomal dominant condition affecting 1 in 500 of the population and is a common cause of sudden cardiac death, particularly in the young. The left ventricular hypertrophy in HCM is usually asymmetrical (in contrast to the concentric left ventricular hypertrophy seen in hypertension or aortic stenosis) and systolic function is preserved but diastolic function is impaired. If the hypertrophy is located in the left ventricular outflow tract it may obstruct the flow of blood out of the left ventricle into the aorta – this is hypertrophic *obstructive* cardiomyopathy (HOCM).

Hypertrophic cardiomyopathy may be asymptomatic, but can present with:

- breathlessness
- chest pain
- palpitations
- pre-syncope/syncope
- (sudden cardiac death).

Ask about any known family history of the condition (or of sudden death) – family screening is important, so compile a list of first-degree relatives. The clinical features include:

- 'jerky' pulse (pulsus bisferiens)

BOX 7.6 CAUSES OF SECONDARY HYPERTENSION
- Renal parenchymal disease (e.g. polycystic kidney disease)
- Renovascular disease (e.g. renal artery stenosis)
- Endocrine/metabolic:
  - phaeochromocytoma
  - acromegaly
  - Conn's syndrome
  - Cushing's syndrome
- Drugs:
  - steroids
  - non-steroidal anti-inflammatory drugs
  - oral contraceptives
  - liquorice
- Coarctation of the aorta

cardiovascular disease. In 95 per cent of cases hypertension is idiopathic ('essential' hypertension), but in 5 per cent there is an identifiable underlying cause (Box 7.6).

Symptoms

Hypertension is usually asymptomatic and discovered as an incidental finding during a 'routine' examination. However, it may present with features resulting from end-organ damage:

- myocardial ischaemia or infarction
- heart failure
- peripheral vascular disease
- aortic dissection
- cerebrovascular disease (e.g. stroke)
- renal failure.

Signs

- Measure blood pressure (p. 49):
  - grade the severity of hypertension (Table 7.10).
- Loud aortic component to second heart sound (A_2).
- Look for evidence of an underlying cause of hypertension:
  - renal parenchymal disease
  - renovascular disease
  - endocrine/metabolic disease
  - coarctation of the aorta.
- Look for evidence of end-organ damage:
  - hypertensive retinopathy

- double impulse apex beat
- fourth heart sound (S_4)
- ejection systolic murmur (if obstruction is present), usually best heard at the lower left sternal edge. The murmur increases in loudness with a Valsalva manoeuvre (in contrast to aortic stenosis, where the murmur becomes quieter).

The diagnosis of hypertrophic cardiomyopathy can be confirmed with echocardiography.

Hypertension

Hypertension is arbitrarily defined as a blood pressure >140/90 mmHg and is a major risk factor for

Table 7.10 British Hypertension Society classification of blood pressure levels

Category	Systolic blood pressure (mmHg)	Diastolic blood pressure (mmHg)
Optimal blood pressure	<120	<80
Normal blood pressure	<130	<85
High-normal blood pressure	130–139	85–89
Grade 1 hypertension (mild)	140–159	90–99
Grade 2 hypertension (moderate)	160–179	100–109
Grade 3 hypertension (severe)	≥180	≥110
Isolated systolic hypertension (Grade 1)	140–159	<90
Isolated systolic hypertension (Grade 2)	≥160	<90

Reprinted by permission from Macmillan Publishers. Williams B, Poulter NR, Brown MJ *et al.* 2004. Guidelines for management of hypertension: report of the fourth working party of the British Hypertension Society 2004 – BHS IV. *Journal of Human Hypertension* **18**: 139–85.

- left ventricular hypertrophy
- heart failure
- cerebrovascular disease (e.g. stroke, transient ischaemic attack, carotid artery bruits)
- hypertensive encephalopathy
- peripheral vascular disease.

Investigations

Investigations in the hypertensive patient should include:

- urine dipstick analysis for protein and blood
- serum urea and electrolytes, glucose, lipid profile
- ECG
- echocardiogram, if left ventricular hypertrophy is suspected.

Ambulatory blood pressure monitoring can be useful in cases of 'white coat' hypertension.

SMALL PRINT

Accelerated ('malignant') hypertension is rare, affecting around 1 per cent of hypertensive patients, but is a medical emergency. It is characterized by severe hypertension and the presence of grade III/ IV hypertensive retinopathy and/or hypertensive encephalopathy (seizures, blurred vision, altered mental state).

Atrial fibrillation

Atrial fibrillation (AF) is the commonest sustained arrhythmia and affects 5–10 per cent of elderly people. It can be classified as paroxysmal, persistent or permanent:

- *paroxysmal AF* – spontaneously terminating episodes of AF on a background of sinus rhythm
- *persistent AF* – continuous AF with no intervening sinus rhythm
- *permanent AF* – continuous AF where there is no expectation of restoring sinus rhythm (e.g. by DC cardioversion).

Symptoms

Atrial fibrillation may be asymptomatic (incidental finding). However, it may present with:

- palpitations (irregular and often fast)
- breathlessness
- fatigue
- dizziness or syncope
- reduced exercise tolerance
- symptoms arising from systemic embolism (e.g. stroke, peripheral embolism)
- symptoms of an underlying cause (see Box 7.7).

BOX 7.7 CAUSES OF ATRIAL FIBRILLATION

- Hypertension
- Ischaemic heart disease
- Hyperthyroidism
- Sick sinus syndrome
- Alcohol
- Mitral or tricuspid valve disease
- Cardiomyopathy
- Atrial septal defect
- Pericarditis
- Myocarditis
- Pulmonary embolism
- Pneumonia
- Cardiac surgery
- Idiopathic ('lone') atrial fibrillation

Systemic embolism is a significant risk in AF and may also be a presenting feature. The risk of stroke can be estimated using the $CHADS_2$ score (see Box 7.8).

Signs

The signs of atrial fibrillation include:

- irregularly irregular pulse, often with tachycardia
- blood pressure:
  - may be high if underlying hypertension
  - may be low if AF is poorly tolerated
- absent 'a' wave in JVP (absent atrial systole)
- variable intensity S_1
- signs of left ventricular failure if AF is poorly tolerated
- signs of underlying conditions (e.g. hyperthyroidism, mitral or tricuspid valve disease).

Investigations

The diagnosis of AF can be confirmed with an ECG, which will show absent P waves and an irregularly

BOX 7.8 PREDICTING STROKE RISK IN AF – THE CHADS$_2$ SCORE

The CHADS$_2$ score predicts stroke risk in patients with non-rheumatic AF (patients with rheumatic valve disease already have a high stroke risk). The CHADS$_2$ score assigns 1 point for each of the following characteristics:

- **C**ongestive heart failure
- **H**ypertension
- **A**ge ≥75 years
- **D**iabetes mellitus

and assigns 2 points for:

- **S**troke or transient ischaemic attack.

Thus patients can have a total CHADS$_2$ score between 0 and 6. A score of 0 is taken to indicate a low risk, 1 a moderate risk, and 2 or more a high risk of stroke.

Reference: Gage BF *et al*. Validation of clinical classification schemes for predicting stroke results from the National Registry of Atrial Fibrillation. *JAMA* 2001; **285**: 2864–70.

irregular rhythm, often with a fast ventricular rate. Ambulatory ECG monitoring may be required if the AF is paroxysmal. An echocardiogram will identify underlying structural heart disease, and thyroid function tests are essential, as AF may be the only sign of a thyroid disorder.

Atrial flutter

Atrial flutter causes similar symptoms to AF and carries similar implications in terms of ventricular rate control, anticoagulation and cardioversion. However, in atrial flutter the underlying atrial rhythm is regular (approximately 300 atrial depolarizations per minute) as opposed to irregularly irregular in AF. Patients with atrial flutter will often have 2:1, 3:1 or 4:1 atrioventricular block, which gives them a ventricular rate of 150 bpm, 100 bpm or 75 bpm respectively. Unlike AF, the pulse will usually be *regular* on examination (unless the patient has variable block). Thus from the pulse alone it can be impossible to distinguish between atrial flutter and sinus rhythm, and an ECG should be recorded to confirm the diagnosis.

Aortic stenosis

Calcific degeneration of the aortic valve is one of the commonest causes of aortic stenosis and is characterized by progressive fibrosis and calcification of the aortic valve. *Bicuspid aortic valve* is also common, and is thought to be responsible for around half of cases of severe aortic stenosis in adults (particularly when aortic stenosis occurs at a young age). *Rheumatic aortic stenosis* is less common than rheumatic mitral stenosis, and the two often co-exist in the same patient. There is fusion of the commissures of the aortic valve cusps and the cusps themselves become fibrotic and eventually calcified.

Symptoms

Aortic stenosis may be asymptomatic (incidental finding) or it may present with:

- exertional chest pain
- exertional dizziness and/or syncope
- exertional breathlessness.

The development of symptoms has prognostic implications: those with chest pain as a result of aortic stenosis have an average life expectancy of 5 years, those with exertional syncope 3 years, and those with heart failure just 1 year.

Signs

The signs of aortic stenosis include:

- slow-rising, small volume pulse
- low systolic blood pressure and narrow pulse pressure
- hyperdynamic apex beat (as a result of left ventricular hypertrophy)
- soft or absent aortic component (A$_2$) to second heart sound
- reversed splitting of S$_2$ (A$_2$ occurring *after* P$_2$)
- ejection click (if cusps remain mobile)
- harsh ejection systolic murmur
  - loudest in the aortic area
  - may cause a systolic thrill
  - may radiate to the carotid arteries
- signs of left ventricular failure (p. 67) in advanced cases.

Indicators of severity

- Slow-rising pulse.
- Presence of a systolic thrill.
- Soft or absent aortic component (A_2) to second heart sound.
- Late peaking in the intensity of the ejection systolic murmur.
- Symptoms and/or signs of left ventricular failure.

Differential diagnosis

An ejection systolic murmur may also be heard with:

- increased flow across a normal valve ('innocent' murmur, e.g. due to fever, anaemia, pregnancy)
- supravalvular aortic stenosis
- subvalvular aortic stenosis
- pulmonary stenosis
- hypertrophic obstructive cardiomyopathy (p. 68).

> **CLINICAL PEARL**
>
> The term 'aortic sclerosis' is often used when there is an ejection systolic murmur and on echo some thickening of the aortic valve cusps is evident, but there is no significant pressure gradient across the valve. Many cases of aortic sclerosis subsequently go on to develop stenosis.

Aortic regurgitation

Aortic regurgitation can result from a problem with the aortic valve itself or from a problem with the aortic root affecting an otherwise normal valve. *Valvular* causes include:

- bicuspid aortic valve, causing incomplete closure of the valve
- calcific degeneration of the aortic valve
- rheumatic aortic valve disease
- infective endocarditis
- connective tissue diseases (e.g. rheumatoid arthritis, systemic lupus erythematosus).

Aortic root causes result from dilatation and/or distortion of the aortic root. These include:

- hypertension
- Marfan's syndrome

- Ehlers–Danlos syndrome
- osteogenesis imperfecta
- aortic dissection
- sinus of Valsalva aneurysm
- cystic medial necrosis
- syphilitic aortitis
- Behçet disease.

Symptoms

Aortic regurgitation may be asymptomatic (incidental finding), or may present with symptoms of left ventricular failure:

- breathlessness
- orthopnoea
- paroxysmal nocturnal dyspnoea.

Symptoms may also indicate the aetiology (e.g. tearing interscapular pain in aortic dissection; fever and sweats in infective endocarditis).

Signs

The signs of aortic regurgitation include:

- collapsing pulse
- low diastolic blood pressure and wide pulse pressure
- prominent arterial pulsation (Table 7.11)
- displaced and hyperkinetic apex beat
- presence of a diastolic thrill in the aortic area/ lower left sternal edge
- soft aortic component (A_2) to second heart sound
- early diastolic murmur in the aortic area and lower left sternal edge.

There may also be additional murmurs:

- an ejection systolic murmur, reflecting hyperdynamic flow across the aortic valve
- an Austin Flint murmur (an apical low-pitched mid-diastolic murmur caused by the regurgitant jet impinging on the anterior mitral leaflet).

Signs of left ventricular failure (p. 67) may be seen in advanced cases. Signs may also indicate the aetiology, such as:

- fever and splinter haemorrhages in infective endocarditis
- clinical features of Marfan's syndrome
- signs of aortic dissection.

Table 7.11 Eponymous signs in aortic regurgitation

Sign	Description
Becker's sign	Prominent retinal artery pulsation
Corrigan's sign	Prominent carotid pulsation
De Musset's sign	Head nodding in time with the heart beat
Duroziez's sign	Systolic and diastolic murmurs heard over the femoral artery while partially compressing the vessel with the diaphragm of the stethoscope
Gerhardt's sign	Pulsation of the spleen in time with the heart beat
Hill's sign	Higher blood pressure (>20 mmHg) in the legs than in the arms
Landolfi's sign	Rhythmic pupillary pulsation in time with the heart beat
Lincoln sign	Excessive pulsation in the popliteal artery
Mayne's sign	A fall in diastolic blood pressure (>15 mmHg) on raising the arm above the head
Müller's sign	Pulsation of the uvula in time with the heart beat
Quincke's sign	Prominent capillary nail bed pulsation
Rosenbach's sign	Pulsation of the liver in time with the heart beat
Traube's sign	A double sound heard over the femoral artery while compressing it distally

Indicators of severity

- Collapsing pulse
- Wide pulse pressure
- Soft aortic component (A_2) to second heart sound
- Presence of a third heart sound (S_3)
- Long diastolic murmur
- Presence of an Austin Flint murmur
- Symptoms and/or signs of left ventricular failure.

Differential diagnosis

An early diastolic murmur may also be heard with pulmonary regurgitation.

Mitral stenosis

Rheumatic valve disease most commonly affects the mitral valve, causing thickening and fusion along the leaflet edges. Other causes of mitral stenosis are rare and include congenital mitral stenosis, mitral annular calcification, systemic lupus erythematosus, rheumatoid arthritis, carcinoid syndrome and infective endocarditis. Some conditions can mimic mitral stenosis by obstructing the mitral orifice, such as left atrial myxoma or infective endocarditis with a large vegetation.

Rheumatic mitral stenosis usually presents 20–40 years after an episode of rheumatic fever and is now relatively uncommon in developed countries. Most patients are female, and most will have other co-existent valve disease. The symptoms can build up insidiously over a long period, but a new event (such as pregnancy or the onset of atrial fibrillation) can cause a sudden deterioration. Once a patient develops symptoms, if left untreated their 10-year survival is around 50–60 per cent.

Symptoms

The symptoms often have a gradual onset and include:

- breathlessness (including orthopnoea and paroxysmal nocturnal dyspnoea)
- cough
- haemoptysis
- peripheral oedema
- peripheral emboli.

Signs

The signs of mitral stenosis include:

- malar flush ('mitral facies')
- low-volume pulse
- AF (is common)
- tapping apex beat (palpable S_1)
- loud S_1
- opening snap
- low-pitched mid-diastolic murmur (with pre-systolic accentuation if in sinus rhythm) loudest at the apex (use the bell of the stethoscope).

If you suspect pulmonary hypertension, look for:

- large 'a' wave in the JVP (but the 'a' wave is absent if in AF)
- left parasternal heave (right ventricular hypertrophy)
- loud P_2.

Indicators of severity

- Low-volume pulse
- Soft S_1
- Early opening snap
- Long diastolic murmur
- Signs of pulmonary hypertension.

Differential diagnosis

A diastolic murmur may also be heard with:

- tricuspid stenosis
- aortic regurgitation (and/or Austin Flint murmur, p. 72)
- pulmonary regurgitation
- left atrial myxoma (listen for a 'tumour plop' as the myxoma obstructs the mitral orifice).

Mitral regurgitation

Mitral regurgitation can result from dysfunction of any part of the mitral valve apparatus: the leaflets, annulus, papillary muscles or chordae tendineae. Causes include:

- myxomatous degeneration/mitral valve prolapse
- rheumatic valve disease
- infective endocarditis
- ischaemic heart disease (papillary muscle dysfunction/rupture)
- mitral annular dilatation ('functional' mitral regurgitation, secondary to left ventricular dilatation).

Symptoms

Mitral stenosis may be asymptomatic. The symptoms may be insidious (chronic MR) or abrupt (acute MR) and include:

- breathlessness (including orthopnoea and paroxysmal nocturnal dyspnoea)
- fatigue.

The symptoms may also indicate the aetiology (e.g. myocardial infarction, infective endocarditis).

Signs

The signs of MR include:

- AF (may be present)
- displaced apex beat with hyperdynamic character
- soft or absent S_1

- S_3 present
- pansystolic murmur
  - loudest at the apex
  - may cause a systolic thrill
  - may radiate to the axilla
- signs of heart failure in advanced (or acute) cases.

> ### CLINICAL PEARL
> Mitral valve prolapse is the single commonest cause of mitral regurgitation in the developed world, and as well as being a result of degenerative valve disease can also occur in collagen disorders such as Ehlers–Danlos syndrome or Marfan's syndrome, or papillary muscle dysfunction/rupture. Characteristic signs of mitral valve prolapse are a mid-systolic click followed by a late systolic murmur.

Indicators of severity

- Displaced apex beat
- Soft or absent S_1
- Loud S_3
- Early A_2
- Loud pansystolic murmur
- Signs of pulmonary hypertension
- Symptoms and/or signs of left ventricular failure

Differential diagnosis

A systolic murmur may also be heard with:

- tricuspid regurgitation
- ventricular septal defect
- aortic stenosis
- pulmonary stenosis.

Atrial septal defect

Atrial septal defect (ASD) can remain asymptomatic for many years and may present late in adult life. It can also be an incidental finding. In advanced cases, the increased pulmonary blood flow eventually leads to pulmonary hypertension and right heart failure.

Symptoms

Atrial septal defect may be asymptomatic or may present with:

- breathlessness
- recurrent respiratory infections

- palpitations (atrial fibrillation)
- paradoxical embolism.

Signs

The signs of ASD include:

- AF – can occur
- fixed splitting of S_2 (p. 56)
- low-pitched diastolic (flow) murmur in tricuspid area
- ejection systolic (flow) murmur in pulmonary area
- pulmonary hypertension and right heart failure (advanced cases).

Ventricular septal defect

A ventricular septal defect (VSD) permits oxygenated blood flow from left ventricle into right ventricle. In advanced cases, the increased pulmonary blood flow eventually leads to pulmonary hypertension and right heart failure. These defects can be congenital or acquired (e.g. post myocardial infarction).

Symptoms

Ventricular septal defect may be asymptomatic or may present with:

- breathlessness
- recurrent respiratory infections.

Signs

The signs of VSD include:

- systolic thrill at lower left sternal edge
- wide splitting of S_2
- loud P_2 if pulmonary hypertension
- harsh pansystolic murmur at lower left sternal edge (louder with *small* defects)
- pulmonary hypertension and right heart failure (advanced cases).

Persistent (patent) ductus arteriosus

A persistent (patent) ductus arteriosus (PDA) is an abnormal connection between the aorta and pulmonary artery, allowing shunting of oxygenated blood to the lungs. The increased pulmonary blood flow eventually leads to pulmonary hypertension and right heart failure.

Symptoms

A PDA may be asymptomatic or may present with:

- breathlessness
- recurrent respiratory infections.

Signs

The signs of PDA include:

- bounding pulses with a widened pulse pressure
- systolic thrill in first left intercostal space
- loud P_2 if pulmonary hypertension
- continuous ('machinery') murmur in first left intercostal space
- pulmonary hypertension and right heart failure (advanced cases).

Eisenmenger's syndrome

The presence of a left-to-right shunt (such as an ASD, VSD or PDA) allows blood to pass directly from the left side of the circulation to the right, increasing the volume of blood flowing through the pulmonary circulation. Over time this leads to pulmonary hypertension and right heart failure. Once right-sided pressures exceed left-sided pressures, the shunt reverses, causing blood to start shunting from right-to-left instead. At this point, the patient is said to have developed Eisenmenger's syndrome (or reaction). Venous (deoxygenated) blood entering the right heart starts crossing directly into the left heart, bypassing the lungs. Clinical signs include:

- cyanosis
- clubbing
- signs of pulmonary hypertension.

Coarctation of the aorta

Coarctation of the aorta is a narrowing that typically occurs just distal to the origin of the left subclavian artery. Patients presenting in adulthood are usually asymptomatic.

Signs

The signs of coarctation of the aorta include:

- radio-femoral delay with weak lower limb pulses
- upper body hypertension (arms but not legs)
- systolic murmur in left infraclavicular area and near left scapula

- continuous murmur may be present if there are large collateral vessels (which cause rib notching on the chest X-ray).

There may be features of associated Turner's syndrome (p. 47) or bicuspid aortic valve (ejection click and possibly murmurs of aortic stenosis and/or regurgitation).

Infective endocarditis

Infective endocarditis refers to an infection of the endocardium (e.g. *Staphylococcus aureus, Streptococcus viridians*) usually on a background of pre-existing structural heart disease (e.g. valve disease or valve prosthesis, congenital heart disease). In the past, infective endocarditis has been classified as acute or subacute ('SBE', subacute bacterial endocarditis) but this terminology is outdated and should no longer be used.

Symptoms

The symptoms of infective endocarditis include:

- fever
- fatigue
- anorexia
- weight loss
- 'flu-like symptoms.

Signs

The signs of infective endocarditis include:

- anaemia
- fever
- clubbing
- splinter haemorrhages
- Janeway lesions
- Osler's nodes
- Roth spots
- evidence of underlying structural heart disease, and there may be a new or changing heart murmur
- splenomegaly
- peripheral emboli.

Pericarditis

Acute pericarditis

Acute inflammation of the pericardium can result from viral infection (e.g. Coxsackie), tuberculosis,

myocardial infarction (early or late – Dressler's syndrome), autoimmune disorders (e.g. rheumatoid arthritis), uraemia, malignancy and following cardiac surgery.

Symptoms

The symptoms of pericarditis include:

- chest pain
  - sharp or 'raw'
  - worsened by lying flat
  - eased by sitting forwards
  - varies with respiration
- cough
- breathlessness
- fatigue.

Signs

The signs of pericarditis include:

- fever
- tachycardia
- pericardial friction rub.

IMPORTANT *i*

A pericardial effusion can exert sufficient pressure on the heart to cause haemodynamic compromise – this is called *cardiac tamponade*. The three 'classical' signs of tamponade – known as Beck's triad – comprise: hypotension; raised JVP; and quiet heart sounds.

Cardiac tamponade also causes: tachycardia; pulsus paradoxus (p. 49); prominent x descent in the JVP; and an impalpable apex beat.

The diagnosis can be confirmed by echocardiography. Cardiac tamponade is a medical emergency, requiring urgent drainage of the pericardial effusion.

Constrictive pericarditis

Thickening and fibrosis of the myocardium may follow an episode of acute pericarditis, and this can constrict the heart, restricting the filling of the cardiac chambers. It is particularly common after tuberculous pericarditis.

Symptoms

The symptoms of constrictive pericarditis include:

- history of prior acute pericarditis
- fatigue
- breathlessness
- abdominal swelling
- peripheral oedema.

Signs

The signs of constrictive pericarditis include:

- pulsus paradoxus
- raised JVP
  - prominent x and y descents (the sudden 'collapse' of the raised JVP is termed Friedreich's sign)
  - Kussmaul's sign (p. 54)
- quiet heart sounds
- early S_3
- pericardial 'knock'
  - due to sudden termination of ventricular filling
  - heard early in diastole, after S_2
  - occurs earlier, and is a higher pitch than, an S_3 added sound
- hepatomegaly
- splenomegaly
- ascites
- peripheral oedema.

Constrictive pericarditis or restrictive cardiomyopathy?

The diagnosis of constrictive pericarditis is notoriously difficult to make, and is often missed. It can be particularly difficult to distinguish between constrictive pericarditis and restrictive cardiomyopathy. Clinical features in favour of constrictive pericarditis include:

- history of prior pericarditis
- early S_3
- pericardial 'knock'
- absence of mitral or tricuspid regurgitation.

Echocardiography can be very useful in making the distinction between constrictive pericarditis and restrictive cardiomyopathy.

PERIPHERAL ARTERIAL DISEASE

Clinical history

Peripheral arterial disease is usually a consequence of atherosclerosis. The cardinal symptom is intermittent claudication – a sensation of aching, cramping or pain, most commonly in the calf muscle, which is brought on by exercise and relieved by rest. Less commonly, claudication affects the thigh muscles or the buttocks.

Ask the patient about the character and location of their symptoms, and enquire about functional limitation – how far can they walk before the symptoms occur, and what impact does this have upon their activities of daily living?

More severe limb ischaemia causes rest pain, often described as a burning discomfort in the foot and toes particularly when lying in bed at night. The patient may also present with non-healing wounds and gangrene.

Ask about cardiovascular risk factors (p. 45), particularly diabetes mellitus, and any history of other cardiovascular conditions such as ischaemic heart disease or cerebrovascular disease.

Physical examination

Perform a full cardiovascular examination, with a particular emphasis on the arterial pulses. Record the presence or absence of each pulse, and if a pulse is present describe whether it is normal, diminished or aneurysmal. With the patient lying supine on an examination couch, assess the:

- radial pulse
- brachial pulse
- carotid pulse
  - auscultate for bruits
- abdominal aorta:
  - inspect the abdomen for obvious aortic pulsation
  - palpate the abdomen for the presence of a pulsatile mass – in thin patients a normal aorta may be palpable
  - auscultate for bruits
- femoral pulse:
  - palpate with your fingertips in the inguinal crease, midway between the pubic tubercle and anterior superior iliac spine

- auscultate for bruits
- popliteal pulse:
  - flex the knee and reach behind, with your thumb on the patella, to palpate the popliteal pulse with your fingertips
- posterior tibial pulse:
  - palpate with your fingertips just posterior to the medial malleolus
- dorsalis pedis pulse:
  - palpate with your fingertips on the dorsum of the foot lateral to the tendon of extensor hallucis longus.

Inspect the legs for general signs of chronic ischaemia:

- cool feet/toes
- shiny, hairless skin
- toenail dystrophy
- arterial ulceration, most commonly found on the foot and the mid-shin
  - commoner in men
  - painful
  - has a regular margin
- gangrene (tissue necrosis, usually affecting the toes).

Look for evidence of co-existent peripheral venous disease (p. 79).

CLINICAL PEARL

Buerger's test is used to assess the arterial supply to the leg.

1. With the patient lying supine on an examination couch, raise both legs to an angle of 45° for 1–2 minutes.
2. Observe the colour of the feet – pallor while elevated indicates ischaemia.
3. Ask the patient to sit upright on the edge of the couch, with their legs hanging over the side.
4. Observe the colour of the feet again. Normally the feet should turn pink. Redness (reactive hyperaemia) indicates peripheral arterial disease.

Investigations

The ankle:brachial pressure index (ABPI) is a simple method for assessing the peripheral arterial circulation. A blood pressure cuff is applied around the lower calf (above the ankle) and inflated while a Doppler ultrasound probe is applied to the dorsalis pedis and posterior tibial artery in turn. Record the maximum cuff pressure at the point at which flow in each artery is detected. Then, use the cuff to measure systolic blood pressure at the brachial artery in the right and left arms. Calculate the ratio between the highest pedal artery pressure (dorsalis pedis or posterior tibial) and the highest brachial artery pressure (right or left arm) – this is the ABPI and is normally >1.0. An ABPI <0.9 indicates some degree of arterial disease, and typical values in intermittent claudication lie in the range 0.5–0.8. An ABPI <0.5 indicates severe ischaemia and can be associated with rest pain, arterial ulcers and gangrene. Arterial calcification causes spuriously high ABPIs, often >1.3.

Other important investigations in peripheral arterial disease are:

- arterial ultrasound scan (e.g. carotid artery stenosis)
- CT scan (e.g. abdominal aortic aneurysm)
- MRI scan (e.g. renal artery stenosis)
- angiography (e.g. limb ischaemia).

Common diagnoses

Acute limb ischaemia

Acute limb ischaemia is an emergency and commonly results from thrombosis or peripheral embolism. It requires urgent assessment and intervention. The clinical features are summarized by the 'rule of Ps':

- painful (but becoming painless later)
- paraesthesiae
- paralysed
- pale
- pulseless
- perishing cold.

As time passes, the initially pale limb becomes mottled and then dark purple or black.

Chronic limb ischaemia

The key features of chronic limb ischaemia are discussed above (see p. 77).

Mesenteric ischaemia

See Chapter 9, p. 112.

Stroke and transient ischaemic attack

See Chapter 12, p. 203.

Raynaud's phenomenon

Raynaud's phenomenon occurs when there is an exaggerated vasomotor response, primarily affecting the fingers, in cold weather or as a response to emotional stress. A sequence of changes affects the fingers:

1. on exposure to cold, the fingers turn pale (*white*) and become numb due to digital arterial spasm
2. next, the fingers turn blue (*cyanosis*) as the blood in the fingers becomes desaturated
3. on re-warming, the fingers turn red due to a reactive hyperaemia, and this phase can be associated with finger paraesthesiae and swelling, before eventually returning to normal.

Primary Raynaud's phenomenon (sometimes termed Raynaud's *disease*) is idiopathic and is most commonly seen in young women. Secondary Raynaud's phenomenon is seen in association with such conditions as systemic lupus erythematosus, systemic sclerosis or rheumatoid arthritis.

PERIPHERAL VENOUS DISEASE

The commonest peripheral venous disorders are:

- varicose veins
- superficial thrombophlebitis
- deep vein thrombosis (DVT)
- chronic venous insufficiency (including ulceration).

Varicose veins

Normally the superficial veins of the leg drain into the deep veins via communicating veins. Incompetence of the valves within these communicating veins leads to retrograde filling of the superficial veins, causing the veins to become dilated and tortuous (varicose veins). Varicose veins can be painful (usually an aching or heavy discomfort) and cause itching. Enquire about ankle swelling or any history of leg ulceration or DVT. Ask if the patient has previously had any varicose vein surgery (e.g. sclerotherapy, vein stripping).

Examine the legs while the patient is standing as well as lying supine. Look for:

- dilated, tortuous superficial veins
- ankle swelling
- venous eczema (also known as gravitational, stasis or varicose eczema), a red-brown discoloration of the skin, often scaly, mainly around the ankle but sometimes more widespread
- venous ulceration.

Trendelenburg's test

Trendelenburg's test assesses the competency of the valves in the communicating leg veins. Ask the patient to lie supine on an examination couch, and then raise the leg as far as practical to empty the superficial veins. Keeping the leg elevated, apply a tourniquet around the upper thigh (compressing the superficial veins) and ask the patient to stand. Normally, the superficial veins will refill slowly from below. If however, there is incompetence of a valve in a communicating vein below the level of the tourniquet, the superficial veins will fill more quickly. If the superficial veins fill rapidly on removal of the tourniquet, the incompetence is above the tourniquet at the level of the sapheno-femoral junction. The test can be repeated with the tourniquet applied at different levels of the leg to precisely locate incompetent valves.

Superficial thrombophlebitis

Superficial thrombophlebitis is inflammation of a superficial vein, often with associated thrombosis, causing pain. It most commonly occurs in leg veins (especially varicose veins) but any vein can be affected. Examine the affected vein(s) for redness, swelling, warmth and tenderness. Superficial thrombophlebitis can infrequently lead to deep vein thrombosis and pulmonary embolism. Migratory thrombophlebitis is recurrent, affects otherwise normal veins, and can be associated with underlying malignancy (Trousseau's sign of malignancy).

Deep vein thrombosis

Deep vein thrombosis can be asymptomatic, but commonly presents with pain and swelling in the affected leg. It is usually unilateral and most commonly affects the calf veins, but may extend more proximally. It can also affect the arm (axillary or subclavian vein thrombosis), particularly in patients with a central venous catheter *in situ*. The main acute risk of a DVT is that the clot embolizes to the lungs, causing pulmonary embolism (p. 106). In the long term, DVT can result in chronic venous insufficiency (post-thrombotic syndrome).

Risk factors for DVT include:

- immobility
  - recent surgery
  - bed rest
  - prolonged travel
- age >60 years
- acute medical illness
- pregnancy
- obesity
- malignancy
- thrombophilia
- personal or family history of venous thromboembolism
- oral contraceptives or hormone replacement therapy.

When examining a patient with suspected DVT, look for swelling in the affected limb – measure the limb circumference with a tape measure and compare it with the opposite side. Examine for tenderness and assess whether the limb looks red or feels warm. The clinical appearance of a DVT can be mimicked by a ruptured Baker's (popliteal) cyst – the two conditions can be distinguished with an ultrasound scan.

Chronic venous insufficiency (including ulceration)

Chronic venous insufficiency can result from previous DVT, varicose veins or reduced contraction of leg muscles (chronic immobility). It may be asymptomatic, but can cause a feeling of aching and 'heaviness' in the legs. Examine the patient for evidence of:

- varicose veins
- ankle swelling (which may be only slightly pitting)
- venous eczema
- lipodermatosclerosis (fibrosis of subcutaneous fat, leading to 'tightening' of the skin and narrowing of the leg just above the ankle – the so-called 'beer bottle leg')
- venous ulceration.

Venous ulcers are most commonly found above the medial malleolus, and can occur following trauma or spontaneously (see Fig. 18.14, p. 312). Venous ulcers:

- are commoner in women and the elderly
- have an irregular margin
- have a pink (granulation tissue) base, with green slough.

In contrast to arterial ulceration, the leg is usually warm with palpable pulses in the presence of venous ulceration.

SUMMARY

Key features of the presenting history are:

- chest discomfort
- breathlessness
- palpitation
- pre-syncope and syncope
- peripheral oedema.

Include the following in your physical examination:

- general examination
- the hands
- arterial pulses
  - rate
  - rhythm
  - character and volume
- blood pressure
- face and eyes
- jugular venous pressure
  - height of the JVP
  - character of the JVP
- praecordium
  - inspection
  - palpation
    - apex beat
    - left parasternal heave
    - thrills

- auscultation
  - heart sounds
  - heart murmurs
- chest and back
- abdomen
- lower limbs
  - arterial circulation
  - venous circulation
  - peripheral oedema.

FURTHER READING

Brostoff JM. 2009. Re-examining examination: misconceptions in clinical medicine. *Journal of the Royal Society of Medicine* **102**:11–15.

Houghton AR. 2009. *Making sense of echocardiography*. London: Hodder Arnold.

Houghton AR, Gray D. 2008. *Making sense of the ECG*, 3rd edn. London: Hodder Arnold.

O'Brien E, Asmar R, Beilin L, *et al*. 2003. On behalf of the European Society of Hypertension Working Group on Blood Pressure Monitoring. European Society of Hypertension recommendations for conventional, ambulatory and home blood pressure measurement. *Journal of Hypertension* **21**:821–848.

Perloff JK. 2009. *Physical examination of the heart and circulation*, 4th edn. New York: McGraw-Hill Medical.

Ramrakha P, Hill J (eds). 2006. *Oxford handbook of cardiology*. Oxford: Oxford University Press.

8

THE RESPIRATORY SYSTEM

David Baldwin

INTRODUCTION

Respiratory medicine comprises a large part of everyday clinical practice for two reasons:

- respiratory conditions are common – accounting for more than 13 per cent of all emergency admissions and more than 20 per cent of general practitioner consultations
- respiratory symptoms and signs as elicited by respiratory history and examination are often present in non-respiratory conditions as well as respiratory conditions.

CLINICAL HISTORY

The six key symptoms of respiratory disease are:

- chest pain (that may be extended to chest sensations)
- dyspnoea
- cough
- wheeze
- sputum production
- haemoptysis.

In a respiratory clinic it would be routine as well to ask about snoring and excessive daytime sleepiness, especially in patients who are overweight, because this might lead to a diagnosis of obstructive sleep apnoea syndrome. Other more generic symptoms are also common in respiratory disease and should be covered elsewhere in the history. Enquire about weight loss, anorexia and headache, as these may all be part of common respiratory illnesses. Once the patient has given their account, prompted by open-ended questions, go on to examine the nature of the symptoms in more detail.

Chest pain

Ask about the onset, character, severity, duration, radiation, and any previous history of chest pain.

Pleuritic chest pain (Box 8.1) is pain that is made worse by breathing and is often sharp and stabbing in nature, commonly when the patient takes a breath in. In these circumstances it is important to ask about the onset of the chest pain and how it relates to other symptoms, and also bear in mind other risk factors for illnesses.

BOX 8.1 COMMON CLINICAL DILEMMA: IS IT A PULMONARY EMBOLISM (PE)?

Initial history: sudden onset of pleuritic chest pain and dyspnoea ?PE.

Detail of onset 1: febrile illness for 2 or 3 days beforehand with cough productive of purulent sputum, *then* pleuritic chest pain developed.

You conclude: pleurisy secondary to chest infection most likely – correlate with other tests for infection.

Detail of onset 2: sudden onset of pleuritic chest pain; no other explanation for this.

You conclude: pulmonary embolism must be excluded – do a D-dimer assay, and if elevated do a CT pulmonary angiogram (may be indicated even if D-dimer level normal).

A history of chronic pleuritic chest pain going back several months or years could indicate an inflammatory disorder resulting in pleurisy. This can occur in a variety of collagen vascular disorders but is a relatively rare cause of pleuritic chest pain. Chest pain that is dull and persistent in one area, and especially if it is keeping the patient awake at night, could indicate a malignant process within the chest that is affecting the chest wall. Such pains have usually been going on for weeks or more and get progressively worse, and may or may not be augmented by palpation of the chest.

Dyspnoea

Analysis of dyspnoea should be approached in a similar way to that of chest pain, so ask about severity, duration, onset, precipitating factors, and previous history. It is absolutely crucial to ask about the onset. Ask the patient what they were doing at the time when the breathlessness started in order to jog their memory and give you some idea as to how sudden the onset was.

- Shortness of breath that has appeared out of the blue with no apparent precipitating factor should make you search for other risk factors for thromboembolic disease and suggest appropriate tests.
- In contrast, a slow onset of gradually increasing shortness of breath over many months may indicate a more chronic condition such as chronic obstructive pulmonary disease (COPD) or interstitial lung disease.
- A previous history of episodes of shortness of breath is often very useful in determining a diagnosis.
- Conditions that have exacerbations of breathlessness such as COPD, asthma or bronchiectasis have often already been diagnosed and may have important clues in the rest of the history.

Relate dyspnoea to other symptoms (see Box 8.2). Patients with asthma and COPD may have associated wheeze, and in bronchiectasis there may be a history of chronic high volume sputum production. Ask about whether the breathlessness is present at rest or whether it is only exercise-related.

- Breathlessness that comes on repeatedly at rest implies different pathophysiology in that there is some sort of disturbance that is causing the sensation of breathlessness and it does not depend on physical activity. This could include pulmonary thromboembolism, cardiac arrhythmias, cardiac ischaemia or spontaneous pneumothorax.
- Breathlessness that is usually precipitated by physical exertion implies that there is some deficiency in the body's ability to cope with the extra exertion and this might occur in conditions such as asthma, COPD, heart failure and interstitial lung disease. All of the latter conditions can of course, in their most severe forms, produce breathlessness at rest. On its own, it is a relatively non-specific symptom.

Wheeze

You must ensure that you understand what your patient means when they answer positively to your

---

> **BOX 8.2** CHEST PAIN AND DYSPNOEA OVERLAP WITH OTHER SYSTEMS
>
> **Example A:** History of crushing central chest pain radiating to the arm and associated with nausea and vomiting and a feeling of dread.
>
> *Conclusion*: Myocardial ischaemic pain.
>
> **Example B:** Progressive dyspnoea and fatigue over several months. Pallor, but no other symptoms or signs; haemoglobin 6.0 g/dL.
>
> *Conclusion*: Anaemia.
>
> Dyspnoea and chest pain are symptoms that can be present in many conditions – usually related to either the heart or the lungs (example A), but occasionally more generic (example B).

---

direct question: 'Do you wheeze?' This question is useful because it will encourage the patient to describe any noises that they make with their breathing. Then, by further questioning, you can clarify exactly what is meant. From a medical perspective, a wheeze is a musical note generated from the lungs that may be a single note (monophonic wheeze) or multiple different notes (polyphonic wheeze). This will be clarified by auscultation. Patients find it difficult to describe the noises that they are making but you should attempt to get them to do so. Prompting them with suggestions that the sound might be musical or a squeaking sort of sound often helps them. If the patient appears to be describing a monophonic wheeze or stridor (see 'Physical examination', p. 87), then ask on which side the patient experiences this and whether the noise is worse when lying on the left or right side. This can indicate large airway obstruction, of which lung cancer is the most serious cause.

Ask about the onset, duration and periodicity of wheeze. Wheeze that occurs more at night and first thing in the morning, and that may be exacerbated by exercise, is suggestive of asthma and COPD. A pronounced variation in the severity of wheeze (worse at night and in the morning compared to daytime) is more suggestive of asthma, but by no means excludes COPD. Ask about the relationship between other respiratory symptoms and precipitating factors, specifically asking about exercise and cold or foggy weather. This will give you an idea about whether the wheeze is variable rather than fixed and this may be important in relation to the differential diagnosis of asthma or COPD. During this direct questioning, you may identify that the patient experiences a rattling sort of sound that is not a wheeze but nevertheless one that may be important in the differential diagnosis. For example, some patients are aware of a crackling sound that is often generated by the movement of mucus in the lungs and may be accompanied by coarse crackles on physical examination.

Cough

Cough is the commonest symptom that is associated with pure respiratory disease. The function of cough is to expel unwanted elements from the respiratory tract; that includes both foreign elements and substances generated by the host. Thus cough is a prominent feature of upper respiratory infections, inhalation of irritants such as dusts and chemicals, as a result of lower respiratory infections, and the result of accumulation of products within lung (e.g. in pulmonary oedema). In addition to this, cough receptors within the lung can be stimulated as happens in interstitial lung disease or in endobronchial sarcoidosis.

One of the key factors, therefore, is to determine the onset and duration of the cough and its relation to other symptoms. A cough that has been present for a couple of weeks and has been associated with a coryzal illness is easily put down to an upper respiratory tract infection that may be caused by the rhinovirus. Cough of medium duration (3 weeks to 3 months) is more likely to have a non-self-limiting cause – lung cancer fits into this category, as well as the causes of chronic cough shown in Table 8.1. A tickly, irritating cough is often associated with upper respiratory pathologies and the most common causes of this are upper respiratory tract infections, rhinosinusitis, oesophageal reflux and laryngeal dysfunction syndrome. Ask about whether the cough is productive; this leads to a discussion about sputum production.

Sputum

Establish whether sputum production is a new symptom, whether it is produced most days or intermittently. Sputum produced on a daily basis will be

Table 8.1 A quick guide to the causes of chronic cough (more than 6 months)

Asthma	Worse at night/early morning History of chestiness as a child Family history of atopy Relief by salbutamol (not always)
Chronic obstructive pulmonary disease	Longstanding smoking Chronic bronchitis
Rhinosinusitis	Tickly, irritating cough Post-nasal drip sensation History of sinusitis – frontal headache, nasal discharge History of recurrent rhinitis – nasal discharge and blockage
Gastro-oesophageal reflux	Tickly, irritating cough Acid reflux symptoms Response to proton pump inhibitor
Laryngeal hypersensitivity	Tickly, irritating cough Voice disturbance Cough precipitated by talking No nocturnal symptoms Vigorous cough Unresponsive to medication
Other	Includes lung cancer, bronchiectasis, interstitial lung disease, eosinophilic bronchitis Requires specialist investigation

due to a condition that is present on a daily basis, i.e. a chronic condition. The two commonest conditions that do this are COPD (*chronic bronchitis* – 'a productive cough which occurs for more than 3 months of the year in each of two successive years' (Medical Research Council (MRC, criteria)) and bronchiectasis. Get an idea of exactly how much sputum is produced by asking if they are coughing up a thimbleful or an egg-cupful or more each day. The higher volume favours bronchiectasis more than COPD, but in practice there are many patients with bronchiectasis who produce very little sputum. It is relatively unusual to find a patient with chronic bronchitis who is coughing up more than an egg-cupful a day. Lastly, the type of sputum that is coughed up is important. Enquire whether the sputum is clear or cloudy, and what colour it is. Purulent sputum is generally coloured yellow or varying shades of green, and importantly it is cloudy denoting its content of inflammatory cells and pus cells. Enquire about

Table 8.2 Characteristics of sputum production in relation to diagnosis

Characteristic	Likely diagnosis
Acute onset, purulent sputum, clearing after 1–3 weeks	Acute bronchitis Pneumonia
Regular sputum production, more than a half egg-cupful, varying in purulence	Bronchiectasis Occasionally chronic bronchitis
'Chronic productive cough for more than 3 months in each of 2 consecutive years...'	Medical Research Council criteria for definition of chronic bronchitis
Clear or slightly opaque sticky sputum, white yellow or green	Asthma
Colour of purulent sputum and organism	Lime green – *Haemophilus influenzae* 'Rusty' – *Streptococcus pneumoniae* Dark green – *Pseudomonas aeruginosa*
Foul smell and taste	Chronic pulmonary sepsis with cavities in the lung Infection from rotting teeth and associated gum disease

the sputum colour and purulence when the patient is well compared with what it is like when they are poorly with other symptoms. Clear, almost colourless, or white sputum may be a normal phenomenon in small amounts and is the sort of sputum that is produced by patients with chronic bronchitis when they do not have an infective exacerbation. Sputum that becomes yellow and cloudy in relatively small volumes would be consistent with an infective exacerbation of chronic bronchitis or COPD. Some organisms are associated with particular features of the sputum (Table 8.2). *Pseudomonas aeruginosa* produces brown and green pigments called pyocyanins. When patients with bronchiectasis are colonized with *Pseudomonas* their lung function may deteriorate much more rapidly.

Haemoptysis

Haemoptysis is an alarming symptom and if not mentioned in the initial history it is very important that you enquire about this as patients may choose to avoid mentioning it. When a patient says that they have haemoptysis, you need to ask about whether this is in the form of small clots or little lines in the sputum, and you will know by then about the context of the haemoptysis. Larger volumes of bright red blood that persist for many days are more often associated with malignant lesions in the chest, but most studies that have looked at symptoms have shown that any haemoptysis may indicate a diagnosis of

malignancy and therefore it should always be treated seriously.

Whether one goes forward to investigate patients for suspected lung cancer will depend not only on the history that you elicit about the type of haemoptysis, but also the risk factors that the patient has for developing lung cancer. The two most important risk factors are:

- the age of the patient
- whether they have ever been a smoker.

> **IMPORTANT** *i*
>
> Current recommendations indicate that urgent referral to a hospital clinic should be made when patients have haemoptysis, are over the age of 40, and are current or ex-smokers. However, a young patient who has a small amount of streak (lines in sputum) haemoptysis in the context of an upper respiratory tract infection usually will not require referral. Larger volumes of haemoptysis normally have a cause and even young patients will require referral.

Snoring and sleep disturbance

These are common symptoms of sleep apnoea syndrome. Snoring is a sign of upper airway obstruction and while it is present in 25 per cent of the normal population, in patients who are overweight the severity of snoring can be much worse. These patients will often give a history of snoring being audible outside the bedroom or even downstairs (and occasionally outside the house!). These patients also often give a history of excessive daytime sleepiness and will be unable to stay awake at certain times despite wishing to. We now include these symptoms in the respiratory history as they are often not included elsewhere. Sleep apnoea syndrome is a common condition, being present in about 5 per cent of middle-aged men, and is responsible for a good deal of morbidity.

Past medical history

In the past medical history always enquire about childhood infections including pneumonia, previous thoracic operations (it is surprising what patients may forget), and any history of tuberculosis. Childhood infections and pneumonia may give a clue as to the cause of bronchiectasis, or may indeed signify the fact that lungs were abnormal from a very early age, which may point to a congenital cause of chronic lung disease. A history of frequent childhood chest infections, or just being chesty as a child, may add supportive evidence towards a diagnosis of asthma if the rest of the history fits with that.

Family history

In the family history, it is again important to enquire about tuberculosis. Ask whether any of the family members have had tuberculosis and in particular whether there was any contact with them. Patients will often volunteer that they were screened after contact with tuberculosis and may even tell you about whether they had a Bacille Calmette Guérin (BCG) vaccination or not. Usually patients will have had a Mantoux test or Heaf test to look for any pre-existing immunity to tuberculosis and they will often remember that they did not need a vaccination after this test whereas other peers at the time did.

Note any family history of bronchiectasis, but if there is cystic fibrosis in the family, patients will usually be well aware of this. A strong family history of lung cancer in an elderly patient is important not only because the risk of lung cancer in the individual is increased slightly, but also as they will be very much aware of what a horrible illness lung cancer is

and this will give you some insight into their understanding of the condition.

Social history

Record an accurate smoking history (as described on p. 7). For ex-smokers, record the time that they have stopped smoking as the chances of smoking-related illness diminish somewhat after cessation of smoking. Enquire about passive smoking as this is known to at least double the risk of lung cancer and ischaemic heart disease.

In the social history, enquire about any relevant exposures. The most important is exposure to asbestos, which overlaps with the occupational history (see below), and also enquire about anything that may cause hypersensitivity pneumonia (extrinsic allergic alveolitis). This includes a variety of moulds (mouldy hay, certain moulds growing on hard woods, and occasionally even in the house). Enquire about exposure to birds and whether any symptoms are related to cleaning the cage. Hypersensitivity pneumonia (Fig. 8.1) results in a type III immune response with symptoms appearing about 6 hours after exposure and continuing for 3 days. Symptoms include shortness of breath and flu-like symptoms.

In the more general social history, try to get an idea of the limitation that the illness is producing in

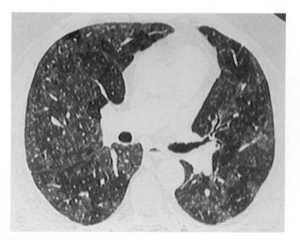

Figure 8.1 High resolution computed tomography (CT) scan of the thorax showing multiple small nodules and patches of dark and lighter lung in the distribution of the secondary pulmonary lobule. The diagnosis was bird fancier's lung, a form of hypersensitivity pneumonitis.

the patient's activity and an idea of the level of support that is around in the home. When patients are developing an illness that may result in them becoming dependent, it is important to enquire about how local their children are and about whom they regard as helping them most in the home environment.

Occupational history

In the occupational history, record occupations that are known to relate to respiratory disease. Thus electricians, plumbers, power station workers, etc., will have some risk of being exposed to asbestos. These occupations have a markedly raised standardized mortality ratio for mesothelioma and asbestosis. (The standardized mortality ratio is the ratio of observed deaths to expected deaths in a population.) Lesser exposure to asbestos may have occurred in garage mechanics when cleaning out brake-linings (that used to be asbestos lined) and even in teachers who used to conduct science lessons when asbestos sheets were used to insulate desks against the Bunsen burners.

The detail of the occupational history will depend on whether you are considering an occupation-related condition, but it would be important to ask about whether symptoms are worse at work and better away from work if you are considering occupational asthma. There are many agents that have been identified as sensitizers and which may induce asthma, and those present in glues and paints are most prevalent.

> **SMALL PRINT**
>
> There are a number of interesting and much rarer causes, for example some laboratory workers can develop asthma as a result of exposure to animal urine. In these circumstances a detailed occupational history including the names of employers will be required.

Systems enquiry

Respiratory illness may produce symptoms in other systems. Patients with cystic fibrosis may have symptoms of malabsorption which will be revealed on direct questioning about the characteristics of the stool. If you are suspecting collagen vascular disorders, ask about arthropathy or skin rashes and whether the patient has ever had iritis. Occasionally patients will develop blackouts because of hypoxic episodes after a bout of coughing (cough syncope). Remember also that many patients (especially the elderly) with respiratory illness will have co-existent illness in other systems and it is essential that the illnesses are managed together if you are to have any success in alleviating symptoms. Cardiovascular and respiratory illnesses are responsible for the vast majority of deaths in elderly patients and they commonly co-exist.

PHYSICAL EXAMINATION

General observations

Begin by introducing yourself. Next look from the end of the bed and take in all of the patient's surroundings, including whether or not they have oxygen, a nebulizer, a sputum pot, and many other observations which may have already been recorded, such as are present on an observation chart. Look closely at the patient and observe whether there are any signs of respiratory distress. These signs include cough, wheeze or stridor, and any signs of laboured breathing. At this point count the respiratory rate and try to characterize any abnormalities noted. Look to see whether the breathing is shallow.

> **CLINICAL PEARL**
>
> Rapport is important because it ensures that the patient is cooperative and therefore improves the physical examination and also of course puts the patient at ease in what are often stressful circumstances for them.

Note any abnormality of the voice and look generally to see whether the patient is anaemic, cyanosed or plethoric (as may occur in polycythaemia). Fetor (unpleasant breath) may indicate an anaerobic infection of the lung.

The hands

Ask the patient to put their hands out in front of you and cock the wrists back, showing them how to do

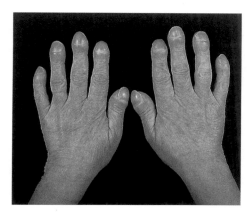

Figure 8.2 Clubbing of the fingers. From: Gray D, Toghill P. (eds), *An introduction to the symptoms and signs of clinical medicine*, with permission. © 2001 London: Hodder Arnold.

this yourself, and make sure they put a lot of effort into trying to extend the wrist. A proper examination for a flapping tremor would require about a minute of this, but usually if a flap is going to occur it does so in the first 10 seconds.

Next, scrutinize the hands themselves and look for clubbing of the fingers (Fig. 8.2). The first sign of clubbing is loss of the angle between the nail bed and the nail. It is important that you get an idea of

the look of normal nails so as to recognize early clubbing of the fingers. The angle of the nail to the nail bed is lost because of increased swelling beneath the nail. This leads on to the development of fluctuation of the nail bed. To elicit this, you need to fix the finger while wobbling the nail bed from side to side. This is done by placing the middle fingers on the middle phalanx of the finger and the thumbs on the proximal interphalangeal joint from beneath, then using the index fingers to test for fluctuation of the nail bed by wobbling from side to side (Fig. 8.3). It is important that you practise this on normal nails to get an idea of the normal range. Later, in more advanced swelling, there is increased curvature of the nails in short and long axes.

Respiratory causes of finger clubbing

- Bronchial carcinoma (non-small cell)
- Intrathoracic suppuration
  - Bronchiectasis
  - Empyema
  - Cystic fibrosis
  - Pulmonary abscess
- Fibrosing alveolitis (usual interstitial pneumonia).

Rare causes include tuberculosis, sarcoidosis, pleural mesothelioma, pleural fibroma, lipoid pneumonia,

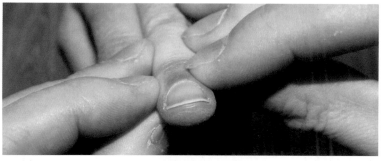

(a)

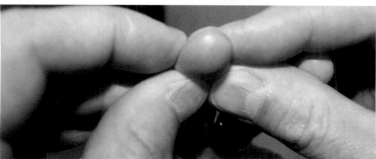

(b)

Figure 8.3 Testing for excessive fluctuation of the nail bed. (**a**) The middle fingers fix the patient's middle phalanx and the thumbs fix the interphalangeal joint. (**b**) The index fingers are used to wobble the base of the nail from side to side.

pulmonary artery sarcoma, pulmonary metastases, Castleman's disease, pulmonary lymphoma, idiopathic pulmonary haemosiderosis.

> ### CLINICAL PEARL
> When checking for clubbing, ask the patient to hold the distal phalanx of one finger 'back to back' against the distal phalanx of the same finger on the opposite hand, such that the two fingernails are touching. Normally there is a small 'window' separating the two nail beds – loss of this 'window' indicates clubbing. This is known as Schamroth's test.

Occasionally gross clubbing is associated with painful wrists and lower legs. Radiographs may show periosteal new bone formation (Fig. 8.4). This is hypertrophic pulmonary osteoarthropathy (HPOA) and is most commonly associated with non-small cell lung cancer.

The temperature and colour of the hands may give a clue as to whether the patient has features of

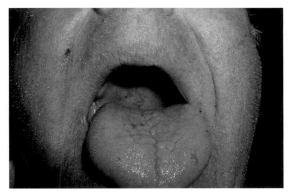

Figure 8.5 Central cyanosis.

carbon dioxide retention or central cyanosis. Hands that are abnormally blue but warm indicate that the patient is centrally cyanosed and this can be confirmed by looking centrally at the tongue (Fig. 8.5). Hands that are cool and blue may either indicate that there is peripheral cyanosis or combined central and peripheral cyanosis. Warm, well-perfused hands along with a flapping tremor indicate carbon dioxide retention.

Look for other signs of systemic disease, for example joint abnormalities may suggest a diagnosis of rheumatoid arthritis as a cause of bronchiectasis or telangiectasis a diagnosis of systemic sclerosis (Fig. 8.6).

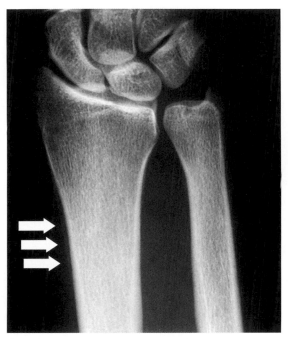

Figure 8.4 Radiograph of the distal radius and ulna showing periosteal new bone formation in hypertrophic pulmonary osteoarthropathy (arrows).

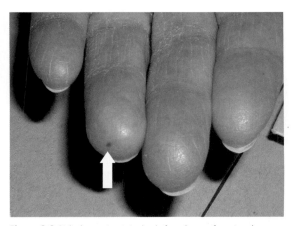

Figure 8.6 It is important to look for signs of systemic disease that may cause lung disease. A telangiectasis such as this may suggest a diagnosis of systemic sclerosis or CREST syndrome. These can cause pulmonary fibrosis or pulmonary hypertension.

Head and neck

Next, begin a closer inspection of the head and neck. Look for any evidence of distended veins in the neck before doing a formal examination of the jugular venous pressure. Also look at the upper thorax for any distended veins that may indicate superior vena cava obstruction. This condition occurs when there is lymphadenopathy within the mediastinum that is occluding the superior vena cava. This produces fixed elevation of the jugular venous pressure and distended external jugular veins as well as evidence of collateral venous return on the upper thorax. The face becomes a dusky grey colour in severe cases and there is some swelling of the face. This may include some periorbital (Fig. 8.7) and conjunctival oedema (chemosis). Rarely there is oedema of the hands and forearms.

Look for central cyanosis by asking the patient to put out their tongue and raise it upwards. Minor degrees of central cyanosis are difficult to detect and you need to have good light. Peripheral cyanosis is detected when approximately 1.5 g/dL of deoxyhaemoglobin is present in the blood. Thus, the chance of detecting cyanosis is greater if the haemoglobin concentration is higher. Cyanosis is usually detected when the oxygen saturation is around 90 per cent. This means that 10 per cent of the haemoglobin in the blood is desaturated and if the haemoglobin is 15 g/dL, then there is 1.5 g/dL of deoxyhaemoglobin. If the patient is polycythaemic with a haemoglobin of 20 g/dL, then central cyanosis would be detected at higher levels of saturation (approximately 93 per cent in this case). The converse is that when people are anaemic it will be much more difficult to detect significant hypoxia. Take, for example, a patient with a haemoglobin of only 5 g/dL who has an oxygen saturation of 80 per cent and still only has 1.0 g/dL of deoxyhaemoglobin. This demonstrates why, as part of the routine respiratory examination, an oxygen saturation monitor should be placed on the patient as soon as possible. It is also a very good way of learning how good you are at detecting cyanosis!

Look for signs of anaemia by inspecting the conjunctivae. Anaemia is usually detected when the haemoglobin has fallen to around 8 g/dL. While looking for anaemia, take a general look at the eyes. Look to see if there is any partial ptosis (indicative of Horner's syndrome). Look at the eyes in general for any signs of previous iritis (a manifestation of sarcoidosis and rarely tuberculosis) and note any evidence of chemosis. Patients with severe and chronic hypocapnia may develop papilloedema so it is important to look in the fundi, especially if the patient is complaining of headaches.

Begin a systematic examination of the neck feeling for supraclavicular and cervical lymph nodes. For this you need to know the position of the lymph nodes and get an idea of what a normal neck feels like. If you find a lymph node, note:

- its size and position
- whether it is fixed or mobile
- whether it is hard or rubbery.

Rubbery lymph nodes are more common in patients who have reactive lymphadenopathy to an infection or in patients with lymphoma. Hard, fixed and craggy lymph nodes are more common in patients with metastases from solid tumours such as carcinoma of the lung or gastro-oesophageal carcinoma. It is best to examine the lymph nodes from behind the patient and to use a gentle probing technique to ensure that the patient stays relaxed. Look for evidence of any thyroid enlargement and note any previous scars including any scars that may indicate a previous tracheotomy or tracheostomy which are present just beneath the thyroid cartilage.

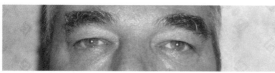

(a)

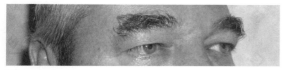

(b)

Figure 8.7 Periorbital oedema in superior vena cava obstruction. Note the oedema of the eyelids leading to obscuration of the root of the eyelash.

Upper respiratory tract

Look in the mouth, checking for any evidence of swelling at the back of the mouth. In patients with

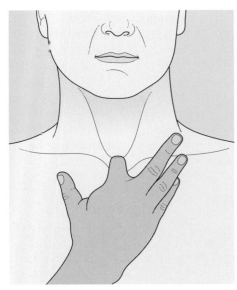

Figure 8.8 Checking the position of the trachea. From: Gray D, Toghill P. (eds), *An introduction to the symptoms and signs of clinical medicine*, with permission. © 2001 London: Hodder Arnold.

sleep apnoea syndrome, there is often marked oedema in this area and the posterior wall of the pharynx may be obscured. Patients who present with difficulty breathing and stridor may exhibit swelling of the lips, tongue and other tissues indicating angio-oedema. Look at the nose, asking the patient if they can breathe in through their nostrils while occluding the opposite nostril to get an idea of nasal patency. Use a pen-torch to look up the nose and check whether there is any nasal mucosal inflammation. Further examination of the nose and larynx is usually the domain of an ear, nose and throat specialist (Chapter 20).

Check the position of the trachea (Fig. 8.8). The trachea is deviated when the lungs and mediastinum are pushed over to one or other side of the thorax due to a lesion causing reduction in volume on one side, e.g. collapse of the lung, or a lesion producing expansion on one side of the lung (massive pleural effusion or tension pneumothorax) (Fig. 8.9). Examining the trachea is a real skill and does require a lot of practice. The key is to *gently* place the tip of your finger in the suprasternal notch and move it from side to side to get an idea of the curvature of the trachea. Once you have a firm idea of where the apex of the curvature is, then that is the centre point of the trachea. You then look to see its relationship to the insertion points of the sternal heads of the sternocleidomastoid muscle.

Once you have perfected the technique you will note that in a proportion of patients, the trachea is very slightly deviated to the right (a matter of 1–2 mm). Remember that it is important to detect deviation just above the very lowest point of the trachea that you can feel in the sternal notch. If you go any higher you will miss tracheal deviation. You also need to notice the distance between the sternal notch and the thyroid cartilage. This will give you an idea whether there is shortening of the palpable trachea, which happens in COPD due to hyperexpansion of the chest. The dis-

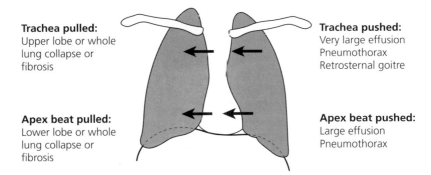

Trachea pulled:
Upper lobe or whole lung collapse or fibrosis

Trachea pushed:
Very large effusion
Pneumothorax
Retrosternal goitre

Apex beat pulled:
Lower lobe or whole lung collapse or fibrosis

Apex beat pushed:
Large effusion
Pneumothorax

Figure 8.9 Movement of the mediastinum (trachea and heart) as the result of various pathologies. The trachea may remain central despite collapse/effusion if fixed by mediastinal cancer. From Gray D, Toghill P (eds), *An introduction to the symptoms and signs of clinical medicine*, with permission © 2001 London: Hodder Arnold.

tance should be around 2 cm. You may also note quite a pronounced downward movement of the trachea on inspiration ('tracheal tug'). Note any thyroid enlargement that may produce deviation of the trachea.

The chest

Skin

Take note of any abnormality of the skin, both on the chest wall and more widely. Although rare, skin abnormalities are often diagnostic. They include evidence of metastatic tumour nodules, manifestations of sarcoidosis that might include erythema nodosum, cutaneous sarcoid, and any systemic features of collagen vascular disorders such as the rash of lupus erythematosus, livedo reticularis, and features of rheumatoid arthritis. If there is unilateral chest pain, then look for any herpetic vesicles that might indicate herpes zoster, or any depigmented scars in the distribution of a dermatome that may indicate previous herpes zoster.

Abnormalities of chest shape

To observe the chest for any abnormalities of shape you will need full exposure of the thorax. The commonest abnormality of shape occurs in patients with severe COPD, where the term applied is 'barrel-chested'. This indicates that the lateral and anteroposterior (AP) diameters approximate. It is important, therefore, to look for this and, if you are unsure, to place your hands on either side of the thorax in the lateral plane and then move them in the anteroposterior (AP) plane and see whether there is any evidence of an increase in AP diameter. Chest deformity in COPD is not a reliable measure of functional deficit, as it may not present in patients with moderate disease.

In normal subjects, the ratio between the AP diameter and lateral diameter is 5:7 and may be as low as 1:2 in normal subjects. Pigeon chest deformity (pectus carinatum) is present when there is a localized prominence of the sternum and costal cartilages with indrawing of the ribs producing Harrison's sulci (symmetrical horizontal grooves above the costal margins). The costal margins themselves may be everted. Pigeon chest deformity is often a result of early respiratory disease producing increased respiratory effort that distorts the development of the chest when it is in a relatively pliable state (Fig. 8.10). Deformity also may

be caused by rickets. Funnel chest deformity (pectus excavatum, Fig. 8.11) is present when there is a localized depression of the lower end of the sternum with the attached costal cartilages. It usually produces no respiratory defect but can cause what appears to be displacement of the heart on the chest X-ray, and in very severe abnormalities can cause some compression of the heart between the sternum and the vertebral bodies. On examination the apex beat may be

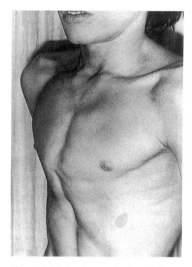

Figure 8.10 Pectus carinatum (pigeon chest) in a teenage boy with asthma since infancy. From: Ogilvie C, Evans CC (eds), *Chamberlain's symptoms and signs in clinical medicine* (12th edition), with permission. © 1997 London: Hodder Arnold.

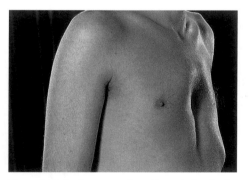

Figure 8.11 Pectus excavatum (funnel chest). From: Gray D, Toghill P (eds), *An introduction to the symptoms and signs of clinical medicine*, with permission. © 2001 London: Hodder Arnold.

displaced and lung function may show a reduced total lung capacity.

Look for evidence of thoracic operations (see also Box 8.3). In older patients, there may be evidence of thoracoplasty where the chest has been surgically collapsed to compress the lung beneath, which often results in a reduction in ventilatory capacity and can lead to respiratory failure in later life. Look for any evidence of curvature of the spine, in both the AP and lateral planes. This would indicate kyphoscoliosis (Fig. 8.12). This can not only produce a hunchback deformity but also the twisting of the spine may produce some profound effect on pulmonary function by reducing lung capacity and increasing the work of breathing. Severe kyphoscoliosis may result in early respiratory failure presenting as hypercapnia and hypoxia. Note any protrusion of the ribs on one side of the body – a common feature of kyphoscoliosis and indicative of a more severe defect (Fig. 8.12b).

> ### BOX 8.3 LESIONS OF THE CHEST WALL ON INITIAL OBSERVATION
> - Cutaneous lesions, e.g. bruises, scars, sinuses, nodules (e.g. sarcoid), skin eruptions.
> - Subcutaneous lesions, e.g. metastatic tumour rodules, lipomas, inflammatory swellings.
> - Subcutaneous emphysema (air in the subcutaneous tissues causing diffuse swelling of the chest wall and neck, and recognized by palpating the area for a crackling sensation). Subcutaneous emphysema is usually a result of pneumothorax or the treatment of pneumothorax with intercostal chest drainage. Occasionally it can be due to rupture of alveoli into the mediastinum resulting in mediastinal emphysema. In this circumstance the heart sounds may change considerably reflecting air in the pericardium.
> - Abnormal blood vessels, e.g. superior vena caval obstruction.
> - Bony prominences, e.g. sternum, ribs, scapula, costochondral junctions.
> - Axillary lymphadenopathy.
> - Breast lesions (Chapter 16).
> - Localized areas of tenderness that may result from tumour invasion or fractures.

Depth and regularity of breathing

You will have already counted the respiratory rate, the normal being around 14 breaths per minute. Also note the depth and regularity of breathing.

The depth of breathing is increased in states producing metabolic acidosis such as diabetic ketoacidosis or uraemia, and is decreased in patients with type 2 respiratory failure. Periodic, or Cheyne–Stokes, breathing is characterized by a cyclical variation in the depth of respiration with the depth slowly

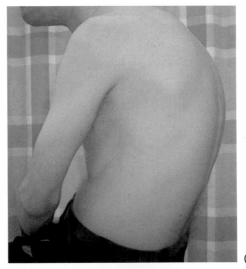
(a)

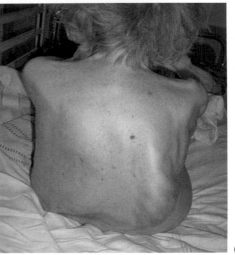
(b)

Figure 8.12 Kyphosis (a) and kyphoscoliosis (b). Note the prominence of the ribs on the right of the chest in (b). Such deformities can produce abnormalities of respiratory function including respiratory failure.

decreasing until there is a period of apnoea followed by a sudden increase in the depth of breathing. This occurs in a variety of neurological conditions, especially those involving the medulla oblongata, and occasionally in cardiac failure.

Hyperventilation (see Box 8.4) may occasionally occur in patients with severe brain damage caused by trauma, haemorrhage or infarction. Irregular, gasping or sighing respiration is characteristic of patients who are hyperventilating for non-organic causes. This may be associated with symptoms related to a drop in ionized calcium in the bloodstream due to a reduction in the partial pressure of carbon dioxide. There may be a light-headed feeling and tingling in the fingers and toes. However, it should be noted that hyperventilation is often a co-existing factor in organic disease and it is here that a calm manner in the doctor can improve the symptoms of breathlessness markedly.

Mode of breathing

Note the mode of breathing. In healthy females, more use is made of the intercostal muscles in passive breathing and therefore they appear to be breathing more with their 'thorax' rather than their 'abdomen'. Males use their diaphragms proportionally more and therefore the respiratory movements are mainly abdominal as the diaphragm descends.

Patients with **respiratory distress** use their accessory muscles for respiration, which include the sternocleidomastoid and intercostal muscles. Patients with severe airflow obstruction will sit forwards, often holding onto something to brace the thorax and improve the mechanical function of the diaphragm and chest wall. This might be accompanied by pursed lip breathing, which works by increasing the air pressure within the airways and preventing them collapsing as the patient exhales.

Note any indrawing of the suprasternal and supraclavicular fossae, intercostal spaces and epigastrium with inspiration. This is a further indicator of respiratory distress. During exhalation you may see some contraction of the abdominal muscles and latissimus dorsi. Normally there is no need for this as the elastic recoil of the lung is adequate to achieve exhalation. However, in airflow obstruction as a result of emphysema there is reduced elastic recoil pressure as well as some airflow obstruction, and hence more active exhalation is required.

Chest wall expansion

Measuring of the expansion of the chest wall is important, especially in examinations as it will give you an immediate clue as to which side the abnormality is on. Even conditions that produce hyperinflation on one side of the chest (pneumothorax) will also produce reduction in expansion on the same side (hyperinflation indicates that the lung is larger than it should be in a static sense, whereas expansion refers to the differences in lung volumes between inhalation and exhalation). Chest expansion in normal individuals varies from 2 cm to more than 5 cm. The majority of the chest wall expansion occurs at the lower chest anteriorly. The ribcage swings upwards and outwards on inspiration; therefore this is the point where most of the expansion will be detected.

The measurement of expansion is often done badly and requires some practice. You need to imagine that your hands are separated from your body and merely glued onto the chest very firmly, but not so firmly that you restrict chest wall expansion. The thumbs project horizontally from your hands and

---

BOX 8.4 THE SENSATION OF BREATHLESSNESS

Almost every condition that produces breathlessness can be explained on the basis of one or more of the following three components:

- **Increased work of breathing**: Many patients with airflow obstruction (asthma, COPD) or patients who have stiffer lungs that are therefore less compliant (pulmonary oedema, pulmonary fibrosis) will have an increased work of breathing. This leads directly to a sensation of breathlessness.
- **Chest wall restriction**: Anything that restricts expansion of the chest wall will lead to a sensation of breathlessness.
- **Hyperventilation**: Increased rate and depth of breathing activate the pulmonary stretch receptors and thereby cause a sensation of breathlessness.

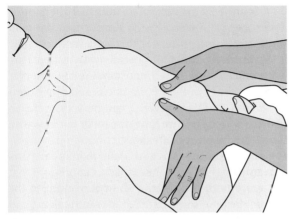

Figure 8.13 Assessing chest expansion.

almost touch. In practice, your elbows need to be at the sides of your body (not protruding out horizontally). Then, observe the movement of your thumbs while the patient is breathing normally. With good technique you will often see a reduction in expansion on the affected side at this time. Ask the patient to take a breath in and look to see what happens (Fig. 8.13).

In a patient with severe COPD, do not be dismayed if you notice that after a small initial expansion your thumbs then cross over in the midline. This can happen because their diaphragm is so flat that after a little initial chest expansion, they then pull horizontally resulting in inward movement of the lower thorax. This shows you have the correct technique. Placing your hands on the middle of the anterior chest and looking for upwards and outwards movement of the thumbs (towards the respective shoulders) is a very good way of looking for expansion and this can be repeated at the top of the chest just below the clavicles.

Measurement of expansion at the back of the chest is always difficult in clinical situations as you need to get the patient to sit on the end of the bed, facing away from you, and then place your hands in a similar fashion to the anterior chest. In practice it is much more informative to do this from the front of the chest, but it is often done extremely badly from the back of the chest and therefore is likely to be misleading. While palpating the chest, you should also check vocal fremitus (Box 8.5): place the sides of your hands on both sides of the chest simultaneously at the top, mid-zone and lower zone anteriorly and posteriorly, and ask the patient to say 'one one one'.

Percussion

You will need to practise the technique of percussion. Place one hand firmly on the chest wall with the fingers separated and then use the middle finger of your dominant hand to tap the finger with a hammer effect (Fig. 8.14).

When percussing, your aim should be to compare equivalent sites on both sides of the chest for the degree of resonance. It is therefore important that you are clear about the surface anatomy (see below) so that you truly do compare both the sides. Anteriorly this should be done with respect to the mid-clavicular line and mid-axillary line on both sides. It is quite common to see people percussing more laterally over the nearer lung compared with the

Correct method of percussion

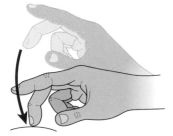

Figure 8.14 Correct method of percussion. Note the movement at the *wrist* and the *vertical* position of the terminal phalanx of the percussing finger as it strikes the other. From: Ogilvie C, Evans CC (eds), *Chamberlain's symptoms and signs in clinical medicine* (12th edition), with permission. © 1997 London: Hodder Arnold.

lung furthest away from them, purely because they are having to stretch a little over the patient. This can lead to inaccurate physical signs.

Dullness to percussion occurs in patients with consolidation or pulmonary collapse and a raised hemidiaphragm, stony dullness (akin to percussing on the head) in pleural effusion, and hyperresonance in patients with severe hyperinflation such as marked emphysema and pneumothorax. You will normally be able to detect some dullness to percussion over the third to fifth interspaces anteriorly, indicating cardiac dullness, and loss of this usually indicates hyperinflation.

A knowledge of surface anatomy of the lung is always useful. Anteriorly, the lungs come down to the sixth rib, and posteriorly to the eleventh rib (Fig. 8.15). It can be difficult to decide when patients are hyperinflated and more important are the observations of change in the AP diameters and other signs of severe COPD. However, it can be very useful in patients with restrictive lung disease or patients who have bilateral pleural effusions (common in congestive cardiac failure). It is also useful to know the surface markings of the lobes so as to appreciate that the majority of the anterior chest is relevant to the upper lobe (and some middle lobe on the right) and halfway up the thorax at the back is relevant to the lower lobe. The area of dullness to percussion will generally be much smaller than the surface anatomy of any lobe due to some reduction in the size of the affected lobe and also a reduction in the size of its surface representation.

Auscultation

In clinical practice, you will find that auscultation is the most helpful part of the respiratory examination except for the respiratory rate. It is important, therefore, that you familiarise yourself with normal vesicular breath sounds. These have a rustling quality and are louder during inspiration and usually only the first third of expiration is audible. There is no gap between inspiration and expiration. This is in contrast with bronchial breath sounds where the sound is much harsher, there is a pronounced gap between

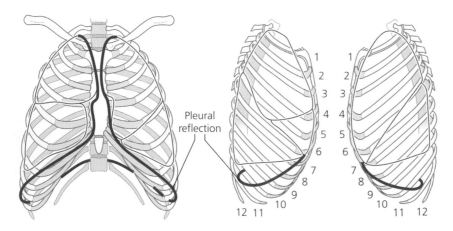

Figure 8.15 Lung margins in relation to ribs. Note that from the front of the chest the lower lobes have no significant surface reflection.

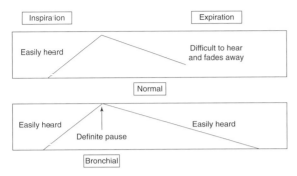

Figure 8.16 Normal and bronchial breath sounds. From: Gray D, Toghill P (eds), *An introduction to the symptoms and signs of clinical medicine*, with permission. © 2001 London: Hodder Arnold.

inspiration and expiration, and you can usually hear the whole of expiration (Fig. 8.16).

Normal breath sounds originate from the larynx so listening to your larynx is a good way of getting used to bronchial breath sounds. To do this you will need to attempt to breathe normally – a difficult thing to do when you are trying to listen to your own breathing. When the sound leaves the larynx it travels down the trachea and then divides when the airway divides. Some sound must be transmitted through the lung parenchyma but most travels down the airway. Eventually the sound travels along airways of different lengths and therefore becomes out of phase. Next it arrives in the respiratory bronchioles and alveoli and then gets transmitted through the chest wall to your stethoscope. The fat layer filters out much of the high frequency sound (above 4 kHz). The resulting sounds are much softer (because the sound has effectively been diluted throughout the whole of the lungs). There is no gap

between inspiration and expiration (because all of the sound has become out of phase and therefore 'filled in' the gap. Finally, the first third of expiration is now the only part that is audible because the latter two-thirds are much quieter (you will know this from listening to your own laryngeal breath sounds; see Table 8.3).

It is important to understand this because you can then understand why breath sounds differ. For example, if you are listening to an area of consolidation and you have your stethoscope directly over the consolidation, you will hear pure bronchial breath sounds. As you move away from this, you will begin to hear a mixture of vesicular breath sounds and bronchial breath sounds so that the breath sounds will be less harsh, there will be a less pronounced gap, and you may have difficulty hearing all the expiration.

Likewise, in a moderate pleural effusion, breath sounds will be absent directly over the pleural effusion and as you move up towards the top of the effusion, become more distinct. If there is some associated collapse/consolidation at the top of the effusion you may even hear some bronchial breath sounds. As you move up further, the breath sounds will become more vesicular but you may hear a prolonged expiratory phase.

It is important also to understand that this applies to airways that are normal. In patients with COPD, who have fixed narrowing of their airways, a considerable amount of sound is generated from the airways themselves and therefore you can often hear prolonged expiratory breath sounds. In emphysema, the breath sounds will be very much reduced but you may well hear prolonged expiratory breath sounds owing to sound generated in the narrow airways.

Table 8.3 Bronchial versus vesicular breath sounds

	Vesicular	Bronchial
Character	Soft and quiet	Harsh and loud, may be high-pitched (in consolidation) or low-pitched (occasionally heard in pulmonary fibrosis)
Expiration	First third of expiration only heard	All of expiration heard (remember that expiratory time is normally longer than inspiratory time)
Gap	No gap between inspiratory sound and the beginning of the expiratory sound	Clear pause between inspiratory sound and expiratory sound

Lastly, it is important to understand the way in which sound is transmitted through various substances. Although sound is transmitted well through fluid (you can hear someone tapping at the other end of a swimming pool when your head is under water), it is not transmitted well from an air to a fluid interface (you cannot hear someone talking to you from the side of the swimming pool when your head is under water). Thus breath sounds that come from the larynx and hit a pleural effusion are reflected and therefore you are unable to hear breath sounds from the chest wall. Consolidated lung transmits sound very well (especially high frequency sounds). This produces the harsh breath sounds that one hears in bronchial breathing. However, there has to be an airway that goes into the consolidated lung tissue so that the sound is transmitted through into the tissue. Consolidation that is associated with bronchial obstruction will not give bronchial breath sounds but instead breath sounds will be reduced or absent. Asking the patient to whisper 'twenty-two' demonstrates how well high-pitched breath sounds are transmitted in consolidated lung tissue. This is a phenomenon of aegophony.

The common term of 'air entry' is potentially misleading and does not relate to the pathophysiology. For example, over a pneumothorax the breath sounds may be very much reduced but the air entry into the underlying lung is still considerable. In severe emphysema there is still considerable air entry into the lung but the breath sounds may be virtually absent. In consolidated lung, although the breath sounds are increased or even bronchial in nature, there is very little air entry.

Added pulmonary sounds

There are three common added pulmonary sounds:

- rhonchi or wheezes, which are continuous
- musical type sounds, crepitations or crackles, which are distinct clicking sounds and discontinuous
- pleural sounds, which essentially consist of a pleural rub – a leathery or creaking sound produced by the movement of the visceral pleura over the parietal pleura when the surfaces are roughened, usually by fibrinous material.

Occasionally a 'click' is audible synchronous with cardiac systole and is thought to be due to a pneumothorax between the two layers of pleura overlying the heart.

Wheezes can be divided into those resulting from air travelling through narrowed airways from a single airway (monophonic wheeze) or multiple airways (polyphonic wheeze). Polyphonic wheeze is a characteristic of airway narrowing due to COPD or asthma and monophonic wheezes may be a result of large airway obstruction such as occurs in bronchial carcinoma. Crepitations are divided arbitrarily into fine, medium and coarse varieties (Box 8.6).

BOX 8.6 TYPES OF CREPITATIONS

- **Fine crepitations**: Very numerous individual clicks of low amplitude and high pitch.
- **Medium crepitations**: Less numerous individual clicks of lower amplitude and lower frequency.
- **Coarse crepitations**: Infrequent individual clicks (few enough to count during an inspiratory cycle) that are individually much louder (higher amplitude) and of lower frequency.

This classification fits very nicely with what we know about the pathophysiology that generates crackles. In pulmonary oedema, alveoli are collapsed due to excess water impeding the role of surfactants keeping them open during expiration. During inspiration, these highly mobile structures snap open very quickly thus producing a very high-pitched sound. They are also very small structures and very numerous hence there is very little sound coming from them (low amplitude) and very many individual clicks. Coarse crackles are commonly due to secretions moving around in airways. Here you can imagine sputum in an airway that, as the patient breathes in, moves or bubbles. There is a comparatively large amount of fluid moving and it moves relatively slowly thus producing a low-pitched sound of considerable volume (amplitude).

Pulmonary fibrosis produces fine to medium crackles depending on the pathophysiology. If there is prominent alveolitis, then numerous alveoli are affected and again these structures snap open, although because they are thickened they snap

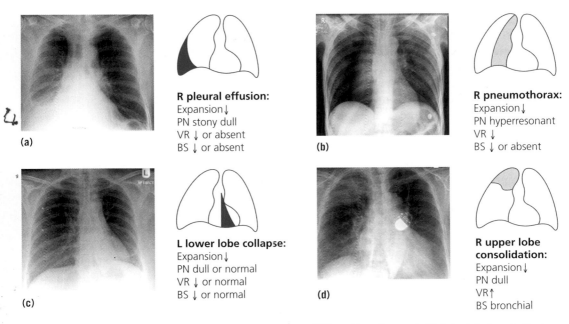

R pleural effusion:
Expansion↓
PN stony dull
VR ↓ or absent
BS ↓ or absent

(a)

R pneumothorax:
Expansion↓
PN hyperresonant
VR ↓
BS ↓ or absent

(b)

L lower lobe collapse:
Expansion↓
PN dull or normal
VR ↓ or normal
BS ↓ or normal

(c)

R upper lobe consolidation:
Expansion↓
PN dull
VR↑
BS bronchial

(d)

Figure 8.17 Expansion, percussion note (PN), vocal resonance (VR) and breath sounds (BS) in: (**a**) pleural effusion, (**b**) pneumothorax, (**c**) lobar collapse and (**d**) lobar consolidation.

open slightly less quickly and with a bit more force, hence the crackles are a bit louder and slightly lower pitched. When there is an established fibrosis, the alveoli are much stiffer and more difficult to snap open, thus even louder and lower pitched because of their increased inertia.

Medium crackles may also be caused by numerous secretions being present as is the case in patients with severe bronchiectasis, especially during an infective exacerbation. These might be termed 'medium to coarse crackles' and those resulting from pulmonary fibrosis 'medium to fine'. Sometimes the crackles of pulmonary fibrosis are akin to the sensation one gets when pulling apart Velcro.

Lastly, decide whether crackles are fixed or not. Crackles that are fixed are those that do not change their pattern during an inspiratory cycle after a period of coughing. It is important, however, to have a good technique here because if you test different depths of inspiration after coughing you will mislead yourself, and likewise if you move your stethoscope from the position that it was in for the first inspiration prior to coughing you will again mislead yourself. So it is important to ensure that the patient takes a full breath in each time and the stethoscope does

not move. This is in contrast to crackles that are as a result of sputum where these commonly change. It is very difficult to detect any change in very fine crackles such as those heard in pulmonary oedema because there are simply too many.

Once you have examined the respiratory system, it is important that you pause to think and decide what pathological process would fit the signs. It is important to be clear in your mind about the signs you feel are most prominent and therefore most important, and give these more emphasis than the ones that are perhaps a little less certain. Four common conditions and physical signs are shown in Fig. 8.17.

INVESTIGATION OF RESPIRATORY DISEASE

Investigations form an extension of the diagnostic process that has started with the history and physical examination, but they also serve to define the level of respiratory function and give a clue as to the likely treatment. You will usually have a good idea as to the diagnosis and initial investigations are done to confirm the diagnosis or to detect any co-existing abnormalities. For example, you may have a history of new-onset haemoptysis in a heavy smoker and on examination a monophonic wheeze is audible. The strong suspicion of bronchial carcinoma is confirmed by a chest X-ray that shows an enlarged right hilum. The rest of the investigations then confirm the diagnosis (obtaining samples for histological examination by bronchoscopy), stage the cancer (computed tomography (CT) scan) and measure fitness for treatment (lung function tests etc.).

As well as targeted investigations, generic tests are very useful.

- The full blood count will detect anaemia, and a differential white cell count may show an increased eosinophil count in asthma and other allergic diseases.
- The lymphocyte count may be depressed in some collagen vascular disorders and sarcoidosis.

Also check the renal, liver and bone profiles.

- Renal function would be important if the patient is to undergo any further tests, especially those relying on a contrast injection such as CT scanning and positron emission tomography (PET) as patients with abnormal renal function may have a deterioration following contrast injection.
- The liver and bone profiles are important mainly in patients who are suspected of having lung cancer as these organs may be affected as a result of metastases, or hypercalcaemia may be present due to ectopic parathyroid hormone (PTH) secretion.

In patients who may be undergoing biopsies, it is important to check the clotting time. The sequence of investigations may vary depending on the prospective diagnosis.

COMMON DIAGNOSES

Asthma and COPD

These diagnoses are commonly used incorrectly, and interchangeably, in the context of airflow obstruction and this is usually due to the lack of a systematic approach. Table 8.4 shows what to look for when deciding whether a patient has asthma or COPD. Sometimes the differentiation between the

two remains difficult and in these circumstances it is best to manage the patient as if they have reversible airflow obstruction as this is the treatment most likely to produce benefit – inhaled or oral steroids and bronchodilators.

Investigation of the peak flow can help in distinguishing the two conditions – marked diurnal variation is much more common in asthma than COPD. A forced expiratory volume in 1 second (FEV1) that increases by more than 15 per cent or 200 mL after a bronchodilator is by definition significant reversibility and much more common in asthma. Similarly, asthma can be defined by inhalation of progressively stronger concentrations of irritants such as methacholine or histamine. An abnormally vigorous response to relatively low concentrations is used to define bronchial hyper-reactivity. This is a much more common finding in asthma than in COPD.

In severe airflow obstruction, a patient may be in danger of going into respiratory failure and so in patients with asthma look for their ability to speak without stopping – an asthmatic person who is unable to speak is in trouble. Measuring the respiratory rate is important as this again suggests the severity of the condition, and record the pulse rate – the greater the pulse rate, the more severe the compromise. COPD patients may be cyanosed in their stable state but it would be unusual for a patient with very good functionality beforehand (who can walk up hills, etc.) to be cyanosed on presentation in an admissions unit. It is important, therefore, to correlate the clinical history with the respiratory examination when assessing severity in COPD. Patients with asthma should not be cyanosed on examination and if they are, this is usually a sign of a very severe acute asthma attack and requires immediate expert intervention with the use of high percentage oxygen, bronchodilators, steroids, and management in a safe environment in the hospital.

Pneumonia

Pneumonia is broadly divided into community-acquired pneumonia (CAP) and hospital-acquired pneumonia (HAP). The clinical features are the same – fever, cough, sputum, dyspnoea, pleuritic chest pain and systemic symptoms that may include malaise and confusion. On examination there is a

Table 8.4 Asthma versus chronic obstructive pulmonary disease (CCPD)

	Asthma	COPD
Age of onset	May give a history of recurrent chest 'infections' as a child, treated with bronchodilators. In late-onset asthma, symptoms begin in adult life at any age (can cause confusion with COPD)	Symptoms usually begin after the age of 50 but can present in the late 30s and early 40s
Smoking history	A history of non-smoking or minimal smoking history (less than 10 pack-years) is strongly in favour of asthma rather than COPD	Mandatory. COPD without a smoking history is very rare
History of other allergic phenomena	Present in asthma, e.g. rhino-sinusitis and nasal polyps, eczema, hay fever	Not a feature of COPD (but may co-exist so can be a cause of confusion)
Diurnal variation	Nocturnal symptoms and increased severity of symptoms on waking/early morning are more characteristic of asthma	COPD symptoms tend to be of similar severity throughout the day and breathlessness may be exercise-related. In severe COPD, nocturnal symptoms can be commoner
Exacerbations	Often triggered by viral infections. Very little difference from COPD	Often triggered by viral infections. Very little difference from asthma
Response to irritants	Symptoms of wheeze and cough often triggered by inhaled irritants. This may include dusts, perfumes, animal fur, exercise, and a change in temperature. May lead to persistent symptoms relieved by bronchodilator medication	Response to irritants less prominent. Exercise main precipitant
Sputum production	In asthma, sputum production is usually minimal, however small amounts of quite viscid green sputum may be coughed up or even some mucus plugs which tend to be semi-transparent and green	There may be a history of chronic bronchitis (daily sputum production for more than three months of the year for two consecutive years). Sputum often turns purulent during exacerbations
Chest examination	During an asthma attack/exacerbation, there is prominent wheeze audible. Cyanosis is unusual and except in severe asthma the chest wall shape is normally unaffected although there might be evidence of hyperinflation	Wheeze is usually less prominent than asthma (although present), the breath sounds are reduced and there is evidence of hyperexpansion. In moderate to severe COPD there may be considerable increase in the anteroposterior diameter of the chest as well as other features described above in respiratory examination
Peak flow measurement	Marked diurnal variation	Little evidence of variation and bronchial hyper-reactivity
Bronchial hyper-reactivity	Abnormal reaction to inhaled histamine or methacholine	Normal reaction to inhaled histamine or methacholine

raised respiratory rate and tachycardia. Signs of consolidation may be present. The commonest finding on auscultation is of localized crackles that are usually coarse to medium. The patient is usually pyrexial but not always. Occasionally elderly patients may present with confusion and immobility ('off legs'). Apart from a rapid respiratory rate there may be no other specific signs. A chest X-ray is most important for diagnosis. Symptoms and signs are used to assess the severity of CAP (Table 8.5).

Hospital-acquired pneumonia (see Box 8.7) is defined as features of pneumonia set out above with the onset at least 72 hours after a hospital admission. Two further forms of pneumonia exist (ventilator-

Table 8.5 Severity markers in community-acquired pneumonia

Clinical feature	Indicator of severity
Confusion (*C)	Mental test score ≤8/10 or new disorientation in person, place or time
Urea (*U)	>7 mmol/L
Respiratory rate (*R)	≥30 per minute
Blood pressure (*B)	Systolic <90 mmHg or diastolic ≤60 mmHg
Age (*65)	≥65 years
Co-morbidity	COPD, cardiac disease, diabetes, stroke
Hypoxaemia	PaO_2 <8kPa
Albumin	<35 g/L
White cell count	<4 or >20 × 10^9/L
Radiology	Bilateral or multilobe involvement
Microbiology	Positive blood culture

Items marked * are components of the CURB-65 risk score: 1 point is scored for each item present, and a score ≥3 indicates severe pneumonia. CURB-65 score reproduced from *Thorax*, Lim WS, van der Eerden MM, Laing R, **58**: 377–82 © 2003 with permission from BMJ Publishing Group Ltd.

BOX 8.7 RISK FACTORS FOR HOSPITAL-ACQUIRED PNEUMONIA

- Age >70 years
- Chronic lung disease/co-morbidity
- Reduced conscious level/stroke
- Chest/abdominal surgery
- Mechanical ventilation
- Nasogastric feeding
- Previous antibiotic usage
- Poor dental hygiene
- Steroids or cytotoxic drugs

acquired pneumonia and aspiration pneumonia). These conditions arise in different contexts and have the same examination findings.

Lung cancer and mesothelioma

Lung cancer is broadly divided into non-small cell and small cell lung cancer. The clinical features are similar but small cell lung cancer, being of neuro-endocrine origin, is more commonly associated with paraneoplastic syndromes. Table 8.6 summarizes the symptoms and signs that may be present. It should be noticed that some patients have remarkably few signs. The commonest presenting symptom is cough, followed by persistent 'chest infection' and haemoptysis.

Horner's syndrome (due to damage to the sympathetic chain due to an apical or Pancoast's tumour) is important to look for as it can be missed. It is easily remembered by its four features, all of which get smaller:

- myosis (smaller pupil on the affected side)
- ptosis (smaller palpebral fissure). Remember that the ptosis is due to autonomic paralysis – the sympathetic supply to the superior tarsal muscle. It is not, as is commonly reported in error, due to paralysis of the levator palpebrae superioris
- enophthalmos, where the eye is more sunken into the socket (and effectively smaller)
- anhydrosis – where the sweating becomes 'smaller'. The best way to detect this is to run the back of your index finger gently over the person's forehead above the eye. Your finger will slip much more easily over the dryer skin than on the unaffected side.

Horner's syndrome may be caused by Pancoast's tumour and therefore it is important also to look for any evidence of weakness of the small muscles of the hand and any other motor loss, and also to ask about shoulder pain. About 10 per cent of patients with lung cancer present with metastatic disease, this being more common in non-small cell lung cancer. This may lead to cervical or supraclavicular lymphadenopathy and an enlarged liver, symptoms of bone pain or pathological fracture, evidence of neurological deficit due to cerebral metastases, or symptoms related to hypercalcaemia (confusion, generalized weakness and malaise, nausea, constipation).

Paraneoplastic syndromes (excluding cachexia, wasting and clubbing; Box 8.8) cause symptoms in about 5 per cent of patients with small cell lung cancer, and about 1 per cent in non-small cell lung cancer. Clubbing does not occur in small cell lung cancer and can be a useful distinguishing feature.

Mesothelioma presents with persistent chest wall pain or breathlessness due to the development of a

Table 8.6 Tumour symptoms

Symptoms due to endobronchial tumour	Cough, haemoptysis, persistent chest infection Lobar or lung collapse (due to airway obstruction) Monophonic wheeze Dyspnoea
Symptoms due to other mass effect of tumour	Chest pain (chest wall invasion or sometimes due to lung collapse) Shoulder pain (diaphragmatic involvement) Development of pleural effusion (signs reviewed in respiratory examination) Hoarse voice with characteristic bovine cough (due to tumour invasion of the left recurrent laryngeal nerve) Dysphagia (due to mass effect in the mediastinum) Raised hemidiaphragm (due to phrenic nerve paralysis – can be difficult to distinguish from pleural effusion) Superior vena caval obstruction (due to tumour or lymphadenopathy in the mediastinum – signs reviewed in respiratory examination) Horner's syndrome (myosis, ptosis, enophthalmos, anhydrosis) Weakness of small muscles of hands (C5/C6/T1, may result from invasion of the brachial plexus in Pancoast's tumour)

BOX 8.8 PARANEOPLASTIC SYNDROMES

- Syndrome of inappropriate antidiuretic hormone secretion (SIADH)
- Ectopic adrenocorticotropic hormone (ACTH) secretion – features of Cushing's syndrome but often with weight loss rather than weight gain
- HPOA. This produces painful wrists and shins and is characterized by periosteal new bone formation on X-ray (see Fig. 8.4, p. 89). It is usually associated with marked clubbing of the fingers and toes (more common in squamous cell carcinoma and adenocarcinoma)
- Cerebellar syndrome
- Limbic encephalitis
- Eaton–Lambert syndrome

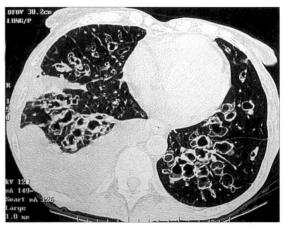

Figure 8.18 High-resolution computed tomography (CT) scan of the thorax showing multiple medium-sized cysts. The patient produced a cupful of sputum per day and had bilateral coarse crackles. The diagnosis is bronchiectasis (in this case saccular).

pleural effusion. In about 50 per cent of people you will find a history of asbestos exposure. Rarely, where there is invasion of the intercostal space, it is possible to palpate filling-in of the space with hard tumour.

Bronchiectasis and cystic fibrosis

Bronchiectasis is characterized by cough productive of large volumes of sputum. When you elicit a history of productive cough, quantify it by asking if the patient is coughing a thimbleful, an egg-cupful or a cupful per day. If the patient is coughing an egg-cupful per day, this is strongly suggestive of bronchiectasis. Bronchiectasis may also produce

recurrent haemoptysis and as lung function deteriorates the patient may be breathless. Occasionally there is some intermittent polyphonic wheeze but the wheeze is not usually that prominent. There may be focal areas of coarse to medium crackles that may be inspiratory or expiratory. During infections, there may be intermittent pleuritic chest pain and lethargy or malaise. The history and examination may help to suggest an underlying cause of bronchiectasis. High-resolution CT scan confirms the diagnosis (Fig. 8.18).

In cystic fibrosis, the history often goes back to childhood (although occasionally patients do present with almost no symptoms in adult life). There may be symptoms of malabsorption.

Tuberculosis

Pulmonary tuberculosis presents with a productive cough, haemoptysis and systemic symptoms of weight loss, night sweats and malaise. It may also produce breathlessness and chest pain. Haemoptysis is more common with cavitatory disease. The signs are non-specific and may include coarse crackles and signs of a pleural effusion or signs of consolidation. There may be cervical lymphadenopathy. Symptoms and signs may arise from the complications of tuberculosis that may include bronchiectasis and upper lobe fibrosis. Localized crackles over the affected area may be heard. Occasionally endobronchial disease produces stenosis of the airways and a monophonic wheeze is audible. Recurrent collapse of the right middle lobe may be caused by enlarged hilar lymph nodes compressing the right middle lobe bronchus. Occasionally patients will have had treatment for tuberculosis by thoracoplasty, resulting in marked chest wall deformity (see Respiratory examination, p. 87). Extrapulmonary tuberculosis may produce some specific signs (Table 8.7).

Sarcoidosis

Sarcoidosis may present as a mild but acute illness which is usually non-progressive (Löefgren's syndrome). The symptoms are fever, arthralgia and painful erythema nodosum. The chest X-ray shows bilateral hilar lymphadenopathy. This occurs more commonly in Caucasians. Heerfordt's syndrome is a similar acute illness with fever, arthralgia, and bilateral parotid enlargement. Again this condition usually responds quickly to treatment with steroids or resolves spontaneously. In other forms of sarcoidosis (and in the minority that present with Löefgren's syndrome or Heerfordt's syndrome) there is involvement of the lung parenchyma and airways. Bilateral hilar lymphadenopathy is present. Symptoms are of malaise and arthralgia and respiratory symptoms are usually cough or occasionally chest pain. In a minority of patients (15 per cent) there is progressive interstitial lung involvement causing dyspnoea, continued cough and chest pain. Occasionally lung disease progresses to pulmonary fibrosis. Sarcoidosis is a systemic disease and may affect the heart, central nervous system, spleen, liver and kidneys. The skin and eyes may also be affected. Classic skin rash is lupus pernio, and episodes of iritis may occasionally lead to blindness. Sarcoidosis may also cause hypercalcaemia resulting in the symptoms set out above under lung cancer.

Interstitial lung disease

Table 8.8 gives an overview classification of the interstitial lung diseases with particular features on history and examination. Symptoms and signs will depend on the area of the lung that is affected and any associated systemic features. Interstitial lung disease that produces prominent fibrosis will lead to fine to medium crackles that do not change on coughing. Lung diseases that produce some airway narrowing may lead to wheezes or squeaks.

Table 8.7 Extrapulmonary tuberculosis

Spinal tuberculosis	Pott's disease of the spine with involvement of the thoracic vertebrae which may produce an angular kyphosis or 'gibbus'. It is important to look for signs of spinal cord compression
Central nervous system disease	This may include tuberculous meningitis, which presents with fever, headaches and altered conscious level with or without focal neurological signs. Tuberculomas may act as space-occupying lesions producing a variety of neurological signs
Pericardial disease	Occasionally large pericardial effusions may lead to cardiac tamponade
Renal and genitourinary tract tuberculosis	Rarely presents with symptoms, but when it does it may cause prostatitis and epididymitis

Table 8.8 Features of interstitial lung diseases

Interstitial lung disease	Common feature in the history or examination
Idiopathic interstitial pneumonia	
• Usual interstitial pneumonia (UIP)	Prominent fine to medium basal inspiratory crackles. Clubbing in 50 per cent. Long history onset over years. Cough and shortness of breath progressive
• Non-specific interstitial pneumonia (NSIP)	Possibly shorter onset over months to years. Clubbing less common. Cough and shortness of breath progressive
• Cryptogenic organizing pneumonia (COP)	Onset over months. Breathlessness, dry cough, fever, myalgia, weight loss (may present as persistent chest infection). Clubbing absent. Localized inspiratory crackles
• Acute interstitial pneumonia (AIP)	Fevers, tiredness, myalgia, followed by rapid onset (over days). Widespread crackles on examination (Velcro). Mortality >50 per cent
• Respiratory bronchiolitis interstitial lung disease (RBILD)	Occurs in smokers. Mild breathlessness and cough. Scanty crackles on examination
• Desquamative interstitial pneumonia (DIP)	Occurs in smokers. Onset of breathlessness and cough over weeks to months. Clubbing common
• Lymphoid interstitial pneumonia (LIP)	Onset of cough and breathlessness over several years. Fever, weight loss, scanty crackles
Hypersensitivity pneumonitis	History of exposure to appropriate allergen (moulds, animal droppings, birds, etc). Symptoms acute with breathlessness, dry cough, fever, arthralgia, myalgia and headache 6 hours after exposure. Crackles and squeaks on auscultation. Symptoms settle after 3 days (type III immune reaction). Chronic progressive breathlessness, dry cough, crackles and squeaks on examination
Bronchiolitis	Proliferative bronchiolitis may be caused by COP, hypersensitivity pneumonitis, bone marrow, heart and lung transplant, acute infections such as *Mycoplasma*, *Legionella* and influenza. Symptoms are of progressive breathlessness and dry cough. Constrictive bronchiolitis rare. Connections with connective tissue disease, particular rheumatoid arthritis. Occasionally triggered by infection — viral adenovirus, respiratory syncytial virus, influenza. Cough and progressive dyspnoea
Eosinophilic lung disease	
Asthma and allergic bronchopulmonary aspergillosis (ABPA)	Severe asthmatic symptoms
Simple pulmonary eosinophilia (Löeffler's syndrome)	Cough, malaise, rhinitis, fever, night sweats, dyspnoea, wheeze, exposure to parasites (foreign travel)
Tropical pulmonary eosinophilia	As per Löeffler's syndrome, except symptoms over weeks to months, rather than days to weeks
Chronic eosinophilic pneumonia	Episodic episodes of cough, malaise, dyspnoea and fever
Acute eosinophilic pneumonia	Similar presentation to community-acquired pneumonia
Hyper-eosinophilic symptoms	Symptoms for weeks/months, fever, weight loss, cough, night sweats, pleuritic, Churg–Strauss syndrome, rhinitis, past history of asthma, other organ involvement including vasculitic rash
Drug-inducted pulmonary eosinophilia	History of recent new drug. Cough, dyspnoea, fever — spectrum of severity

Pulmonary embolism

In acute pulmonary embolism symptoms depend on the size of the clot. In approximately 60 per cent of patients there is an acute onset of pleuritic chest pain with or without haemoptysis. A pleural rub may be heard on examination. The pathophysiology is pulmonary infarction with obstruction of a peripheral vessel. In 25 per cent of patients there is sudden onset of acute breathlessness. Here the clot tends to be larger and more central. With massive pulmonary embolism there may be sudden circulatory collapse resulting in hypotension, loss of consciousness, or immediate cardiac arrest. In these circumstances there will be evidence of acute right heart failure with elevation of the jugular venous pressure. There will be sinus tachycardia and hypotension with signs of peripheral vasoconstriction. The patient will be cyanosed clinically and there will be reduced oxygen saturation on pulse oximetry. Occasionally in patients with pre-existing lung or heart disease, a relatively small pulmonary embolism will produce symptoms of severe breathlessness. Pulmonary embolism can also be a cause of acute atrial fibrillation. Other examination findings might include a loud pulmonary second sound and splitting of the second heart sound with a gallop rhythm, or a low-grade fever. See Box 8.9 for risk factors of pulmonary embolism.

BOX 8.9 RISK FACTORS FOR PULMONARY EMBOLISM

- Recent surgery, especially major surgery
- Late pregnancy
- Malignancy, especially pelvic/abdominal and advanced cancer
- Lower limb fracture
- Reduced mobility (especially hospitalization)
- Previous proven venous thromboembolism
- There are also a variety of minor risk factors, including the contraceptive pill, long-distance air travel, thrombotic disorders, obesity, inflammatory bowel disease and nephritic disease.

Pneumothorax

Pneumothorax presents with acute onset of pleuritic chest pain and/or breathlessness, which may be mild or absent in patients with prior normal lung function. The patient may feel bubbles or crackles under the skin and on examination you may feel subcutaneous emphysema. There may be tachycardia and chest signs (as discussed in 'Physical examination', p. 87). Hammond's sign refers to a click on auscultation in time with the heart sounds and is usually in association with a left-sided pneumothorax only.

SUMMARY

The six key symptoms of respiratory disease are:

- chest pain (that may be extended to chest sensations)
- dyspnoea
- cough
- wheeze
- sputum production
- haemoptysis.

When examining the respiratory system, assess:

- general observations
    - oxygen, a nebulizer, a sputum pot
    - observation chart
    - signs of respiratory distress
    - respiratory rate and characterize any abnormalities noted
    - any abnormality of the voice
    - anaemic, cyanosed or plethoric
- hands
    - flapping tremor
    - clubbing of the fingers
    - peripheral cyanosis
    - other signs of systemic disease
- head and neck
    - distended veins/jugular venous pressure
    - central cyanosis
    - anaemia
    - partial ptosis (indicative of Horner's syndrome)

- papilloedema
- supraclavicular and cervical lymph nodes
- thyroid enlargement
- scars that may indicate a previous tracheotomy or tracheostomy
- upper respiratory tract
  - look in the mouth
  - look at the nose
  - check the position of the trachea
- the chest
  - skin
  - abnormalities of chest shape
  - evidence of thoracic operations
  - depth and regularity of breathing
  - mode of breathing
  - chest wall expansion
  - vocal fremitus and vocal resonance
  - percussion
  - auscultation
  - rhonchi or wheezes
  - musical type sounds, crepitations or crackles
  - pleural rub.

FURTHER READING

Chapman S, Robinson G, Stradling J, *et al.* 2009. *Oxford handbook of respiratory medicine*, 2nd edn. Oxford: Oxford University Press.

9

THE GASTROINTESTINAL SYSTEM

Venkataraman Subramanian and Guruprasad P Aitha

INTRODUCTION

The gastrointestinal system includes the alimentary tract from mouth to anus, the liver, hepatobiliary structures including the gallbladder, pancreas and the biliary and pancreatic ductal systems. Effective clinical evaluation of gastrointestinal system relies upon recognizing the pattern of symptoms and signs. This is made more challenging because these occupy a small abdominal cavity, shared with parts of genitourinary system and vascular tree, with symptoms conveyed in unmyelinated afferent C fibres located on the walls of hollow viscera and capsules of solid organs to a relatively small area on the sensory cortex.

CLINICAL HISTORY

Almost half of gastrointestinal problems are not associated with physical signs or positive test results. Hence, the diagnosis and management is often based entirely on the inferences drawn from a patient's symptoms. In addition, as sets of symptoms are common to both 'medical' and 'surgical' conditions, identifying subtle variations in these patterns is critical for appropriate and timely clinical management.

When taking the history, you must ask about the following:

- accurate description of the symptom(s)
- time of onset
- occurrence and reoccurrence
- location and radiation
- aggravating and relieving factors
- relationship to other symptoms
- any previous abdominal or pelvic surgery
- history of travel and laxative misuse if there is diarrhoea
- presence of other systemic illnesses such as diabetes or cardiovascular disease that might affect the digestive system or share similar risk factors

- history of alcohol excess, peptic ulcer or liver disease
- family history of inflammatory bowel disease, coeliac disease, liver disease or bowel cancer
- risk factors:
  - smoking and alcohol consumption may impact on diagnosis and management, particularly of inflammatory bowel disease and chronic liver disease
  - alcohol excess, non-steroidal anti-inflammatory drugs (NSAIDs), antiplatelet agents and anticoagulants increase the risk of gastrointestinal haemorrhage
  - alcohol excess, intravenous drug misuse, risk behaviour and metabolic syndrome increase the risk of chronic liver disease.

CLINICAL PEARL

Symptoms suggestive of systemic inflammatory response, anaemia and weight loss generally indicate organic diseases and not functional disorders.

Dysphagia

Difficulty in swallowing is often described as food 'sticking' or 'not going down'. The sensation of a lump in the throat or retrosternal area (globus) is not true dysphagia, rather a perceived inability to swallow unrelated to eating, often associated with psychiatric comorbidities especially in females – when the term 'globus hystericus' is used.

Dysphagia is a 'red flag' symptom, as many patients with this symptom will have clinically significant pathology.

- In mechanical obstruction, solids 'stick' more than liquids.
- In neuromuscular causes, liquids 'stick' more than solids.

The history and associated symptoms may give a clue to the aetiology:

- weight loss and worsening dysphagia – oesophageal cancer is likely
- pain on swallowing (odynophagia) that is sharp and burning suggests mucosal inflammation (oesophagitis, infections or radiation), but a crampy or squeezing pain suggests a neuromuscular cause
- difficulty in *initiating* swallowing is suggestive of oropharyngeal dysphagia
- regurgitating old food is suggestive of pharyngeal pouch (Zenker's diverticulum)
- cough associated with swallowing suggests neuromuscular abnormalities
- acute onset is characteristic of bolus obstruction.

Dyspepsia or reflux

Heartburn (pyrosis) is a retrosternal burning sensation commonly experienced by up to 45 per cent of the population in the past 12 months. This characteristically occurs, or worsens, when bending over, straining or lying down, especially after a meal. Heartburn can often be associated with chest pain secondary to oesophageal spasm, which may be relieved by nitroglycerin, a smooth muscle relaxant. Unlike angina, it is unrelated to exertion and often occurs at rest. Its presence implies gastro-oesophageal reflux disease (GORD) and acid regurgitation.

> **CLINICAL PEARL**
> The word heartburn is poorly understood by patients so you may need to ask about 'a burning feeling rising from the stomach or lower chest up toward the neck'.

Waterbrash, the spontaneous flooding of the mouth with salivary secretions, accompanies heartburn. *Rumination*, in which meals are routinely regurgitated and swallowed, usually has no long-term consequences. *Regurgitation* is a passive process of retrograde flow of oesophageal contents into the mouth. Acid regurgitation is a cardinal symptom of GORD; some patients may have 'bolus reflux', which responds poorly to treatment with proton pump inhibitors.

Dyspepsia or 'indigestion' includes a group of symptoms believed to originate in the foregut. The main symptom is usually upper abdominal pain or discomfort, often associated with heartburn, bloating, belching, early satiety and nausea or vomiting. It is often caused by peptic ulcer, inflammation in the stomach and/or duodenum secondary to *Helicobacter pylori* infection or use of NSAIDs, presence of GORD and even functional bowel disorders. No symptom pattern reliably distinguishes the causes of dyspepsia, nor are there any symptoms that distinguish duodenal from gastric ulcers.

Nausea and vomiting

Nausea is an unpleasant, queasy feeling in the throat or stomach that usually precedes vomiting. *Vomiting*, in contrast, is a highly specific physical event that results in the rapid, forceful evacuation of gastric contents in retrograde fashion from the stomach up to and out of the mouth. It may be accompanied by tachycardia, hypersalivation, waterbrash and excessive perspiration. Vomiting must be distinguished from rumination and regurgitation. Nausea and vomiting are considered chronic if they last for more than 1 month.

Acute nausea and vomiting is usually due to:

- gastrointestinal infection
- ingestion of toxins (food poisoning)
- drugs
- head trauma
- abdominal visceral pain
- pregnancy.

Chronic nausea and vomiting usually suggests:

- motility disturbance
- endocrine or metabolic disorder
- intracranial pathology such as a space-occupying lesion
- partial mechanical obstruction of the gastrointestinal tract.

Vomiting during or soon after a meal is often functional but can occur with pyloric ulcers. Stale food in the vomitus 1–3 hours after a meal suggests gastric outlet, high small-bowel obstruction or gastroparesis. Feculent odour usually represents distal small-bowel or colonic obstruction, but can be due to gastrocolic fistulas, peritonitis with ileus, or bacterial overgrowth of the proximal small bowel/stomach.

Gastrointestinal bleeding

Gastrointestinal bleeding is a medical emergency requiring rapid evaluation and treatment. Distinguishing between upper gastrointestinal bleed (Box 9.1) and lower gastrointestinal bleed is important as their differential diagnoses and treatment differ.

Haematemesis is the vomiting of either bright red blood or 'coffee grounds' material (blood altered by exposure to acid). It almost always denotes an upper gastrointestinal bleed proximal to the ligament of Treitz (at the end of the duodenum).

Melaena is the passage of blood gradually degraded to haematin or other haemachromes by bacteria to produce a black tarry offensive stool. It requires at least 50 mL of blood delivered into the upper gastrointestinal tract, although up to 100 mL may be clinically silent. The source of bleeding may be the upper gastrointestinal tract, distal small bowel or ascending colon.

Approximately 10 per cent of all patients with rapid bleeding from an upper source present with *haematochezia*, the passage of bright red, maroon stool or clots per rectum, usually from a lower gastrointestinal bleed.

Occult bleeding, bleeding that is not apparent to the patient, usually results from small bleeds. It often presents with iron deficiency anaemia.

A non-bloody nasogastric aspirate suggests bleeding from a source outside the upper gastrointestinal

---

BOX 9.1 COMMON CAUSES OF UPPER GASTROINTESTINAL BLEEDING
- Peptic ulcer (40–50 per cent)
- Gastroduodenal erosions (10 per cent)
- Oesophagitis (5–10 per cent)
- Mallory–Weiss tear (10 per cent)
- Varices (5–10 per cent)
- Vascular malformations (5 per cent)
- Malignancy (4–5 per cent)
- Unidentified (20 per cent)

IMPORTANT   *i*

Acute upper gastrointestinal haemorrhage is a common, life-threatening medical emergency with an annual incidence of 50–150/100 000 population and 10 per cent mortality in the UK.

Table 9.1 Rockall score

Initial Rockall score calculated from clinical criteria pre-endoscopy (maximum total score 7). An initial Rockall score of 0 is regarded as low risk				
Criterion	**Score 0**	**Score 1**	**Score 2**	**Score 3**
Age	<60	60–79	≥80	–
Shock	SBP >100; HR <100	SBP >100; HR >100	SBP <100; HR >100	–
Co-morbidity	None	–	Cardiac disease, any other major co-morbidity	Renal/liver failure, disseminated malignancy
A *full* Rockall score can be calculated *after* endoscopy by adding score for the following criteria to the pre-endoscopy score (maximum total score 11). A full Rockall score of ≤2 is regarded as low risk				
Criterion	**Score 0**	**Score 1**	**Score 2**	**Score 3**
Endoscopic diagnosis	Mallory–Weiss tear, no lesion	All other diagnoses	Malignancy of the upper GI tract	–
Major stigmata of recent haemorrhage	None or dark spot only	–	Blood in upper GI tract, adherent clot, visible or spurting vessel	–

GI, gastrointestinal; HR, heart rate (beats per minute); SBP, systolic blood pressure (mmHg).
Reproduced from *Gut*, Rockall TA, Logan RF, Devlin HB, Northfield TC, **38**: 316–21, © 1996 with permission from BMJ Publishing Group.

tract, but is normal in up to 25 per cent of cases with upper gastrointestinal bleeding. Even a bile-coloured aspirate, which signifies sampling of the duodenum, does not exclude an upper gastrointestinal source of bleeding.

Assessment of the severity of gastrointestinal bleeding

Scoring systems to risk stratify patients with upper gastrointestinal bleeding have been developed, based on a combination of clinical, laboratory and endoscopic features, two of which are the widely used Rockall scoring system (Table 9.1), which predicts mortality, and the Glasgow–Blatchford scoring system (Table 9.2), which predicts need for intervention and identification of patients with low risk bleeding.

Abdominal pain

Abdominal pain can be classified into three categories:

- *Visceral*: a dull poorly localized pain in the abdominal wall experienced when noxious stimuli trigger visceral nociceptors. The site of pain corresponds roughly to the dermatomes appropriate to the abdominal organ from which the pain originates. It is often associated with autonomic features such as sweating, nausea, vomiting and pallor. Poor localization is believed to be due to visceral multisegmental innervation and, compared with skin, fewer visceral nerve endings.
- *Somato-parietal*: This pain originates from parietal peritoneum so is better localized than visceral pain, for example pain at McBurney's point in appendicitis.
- *Referred*: This is pain felt remote to the diseased organ, believed to be due to convergence of visceral and somatic afferent neurones from different areas in the spinal cord.

Box 9.2 summarizes the localization of common causes of acute abdominal pain.

Table 9.2 Glasgow–Blatchford scoring system

Admission risk marker	Criterion	Score
Blood urea (mmol/L)	≥6.5 and <8	2
	≥8 and <10	3
	≥10 and <25	4
	≥25	6
Haemoglobin (dg/L) *for men*	≥12 and <13	1
	≥10 and <12	3
	<10	6
Haemoglobin (dg/L) *for women*	≥10 and <12	1
	<10	6
Systolic blood pressure (mmHg)	100–109	1
	90–99	2
	<90	3
Pulse (bpm)	>100	1
Melaena	Present	1
Syncope	Present	2
Hepatic disease	Present	2
Cardiac failure	Present	2
A patient with a Glasgow–Blatchford score (GBS) of 0 is regarded as low risk and suitable for outpatient management		

Reproduced from *The Lancet*, **356**, Blatchford O, Murray WR, Blatchford M, A risk score to predict need for treatment for upper-gastrointestinal haemorrhage, 1318–21, © 2000, with permission from Elsevier.

BOX 9.2 LOCALIZATION OF COMMON CAUSES OF ACUTE ABDOMINAL PAIN
- Right upper quadrant:
  - biliary obstruction
  - acute cholecystitis
  - hepatomegaly.
- Left upper quadrant:
  - splenic infarct
  - acute focal pancreatitis
  - ischaemic colitis at watershed zone near splenic flexure.
- Right lower quadrant:
  - appendicitis
  - terminal ileitis
  - Crohn's disease
  - typhlitis.
- Left lower quadrant:
  - diverticulitis
  - infectious colitis (amoebic, bacterial)
  - inflammatory bowel disease.
- Either left or right lower quadrant:
  - tubo-ovarian disease in women
  - ectopic pregnancy
  - salpingitis

continued

- pyelonephritis
- ureteric stone.
- Central abdominal pain:
  - gastritis/peptic ulcer
  - small intestinal ischaemia (abdominal angina)
  - acute pancreatitis (often referred to the back)
  - gastroenteritis.
- Diffuse:
  - peritonitis due to perforated viscus
  - inflammatory bowel disease with toxic megacolon
  - haemorrhagic pancreatitis
  - spontaneous bacterial peritonitis (in patients with ascites)
  - postoperative (after abdominal surgery).

It is important to ask about aggravating and relieving factors.

- Classical biliary colic can be exacerbated by fatty foods and the pain of chronic mesenteric ischaemia is worse after a meal.
- Associated symptoms such as fever, right upper quadrant pain and jaundice (Charcot's triad) occur in 50–75 per cent of patients with cholangitis.
- Mesenteric ischaemia typically presents with pain after meals, and pain associated with duodenal ulcer wakes the patient up from sleep but is rarely present in the morning.
- Associated symptoms such as fever, right upper quadrant pain and jaundice (Charcot's triad) occur in 50–75 per cent of patients with cholangitis.

The severity of abdominal pain can be underestimated in patients with diabetes or those who are immunocompromised and elderly or very young patients. Symptoms and signs of acute abdominal pain can change over minutes to hours and serial examination often can improve the diagnostic yield.

Change in bowel habit (diarrhoea and constipation)

Diarrhoea

Many patients use the term 'diarrhoea' when they experience increased stool fluidity. Stool frequency of three or more bowel movements per day and stool

CLINICAL PEARL

While evaluating patients with abdominal pain, asking about rapidity of onset and duration of symptoms is of prime importance.

- Sudden onset of well-localized severe pain is likely to be due to catastrophic events such as a perforated viscus, ruptured aneurysm or mesenteric ischaemia.
- Pain present for weeks to months is often less life-threatening than pain presenting within hours of symptom onset.

weight greater than 200 g is considered abnormal in Western countries, though patients with increased fibre intake may exceed this. Diarrhoea is (see Box 9.3):

- *acute*: if it lasts less than 2 weeks (mostly due to infection)
- *persistent*: if it lasts more than 2 but less than 4 weeks (usually an atypical presentation of acute diarrhoea)
- *chronic*: if it has been present for more than 4 weeks.

Dysentery is the passage of bloody stools and is often associated with tenesmus or spasm of the anal

BOX 9.3 A CLINICAL CLASSIFICATION OF DIARRHOEAL DISEASES

Acute infective diarrhoea:
- watery diarrhoea:
  - enterotoxin associated: cholera toxin, heat labile enterotoxin of *Escherichia coli*, heat stable enterotoxin of *E. coli*, zonula occludes toxin, accessory cholera exterotoxin, etc.
  - enteroadhesive associated: aggregative, adherent *E. coli*
  - cytotoxin associated: enteropathogenic *E. coli*, Shiga-like toxin, etc.
  - viral diarrhoeas: rota, adeno, Norwalk, etc.
  - parasite associated: *Giardia, Cryptosporidium, Isospora*
  - unknown mechanism: anaerobes, *Giardia*.

continued

- dysentery
  - invasive bacteria: *Shigella, Salmonella, Campylobacter*
  - parasites: *Entamoeba histolytica*
- mucoid diarrhoea: any of the pathogens that cause watery diarrhoea or dysentery
- antibiotic-associated diarrhoea: *Clostridium difficile*
- parenteral diarrhoea
- travellers' diarrhoea.

Persistent diarrhoea.

Chronic diarrhoea:

- malabsorption syndromes:
  - secondary malabsorption syndromes
  - luminal factors
  - mucosal factors
  - interference with vascular and lymphatic transport
  - pancreatic and biliary deficiency
  - primary malabsorption syndrome: tropical sprue
- inflammatory bowel diseases
- diarrhoea of the immunocompromised
- irritable bowel syndrome.

Modified from: Mathan VI. 1998. Diarrhoeal diseases. *British Medical Bulletin* **54**: 407–19, by permission of Oxford University Press.

CLINICAL PEARL

Stool gazing:

- The recto-sigmoid colon acts as a storage reservoir for stool. So with distal colonic inflammation or motility disturbances, frequent small bowel movements ensue.
- Larger bowel movements are seen with lesions in the right colon and small bowel.
- Presence of blood in the stool points towards either inflammatory bowel disease or malignancy, but in those with *infective* diarrhoea it is highly specific for infections with a invasive organism.
- Presence of oil or food suggests either malabsorption or rapid intestinal transit.
- Urgency and incontinence suggests a problem of rectal compliance or loss of tone in the sphincters.
- Excessive flatus is often due to fermentation of carbohydrates by colonic bacteria either due to ingestion of poorly absorbed carbohydrates or malabsorption of carbohydrates by the small intestine.

---

sphincter associated with cramping and ineffective straining at stool.

Constipation

Constipation (Box 9.4) is a common complaint. It is associated with inactivity, low calorie intake, the number of medications being taken (independent of their side effects), low income, low education level, depression and physical and sexual abuse. Patients may interpret the term 'constipation' differently – a formal definition is given in Box 9.4.

Acute constipation may be due to:

- a sudden decrease in physical activity
- a change in diet, particularly reducing fibre
- use of medications (such as opiates, calcium channel blockers, anticholinergic drugs)
- anal pain
- in the over 40s – a colonic neoplasm.

BOX 9.4 DEFINITION OF CONSTIPATION

At least 12 weeks, which need not be consecutive, in the preceding 12 months, of two or more of:

- Straining during >1 in 4 defecations
- Lumpy or hard stools in >1 in 4 defecations
- Sensation of incomplete evacuation in >1 in 4 defecations
- Sensation of anorectal obstruction/blockade in >1 in 4 defecations
- Manual manoeuvres to facilitate >1 in 4 defecations (e.g. digital evacuation, support of the pelvic floor); and/or <3 defecations/week.

Loose stools are not present, and there are insufficient criteria for IBS.

Reproduced from *Gut*, Thompson WG, Longstreth GF, Drossman DA *et al.* **45** (Suppl 2): II43–7, 1999 with permission from BMJ Publishing Group Ltd.

A third of patients with *chronic constipation* have a functional disorder (some with a medical condition such as diabetes, Parkinson's disease, multiple sclerosis or on medication contributing to constipation), a third have a defecatory disorder, one sixth have irritable bowel syndrome (IBS) and a quarter have combined IBS and outlet-type defecatory disorder or took a medication that could have caused or contributed to the condition.

Faecal impaction is accumulation of a large amount of hard stool in the rectum that cannot be passed because of its size and consistency.

Remember that history alone is not useful in distinguishing functional from organic causes of constipation. Constipation associated with abdominal pain and bloating is more likely to be due to mechanical obstruction (cancer, stricture or faecal impaction). However, IBS itself can present with abdominal pain and a subjective sensation of bloating. Acute onset of symptoms suggests the cause to be mechanical obstruction. Symptoms of pain, bloating, and incomplete defecation predominate in constipation associated with IBS.

Jaundice

'Icterus', a yellow discoloration of tissues, may be due to:

- carotenoderma: excess consumption of carotene containing foods like carrots and leafy vegetables stains the palms, soles, forehead and nasolabial creases but spares the sclera
- drugs: such as quinacrine and exposure to phenols
- jaundice: characterized by yellow discoloration of the skin and mucous membranes due to abnormal increase in serum bilirubin >35 mmol/L (2 mg/dL). The sclera appear yellow first, as bilirubin has a high affinity to elastin in scleral tissue. Bilirubin gives urine a brown ('tea' or 'cola') colour.

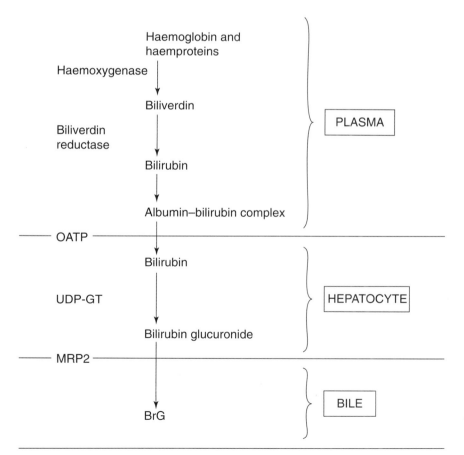

Figure 9.1 Overview of bilirubin metabolism and transport. OATP, organic anion transporter; UDP-GT, uridine diphosphoglucuronyl transferase; MRP2, multidrug resistance protein.

Serum bilirubin level rises when the balance between production and clearance is altered and thus the evaluation of a jaundiced patient requires an understanding of bilirubin production, metabolism and excretion (Fig. 9.1).

Problems in the pre-hepatic phase

Over-production of bilirubin

Inherited and acquired haemolytic disorders lead to excessive haem production and an unconjugated hyperbilirubinaemia (see Box 9.5), which is not excreted in the urine. Serum bilirubin rarely exceeds 86 mmol/L (5 mg/dL) so jaundice tends to be mild and recurrent and associated with symptoms of anaemia. Accelerated haemolysis, especially in inherited conditions, is associated with the formation of pigment gallstones which may obstruct the biliary tree and lead to conjugated hyperbilirubinaemia.

Impaired uptake and conjugation

Drugs such as rifampicin cause unconjugated hyperbilirubinaemia by reducing hepatic uptake. Rare inherited syndromes such as Crigler–Najjar syndromes I and II and Gilbert's syndrome are caused by dysfunction or absence of the enzyme uridine diphosphoglucoronyl transferase (UDP-GT), which mediates conjugation of the hydrophobic bilirubin to hydrophilic bilirubin monoglucoronide and diglucoronide conjugates that are suitable for excretion.

- Crigler–Najjar I is very rare and is characterized by complete absence of the enzyme UDP-GT leading to neonatal kernicterus and death.
- Crigler–Najjar II is more common and there is reduced activity of the enzyme and patients live to adulthood.
- Gilbert's syndrome is quite common and is due to reduced enzyme activity and manifests clinically as very mild jaundice especially in times of physiological stress such as periods of fasting or unrelated viral infections.

Problems in the hepatic phase

The UDP-GT activity is well maintained in both acute and chronic hepatocellular damage and even

---

BOX 9.5 CAUSES OF UNCONJUGATED HYPERBILIRUBINAEMIA

Haemolytic disorders:
- inherited:
  - spherocytosis, elliptocytosis
  - glucose 6-phosphate dehydrogenase and pyruvate kinase deficiency
  - sickle cell disorder
- acquired:
  - immune haemolysis
  - microangiopathic haemolytic anaemia
  - paroxysmal nocturnal haemoglobinuria.

Ineffective erythropoiesis:
- vitamin B_{12} deficiency
- folate deficiency
- thalassaemia
- severe iron deficiency anaemia.

Drugs

Inherited conditions;
  - Crigler–Najjar syndrome types I and II
  - Gilbert's syndrome

---

increased in cholestasis. Impaired secretion in association with parenchymal liver disease leads to 'regurgitation' of conjugated bilirubin from liver cells into the bloodstream. Deep yellow urine suggests a possibility of concentrated urine in dehydration rather than bilirubinuria. Some hepatocellular causes of jaundice are listed in Box 9.6.

BOX 9.6 HEPATOCELLULAR CONDITIONS CAUSING JAUNDICE

Viral hepatitis:
  - hepatitis A, B, C and E
  - Epstein–Barr virus (EBV)
  - cytomegalovirus (CMV).

Alcohol.

Autoimmune hepatitis.

Medications/drugs;
  - dose dependent, e.g. paracetamol overdose
  - idiosyncratic, e.g. isoniazid.

Environmental toxins:
  - Bush tea

continued

- Kava Kava
- mushrooms.

Metabolic causes:
- Wilson's disease
- Haemochromatosis
- Non-alcoholic fatty liver disease (NAFLD)
- α-1 antitrypsin deficiency.

Vascular causes:
- Budd–Chiari syndrome
- ischaemic hepatitis.

SMALL PRINT

In cirrhosis, two-thirds of patients with alcoholic liver disease and 25 per cent of those with other aetiologies report impotence. Reduced desire, difficulty in arousal and dyspareunia are described in 20–33 per cent of women with chronic liver disease.

Problems in the post-hepatic phase

Differentiating hepatocellular from cholestatic jaundice (due to biliary or impaired bile flow) is not straightforward – changes in bile pigment metabolism are the same in both, so dark brown urine due to bilirubinuria does not help, nor does spontaneous (or easily induced) bleeding (from nose or gums) or bruising, which may occur in both acute or chronic liver disease (often related to thrombocytopenia) and following malabsorption of fat-soluble vitamin K in cholestatic disease.

Itching (pruritus) in cholestasis may be due to high plasma concentrations of bile salts. In liver disease it is of variable severity, can be more prominent in the extremities rather than the trunk (and rarely affects the face and neck), especially after a hot bath or at night when the skin is warm. Impaired excretion of the bile is also associated with reduced stercobilinogen in the stool giving a clay colour to the stool. Frank fat malabsorption in complete biliary obstruction may lead to offensive fatty stools (*steatorrhoea*).

Right upper quadrant pain from distension and increased pressure within the bile duct in cholestatic jaundice may distinguish patients with obstructive jaundice from those with other cholestatic conditions. Pain due to obstruction from bile duct stones is not a consistent feature except in acute obstruction; although described as 'biliary colic', the pain does not wax and wane. Biliary pain is absent in most pancreatic tumours where obstruction is gradual yet complete, although the bile duct may be markedly dilated, presumably due to relatively low wall tension.

BOX 9.7 CHOLESTATIC CONDITIONS CAUSING JAUNDICE

Non-obstructive:
- viral hepatitis
  - fibrosing cholestatic hepatitis – hepatitis B and C
  - cholestasis with hepatitis – hepatitis A and E, CMV, EBV
- drugs:
  - pure cholestasis – anabolic steroids, pill
  - cholestatic hepatitis – co-amoxiclav, flucloxacillin, erythromycin esteolate
  - chronic cholestasis – chlorpromazine
- primary biliary cirrhosis
- primary sclerosing cholangitis
- inherited conditions:
  - Dubin–Johnson syndrome
  - Rotor's syndrome
  - Progressive familial intrahepatic cholestasis
- miscellaneous:
  - cholestasis of pregnancy
  - sepsis
  - total parenteral nutrition
  - paraneoplastic syndrome

Obstructive:
- malignant
  - cholangiocarcinoma
  - pancreatic cancer
  - periampullary cancer
  - malignant involvement of the porta hepatis lymph nodes
- benign
  - choledocholithiasis
  - primary sclerosing cholangitis
  - chronic pancreatitis
  - acquired immune deficiency syndrome (AIDS) cholangiopathy

The functional reserve of the liver is so great that occlusion of intrahepatic ducts does not give rise to jaundice until ducts draining up to 75 per cent of the liver parenchyma are occluded. Some causes of cholestatic jaundice are listed in Box 9.7.

PHYSICAL EXAMINATION

Clinical signs help refine the estimates of pre-test probability of a condition and should be put in context of patients' symptoms and presentations. Their negative predictive value may be low, for example a patient with compensated cirrhosis may have no clinical signs. Clinical signs may be:

- very specific (e.g. a Kaiser–Fleischer ring, a brown ring at the periphery of the cornea due to deposition of copper in Descemet's membrane in Wilson's disease)
- non-specific (e.g. clubbing)
- epiphenomena (e.g. spider naevi (Fig. 9.2) – vascular abnormalities with central arteriole and radiating blood vessels like spider legs that point to chronic liver disease in someone with appropriate risk factors)
- useful pointers to disease severity (e.g. portal hypertension and hepatic encephalopathy are markers of decompensated cirrhosis)
- 'complementary' – multiple signs pointing to the same abnormality are valuable only when the initial findings are equivocal.

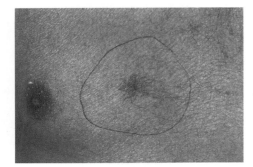

Figure 9.2 Spider naevus. From: Gray D, Toghill F (eds), *An introduction to the symptoms and signs of clinical medicine*, with permission. © 2001 London: Hodder Arnold.

The general examination

In patients presenting with acute onset of symptoms, you must include clinical evidence of systemic inflammatory response such as tachycardia (heart rate >90 bpm), body temperature <36 or >38 °C or tachypnoea (respiratory rate >20/minute) in your initial observations. Hypotension (systolic BP <90 mmHg) with signs of shock (cold, clammy extremities in hypovolaemic shock or warm, sweaty skin in septic shock) should prompt immediate resuscitation.

Signs of dehydration

About 2 L of fluids are consumed daily and 7 L secreted into the gastrointestinal tract, so it is not surprising that dehydration is an important marker of severity in several digestive diseases. You must look for signs of dehydration in patients with diarrhoea. Simple indicators of mild dehydration (5 per cent), especially in children, include:

- skin turgor: checked by pulling up the skin on the back of an adult's hand or child's abdomen for a few seconds and checking how quickly it returns to the original state
- capillary refill: measured by pressing a fingernail until it turns white, and taking note of the time needed for colour to return on release – normally less than 2 seconds.

Assessment of nutritional status

The 'subjective global assessment rating' (Detsky *et al.*, 1987) has a high degree of interobserver agreement combining information regarding amount of weight loss in the last 6 months, functional capacity, gastrointestinal symptoms such as anorexia, nausea, vomiting, diarrhoea and their relation to nutrition with the elements of the physical examination (loss of subcutaneous fat, muscle wasting and ankle or sacral oedema). Patients are classified as *well nourished*, *moderately* or *severely malnourished*.

There may be signs of specific deficiencies such as:

- flat angle or spooning of nails in iron deficiency
- glossitis in iron and B_{12} deficiency
- angular stomatitis (redness and cracks at the angles of the mouth (Fig. 9.3)) in association with deficiency of iron, riboflavin, folate and cobalamin (vitamin B_{12}).

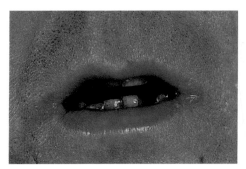

Figure 9.3 Angular stomatitis. From: Gray D, Toghill P (eds), *An introduction to the symptoms and signs of clinical medicine*, with permission. © 2001 London: Hodder Arnold.

Body mass index (BMI) is the patient's weight in kilograms divided by the square of the height in metres. An individual is considered overweight if BMI exceeds $25\,kg/m^2$, or obese if over $30\,kg/m^2$. **Waist hip ratio** (WHR) is the circumference of the waist (measured at the midpoint between the lower costal margin and the iliac crest) and the hip circumference (measured at the widest part of the gluteal region). **Abdominal obesity** (commoner in men) carries a poorer prognosis than gluteofemoral obesity (commoner in women). WHR of >1.0 in men and >0.85 in women has been shown to be associated with adverse health outcomes.

Appearance and cutaneous signs

Some diseases can be spotted straightaway, such as hyper- and hypothyroidism, acromegaly and Addison's disease. Perioral melanin deposition (Fig. 9.4) suggests *Peutz–Jeghers syndrome* which is associated with generalized gastrointestinal hamartomatous polyps most commonly in the jejunum. Oral and tongue telangiectasia are a hallmark of the *Osler–Weber–Rendu syndrome*; lesions in the gastrointestinal tract can result in iron deficiency anaemia.

Erythema nodosum, a type of inflammation in the fatty layer of skin, results in reddish, painful, tender lumps (1–5 cm), most commonly located in the lower leg. This may occur as an isolated condition or in association with:

- inflammatory bowel disease
- oral contraceptive pills
- pregnancy

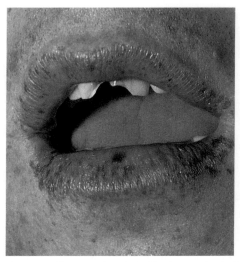

Figure 9.4 Pigmentation of the lips in a patient with colonic polyps (Peutz–Jeghers syndrome). From: Ogilvie C, Evans CC (eds), *Chamberlain's symptoms and signs in clinical medicine* (12th edition), with permission. © 1997 London: Hodder Arnold.

- streptococcal infections
- sarcoidosis
- Behçet's disease.

Tender necrotic undermined skin ulcerations are suggestive of *pyoderma gangrenosum* (Fig. 9.5) typically associated with inflammatory bowel disease (especially ulcerative colitis) or systemic inflammatory conditions including rheumatoid arthritis and chronic myeloid leukaemia.

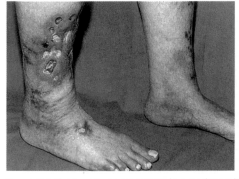

Figure 9.5 Pyoderma gangrenosum in a patient with ulcerative colitis. From: Ogilvie C, Evans CC (eds), *Chamberlain's symptoms and signs in clinical medicine* (12th edition), with permission. © 1997 London: Hodder Arnold.

Signs of liver disease

Parotid enlargement, Dupuytren's contracture, hepatitis C infection (look for tattoos, needle tracks), gynaecomastia (see below) and spider naevi may point to chronic liver disease. Jaundice, bruising and flapping tremor may indicate decompensation. Primary or secondary biliary cirrhosis, causes of chronic cholestasis, may be associated with symmetrical yellowish plaques around the eyelids (xanthelasmas). Persistent intrahepatic cholestasis in childhood has been associated with a characteristic facial appearance of widely set eyes, a prominent forehead, flat nose and small chin.

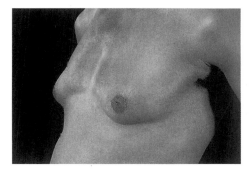

Figure 9.6 Gynaecomastia in a West Indian patient with chronic active hepatitis. From: Gray D, Toghill P (eds), *An introduction to the symptoms and signs of clinical medicine*, with permission. © 2001 London: Hodder Arnold.

- *Jaundice* is apparent in adults when serum bilirubin level exceeds 2.5–3.0 mg/dL (42.8–53 mmol/L).
- *Subconjunctival haemorrhage* is often seen in leptospirosis and with acute liver failure from any cause, while bruising of periorbital skin raises a possibility of amyloid.
- Increased *pigmentation* is seen with chronic cholestatic conditions, haemochromatosis and porphyria cutanea tarda.
- *Vitiligo*, a common patchy depigmentation due to autoimmune destruction of melanocytes (seen in 1 per cent of the population) is also associated with primary biliary cirrhosis and autoimmune hepatitis.
- *Enlarged parotids* are seen in patients with cirrhosis due to alcohol misuse and/or malnutrition; these are painless and non-tender with patent ducts and increased secretion.
- *Spider naevi* may be observed anywhere above the umbilicus. They may be seen in women taking oral contraceptives or during pregnancy, or in chronic liver disease, especially in men. In alcoholic liver disease, they are large and numerous, often in association with redness of thenar and hypothenar eminences (palmar erythema).
- *Gynaecomastia* (Fig. 9.6), a tender palpable enlargement of glandular breast tissue under the areola, should be distinguished from breast enlargement due to obesity (lipomastia), which may be seen in normal men due to the conversion in peripheral tissue of circulating androgens to oestrogen. Feminization, manifesting as gynaecomastia and thinning of body hair, occurs when the testosterone:oestradiol ratio is less than the normal 100:1. Except for physiological states (adolescence and ageing), gynaecomastia occurs in some males with liver disease and with drugs such as spironolactone.
- *'Flapping tremor'* (asterixis) describes brief, intermittent flexion of fingers or wrists, with a rapid return to the original position, affecting the shoulders and head when severe. Flaps are not specific for hepatic encephalopathy, and occur in uraemia, respiratory failure and hypokalaemia.
- *Dupuytren's contracture*, thickening and shortening of palmar fascia causing fixed flexion deformity of fingers, affects up to 20 per cent in men over 65 years, perhaps due to free radical formation from the action of xanthine oxidase on hypoxanthine. It is more frequently seen in individuals with history of alcohol excess.
- White nails, transverse white lines and clubbing are too non-specific to be helpful in diagnosis.
- *Testicular atrophy* is common in cirrhotic males, particularly with alcoholic liver disease or haemochromatosis.

Abdominal examination

Figure 9.7 shows the four abdominal quadrants used for descriptive purposes and Table 9.3 lists the organs within each quadrant.

Inspection

Stand on the patient's right side with the patient supine and the bed or couch at a comfortable height.

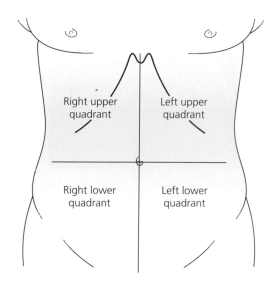

Figure 9.7 The four quadrants of the abdomen.

Ideally, the entire abdomen from xiphisternum to symphysis pubis should be exposed, but you may need to adapt the clinical examination to respect patients' sensitivity and cultural differences.

The *abdominal contour* is normally flat or slightly concave. A scaphoid abdomen with marked concav-ity may correlate with weight loss. *Abdominal distension* may be due to:

- obesity (**f**at)
- gaseous distention (**f**latus)
- ascites (**f**luid)
- abdominal mass (**f**atal if cancerous)
- in women, pregnancy (**f**etus).

As fluid accumulation in *ascites* starts in the pelvis and extends along the paracolic gutters, character-istic bulging at the flanks appear in moderate and large ascites. *Obesity* usually causes a more uni-formly rounded abdomen with a deep umbilicus (as it is adherent to the peritoneum). Asymmetry of the abdominal contour may indicate the presence of a mass in the abdomen. An everted umbilicus indi-cates increased intra-abdominal pressure due to ascites (Fig. 9.8) or an intra-abdominal mass.

An *umbilical hernia* can also cause the umbilicus to be everted. Umbilical hernias protrude through a defective umbilical ring; they are commoner in infants than adults. *Incisional hernia* protrudes through an operative scar and an *epigastric hernia* is a small midline protrusion through a defect in the linea, best noticed with the patient flexing the head. Ascites, obesity, previous surgeries and multiparous

Table 9.3 Abdominal organs and the quadrants they are usually present in

Upper–right	Upper–left
Liver	Left lobe of liver
Gallbladder	Spleen
Stomach (pyloric area)	Stomach (fundus and body)
Duodenum	Body and tail of pancreas
Head of pancreas	Upper pole of left kidney and adrenal gland
Upper pole of right kidney and adrenal gland	Splenic flexure
Hepatic flexure	Part of transverse and descending colon
Part of ascending colon	
Lower–right	**Lower–left**
Lower pole of right kidney	Lower pole of left kidney
Caecum and appendix	Sigmoid colon and part of descending colon
Part of ascending colon	Left ovary and fallopian tube
Right ovary and fallopian tube	Uterus or bladder if enlarged
Uterus/bladder if enlarged	

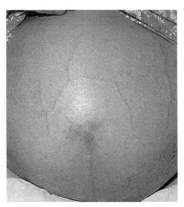

Figure 9.8 Eversion of the umbilicus in ascites. From: Ogilvie C, Evans CC (eds), *Chamberlain's symptoms and signs in clinical medicine* (12th edition), with permission. © 1997 London: Hodder Arnold.

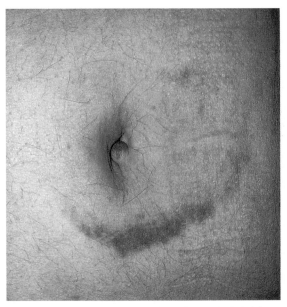

Figure 9.10 Cullen's sign. From: Gray D, Toghill P (eds), *An introduction to the symptoms and signs of clinical medicine*, with permission. © 2001 London: Hodder Arnold.

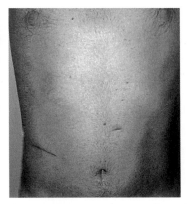

Figure 9.9 Laparoscopic scars. From: Ogilvie C, Evans CC (eds), *Chamberlain's symptoms and signs in clinical medicine* (12th edition), with permission. © 1997 London: Hodder Arnold.

women may cause a midline ridge due to separation or divarication of the rectus abdominis muscles.

Note the location of *postoperative scars* (Fig. 9.9) and any surgically created scar from an ileostomy, jejunostomy or colostomy. Silvery striae ('stretch marks') are normal in parous women and in the obese, and reddish-purple striae occur in many with Cushing's syndrome and obesity.

Abdominal wall *bruising* (ecchymosis) is considered a sign of intraperitoneal or retroperitoneal haemorrhage; ecchymosis in the periumbilical area (Cullen's sign (Fig. 9.10)) or in the flanks (Grey Turner's sign) occurs in less than 3 per cent of patients with acute pancreatitis. *Erythema ab igne*, areas of reticular erythema, are due to repeated exposure to moderate heat (e.g. from a hot water bottle).

A hard subcutaneous nodule (*Sister Mary Joseph's nodule*) may represent metastatic carcinoma of the umbilicus; it is important to differentiate this from a hardened concretion of keratin and sebum due to poor hygiene (omphalolith) – most of the former have stomach, colonic, pancreatic or ovarian malignancy with a median survival of less than a year. Visible intestinal peristalsis rolling across the abdomen may be a sign of intestinal obstruction but is not diagnostic.

In fetal life umbilical veins terminate in the left branch of portal vein; high portal pressure may open these, seen as *dilated veins* that radiate away from the umbilicus, popularly termed 'caput medusae'. Dilated veins may also be seen in inferior vena cava obstruction (Fig. 9.11) and in superior vena cava obstruction involving the azygous veins. In theory, blood should flow downwards from the umbilicus

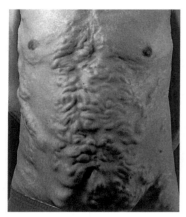

Figure 9.11 Dilated abdominal veins in inferior vena cava obstruction. From: Ogilvie C, Evans CC (eds), *Chamberlain's symptoms and signs in clinical medicine* (12th edition), with permission. © 1997 London: Hodder Arnold.

in portal hypertension and upwards in vena caval obstruction (but most dilated abdominal veins do not have any competent valves and flow can usually be demonstrated in both directions).

Palpation and percussion

Avoid palpation when your hands are cold as this could trigger involuntary abdominal muscle contraction (guarding). Ask if anywhere is painful or tender – defer palpating these areas to the end of the examination. Palpate lightly in all four quadrants with a slight 'dipping' motion, assessing for tenderness and areas of guarding. Then palpate more deeply, depressing the abdomen about 3–5 cm to delineate abdominal masses, their location, shape, size and consistency and detect the presence of tenderness, pulsations and movement with respiration. Traditionally, many eponymous signs have been considered 'diagnostic', but their specificity and sensitivity has been found to be too low for these signs to be considered reliable.

Auscultation

The biological variation in normal *bowel sounds* is immense with changes in pitch, tone and frequency from moment to moment. Bowel sounds are not a good indicator of recovery from postoperative ileus.

In peritonitis, bowel sounds may be diminished or absent but are too unreliable for clinical practice. There are no reliable auscultatory sounds in the diagnosis or surveillance of liver tumours.

Abdominal *epigastric bruits* caused by turbulent flow of blood though intra-abdominal or abdominal wall vessels are common. A short faint mid-systolic bruit in an asymptomatic patient is of no consequence and does not warrant investigation. Abdominal bruits are more frequent in hypertension (especially those with renal artery stenosis) and aortic aneurysms, although sensitivity is too low for screening purposes. Bruits from hepatocellular carcinoma and cirrhosis are best heard in the right upper quadrant and from splenic arteriovenous fistulas and carcinoma of the body of the pancreas in the left upper quadrant. Periumbilical bruits can be heard occasionally in the setting of mesenteric ischaemia.

Venous hums are low pitched, soft and continuous, and are sometimes heard in portal hypertension.

Specific aspects of the abdominal examination

Liver and gallbladder

Normal livers are not as easy to feel as diseased, firm enlarged livers. The liver is pulsatile in tricuspid regurgitation; however, expansile pulsations are difficult to distinguish clinically from transmitted aortic pulsations.

Start the examination over the right lower quadrant. Place your hand parallel to the costal margin lateral to rectus and press gently and firmly, moving the palm upward 2–3 cm at a time towards the lower costal margin. During inspiration, the liver is moved downward by the diaphragm and may 'flip' over the index finger; note the lowest point below the costal margin and its consistency (soft/firm/hard) and texture (smooth/nodular). Its upper border can be established later by percussing in the mid-clavicular line – the resonant note over the air-filled lung contrasts with the dullness over the liver – the liver is generally less than 12 cm from upper to lower border (Fig. 9.12).

The normal gallbladder is not palpable unless enlarged; if *painless*, this is often associated with malignant obstruction of the common bile duct,

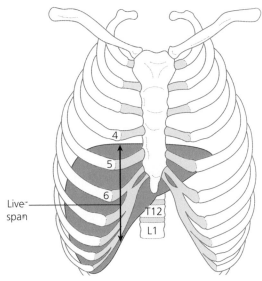

Figure 9.12 The surface markings of the liver, showing the site at which the span is measured. From: Gray D, Toghill P (eds), *An introduction to the symptoms and signs of clinical medicine*, with permission. © 2001 London: Hodder Arnold.

while *painful* enlargement is usually due to inflammation (empyema or cholecystitis). Gallstones are an unlikely cause of enlarged gallbladder in a jaundiced patient (Courvoisier's law). Periampullary cancer or carcinoma of the head of pancreas may present as painless jaundice with a palpable gallbladder.

> **SMALL PRINT**
>
> Some patients with cholecystitis may have tenderness that is triggered during palpation as the gallbladder descends on inspiration (called *Murphy's sign*) but this sign is not diagnostic. *Courvoisier's sign* is jaundice with a palpable, non-tender gallbladder; early presentation and easily available imaging mean the high intraductal pressure of biliary obstruction needed to enlarge the gallbladder is rarely seen, so this sign is of purely historical interest.

The spleen

The spleen is a curved wedge, about 12 cm long, that follows the course of the bony portion of the left tenth rib. It enlarges in the same line, descending below the ribs across the abdomen to the right iliac fossa. An enlarged spleen (*splenomegaly*, Box 9.8) may be felt as a mass in the left upper quadrant moving downwards and inwards during inspiration.

In the supine patient, palpate gently first in the right iliac fossa, proceeding diagonally past the umbilicus to the left costal margin as the patient inspires deeply. The spleen may be easier to feel with the patient in right lateral decubitus position, so that the spleen shifts a little due to gravity. The percussion note is always dull, as the spleen is anterior to the bowel, distinguishing this from other abdominal structures.

> **BOX 9.8** DISEASES ASSOCIATED WITH SPLENOMEGALY
> - Infections: infectious mononucleosis, infective endocarditis, malaria, leishmaniasis, viral hepatitis.
> - Disorders of immune system: immune thrombocytopenia, systemic lupus erythematosus.
> - Disordered splenic blood flow: portal hypertension, splenic vein thrombosis.
> - Haemolytic anaemias: spherocytosis, thalassaemia.
> - Infiltrative diseases:
>   - benign: amyloidosis, Gaucher's disease
>   - malignant: lymphomas, myeloproliferative disorders.

Kidneys

The kidneys may be palpable in thin normal individuals especially women. The kidneys are palpated bimanually using the technique of ballottement.

To palpate the right kidney stand to the right side of the abdomen, with your left hand behind the right flank between the costal margin and the iliac crest with the tips of your fingers lateral to the sacrospinalis muscle mass. Your right hand is placed anteriorly across the abdomen just below the costal margin. Exert firm pressure downward with the fingers of your right hand. With the patient taking deep breaths, flip the fingers of your left hand a few times upwards. The kidney is felt to bump against the fingers of your right hand. Similarly, the left kidney is felt by placing your left hand under the left flank and your right hand is placed anteriorly on the abdominal wall. Occasionally the spleen may be mistaken for an enlarged left kidney. See Box 9.9 for a list of points that help differentiate between an enlarged left kidney and a spleen.

> **SMALL PRINT**
> *Renal angle tenderness* is pain elicited on striking the patient firmly with the heel of a closed fist over the acute angle formed between the twelfth rib and the vertebral column (costovertebral angle). A finding of costovertebral angle tenderness is suggestive of pyelonephritis. This has not, however, been formally studied and no firm recommendations can be made.

BOX 9.9 DIFFERENTIATING BETWEEN SPLEEN AND LEFT KIDNEY

- Presence of a notch on the medial surface of the spleen.
- Can go above the upper margin of the mass (if left kidney).
- Direction of the mass would be oblique along the left tenth rib (if spleen).
- The kidney would be ballottable and bimanually palpable (massive spleen may also be bimanually palpable).
- Cannot insinuate fingers between the mass and the costal margin in splenomegaly.
- Lobulated or irregular mass more likely to be kidney.
- The splenic mass will move appreciably with respiration.

Ascites

Accumulation of free fluid in the abdomen is ascites; its development carries an adverse prognosis. It can be due to:

- cirrhosis
- malignancy
- heart failure
- tuberculosis
- nephrotic syndrome
- other rarer causes (e.g. myxoedema, vasculitis).

When supine, fluid gravitates to the flanks and the air-filled intestines float on top, causing:

- bulging flanks (often difficult to distinguish from obesity just on inspection)
- flank dullness as the air-filled intestines float to the top (percussion note is tympanic centrally over air and dull over bowel in the flanks)
- shifting dullness – identify in the supine patient where fluid is (the percussion note is dull) and where bowel is (the percussion note is resonant); position the hand over the fluid–air interface (part of the hand is over fluid and part over air), roll the patient onto the side, wait for the fluid to settle and percuss again – if there is a significant amount of fluid, the gas-filled bowel will have been lifted by the ascitic fluid so that the percussion note is now resonant
- fluid thrill – the patient (or an assistant) places the edge of a hand firmly down the midline of the abdomen as you tap one flank sharply (Fig. 9.13); if there is ascites, your other hand will feel a transmitted impulse in the opposite flank.

Along with these signs, most patients with ascites have peripheral oedema – due to hypoalbuminaemia and probably from pressure of the peritoneal fluid compressing the veins draining the legs.

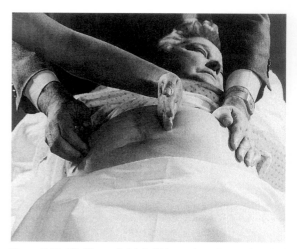

Figure 9.13 Eliciting a fluid thrill in ascites. From: Ogilvie C, Evans CC (eds), *Chamberlain's symptoms and signs in clinical medicine* (12th edition), with permission. © 1997 London: Hodder Arnold.

Examination of the abdominal aorta

The normal aorta bifurcates at the umbilicus and therefore palpable aortic aneurysms are typically found in the epigastrium. It is often readily palpable in thin individuals and those with lax abdominal vasculature and is usually less than 2.5 cm in estimated diameter. With the patient supine, the aortic pulsation is usually felt a few centimetres above the umbilicus and slightly to the left of the midline.

An estimated aortic diameter (by placing one hand on each side of pulsations) greater than 3 cm is considered to be a positive finding. Although Sir William Osler emphasized the expansile pulsation more than 100 years ago, it is the width and not the intensity of the pulsation that that determines the diagnosis of abdominal aortic aneurysm (AAA).

> **IMPORTANT**
> Obesity limits the effectiveness of abdominal palpation in detecting AAA. Hence physical examination cannot safely exclude a diagnosis of AAA and ultrasound should always be done in patients in whom there is a high index of suspicion regardless of the physical findings.

Examination of hernial orifices

The inguinal canal extends from the pubic tubercle to the anterior superior iliac spine and carries the spermatic cord in the male and the round ligament in the female. The internal ring is an opening in the transversalis fascia and lies in the mid-inguinal point halfway between the pubic symphysis and the anterior superior iliac spine. The external ring is an opening of the external oblique aponeurosis and lies immediately above and medial to the pubic tubercle. A direct inguinal hernia is herniation through the external ring and is uncommon, while indirect inguinal hernia is common (85 per cent of all hernias) and is more likely to strangulate, as the bowel and omentum can travel down the canal and protrude through the internal ring into the scrotum.

Examination for inguinal hernias is best done with the patient standing up and undressed from the waist down. An expansile cough impulse is diagnostic of a hernia. Table 9.4 lists the points that differentiate an indirect from a direct inguinal hernia.

Digital examination of the rectum

The routine examination of the abdomen usually concludes with the digital examination of the rectum. The importance of the rectal examination is stressed by the surgical aphorism attributed to Hamilton Bailey – 'if you don't put your finger in it, you might put your foot in it.'

The examination of the rectum can be done with the patient in the left lateral position with the right knee flexed and the left knee semi-extended, or in the standing position bent over with the shoulders and elbows supported on the examination table. Your gloved right hand is used to examine the anus and your gloved left hand spreads the buttocks for better visualization.

Inspect the anal skin for fissures, excoriation, signs of inflammation, warts, fistulae, haemorrhoids, scar and tumours. Visualization of fissures and haemorrhoids improves when the patient is asked to strain. After informing the patient that the rectal examination is going to be done, place your lubricated (with KY jelly) right gloved index finger on the anal verge; the sphincter relaxed by gentle pressure of the palmar surface of the finger. As the sphincter relaxes insert your index finger into the anal canal (Fig.

Table 9.4 Differences between direct and indirect inguinal hernias

Indirect	Direct
Can descend into scrotum	Rarely descends into scrotum
Reduces upwards laterally and backwards	Reduces upwards and backwards
Remains reduced with pressure on internal ring	Not reduced
Defect not palpable	Defect palpable
Reappears at the internal ring and flows medially	Reappears at the same position after reduction

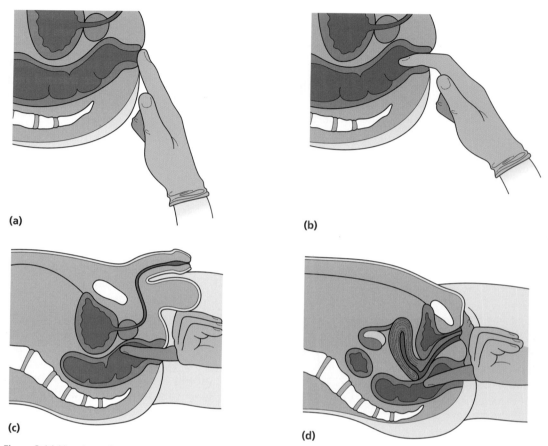

Figure 9.14 How to perform a rectal examination (a, b). (c) The position of the prostate gland. (d) The position of the cervix. From: Gray D, Toghill P (eds), *An introduction to the symptoms and signs of clinical medicine*, with permission. © 2001 London: Hodder Arnold.

9.14). Assess the sphincter tone and then insert your finger as far up the rectum as possible (depending on the length of the examining finger). Feel the lateral walls of the rectum by rotating your index finger along the sides of the rectum. Palpate the posterior and anterior walls as well, for polyps, irregularities or tenderness.

Intraperitoneal metastasis may be felt anterior to the rectum as a hard and shelf-like structure protruding into the rectum, resulting from malignant deposits in the pouch of Douglas. This has been referred to as Blumer's shelf.

Assess the size, shape and consistency of the prostate gland, which lies anterior to the rectum. Only the lower apical portion of the gland is usually palpable. The presence of a hard nodule making the prostate asymmetrical is likely to be malignant, and a symmetrically enlarged soft gland is likely to be due to benign prostatic hypertrophy.

Withdraw your examining finger and inspect it for faecal matter (colour and presence of blood). Finally, tests of faecal occult blood can be performed on the faecal matter sticking to the gloved index finger.

Tenderness and fullness on the right but not on the left side on rectal examination is believed to be indicative of pelvic appendicitis. The utility of the rectal examination in patients with acute appendicitis is questionable, as some studies have shown that abdominal signs are better predictors of appendicitis than rectal examination. If patients presenting with pain in the right lower quadrant of the abdomen are tested for rebound tenderness then rectal examination does not give any further diagnostic information.

CLINICAL PEARL

- The left lobe of an enlarged liver may be mistaken for the spleen, especially when there is a deep fissure between two lobes of the liver. Carefully mapping the lower border of the liver may help in making the distinction.
- Liver pulsatility may be due to tricuspid regurgitation or transmitted from the aorta. In the former, expect a raised jugular venous pressure and peripheral oedema.
- The left kidney may be mistaken for an enlarged spleen – the clue is in the percussion note – the kidney is usually resonant, the spleen dull. It is sometimes possible to get above the renal mass and to insert the hand between the renal mass and left costal margin (unlike the spleen).

INVESTIGATIONS

Commonly used investigations in gastroenterology and their indication and positive findings and interpretation are outlined below. Note that many of these tests are used in other specialities as well, but their uses in the setting of purely gastrointestinal disorders are described here.

Radiological investigations

Table 9.5 summarizes the common investigations, findings and their interpretation in patients with gastrointestinal diseases.

Chest X-ray (erect)

- **Indication:** To assess for perforation of the intestine.
- **Positive findings:** Sliver of air under the diaphragm, air in the mediastinum and/or pleural effusion.
- **Interpretation:** Perforation of the intestine either as a result of a peptic ulcer or diverticular perforation or secondary to an endoscopic procedure. Air in the mediastinum usually indicates oesophageal perforation and occasionally this can be associated with pleural effusions. Pleural effusions can also be seen in patients with ascites (hepatic hydrothorax) and in some patients with

acute pancreatitis who typically have left-sided pleural effusions.

Abdominal X-ray

- **Indications:** To look for intestinal obstruction, for the presence of toxic megacolon in patients with inflammatory bowel disorders.
- **Positive findings:** Dilated fluid filled intestinal loops with air fluid levels, faecal loading in patients with constipation.

Ultrasound

Ultrasound is a useful test in assessing the liver, spleen, portal and hepatic venous blood flow especially when combined with Doppler. In patients with suspected liver cirrhosis, portal hypertension is associated with splenomegaly, ascites and occasionally collaterals. Portal and hepatic vein flow can be assessed using a Doppler study.

Ultrasound is the test of choice for the detection of gallbladder stones as the majority of these are radiolucent and not seen on computed tomography (CT) scans.

In the assessment of patients with jaundice, ultrasound can detect intrahepatic biliary dilation and dilated common bile ducts (indirect evidence of biliary obstruction) as well as the presence of liver metastasis. However, it is quite insensitive for the detection of stones in the common bile duct (other modalities such as endosonography (EUS), magnetic resonance cholangiopancreatography (MRCP) and endoscopic retrograde cholangiopancreatogram (ERCP) are necessary for the diagnosis when bile duct stones are suspected).

Ultrasound is also useful in assessment of intraabdominal (especially liver) abscesses and cysts. Liver biopsies and aspiration of liver abscesses are usually performed under ultrasound guidance.

Barium studies

Barium swallow

This is mainly used for assessment of dysphagia, and is useful for the demonstration of strictures, diverticula and a pharyngeal pouch. The barium swallow has been largely superseded by the use of endoscopy for other indications. Video fluoroscopy for assessment of swallowing is, however, still widely used. Water-soluble contrast such as Gastrografin can be used when perforation is suspected.

Table 9.5 Common findings on chest X-ray, abdominal X-ray and abdominal ultrasound in patients with gastrointestinal diseases

Investigation	Indication	Findings	Interpretation
Chest X-ray (erect)	Suspected intestinal perforation	Sliver of air under the diaphragm	Intra-abdominal hollow viscus perforation most commonly peptic ulcer, diverticular or iatrogenic
	Suspected oesophageal perforation	Air in the mediastinum and/or pleural effusion or hydro-pneumothorax	Oesophageal perforation most commonly due to spontaneous perforation (Boerhaave's syndrome) or iatrogenic
	In patients with ascites and acute pancreatitis	Pleural effusions	Left-sided pleural effusions are typically associated with acute pancreatitis and right-sided ones with ascites (hepatic hydrothorax)
Abdominal X-ray (and kidney, ureter or bladder (KUB) film in suspected renal colic)	Abdominal pain and/or severe constipation and vomiting	Radio-opaque stones in the kidney, ureter or bladder, and rarely gallbladder	90 per cent of kidney stones are radio-opaque (uric acid stones are translucent) and less than 10 per cent of gallbladder stones are radio-opaque
		Dilated loops of bowel with air–fluid levels in a step ladder pattern (in an erect film)	Intestinal obstruction (usually small bowel or proximal colon) or paralytic ileus; very large bowel loops more peripherally located usually suggests colonic obstruction
		Thumb printing	Ischaemic, infective or inflammatory bowel disease and abdominal trauma
	Inflammatory bowel disease (colonic)	Dilated colonic loops (>5.5 cm in transverse colon) usually with mucosal oedema	Toxic megacolon if patient has abdominal pain and systemic signs in the presence of active inflammatory bowel disease
Ultrasound abdomen	Investigate abdominal pain, jaundice, liver disease, ascites	Discrete echogenic areas with focal hypoechoic lesions	Liver metastasis (ultrasound is 80–90 per cent accurate in picking up liver metastasis). Hepatocellular carcinoma can be either a single lesion or diffuse with multiple small abnormal areas
		Discrete anechoic lesions	Cysts or abscess (aspiration of abscess can be done under ultrasound guidance)
		Dilated intrahepatic ducts and/or dilated common bile duct	Biliary obstruction
		Positive sonographic Murphy's sign with gallstones and peri-cholecystic fluid	Cholecystitis
		Diffuse bright echotexture of the liver	Fatty liver

Barium meal follow through and small-bowel enema

The use of barium tests for assessment of the stomach and duodenum has been supplanted by endoscopy. Barium meal follow-through and small-bowel barium enema are now mainly used for the assessment of small-bowel strictures and masses in patients with Crohn's disease, NSAID and radiation enteropathy and small-bowel lymphomas.

More recently, CT and MRI enterography have been shown to be better at assessing the small bowel. As they can provide information on luminal as well as extraluminal pathology, these techniques are replacing barium-based tests for assessment of small intestinal disease.

Double contrast barium enema

Air contrast barium enemas have also been largely supplanted by colonoscopy for assessment of large-bowel symptoms. Colonoscopy has the advantage of being superior at detection of polyps and can provide tissue for diagnosis. Also polyps can be excised via the colonoscope and therefore barium enemas are now frequently used either because of an incomplete colonoscopy (caecum not visualized) or when colonoscopy carries an increased risk. Barium enema is, however, useful in the detection of colonic diverticula as these can be overlooked at colonoscopy. CT scans have become the preferred modality for assessment of diverticular disease are they can accurately detect diverticula as well as provide information on the presence of complications such as diverticular abscesses and perforation at the same time.

Computed tomography

Computed tomography has increasingly become the diagnostic modality of choice for the assessment of patients with acute abdominal pain. Spiral CT avoids artefacts from multiple breath-holds and has become the standard choice. When combined with oral and intravenous contrast it is useful in the assessment of liver disease, luminal and extraluminal pathology. It can provide information on the presence of ischaemia (absence of intravenous contrast) and inflammation (increased intravenous contrast reaching the abnormal area causing it to 'light up'). It is also useful in detection and assessment of space-occupying lesions in the liver and to pick up thrombosis of intra-abdominal vasculature. Computed tomography is also the preferred modality to assess patients with pancreatic disease and is routinely used for assessment of patients with intra-abdominal cancers to assess local as well as metastatic spread and lymphomas to look for nodal and splenic disease. It is, however, not useful in the detection of gallstones as these are generally radiolucent.

CT colography or virtual colonoscopy is considered an alternative non-invasive test to look for colorectal polyps, but it is less accurate than colonoscopy at the present time (especially for small polyps).

Magnetic resonance imaging

The most common indication for magnetic resonance imaging (MRI) was in the assessment of the biliary tree for common bile duct stones/strictures and the presence of primary sclerosing cholangitis. MRI, especially with contrast agents (such as gadolinium and ferrite iron-oxide), is now increasingly used in specialist centres for the assessment of liver masses. MR enterography has also been shown useful in the assessment of the small bowel in patients with Crohn's disease and is rapidly replacing barium tests for this indication.

Angiography

Selective mesenteric angiograms are used in patients with gastrointestinal bleeds either refractory to endoscopic therapy or beyond the reach of the endoscope. Bleeding vessels can be embolized at the same time.

Endoscopic investigation

The advantage of endoscopic examination is not only direct visualization of the lumen of the intestine, but also the possibility of taking biopsies for histopathology and brushings for cytology. Also, several therapeutic procedures like polypectomy, stenting and treatment of bleeding ulcers and vessels can be safely performed via the endoscope.

Upper gastrointestinal endoscopy or oesophagogastroduodenoscopy

Upper gastrointestinal endoscopy using a flexible video endoscope can assess the oesophagus, stomach and first and second parts of the duodenum. It is commonly used for the assessment of upper gastrointestinal symptoms.

Lower gastrointestinal endoscopy or colonoscopy

The reach of the colonoscope is from the rectum to the caecum and the terminal 2–3 cm of the ileum. Colonoscopy usually requires prior bowel preparation to cleanse the colon. It is used mainly in the assessment of patients with diarrhoeal disease including ulcerative and microscopic colitis and Crohn's disease as well as screening and assessment of patients with colonic polyps and cancer. Proctoscopy and rigid sigmoidoscopy are often used as outpatient procedures to assess the anal canal and rectum/proximal sigmoid, respectively. A flexible sigmoidoscopy is a limited examination with a flexible endoscope where the left colon (usually up to the splenic flexure) is assessed.

Small bowel examination

Visualization of the small bowel with endoscopy is a more recent innovation and it is thought that these tests will supplant traditional radiological tests as they become more widely available.

Capsule endoscopy

This involves swallowing a small capsule containing a charge-coupled device (CCD) camera, battery and transmitter and transmits images of the intestine captured on a recording device. Capsule endoscopy is used for the assessment of obscure gastrointestinal bleeds and small bowel inflammatory disorders including Crohn's disease.

Push and balloon enteroscopy

Enteroscopy with a long flexible endoscope can assess the upper gastrointestinal tract up to the upper jejunum. Balloon enteroscopes use an overtube with either one or two balloons to facilitate insertion of the enteroscope deeper into the small bowel. These tests are commonly performed to either biopsy or treat lesions detected on capsule endoscopy or radiological investigation of the small bowel.

Endoscopic retrograde cholangiopancreatography

Endoscopic retrograde cholangiopancreatography (ERCP) involves utilizing a flexible endoscope with the camera positioned on the side rather than end-on in order to visualize the ampulla in the duodenum clearly. Through the working channel of this endoscope the bile ducts are cannulated with a catheter and dye injected into the bile ducts to visualize them on fluoroscopy (X-ray). This test is usually performed when bile duct stones are suspected or if there is biliary obstruction due to benign/malignant

stricture. Bile duct stones can be extracted using a variety of techniques including biliary balloons and baskets and bile duct obstruction relieved using plastic and metal stents.

Endoscopic ultrasound

Endoscopic ultrasound (EUS) combines both video endoscopy and sonography in one system and is being increasingly used as a diagnostic and therapeutic procedure in gastrointestinal disease. The main indications for EUS include local staging of oesophageal, gastric and pancreatobiliary malignancies. It is also useful in detection of common bile duct stones and diagnosis of chronic pancreatitis. EUS-guided biopsy and cytology of mediastinal nodes, peri-oesophageal/gastric nodes and pancreatic masses is now routinely performed. EUS-guided coeliac plexus blocks are also used in alleviating pain secondary to pancreatic cancer infiltrating the coeliac plexus of nerves.

Manometry and pH studies

Oesophageal manometry

This is useful in the diagnosis of achalasia cardia and other motility disorders of the oesophagus such as diffuse oesophageal spasm. This can be done using multichannel pressure recorders which are either perfused or solid state systems.

Oesophageal pH and impedance

The 24-hour ambulatory oesophageal pH monitoring test is used for the assessment of gastro-oesophageal reflux disease. A pH sensor is placed about 5 cm above the gastro-oesophageal junction either via a nasal catheter or by an endoscopically or transnasally placed capsule (which transmits the pH to a recorder wirelessly). Oesophageal multichannel intraluminal impedance detects oesophageal bolus transport and can identify weak acid and bilious and non-acid reflux. It is particularly useful in assessing patients with GORD who have symptoms despite medical treatment.

Anal manometry

Anal manometry tests the pressures generated by the anal sphincter and its ability to respond to signals. It also assesses the sensitivity and function of the rectum. In combination with endo-anal ultrasound, which can assess the structure of anal sphincter, anal manometry is useful in assessing patients with faecal incontinence and those with pelvic floor dysfunction.

Breath tests

Urea breath test

This test detects urease produced in the stomach by *Helicobacter pylori*. Patients ingest 13C-labelled urea, which is split up by the urease leading to the production of 13C-labelled carbon dioxide, which is detected in the breath of the patient.

Hydrogen breath test

Malabsorption of sugars such as lactose (lactose intolerance) is detected by measuring breath hydrogen after ingestion of 50 g of the sugar (lactose). The undigested sugars are fermented by anaerobes in the colon to produce hydrogen, which is excreted in the breath.

Lactulose or glucose hydrogen breath tests

These tests are used to investigate small-bowel bacterial overgrowth. Breath hydrogen is measured every 15–30 minutes for 3 hours after ingestion of 50 g glucose, lactulose. A rise in breath hydrogen as the substrate enters the small bowel indicates small-bowel overgrowth.

Tests for *H. pylori*

Besides the urea breath test mentioned above, there are several ways to detect *H. pylori*.

CLO test

The *Campylobacter*-like organism (CLO) test is performed during upper gastrointestinal endoscopy by inoculating a mucosa biopsy from the antrum of the stomach into a medium containing urea and phenol red, a dye that turns pink at a pH of 6.0 or greater. Urease produced by *H. pylori* metabolizes urea to ammonia and raises the pH above 6.

Gastric biopsy

Routine histological analysis of gastric antral biopsies can often detect the presence of *H. pylori*. The sensitivity of this test can be improved by using special stains.

Stool antigen tests

Presence of *H. pylori* antigen in the stool detected by an enzyme immunoassay (EIA) has been shown to be accurate in the detection of *H. pylori*.

Serology for *H. pylori*

Serological testing for antibodies to *H. pylori* (usually IgG) using the enzyme-linked immunosorbent assay (ELISA) has become a widely accepted, simple, inexpensive, and readily available diagnostic test with high sensitivity. The antibody titres decline slowly with time after treatment, but the rate of decline and cut-off values are unclear.

COMMON DIAGNOSES

The 'acute abdomen'

The onset of fairly abrupt abdominal pain and tenderness requires urgent diagnosis and may lead to surgical intervention. The diagnosis of abdominal pain usually combines history, physical examination and laboratory tests; ultrasound and CT imaging have not proven superior to careful evaluation of symptoms and physical examination. Bear in mind that no single test has ideal specificity and sensitivity.

In *peritoneal inflammation* (peritonitis), sudden movements such as coughing elicit pain, so observe the patient during examination. Guarding and rigidity (reflex spasm of the abdominal wall) may occur during examination; distracting the patient can diminish guarding but not rigidity. If during palpation pressure on the abdomen is released suddenly and the patient winces with pain, rebound tenderness is present.

In *appendicitis*, maximal pain and tenderness occurs at McBurney's point, usually about a third of the way up a line joining the right anterior superior iliac spine and the umbilicus. Rovsing's sign may be present – releasing pressure on the *left* lower abdominal quadrant of the abdomen causes pain in the *right* lower quadrant. There may also be localized peritoneal irritation of the psoas muscle – pain increases when the patient lifts the thigh against resistance (psoas sign) or when the obturator muscle is stretched when the right hip and knee are flexed and the hip internally rotated.

Oesophagus

Gastro-oesophageal reflux disease

The reflux of stomach acid into the lower oesophagus is referred to as GORD. Reflux becomes more likely when there is raised intra-abdominal pressure or a hiatus hernia (reducing the pressure at the lower oesophageal sphincter). Endoscopy may reveal erythema, erosions or ulcers in the lower oesophagus or may be normal. Non-erosive reflux disease is the term used to describe patients with typical reflux symptoms but normal endoscopy. Patients with GORD are usually investigated with oesophageal manometry and 24-hour oesophageal pH and impedance monitoring. Lifestyle modification and antisecretory therapy (with either H2-receptor antagonists or proton-pump inhibitors) is the mainstay of therapy. Antireflux surgery (most commonly a laparoscopic Nissen's fundoplication) is reserved for patients refractory to medical therapy.

Barrett's oesophagus

Usually considered a complication of longstanding reflux disease, Barrett's oesophagus is replacement of the squamous epithelium in the oesophagus with columnar mucosa (often with specialized intestinal metaplasia). This is found in approximately 5–15 per cent of patients with GORD; however, large subgroups of patients with Barrett's oesophagus do not have symptoms. About 0.5 per cent of patients with Barrett's oesophagus develop cancer every year.

Achalasia cardia

Failure of a hypertensive lower oesophageal sphincter to relax before the oncoming bolus of food results in achalasia cardia. There is damage to the oesophageal intramural nerve plexuses with denervation of the oesophageal smooth muscle. Progressive dysphagia and regurgitation of food are prominent symptoms and weight loss is common. The diagnosis is made usually by either a barium swallow, endoscopy or oesophageal manometry.

Carcinoma of the oesophagus

Progressive dysphagia initially to solids and later to liquids is the classical history in patients with carcinoma of the oesophagus. Pain and regurgitation of food are frequent, ultimately leading to weight loss and signs of malnutrition. Upper gastrointestinal endoscopy with biopsies is the diagnostic modality of choice. Local staging of the extent of the tumour into the oesophageal wall and mediastinum is best done by endoscopic ultrasound. A CT scan of the chest and abdomen helps assess for distal metastasis prior to considering resectional surgery.

Stomach

Gastritis

Acute gastritis is commonly due to either the use of NSAIDs or alcohol misuse and presents with abdominal pain. Chronic gastritis is most commonly secondary to *Helicobacter pylori* infection, but autoimmune gastritis (pernicious anaemia), NSAID use and bile reflux have all been implicated.

Ulcer diathesis

This is often called peptic ulcer disease (PUD) and is characterized by ulcers or erosions of the stomach and duodenum. A majority of cases are due to *Helicobacter pylori* infection, but NSAIDs and aspirin are also responsible for a increasing number of cases. Gastrin-producing tumours (gastrinomas) are a rare cause for multiple peptic ulcers. Smoking increases the risk of having peptic ulcer disease. Epigastric pain and dyspepsia are common symptoms. Hunger pains are believed to be more typical of duodenal ulcers but symptoms have not been shown to be reliable in predicting the presence of peptic ulcers. Patients with alarm symptoms (bleeding, anaemia, weight loss, epigastric mass, difficulty swallowing) should undergo prompt endoscopy. Peptic ulcers may be complicated by gastrointestinal bleeding, perforation or pyloric stenosis in approximately 10 per cent of patients.

Gastric cancer

Gastric cancer is more often found in patients with alarm symptoms described above. More often than not the diagnosis is made incidentally at endoscopy.

Patients with recent onset of symptoms over the age of 45 and those with a family history of stomach cancer as well as those with alarm symptoms should have prompt endoscopy to exclude cancer of the stomach.

Small and large intestine

Coeliac disease

In coeliac disease sensitivity to gluten (the protein found in wheat, barley, and rye) results in inflammation of the small-bowel mucosa causing blunting of the villi. The reduction in absorptive surface of the small bowel leads to malabsorption of dietary nutrients to a variable degree. Serological tests such as anti-tissue transglutaminase antibodies are very sensitive and antiendomysial antibodies are fairly specific for this condition. Endoscopic mucosal biopsies from the duodenum showing blunted or absent villi with the presence of intraepithelial lymphocytes are confirmatory. The most severe cases are usually diagnosed in childhood with fat malabsorption and diarrhoea. In adults with less severe symptoms, the presence of iron deficiency anaemia and osteoporosis are indicators to test for the possibility of coeliac disease.

Crohn's disease

Crohn's disease is an inflammatory bowel disease that can affect any part of the intestine but mainly affects the distal small bowel and proximal large bowel around the ileocaecal valve. The inflammation in Crohn's diseases is transmural and thickening or fibrosis of the bowel can result in narrowing and strictures. Penetrating ulcers can lead to the formation of fistulae either between the abdominal viscera or to the skin. Presence of skip lesions with normal areas in between diseased areas is characteristic and granulomas are often noted on histology.

Patients typically present with abdominal pain and diarrhoea, but gross bleeding is rare. Systemic symptoms such as fever are common. Patients with perianal disease may present with either perianal abscesses or fistulae that often need surgical drainage. Patients with disease localized to the ileocaecal region may present with colicky abdominal pain, fever and a tender right iliac fossa mass mimicking appendicular mass/abscess. Diagnosis is usually confirmed by typical radiological and endoscopic appearances with the presence of chronic inflammation on mucosal biopsies. The presence of non-caseating granulomas is noted in less than 50 per cent of cases but is characteristic of this disease.

Ulcerative colitis

Ulcerative colitis is a characterized by inflammation limited to the mucosa of the large bowel with recurrent ulceration. The major symptoms of ulcerative colitis include diarrhoea, rectal bleeding, passage of mucus and abdominal pain. The symptom complex tends to differ according to the extent of disease. Rarely patients with proctitis alone may present with marked constipation. Symptoms have usually been present for weeks, or even months; the slow, insidious onset is characteristic of the disease. Acute presentations of ulcerative colitis mimicking an infective aetiology are not uncommon. Acute severe colitis requires inpatient management due to substantial risk of complications such as toxic megacolon and perforation.

Carcinoma of the colon

Large-bowel cancer can be further divided by the anatomical location of the tumour into colon and rectal cancer. This distinction is important as both the operative and adjuvant treatment of these tumours differs. Symptoms often depend on the location of the tumour. Abdominal pain, bleeding per rectum, change in bowel habit and anaemia are characteristic symptoms. Rectal cancer can present with anal pain, tenesmus and rarely incontinence. Right-sided colonic tumours present more insidiously with anaemia and rarely obstruction to the ileocaecal valve. Left-sided colonic tumours are more likely to present with obstruction as the left colon is of narrower calibre, with more circumferential lesions and a firmer stool consistency. With the advent of colon cancer screening, many patients are asymptomatic.

Diverticular disease

Diverticula or outpouchings of the bowel are most commonly seen in the colon, but also rarely in other parts of the gastrointestinal tract. Microperforation of a diverticulum and the resultant extracolonic or intramural inflammation leads to diverticulitis, and erosion into an artery at the diverticular mouth can lead to a diverticular bleed. Diverticulosis is usually asymptomatic and found incidentally at colonoscopy or with a barium enema. Though it is often found in individuals with abdominal pain or a change in bowel habit, a causal relationship has not been implicated. Diverticular bleeding can present with profuse bright red bleeding per rectum occasionally with haemodynamic compromise. Most bleeds resolve spontaneously, but rarely angiography and embolization of the bleeding vessel or surgery are required. Left lower quadrant pain with fever and diarrhoea are typical of diverticulitis.

Liver

Acute hepatitis

The diagnosis implies acute inflammation of the liver. Clinically, the course of acute hepatitis varies widely with non-specific flu-like symptoms at the onset associated with fever, anorexia, nausea and vomiting and jaundice that follows leading to fulminant hepatic failure needing liver transplantation in a small minority. Physical findings are usually minimal, apart from jaundice and tender hepatomegaly.

Common causes of acute hepatitis are hepatitis A, B or E viruses, CMV, and EBV infections. Non-viral infection such as with *Leptospira* and Q fever can also present with acute hepatitis. Other causes of acute hepatitis are drug-induced hepatotoxicity from paracetamol overdose or idiosyncratic adverse hepatic reactions. Although autoimmune hepatitis is a chronic relapsing remitting condition, it presents as acute hepatitis in a third of cases. Ischaemic hepatitis following circulatory shock is a common scenario in hospitalized patients.

Cirrhosis

In cirrhosis, as a response to liver injury, activated stellate cells proliferate and secrete fibrillar collagen, resulting in excess fibrotic matrix. When the injury is recurrent or chronic, liver fibrosis progresses to cirrhosis (see Box 9.10), defined anatomically by the presence of nodules of hepatocytes separated by fibrous septae. These fibrous septae disrupt the architecture of the liver and impair liver function.

Portal hypertension occurs as a consequence of structural changes within the liver in cirrhosis, lead-

ing to the development of portal–systemic collaterals including gastro-oesophageal varices. Portal (sinusoidal) hypertension is also a prerequisite for the development of ascites, and development of ascites is an important landmark in the natural history of cirrhosis.

BOX 9.10 COMMON CHRONIC LIVER DISEASES THAT LEAD TO CIRRHOSIS

Alcohol excess is a common cause of end-stage liver disease, which is part of a huge spectrum of illness caused by alcohol such as alcoholic fatty liver disease, alcoholic hepatitis and cirrhosis. Non-alcoholic fatty liver disease is currently the commonest chronic liver disease in affluent societies where there is a rising incidence of risk factors such as obesity and diabetes. Chronic hepatitis C virus infection acquired by intravenous drug use or through past exposure to blood products, and hepatitis B virus infection, which spreads through vertical transmission mainly (sexually transmitted or acquired by intravenous drug use in some), are common causes of cirrhosis and hepatocellular carcinoma worldwide.

There are three conditions where autoimmunity causes liver injury: autoimmune hepatitis, primary biliary cirrhosis and primary sclerosing cholangitis (PSC). These are diagnosed on the basis of serology and histology, and cholangiography in the case of PSC.

Hereditary haemochromatosis is the most common genetic disorder in the Caucasian population with a prevalence of up to 1 per 200 in those of northern European origin. Wilson's disease is an autosomal recessive inherited disorder of copper metabolism resulting in liver and/or neuropsychiatric disease. It occurs in all ethnic groups with a worldwide prevalence of 3 per 100000 population. α-1 antitrypsin deficiency is the most common genetic cause of liver disease in children. It can present with neonatal hepatitis syndrome or with decompensated liver disease and portal hypertension in older children. In adults, it can present with raised liver enzymes, chronic hepatitis, cirrhosis, portal hypertension or hepatocellular carcinoma of unknown origin.

Pancreas

Acute pancreatitis

This is an acute inflammatory process, with variable involvement of other regional tissues or remote organ systems. It is characterized clinically by the sudden onset of symptoms. About 80 per cent of acute pancreatitis is related to stones in the common bile duct or alcohol excess. About 10–15 per cent of patients have no identifiable causes.

Chronic pancreatitis

Chronic pancreatitis is a progressive inflammatory disease of the exocrine pancreas characterized by severe and recurrent episodes of abdominal pain associated with pancreatic inflammation, progressive loss of acinar tissue and fibrosis. Alcohol accounts for 70–80 per cent of cases of chronic pancreatitis. Pain is the predominant symptom in most patients. Progressive fibrosis leads to loss of both endocrine and exocrine functions of the pancreas. Diabetes develops in a third of patients and exocrine insufficiency could manifest with diarrhoea, steatorrhoea and weight loss. Other complications include portal or splenic vein thrombosis and development of pancreatic cancer.

Pancreatic cancer

Pancreatic cancer accounts for 6700 deaths per year in the UK. Three main symptoms of pancreatic cancer are pain, weight loss and jaundice. The diagnosis of pancreatic cancer should be considered in older patients with type 2 diabetes of recent onset without a family history and in those with an unexplained attack of acute pancreatitis.

SUMMARY

Clinical history

- Dysphagia:
  - In patients with dysphagia the level of perceived obstruction does not correlate well with the site of pathology.
  - Globus is a diagnosis of exclusion and organic abnormalities must be carefully excluded in these patients.
- Dyspepsia:
  - Indigestion is a common symptom, but can mean different things to different patients. It is important to clarify what patients mean by any particular symptom.
  - Heartburn and acid regurgitation are commoner in patients with GORD.
  - No symptom in particular is specific for or reliably excludes the presence of ulcer diathesis.
- Gastrointestinal bleeding:
  - Prompt assessment of severity of gastrointestinal bleeding using validated clinical tools is an essential part of clinical examination.
  - Absence of blood in nasogastric aspirates does not exclude the presence of upper gastrointestinal bleed.
  - Patients with large-volume, rapid bleeding from the upper gastrointestinal tract can present with haematochezia.
- Abdominal pain:
  - Classic descriptions of pain are often the exception rather than the rule in routine clinical practice.
  - Signs and symptoms in patients with acute abdominal pain can change in severity and presentation with time and serial examinations are helpful.
  - Severity of pain can be underestimated in immunocompromised individuals, patients with diabetes and in extremes of age (very young and very old).
  - While evaluating patients with abdominal pain, asking about rapidity of onset and duration of symptoms is of prime importance.
- Diarrhoea:
  - The term diarrhoea means different things to different patients. So seek out specific details of the symptoms.
  - Duration of symptoms is important as acute diarrhoeal illnesses are often self-limiting and have very different causes from chronic diarrhoea.
  - Use of over-the-counter laxatives is often an overlooked cause for diarrhoea.

- Constipation:
  - New-onset constipation is an alarm symptom especially in elderly people.
  - Patients consider infrequent bowel movements as well as difficulty passing stool as constipation and it is important to make the distinction between these two.
  - History alone is insufficient to distinguish between organic and functional causes of constipation.
- Jaundice:
  - Deep yellow urine suggests a possibility of concentrated urine in dehydration rather than bilirubinuria.
  - Bilirubin gives urine brown, tea or cola colour, which the patients commonly describe.
  - History of dark brown urine (due to bilirubinuria) does not differentiate hepatocellular disease from cholestatic jaundice.
  - Cholestasis can occur without anatomical biliary obstruction.
  - History of risk factors for chronic liver disease is important in identifying acute decompensation of chronic liver disease.

Physical examination

- Auscultation is not a useful adjunct in the evaluation of abdominal symptoms.
- In postoperative patients, auscultation for bowel sounds is not useful in predicting the return of colonic motility and ability to tolerate oral feeds.
- Abdominal bruits are heard frequently in normal individuals and have a poor sensitivity with regard to identification of either aortic aneurysms or renal artery stenosis.
- The combination of right lower quadrant pain, migration of initial peri-umbilical pain to the right lower quadrant and rigidity is useful for identifying acute appendicitis.
- In patients with right upper quadrant pain and suspected cholecystitis, Murphy's sign is only modestly sensitive as it is difficult to localize the gallbladder. Sonographic Murphy's sign has a better diagnostic yield.
- Eliciting rebound tenderness depends on causing pain to the patient but the findings are unlikely to change the diagnosis or management of the patient, hence its use should be discouraged.
- Interobserver variation in liver span estimation is too high for it to be of any practical value.
- Palpability of the liver depends on its consistency – 50 per cent of normal livers with soft consistency extending beyond the costal margin are missed on palpation, whereas the majority of diseased enlarged livers which are firm or hard in consistency are detected by palpation.
- When the spleen is not palpable, percussion does not add to the clinical decision-making process.
- About a third of patients with aortic aneurysms are detected during routine physical examination (but, in high-risk individuals an ultrasound should be performed regardless of physical signs).
- Examination techniques that distinguish direct from indirect hernia have poor interobserver agreement and are unreliable for clinical decision making.

FURTHER READING

Bloom S, Webster G. 2006. *Oxford handbook of gastroenterology and hepatology*. Oxford: Oxford University Press.

Detsky AS, McLaughlin JR, Baker JP, *et al.* 1987. What is subjective global assessment of nutritional status? *Journal of Parenteral and Enteral Nutrition* 11: 8–13.

Talley NJ, Segal I, Weltman MD. 2008. *Gastroenterology and hepatology: a clinical handbook*. Edinburgh: Churchill Livingstone.

10

THE RENAL SYSTEM

Peter Topham

INTRODUCTION

The patient with renal disease can present in a number of ways:

- with symptoms or physical signs that are typically associated with renal disease
- no symptoms but an abnormality is detected on clinical or laboratory examination
- with a diagnosis of systemic disease known to be associated with renal disease
- with a family history of inherited renal disease that prompts further assessment
- following exposure to nephrotoxic agents.

Cardinal symptoms suggesting the presence of underlying renal disease include disorders of micturition, disorders of urine volume, alterations in urine composition, loin pain, oedema and hypertension. In addition, a wide variety of symptoms and complications can be associated with advanced renal failure (uraemia).

Renal disease in asymptomatic patients is often detected on dipstick urinalysis, biochemical analysis of the serum (and urine), and blood pressure measurement undertaken during some intercurrent illness or as part of a health screening programme.

CLINICAL HISTORY

Disorders of micturition

Frequency of micturition

Urinary frequency is the urge to empty the bladder more often than normal. It may be associated with nocturia, urgency (a need to pass urine immediately) and incontinence. The causes of urinary frequency are listed in Table 10.1. It is important to determine whether urinary frequency is associated with normal or increased urine volumes. Normal urine volumes imply bladder dysfunction caused by inflammation,

Table 10.1 Causes of urinary frequency

Increased daily urine volume (polyuria)	Normal daily urine volume
Excessive fluid intake, e.g. compulsive water drinking	Bladder irritation Inflammation Tumour Bladder stone
Increased tubular solute load (osmotic diuresis): • Glucose in poorly controlled diabetes mellitus • Immunoglobulin light chains in myeloma • Urea in chronic renal failure	Reduced bladder volume Fibrotic contraction, e.g. after radiotherapy
Reduced ADH production	External bladder compression
Cranial diabetes insipidus	
Reduced medullary concentration gradient	Neuromuscular dysfunction of the bladder
Nephrocalcinosis	Detrusor instability
Analgesic nephropathy	
Renal papillary necrosis	
Medullary cystic disease	
Sickle cell disease	
Reduced renal response to ADH	
Nephrogenic diabetes insipidus	
Hypercalcaemia	
Chronic hypokalaemia	

ADH, antidiuretic hormone.

tumour or stone of the bladder, or reduced bladder capacity. Increased urine volume indicates polyuria.

Night-time frequency may also be caused by sleep disturbance. Sleep normally induces antidiuretic hormone (ADH) secretion, which causes a reduction in urine volumes. Subjects who sleep poorly have no increase in ADH secretion and therefore urine volumes remain high.

Poor urinary stream

A poor urinary stream is typically caused by bladder outflow obstruction from prostate enlargement or urethral disease. The characteristic symptoms are:

- poor urine flow with a weak stream
- difficulty in initiating micturition (hesitancy) and/or in stopping (terminal dribbling).

Urinary frequency is often also present.

Progression of the obstruction may lead to complete failure of micturition (urinary retention). Paradoxically some patients with bladder outflow obstruction produce increased urine volumes due to tubular dysfunction arising from back pressure on the kidneys. Prolonged bladder outflow obstruction can result in progressive renal dysfunction (obstructive nephropathy).

Dysuria

Pain or discomfort during micturition usually results from bladder, prostatic or urethral inflammation. It is described as a burning or tingling sensation in the urethra or suprapubic area during or immediately after micturition. When associated with frequency and urgency of micturition it indicates cystitis (bladder inflammation, usually due to bacterial infection). Perineal or rectal pain on micturition in men suggests prostatic inflammation (prostatitis).

Disorders of urine volume

Disorders of urine volume can be categorized as polyuria (an increase in urine volume), oliguria (a reduction in urine volume), and anuria (a loss of urine output).

Polyuria

This is defined as urine output over 3 L per day. Patients may find it difficult to differentiate polyuria from frequency, and thirst may in fact be the presenting symptom. Measurement of the daily urine volume is therefore helpful. The causes of polyuria are listed in Table 10.1.

Oliguria

This is the reduction in urine volume below the level required for the excretion of normal metabolic byproducts. It is therefore associated with the accumulation of nitrogenous waste products (i.e. an increase in serum urea and creatinine levels) and indicates the development of acute kidney injury (AKI). Practically, oliguria can be defined as a urine volume less than 500 mL/day, less than 30 mL/h, or less than 0.5 mL/kg body weight/h.

Anuria

This is a urine volume of less than 100 mL/day. It is most commonly due to renal tract obstruction, but can also result from vascular catastrophes (e.g. acute renal artery occlusion), acute cortical necrosis, and inflammatory glomerular disease (e.g. Goodpasture's disease).

Disorders of urinary composition

Haematuria

Visible haematuria is a striking symptom that usually prompts the patient to seek urgent medical attention. Haematuria from any cause can be visible or invisible, i.e. apparent only on urine dipstick testing. It can result from bleeding anywhere in the

---

BOX 10.1 CAUSES OF RED/BROWN URINE

Blood (visible haematuria)
Free haemoglobin (haemolysis)
Myoglobin (rhabdomyolysis)
Urates
Porphyrins (porphyria) (urine may darken on standing)
Homogentisic acid (alkaptonuria)
Drugs:
- analgesics: phenacetin
- antibiotics: rifampicin, metronidazole, chloroquine
- anticoagulants: warfarin, phenindione
- anticonvulsants: phenytoin.
Vegetable dyes:
- beetroot and some berries (anthocyanins)
- rhubarb
- carotene
- food-colouring dyes.

urinary tract from the glomeruli to the urethra, the commonest cause being urinary tract infection. It is important to appreciate that *red/brown urine* does not always indicate haematuria (see Box 10.1).

The pattern of visible haematuria gives clues to the underlying cause:

- visible haematuria present at the start of urine flow with subsequent clearing is usually due to urethral bleeding
- haematuria mainly at the end of micturition (terminal haematuria) is indicative of bladder or prostate bleeding
- glomerular haematuria is often red-brown in colour and may be described as 'smoky' or like coca-cola or tea
- visible haematuria that coincides with episodes of mucosal infection (often pharyngitis) or with exercise is frequently due to IgA nephropathy
- blood clots are never caused by glomerular bleeding.

Proteinuria

This is usually asymptomatic and identified by urine dipstick testing followed by more specific laboratory tests (see Investigations section). However, patients with heavy proteinuria (usually nephrotic range proteinuria (>3.5 g/day)) may describe frothing of the urine on micturition.

Pneumaturia

Patients with fistulae between the urinary and alimentary tracts may describe the passage of air or 'fizzing' of the urine on micturition. This usually results from Crohn's disease, diverticular disease or carcinoma of the colon.

SMALL PRINT

Small pieces of tissue may be passed in the urine in patients with malignant disease of the urinary tract or papillary necrosis. In addition, solid material may enter the urinary tract from the bowel via vesicocolonic fistulae. Patients with a predisposition to stone formation may notice sand-like material in the urine.

Pain

Pain is an inconsistent feature of renal disease. When present it is usually the result of renal tract inflammation or obstruction.

- Inflammation of the kidney due to infection (acute pyelonephritis) results in pain localized to the renal angle on the affected side.
- Perirenal abscess formation may lead to diaphragmatic irritation or psoas muscle irritation depending on the direction in which the abscess tracks.
- Glomerular inflammation is usually asymptomatic. Acute and fulminant glomerulonephritis (GN) may cause a dull lumbar ache.
- The loin pain haematuria syndrome is the constellation of dull loin pain, which may be severe, and visible haematuria. It has no known cause and investigation generally reveals no structural or renal histological abnormality apart from complement (C3) deposition in the walls of afferent arterioles.
- The pain of acute renal tract obstruction is sudden in onset, severe and colicky in nature (ureteral colic). The pain often radiates to the groin, scrotum or labia.
- Chronic urinary tract obstruction in contrast is often asymptomatic. Obstruction at the level of the bladder outflow tract may lead to symptoms of hesitancy, poor flow, and terminal dribbling, but obstruction above this level may be completely asymptomatic.

Oedema

Oedema results from the accumulation of salt and water and reflects an increase in the total body sodium content. In renal disease it occurs either as part of the nephrotic syndrome or because of reduced excretory function and subsequent failure to excrete ingested salt and water. Nephrotic oedema is typically first noticed in a periorbital distribution after a period of recumbency. Facial oedema is rare in advanced renal failure, heart failure or cirrhosis because patients with those conditions are unable to lie flat due to either the development of pulmonary oedema, or pressure on the diaphragm from ascites. As the degree of oedema increases, fluid accumu-

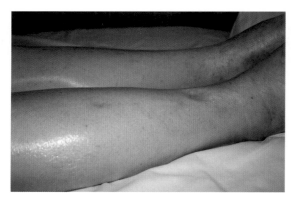

Figure 10.1 Pitting oedema in a patient with nephrotic syndrome.

lates around the ankles, legs, sacrum and elbows in a gravity-dependent manner, and then becomes more generalized (Fig. 10.1). Genital oedema may ensue and cause significant distress.

> **CLINICAL PEARL**
>
> A patient with facial and peri-orbital oedema is very likely to have nephrotic syndrome. This presentation almost never occurs with heart failure, cirrhosis or advanced renal failure because patients cannot lie flat due to the development of pulmonary oedema or because of splinting of the diaphragm from ascites.

Uraemia

In some patients, the underlying renal disease causes no specific symptoms and presentation only occurs once advanced renal failure has developed. The accumulation of nitrogenous waste products leads to the uraemic syndrome (Box 10.2). These symptoms are vague and rarely specific enough to identify renal failure without further investigation.

Symptoms related to systemic disease

Renal disease may be associated with a wide variety of systemic diseases (e.g. systemic lupus erythematosus, multiple myeloma) and therefore the identification of renal disease may be prompted by the development of symptoms of the underlying disease state.

THE REST OF THE HISTORY

Past medical history

Explore all health problems going back to early childhood. A large number of diseases can result in renal dysfunction either directly or as the result of complications during treatment. For example:

- a history of childhood urinary tract infections and late nocturnal enuresis may indicate the presence of vesicoureteric reflux and chronic pyelonephritis
- systemic lupus erythematosus may initially cause symptoms confined to the skin and joints, but later may progress to involve the kidneys
- other chronic inflammatory conditions such as rheumatoid arthritis or Crohn's disease may result in AA amyloidosis with renal involvement
- chemotherapy for malignant disease with cyclophosphamide carries a long-term risk of bladder cancer which may present with haematuria

The medical conditions associated with renal disease are summarized in Table 10.2. You should include a review of previous medical notes with particular emphasis on previous renal function tests.

Gynaecological and obstetric history

In women, seek details of the menstrual history, contraception and pregnancies.

Table 10.2 Conditions associated with renal disease

Condition	Associated renal disease
Hypertension	Hypertensive nephrosclerosis Secondary hypertension due to renal disease
Diabetes mellitus	Diabetic nephropathy Renovascular disease
Gout	Urate nephrolithiasis
Malignancy: • Breast lung, bowel • Myeloma	Membranous nephropathy Myeloma cast nephropathy
Chronic pain	Analgesic nephropathy
Raynaud's syndrome	Systemic sclerosis Systemic lupus erythematosus Cryoglobulinaemia
Recurrent sinusitis or other ENT symptoms	Wegener's granulomatosis
Pleurisy, pericarditis	Rheumatoid arthritis Systemic lupus erythematosus
Haemoptysis	Systemic vasculitis Goodpasture's disease
Recurrent thrombosis and fetal loss	Antiphospholipid antibody syndrome
Deafness	Alport's syndrome
Liver cirrhosis	Hepatorenal syndrome IgA nephropathy
Recurrent urinary tract infection	Reflux nephropathy/chronic pyelonephritis
Tonsillitis	Post-streptococcal glomerulonephritis
Hepatitis B or C	Membranous nephropathy Mesangiocapillary glomerulonephritis Cryoglobulinaemia
Infective diarrhoea	Haemolytic uraemic syndrome
Tuberculosis	Urogenital tuberculosis Amyloidosis Sterile pyuria
HIV infection	HIV associated nephropathy

- A delayed menarche may be caused by chronic kidney disease (CKD).
- Some women with significant renal dysfunction become amenorrhoeic, whilst others develop menorrhagia as a consequence of the associated clotting and platelet abnormalities.
- In women taking the combined oestrogen–progesterone contraceptive pill, renal disease significantly increases the risk of developing hypertension.
- Fertility is impaired in patients with renal disease.
- Renal disease may be exacerbated or initiated by pregnancy. Seek details of pregnancy-associated rises in blood pressure, the presence of proteinuria, and the duration and outcome of pregnancies.
- Although bacteriuria frequently occurs in pregnancy, upper urinary tract infection during pregnancy may indicate a structural abnormality of the upper urinary tract.
- Recurrent fetal loss may suggest the presence of the antiphospholipid antibody syndrome.

Drug history

A variety of drugs may induce or exacerbate renal disease, or may induce circulatory change that adversely affects renal perfusion.

- A single dose of a large variety of drugs may be sufficient to induce an acute allergic interstitial nephritis.
- The interstitial nephritis induced by non-steroidal anti-inflammatory agents may, in contrast, only develop after several months of treatment.
- Hypotensive drugs may cause deterioration in renal function, particularly when the blood pressure is lowered precipitously.
- Angiotensin-converting enzyme inhibitors, angiotensin-receptor blockers, and direct renin inhibitors may cause a profound loss of renal function in patients with significant renovascular disease, or a pre-renal state.
- A number of drugs are also associated with the development or worsening of hypertension which may exacerbate renal disease (Box 10.3).

Determine the *duration* of drug use. Long-term use of certain analgesics (particularly phenacetin and combination analgesics containing caffeine and aspirin) and lithium has been associated with progressive renal impairment. Although now used less commonly in rheumatoid arthritis, prolonged use of gold salts and D-penicillamine may induce membranous nephropathy.

BOX 10.3 DRUGS THAT INDUCE HYPERTENSION
Steroids:
- corticosteroids
- oestrogens
- mineralocorticoids, e.g. fludrocortisone
- androgen derivatives, e.g. danazol.

Calcineurin inhibitors:
- ciclosporin
- tacrolimus.

Erythropoiesis-stimulating agents
- epoetin-α
- epoetin-β
- darbepoetin.

Sympathomimetic agents:
- isoproterenol
- phenylpropanolamine
- monoamine oxidase inhibitors.

Patients may not regard 'over-the-counter' medication and herbal therapies as potentially harmful. It is therefore crucial to specifically ask about such therapies since they may contain potential nephrotoxins (for example aristolochic acid nephropathy caused by the ingestion of 'Chinese herbs').

Finally, some patients take medication surreptitiously. For example, laxatives or diuretics may be used as aids to weight loss, but can lead to severe potassium depletion or rebound oedema.

CLINICAL PEARL
- Obtain a detailed drug history including non-prescribed, over-the-counter drugs and herbal remedies
- Acute tubulo-interstitial nephritis can be induced by one dose of almost any drug or remedy, and herbal medications can contain potential nephrotoxins.

Dietary history

Enquiry into the dietary habits of patients can be informative.

- Excessive salt intake may result in significant hypertension and resistance to antihypertensive therapy. In patients with advanced CKD, significant volume overload and potentially life-threatening pulmonary oedema may be precipitated.
- Patients with renal stones tend to ingest large amounts of animal protein. This results in the increased urinary excretion of calcium, oxalate, and uric acid, and a low urine pH.
- Inadequate fluid intake may promote renal stone formation, particularly in those with an underlying metabolic predisposition to stone disease.
- Excessive alcohol intake leads to an increase in blood pressure and may result in poor concordance with therapy.
- A high intake of fruit juices and other acidic foods increases oxalate intake and may result in calcium oxalate precipitation in the kidney.
- The methylxanthine present in tea and coffee can induce polyuria in those with substantial intakes.

Social history

The socioeconomic and educational status of a patient can have an impact on the development of renal disease:

- The frequency of bacteriuria is much greater in pregnant women from the low socioeconomic group.
- Concordance with therapy is less good in hypertensive patients from the low socioeconomic group.
- Calcium stones form more frequently in men from higher socioeconomic groups, which probably relates to the increased protein intake associated with increasing affluence.
- Tobacco is a significant risk factor for the development and progression of renal disease. It contributes to the accelerated development of atherosclerosis in patients with CKD and is a risk factor for renovascular hypertension, accelerated hypertension, Goodpasture's syndrome, and the development of diabetic nephropathy
- Illicit drug use is associated with a number of renal complications including AKI due to rhabdomyolysis, bloodborne-virus-related renal disease, AA amyloidosis, vasculitis and proliferative glomerulonephritis.

Occupational history

The likelihood of developing renal disease is increased by a number of occupational factors.

- Working in a hot atmosphere results in increased insensible fluid loss, which increases the incidence of renal stone formation.
- The use of aniline dyes in the workplace increases the incidence of urothelial tumours.
- Exposure to inhaled hydrocarbons increases the incidence of Goodpasture's disease.
- A number of infections can also be picked up in the workplace. Miners, sewage workers, and farm labourers are at an increased risk of leptospirosis. Hantavirus infection may arise in laboratory workers handling rodents, or in farmers working in endemic areas.
- Exposure to lead, particularly in a vaporized form (e.g. welding lead pipes), may result in lead nephropathy.

Family history

The exploration of the family history is important for the identification of hereditary renal diseases. It should also be appreciated that a number of other conditions without a clear inheritance pattern, such as systemic lupus erythematosus, IgA nephropathy and diabetic nephropathy, appear to have a genetic predisposition. A classification of inherited renal disease is shown in Table 10.3.

Ethnic and geographical factors

The ethnic background of a patient may impact on the risk of developing certain renal diseases. For example, in the UK:

- African Caribbeans with hypertension or diabetes mellitus: renal failure is more common than in white populations.
- South Asians and African Caribbeans: the incidence of end-stage renal disease is it at least three times higher than in Caucasians.
- White populations and from some parts of Asia: IgA nephropathy is more common than in black populations.
- Oriental, Hispanic and black populations: the incidence and severity of systemic lupus erythematosus is greater than in Caucasians.

Table 10.3 Classification of inherited renal disease

Polycystic kidney disease	
Alport's syndrome and variants (e.g. thin membrane nephropathy)	
Inherited metabolic diseases with renal involvement • With glomerular involvement: • With non-glomerular involvement:	 Fabry's disease, LCAT deficiency cystinosis, hyperoxaluria, inherited urate nephropathy
Other inherited conditions with renal involvement • With glomerular involvement: • With nonglomerular involvement: • With cystic kidney disease:	 congenital nephrotic syndrome nephronophthisis renal angiomyolipoma in tuberous sclerosis, renal cell carcinoma in von Hippel–Lindau disease
Familial IgA nephropathy or focal segmental glomerulosclerosis	
Inherited tubular disorders: • cystinuria • renal tubular acidosis (certain forms) • congenital nephrogenic diabetes insipidus	
Renal diseases with polygenic influences: • diabetic nephropathy • reflux nephropathy • calcium nephrolithiasis	
Unclassified causes	

LCAT, lecithin-cholesterol acyltransferase.

- Arabs, Turks and Sephardic Mediterranean Jews (compared to Sephardic Jews from other regions, Ashkenazi Jews and Armenians): amyloidosis as a complication of familial Mediterranean fever occurs more often.
- Indians or Russians from high tuberculosis prevalence regions: the risk of developing tuberculosis during immunosuppressive therapy (for example after renal transplantation) is higher than in those from low prevalence areas.

PHYSICAL EXAMINATION

General examination

In patients with renal disease, the general examination can provide a wealth of diagnostic information.

Skin

- A decrease in skin turgor is a late sign of volume depletion.
- Uraemic patients frequently have dry and flaky skin with a yellowish-brown hue.
- Scratch marks or reddish-brown papules may indicate pruritus.
- Pallor is common in patients with CKD as a consequence of renal anaemia.
- Diffuse hyperpigmentation of sun-exposed areas may develop in patients with CKD.
- Subcutaneous bruising following minimal trauma is common and reflects disordered platelet activity and fragile cutaneous blood vessels. These lesions often result in discrete areas of hyperpigmentation due to haematin deposition (Fig. 10.2).
- Subcutaneous nodules caused by the deposition of calcium salts within the skin (calcinosis cutis) occur in patients with secondary and tertiary hyperparathyroidism.
- Cutaneous vasculitis can have many appearances including allergic-like exanthema, petechiae and purpura, and lesions with evidence of necrosis and subcutaneous haemorrhage (Figs 10.3 and 10.4).
- Small reddish-purple papules (angiokeratoma) located in the lower abdomen and groin area are suggestive of Fabry's disease.

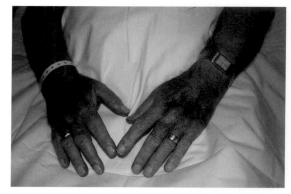

Figure 10.2 Typical skin changes in advanced chronic kidney disease. Note the diffuse hyperpigmentation, focal haemosiderin deposition, and leuconychia.

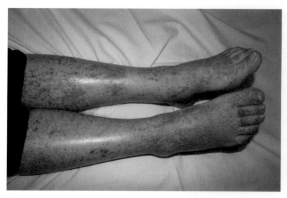

Figure 10.3 Widespread cutaneous vasculitis in a patient with antineutrophil cytoplasmic antibodies (ANCA)-associated vasculitis. Note the associated oedema.

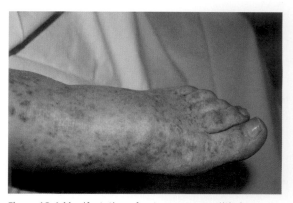

Figure 10.4 Manifestation of cutaneous vasculitis in a patient with antineutrophil cytoplasmic antibodies (ANCA)-associated systemic vasculitis.

- An allergic exanthema may be associated with an allergic interstitial nephritis.
- In advanced renal failure, the accumulation and crystallization of urea and other nitrogenous waste products in sweat results in the deposition of a white crystalline material on the skin, particularly on the face (uraemic frost). This is now very rarely seen.
- Patients on long-term corticosteroids lose subcutaneous tissue and the skin becomes thin, fragile, and prone to low trauma bruising.

Nails

- Transverse ridges (Beau's lines) indicate a serious preceding illness.
- Leuconychia (white nails, Fig. 10.5) can be seen in patients with nephrotic syndrome. If the nephrotic syndrome is transient or recurrent, transverse white bands may be seen (Muehrcke's bands).
- Splinter haemorrhages or nail-fold infarcts are features of vasculitis or infective endocarditis.
- Nail dystrophy can be seen in the nail–patella syndrome and is usually associated with absent or hypoplastic patellae.

Face

- Thickening and rigidity of the facial skin with multiple telangiectasia suggests scleroderma/systemic sclerosis.
- A facial rash with a butterfly distribution may be associated with lupus erythematosus.

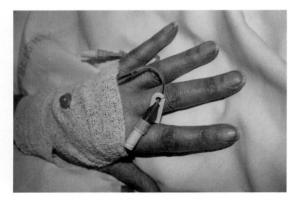

Figure 10.5 Leuconychia in a patient with advanced chronic kidney disease.

- Loss of the nasal cartilaginous septum leading to collapse of the nasal bridge is characteristic of Wegener's granulomatosis.
- Loss of the buccal pad when accompanied by fat loss from the upper part of the body (partial lipodystrophy) is associated with mesangiocapillary glomerulonephritis type 2 (dense deposit disease).
- A moon face may be observed in patients treated with high-dose corticosteroids.

Eyes

- Perilimbal calcification in patients with long-standing uraemia.
- Subconjunctival haemorrhages in patients with vasculitis.
- Lenticonus in patients with Alport's syndrome.
- Cataracts in patients who have had high-dose or prolonged corticosteroid use.
- The characteristic abnormalities of diabetic retinopathy, hypertensive retinopathy or vasculitis on funduscopy.

Chest

Examine the chest to identify:
- pleural effusions – which may arise from volume overload or the nephrotic syndrome
- lung crackles – which may represent volume overload or lung fibrosis
- pleural rubs – which may be caused by uraemia or inflammatory disease such as vasculitis.

Patients with metabolic acidosis may have a Kussmaul's respiratory pattern (deep, sighing breaths).

Praecordium

- Examine the praecordium for the presence of murmurs and a pericardial rub. Carefully document murmurs since an evolving murmur may indicate a diagnosis of infective endocarditis with an associated immune complex-mediated glomerulonephritis.
- Flow murmurs are relatively common in patients with CKD as a consequence of renal anaemia or valvular sclerosis. Aortic, mitral and tricuspid incompetence can be found in patients with autosomal dominant polycystic kidney disease.

- A pericardial rub (pericarditis) can be a manifestation of uraemia (in which case it is an absolute indication to commence dialysis), infection or vasculitis.

Limbs

- Examine for the presence of oedema, which tends to settle in the legs under the effects of gravity. In bedridden patients oedema may be seen in the calves and thighs and also in the presacral area.
- Examine the vascular tree by palpating all pulses and auscultating for vascular bruits.
- Atherosclerotic peripheral vascular disease may be associated with renovascular disease and is also a common complication of CKD. In addition, the identification of peripheral vascular disease is relevant for future vascular access planning (for haemodialysis) and for assessing suitability for renal transplantation.
- Perform a neurological examination to exclude polyneuropathy that may be secondary to uraemia or diabetes mellitus. Polyneuropathy due to renal disease is symmetrical with predominance of the lower limbs. It may cause sensory loss, paraesthesia, dysaesthesia, itch and muscular cramps. A proximal myopathy may also complicate CKD.
- Examine the patellae for abnormalities which may suggest the presence of the nail–patella syndrome – small, poorly developed finger and toe nails and patellae.

Blood pressure

The accurate measurement of blood pressure is a vital part of the clinical evaluation of patients with renal disease. The procedure for measuring blood pressure is as follows.

- Sit the patient quietly for at least 5 minutes. They should be relaxed and not moving or speaking.
- Support the arm at heart level and ensure it is not constricted by tight clothing.
- Use an appropriately sized cuff: the bladder should enclose between 80 per cent and 100 per cent of the arm. If the cuff bladder is too small the blood pressure tends to be overestimated (by up to 30 mmHg in obese patients) whereas a cuff that is too large will underestimate the blood pressure (by 10–30 mmHg).

- When using a mercury manometer ensure that the mercury column is vertical and at the observer's eye level.
- Estimate the systolic blood pressure by palpating the brachial artery, and inflating the cuff until pulsation disappears. Deflate the cuff and then reinflate to 30 mmHg above the estimated systolic pressure needed to occlude the brachial pulse.
- Place the stethoscope diaphragm over the brachial artery and deflate the cuff at a rate of 2–3 mm/second. Record the systolic (first Korotkoff sound) and diastolic (disappearance of sound) pressures to the nearest 2 mmHg. If the Korotkoff sounds do not disappear (e.g. patients with aortic valvular insufficiency or a high cardiac output) record phase IV (muffling of sound) as the diastolic blood pressure.

Increasingly mercury manometers are being replaced by electronic manometers due to concerns over the toxicity of mercury. Ensure that these are validated devices, and that they are calibrated on a regular basis.

Examination of the kidneys and urinary tract

Direct examination of the kidneys is usually not possible so a careful general examination is necessary to identify any abnormalities suggesting underlying renal disease. Nonetheless, an examination of the abdomen can often be informative when significant pathology is present.

Clinical examination of the urinary tract follows the standard pattern of inspection, palpation, percussion and auscultation.

Inspection

On abdominal inspection in thin patients, it may occasionally be possible to see one or both kidneys, particularly if polycystic kidney disease is present. Obstruction of the bladder outflow tract may result in bladder distension which may be visible as a suprapubic mass.

> **SMALL PRINT**
> Rarely, chronic urinary tract obstruction may cause such distension of the ureters that they become visible.

Palpation

Palpation of normal kidneys is usually only possible in thin patients. Palpation is best carried out with the patient in the recumbent position with the head supported on a pillow and the arms resting at the side of the body. To palpate the right kidney, place the left hand posteriorly in the loin and the right hand horizontally on the anterior abdominal wall to the right of the umbilicus. By pushing forward with the left hand and asking the patient to take a deep breath, the lower pole of the kidney may be palpable by pressing the right hand inwards and upwards.

The left kidney is not as readily palpable as the right. To palpate the left kidney, place the left hand posteriorly in the left loin, and the right hand on the anterior abdominal wall to the left of the umbilicus. If the kidney *is* palpable, estimate its size and shape. Normally the surface of the kidney is smooth and relatively hard, but in cystic disease an irregular surface may be appreciated. Note any tenderness on palpation.

Percussion

- In patients with acute pyelonephritis or acute glomerulonephritis, percussion of the renal region may cause severe pain (costovertebral tenderness).
- Pyelonephritis is usually accompanied by fever and dysuria, whereas haematuria, hypertension and oliguria suggest the presence of glomerulonephritis.
- Abdominal percussion may be of value if there is difficulty distinguishing between an enlarged kidney (resonant) and splenomegaly or hepatomegaly (dull).

Auscultation

Abdominal auscultation for vascular bruits is essential in patients with either hypertension or unexplained CKD (particularly if the urinalysis is negative and there is other evidence of atherosclerotic vascular disease). Place the stethoscope posteriorly in the loin, laterally in the flank, and anteriorly, and in each area listen for a bruit.

INVESTIGATIONS

Urinalysis

Urine examination is one of the basic diagnostic tests for patients with renal tract disease. Urine can be evaluated in a number of ways.

Urine dipstick testing

Urine dipstick testing is a widely available bedside test that can provide a wealth of diagnostic information. Dipsticks can detect blood, protein, glucose, ketones, nitrites and leucocyte esterase, and can measure the urine pH. The implications and limitations of dipstick testing are listed in Table 10.4. The key findings of relevance for renal disease are blood and protein. Assuming infection has been ruled out, their presence indicates either structural abnormality in the renal tract or glomerular disease, and therefore persistent abnormalities always require appropriate specialist evaluation. The urine dipsticks are essentially specific for albumin. They therefore do not detect other proteins that may be of relevance to renal disease (e.g. Bence Jones proteins – see below).

> **CLINICAL PEARL**
> - Urine dipstick testing can provide crucial clinical information in the evaluation of patients with suspected renal disease.
> - The finding of blood and protein on urine dipstick testing (in the absence of infection) strongly suggests the presence of glomerular disease and requires early referral of the patient for specialist assessment.

Urine microscopy

In certain circumstances urine microscopy can provide important diagnostic information. The important findings on urine microscopy are shown in Table 10.5.

Specific biochemical tests

In certain situations, undertake specific tests of the urine.

Table 10.4 Implications and limitations of urine dipstick results

	Significance	False negative results	False positive results
pH	Normal pH range 4.8–7.6 Acidic urine: acidosis, high protein intake Alkaline urine: alkalosis, vegetarianism, urine infection, distal renal tubular acidosis	Reduced pH reading in presence of formaldehyde	
Haemoglobin	Dipsticks have high specificity but low sensitivity Persistent positivity on serial urinalyses indicates urinary tract bleeding and further investigation is necessary	Ascorbic acid, concentrated urine, formaldehyde, delayed examination, high nitrite content	Myoglobinuria, bacterial peroxidases, hydrochloric acid
Protein	Dipsticks are essentially specific for albumin A positive result indicates an albumin concentration of at least 250 mg/L and requires formal quantification	Light chains, tubular proteins, hydrochloric acid	pH >9 Quaternary ammonium detergents Chlorhexidine
Glucose	Dipsticks detect glucose concentrations between 0.5 g/L and 20 g/L Glucosuria is usually due to hyperglycaemia, but may be due to proximal tubule dysfunction	Ascorbic acid, bacteria	Oxidizing agents, hydrochloric acid
Leukocyte esterase	A positive result suggests the presence of either neutrophils or macrophages Suggestive of urinary tract infection	Concentrated urine, vitamin C, proteinuria >5 g/L, glycosuria >20 g/L, cephalosporins, 1 per cent boric acid	Oxidizing detergents, bilirubin
Nitrites	Nitrites are formed from nitrates by most Gram negative bacteria and a positive result suggests bacteriuria	No vegetable intake, vitamin C, bacteria that do not reduce nitrates, short bladder incubation	
Ketones	Dipsticks detect both acetone and acetoacetate Positive results indicate diabetic ketoacidosis, fasting, vomiting, or starvation		Drugs that contain free sulphydryl groups (e.g. captopril)

- Quantitative measurement of proteinuria: Until recently, this was performed on 24-hour urine collections. However, these are notoriously unreliable and therefore measurement of the urine albumin (or protein):creatinine ratio (ACR and PCR, respectively) on a spot urine sample is the currently preferred method. A PCR of less than 15 mg/mmol is normal, and equates to less than 150 mg of proteinuria per day. A PCR of greater than 350 mg/mmol represents nephrotic range proteinuria.
- Urine immunoelectrophoresis: This is undertaken to detect immunoglobulin light chains (Bence Jones protein) in patients in whom myeloma is suspected.
- Metabolic screen for stone disease: In patients who form recurrent renal stones, investigate for an underlying metabolic abnormality by measuring calcium, oxalate, urate and cystine excretion in 24-hour urine collections.

Blood

Blood tests are required to:

- assess renal excretory function
- identify the metabolic consequences of CKD
- identify immunological markers of systemic disease that may be associated with renal disease.

To assess renal excretory function, measure the serum creatinine concentration. From this, the estimated glomerular filtration rate (eGFR) can be calculated. The commonly used calculation includes

Table 10.5 Findings on urine microscopy

	Abnormality	Significance
Cells	Erythrocytes	Urinary tract bleeding
	Dysmorphic erythrocytes	Glomerular bleeding, i.e. glomerulonephritis
	Leucocytes	Urinary tract infection Tubulointerstitial nephritis Occasionally acute glomerulonephritis
	Tubular epithelial cells	Tubulointerstitial injury, e.g. acute tubular necrosis
	Atypical urothelial cells	Urothelial malignancy
Casts	Hyaline casts	Normal, or volume depletion
	Granular casts	Rarely of diagnostic use
	Pigmented ('muddy brown') granular casts	Acute tubular necrosis
	Waxy casts	Occur in a wide variety of chronic kidney diseases
	Fatty casts	Nephrotic syndrome
	Red cell casts	Nephritic syndrome/rapidly progressive glomerulonephritis
Lipids	Oval fat bodies	Nephrotic syndrome Sphingolipidoses, e.g. Fabry's
Crystals	Uric acid (large variety of shapes)	Usually no significance
	Calcium oxalate (bipyramidal)	Usually no significance
	Amorphous urates and phosphates (various shapes)	Usually no significance
	Cystine (hexagonal)	Cystinuria
	Cholesterol	Nephrotic syndrome

Table 10.6 Stages of chronic kidney disease

Stage	eGFR (ml/min/1.73 m^2)	Description
1	>90	Normal or increased GFR with other evidence of kidney damage, e.g. proteinuria/haematuria, structural abnormality
2	60–89	Slight decrease in GFR with other evidence of kidney damage (see above)
3A	45–59	Moderate decrease in GFR with or without other evidence of kidney damage
3B	30–44	
4	15–29	Severe decrease in GFR with or without other evidence of kidney damage
5	<15	Established renal failure

Given the important prognostic role of proteinuria, the suffix (p) can be added to each stage to denote the presence of proteinuria (defined as ACR >30 mg/mmol, or PCR >50 mg/mmol.
GFR, glomerular filtration rate.

Table 10.7 Blood tests used in the diagnosis of renal disease

Clinical setting	Tests
Rapidly progressive glomerulonephritis (RPGN)	Antineutrophil cytoplasmic antibody (ANCA) Antiglomerular basement membrane antibody Antinuclear antibody (ANA) Complement C3 and C4
RPGN with suspicion of lymphoproliferative disease or cryoglobulinaemia	Serum and urine protein electrophoresis Cryoglobulins
Nephrotic syndrome	Serum immunoglobulins ANA Complement C3 and C4
Nephrotic syndrome aged over 40 years	Serum immunoglobulins ANA Complement C3 and C4 Serum and urine protein electrophoresis
Unexplained renal failure aged over 40 years	Serum immunoglobulins Serum and urine protein electrophoresis
Thrombotic microangiopathy without infective prodrome	Anti-ADAMSTS13 antibodies

the serum creatinine concentration, age, gender and a correction factor for black subjects. eGFR measurements can be used to categorize the severity of renal disease into CKD stages 1–5 (see Table 10.6).

To assess the complications of CKD, measure the serum phosphate, calcium, bicarbonate, potassium, parathyroid hormone, and haemoglobin. Additional serological tests that are useful in determining the cause of renal disease are shown in Table 10.7.

Imaging

Ultrasound scanning

This is the first-line imaging investigation for the majority of kidney or urinary tract diseases. It is non-invasive, requires no toxic contrast media, requires minimal patient preparation and avoids the use of ionizing radiation. It provides no *functional* information, however. The indications for ultrasound are to:

- assess the size and position of the kidneys
- look for evidence of cortical scarring
- demonstrate and characterize renal masses (solid and cystic)
- demonstrate bladder abnormalities
- identify renal tract obstruction
- demonstrate renal calcification and stone formation.

Intravenous urography

This was commonly used to look for structural abnormalities of the urinary tract and was particularly good for conditions involving the urothelium. Its use, however, has been largely superseded by computed tomography.

Computed tomography

Non-contrast enhanced computed tomography (CT) is the first line investigation for patients with suspected ureteral colic. It has a greater than 95 per cent sensitivity and specificity for stone disease. Contrast-enhanced CT is used to:

- characterize and stage urogenital cancer
- differentiate cystic from solid lesions
- demonstrate soft tissue abnormalities related to the renal tract
- identify collections associated with the renal tract
- evaluate the renal tract after trauma
- identify renal artery stenosis and adrenal tumours in hypertensive patients.

Computed tomography involves a significant radiation dose and also the administration of contrast media which can be nephrotoxic, particularly in patients with impaired renal function.

Magnetic resonance imaging

This is increasingly being used to:

- characterize renal mass lesions
- stage bladder and prostate carcinoma
- assess the presence of tumour thrombus in renal tumours
- detect renal artery stenosis.

It avoids the need for ionizing radiation and the gadolinium-based contrast medium is non-nephrotoxic. However, gadolinium has been associated with a scleroderma-like skin condition (nephrogenic systemic fibrosis) in a small number of patients with significantly impaired renal function. Current guidance is to avoid gadolinium-containing contrast media, if possible, in patients with an eGFR of less than 30 mL/minute.

Renal biopsy

In some patients, examination of blood and urine and imaging investigations are unable to provide a specific diagnosis. Therefore in patients with evidence of glomerular disease (haematuria, proteinuria, impaired renal function) or renal failure of unknown cause, a renal biopsy may be necessary to determine the precise diagnosis. The indications for renal biopsy are shown in Box 10.4.

BOX 10.4 INDICATIONS FOR RENAL BIOPSY
- Nephrotic syndrome
- Acute kidney injury (when pre-renal AKI, obstruction, and acute tubular necrosis are ruled out)
- Systemic disease with renal dysfunction
- Non-nephrotic proteinuria (>1 g/day or > 500 mg/day if associated with haematuria)
- Unexplained chronic kidney disease
- Familial renal disease
- Isolated invisible haematuria (in minority of patients in whom outcome would affect treatment)

Although renal biopsy is a routine investigation for the evaluation of patients with renal disease, it is not without risk and therefore the decision to undertake a renal biopsy should be made by a specialist renal physician. Involve nephrologists early in the management of patients in whom intrinsic renal disease is suspected.

COMMON DIAGNOSES

Nephrotic syndrome

Nephrotic syndrome is the term given to the constellation of:

- heavy proteinuria >40 mg/m^2/h or >50 mg/kg/day; for a 70 kg man, this means more than 3.5 g/day
- hypoalbuminaemia (<25 g/L)
- oedema
- hyperlipidaemia
- lipiduria.

Nephrotic syndrome is a potentially serious condition that is associated with a variety of other complications including hypercoagulability, negative nitrogen balance and infection. The major causes are listed in Table 10.8.

History

Nephrotic patients usually present with oedema which is often first noticed in a peri-orbital distribution after a period of recumbency. This distribution is characteristic of nephrotic syndrome, since patients with oedema due to heart failure or cirrhosis are often unable to lie flat because of pulmonary oedema or pressure on the diaphragm, respectively. As the oedema worsens, fluid accumulates around the ankles, sacrum and elbows in a gravity-dependent manner, and then becomes more generalized. Genital oedema may ensue and cause significant distress. A rapid onset of oedema suggests minimal change disease or focal segmental glomerulosclerosis (FSGS), rather than other causes in which the onset may be more insidious.

Nephrotic patients often describe frothing of the urine on micturition. Visible haematuria in nephrotic patients is rare, but when reported may indicate postinfectious glomerulonephritis, or the development of renal vein thrombosis.

Other key aspects of the history to explore include:

Table **10.8** Common causes of the nephrotic syndrome

Disease	Associations	Diagnostically helpful serological tests
Minimal change disease	Allergy, atopy, NSAIDs, Hodgkin's disease	None
Focal segmental glomerulosclerosis	HIV infection, pamidronate	HIV antibody
Membranous nephropathy	Drugs: gold, penicillamine, NSAIDs Hepatitis B, malaria Lupus erythematosus Malignancy (lung, breast, bowel)	Hepatitis B surface antigen Anti-DNA antibodies
Mesangiocapillary glomerulonephritis (type I)	C4 nephritic factor	C3 low, C4 low
Mesangiocapillary glomerulonephritis (type II)	C3 nephritic factor	C3 low, C4 normal
Amyloidosis	Myeloma Chronic inflammatory and infective disease	Serum and urine protein electrophoresis
Diabetic nephropathy	Other diabetic microvascular disease	None

NSAID, non-steroidal anti-inflammatory drug; HIV, human immunodeficiency virus.

- medication (prescribed or over-the-counter)
- prior acute or chronic infection
- allergies
- features suggestive of a systemic disorder such as lupus erythematosus or diabetes mellitus.

In patients older than 50 years, membranous nephropathy may be associated with epithelial tumours, particularly of the lung, breast or large bowel, therefore enquire about symptoms of malignancy.

A positive family history may indicate Alport's syndrome or an inherited form of focal segmental glomerulosclerosis.

Examination

Severe oedema may be associated with striae even in the absence of steroid therapy. Asymmetrical leg swelling may indicate deep venous thrombosis. Pleural effusion and ascites may be present. The liver may be painlessly enlarged, particularly in children. The jugular venous pressure is usually normal or low, and if elevated co-existent cardiac disease has to be suspected. Amyloidosis may account for both nephrotic syndrome and heart failure in this setting.

White bands (Muehrcke's bands) may be identified on the nails; these correspond to periods of hypoalbuminaemia. Hyperlipidaemia associated with the nephrotic syndrome may result in the formation of xanthoma around the eyes or along tendons.

Investigations

- Urine dipstick will be strongly positive for protein and may also be positive for blood.
- The urine protein:creatinine ratio will be >350 mg/mmol.
- Urine microscopy may demonstrate oval fat bodies and fatty casts.
- Renal function may be normal or impaired.
- Serum albumin concentration will be reduced, usually to less than 25 g/L.
- Cholesterol is usually elevated, often substantially, with 25 per cent of patients having a total cholesterol >10 mmol/L.
- Appropriate immunological investigations include: serum immunoglobulins; antinuclear antibody; and complement components C3 and C4 (Box 10.4 and Table 10.8).
- In patients >40 years send serum and urine for protein electrophoresis.

The majority of patients with nephrotic syndrome will require a renal biopsy to determine the underlying cause. However, in patients with longstanding diabetes mellitus with evidence of retinopathy and peripheral neuropathy a diagnosis of diabetic nephropathy can be assumed.

> **CLINICAL PEARL**
> A presentation with facial oedema usually indicates a diagnosis of nephrotic syndrome.

Nephritic syndrome/rapidly progressive glomerulonephritis

These syndromes result from glomerular inflammation and cause loss of excretory function, fluid retention, and haematuria. Rapidly progressive glomerulonephritis (RPGN) is a severe form of nephritic syndrome which leads to AKI, and may not be self-limiting. Common diseases presenting with the nephritic syndrome/RPGN together with associated features are listed in Table 10.9.

History

The classic nephritic syndrome presentation is:

- oliguria of rapid onset
- weight gain
- generalized oedema, which develops over a few days

- haematuria, which typically manifests as red/brown urine (often described as smoky or cola coloured). Blood clots are never seen.

Other key aspects of the history to explore include:

- a history of prior infection (often pharyngitis or impetigo)
- constitutional symptoms (weight loss, fever, myalgia, arthralgia) which may be associated with vasculitis
- skin rashes which may accompany vasculitis and lupus erythematosus
- respiratory tract symptoms (nasal congestion and bleeding, sinus congestion/infection, deafness, haemoptysis) which are suggestive of Wegener's granulomatosis
- uraemic symptoms.

Obtain a smoking history, and examine the occupational history for exposure to hydrocarbons.

Examination

Examine for volume overload:

- peripheral oedema is usual, but less severe than would be seen in the nephrotic syndrome

Table 10.9 Common causes of the nephritic syndrome/RPGN

Disease	Associations	Diagnostically helpful serological tests
Goodpasture's disease	Lung haemorrhage	Ant glomerular basement membrane antibody; antineutrophil cytoplasmic antibody (ANCA) in some
Vasculitis • Wegener's granulomatosis • Microscopic polyangiitis • Pauci-immune crescentic glomerulonephritis	Respiratory tract involvement Multisystem involvement Isolated renal involvement	cANCA (cytoplasmic) pANCA (perinuclear) pANCA
Immune complex mediated glomerulonephritis: • Lupus erythematosus • Poststreptococcal glomerulonephritis • IgA nephropathy/ Henoch–Schönlein purpura • Infective endocarditis	 Other multisystem features of lupus Pharyngitis, impetigo Purpuric rash, joint and abdominal pain Cardiac murmur, other manifestations of endocarditis	 Ant -DNA antibodies, low C3 and C4 Ant -streptolysin O titre, low C3, normal C4 Serum IgA increased in 30 per cent Positive blood culture, low C3, normal C4

- hypertension is invariable
- pulmonary oedema may develop (combination of hypertension and volume overload)
- elevation of the jugular venous pressure is common.

Other key aspects of the examination include:

- skin rashes
- splinter haemorrhages and nail-fold infarcts
- ENT disease (nasal mucosal inflammation, sinus tenderness, middle ear effusion)
- eyes for subconjunctival haemorrhage and evidence of retinal vasculitis
- lung crackles, pleural rubs
- limbs for neurological deficit which may result from nerve injury due to vasculitis.

Investigations

- Urine examination will demonstrate haematuria and proteinuria (usually subnephrotic).
- Urine microscopy may demonstrate red cell casts.
- Blood tests will show reduced renal function, often an elevated C-reactive protein, and anaemia.
- Additional serological investigations are listed in Tables 10.7 and 10.9.
- A renal biopsy is usually required in patients with RPGN unless an associated infection is identified, in which case a postinfectious glomerulonephritis can be assumed.

> **CLINICAL PEARL**
>
> A patient with acute kidney injury who has haematuria and proteinuria on urine dipstick testing should be considered to have rapidly progressive glomerulonephritis and specialist nephrology input should be sought immediately.

IgA nephropathy/Henoch–Schönlein purpura

IgA nephropathy, characterized by the mesangial deposition of IgA, is the commonest glomerulonephritis in the Western world. The typical clinical presentations are:

- visible haematuria (30–40 per cent of patients) usually 12 to 72 hours after the development of a mucosal infection (usually pharyngitis) or after exercise
- asymptomatic (30–40 per cent of patients) identified on incidental urine testing (haematuria ± proteinuria)
- nephrotic syndrome (5 per cent of patients)
- RPGN (5 per cent of patients)
- severe hypertension (occasional patient)
- loin pain (unilateral or bilateral) (occasional patient).

Henoch–Schönlein purpura is a related disease with the same glomerular abnormalities as IgA nephropathy, but with evidence of systemic vasculitis. This typically presents with:

- a palpable purpuric rash in an extensor surface distribution with sparing of the trunk and face (Fig. 10.6)
- polyarthralgia
- abdominal pain, which in some cases may be severe (presenting as an acute abdomen) and associated with bloody diarrhoea.

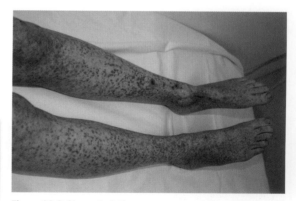

Figure 10.6 Characteristic appearances of the rash of Henoch–Schönlein purpura.

There are no signs that are characteristic of IgA nephropathy, and in Henoch–Schönlein purpura the only specific sign is the characteristic purpuric rash.

There are no specific laboratory investigations that are diagnostic of either IgA nephropathy or Henoch–Schönlein purpura, although up to 30 per cent of patients will have elevated serum IgA levels. A renal biopsy is essential to make a diagnosis of IgA nephropathy.

CLINICAL PEARL

In children, the constellation of haematuria/proteinuria, purpuric rash, arthralgia and abdominal pain is usually sufficient to make a clinical diagnosis of Henoch–Schönlein purpura without the need for renal biopsy.

Diabetic nephropathy

Diabetic renal disease is the commonest cause of end-stage renal disease in the Western world. It accounts for 20–50 per cent of new patients with end-stage renal disease.

Diabetic nephropathy typically presents with a constellation of:

- nephrotic range proteinuria
- hypertension
- progressive renal failure
- overt nephrotic syndrome in some patients (diabetic nephropathy is the commonest cause of nephrotic syndrome).

Key aspects of the history that are useful in making a diagnosis of diabetic nephropathy include:

- diabetes mellitus of long duration (at least 10 years)
- poor glycaemic control
- inadequately controlled hypertension
- microvascular disease in other organ systems, particularly diabetic retinopathy and peripheral neuropathy. Note that some patients with type 2 diabetes can have diabetic nephropathy without retinopathy
- cigarette smoking, ethnicity (Indo-Asians, African Americans), family history of diabetic nephropathy, and socioeconomic factors (poverty) are all risk factors favouring the development of diabetic nephropathy.

Key aspects of the examination are:

- funduscopy for diabetic retinopathy and limb examination for evidence of peripheral neuropathy
- volume state examination for evidence of the nephrotic syndrome
- blood pressure measurement

- examination of the vascular tree for evidence of atherosclerotic vascular disease, including renal bruits.

Investigations

- Proteinuria on urine dipstick.
- Urine protein:creatinine ratio >350 mg/mmol.
- Blood tests will demonstrate impaired renal function, elevated HbA1c, elevated triglycerides.

There are no other specific serological abnormalities diagnostic of diabetic nephropathy. Mostly a diagnosis of diabetic nephropathy can be made confidently on clinical grounds and renal biopsy is reserved for cases with atypical features (haematuria, short duration of diabetes, rapid decline in renal function, rapid onset of nephrosis, abnormal immunological investigations).

Myeloma kidney

Abnormal immunoglobulin proteins produced by malignant plasma cells can produce a variety of renal abnormalities. The commonest renal lesion is myeloma cast nephropathy (myeloma kidney). Patients may present with:

- the systemic effects of the plasma cell malignancy: weight loss, malaise, anaemia (fatigue and exertional breathlessness), bone pain, symptoms of hypercalcaemia (polyuria, thirst, abdominal pain, bone pain), and recurrent infection
- renal dysfunction in patients already known to have myeloma
- isolated renal failure without any associated features. Myeloma kidney is diagnosed on renal biopsy or from the blood and urine investigations undertaken in patients with unexplained renal failure.

Physical examination is usually unhelpful in myeloma patients. Pallor may be present. Bone deposits may cause spine tenderness or deformity. Occasionally mass lesions (plasmacytoma) may be identified.

The diagnosis depends on:

- a serum or urine monoclonal paraprotein with suppression of other immunoglobulin classes (serum and urine protein electrophoresis)
- an excess of plasma cells in the bone marrow (bone marrow biopsy)

- the presence of lytic bone lesions on plain radiography (skeletal survey).

Additional investigations required include full blood count to assess marrow function, and serum biochemistry to assess renal function and to identify hypercalcaemia.

> **CLINICAL PEARL**
>
> If the urine dipstick is negative when other tests (e.g. urine protein:creatinine ratio) indicate significant proteinuria, consider myeloma (dipsticks are albumin-specific and do not detect immunoglobulin light chains).

Autosomal dominant polycystic kidney disease

Autosomal dominant polycystic kidney disease (ADPKD) is a common genetic cause of renal disease with a prevalence of 1:400–1:1000 live births. It accounts for 10 per cent of patients with end-stage renal disease. Patients are often asymptomatic and present with either hypertension, an incidental finding of renal cysts on abdominal ultrasound, or a family history of renal disease.

When specifically questioned, the symptoms at presentation include:

- flank, back or abdominal pain in 60 per cent
- hypertension in 60 per cent
- haematuria in 75 per cent (30–50 per cent visible, 25 per cent invisible)
- a history of urinary tract infection
- uraemic symptoms in a minority. This is most likely with late presentation in the fourth to sixth decades of life.

A family history of renal failure or cystic renal disease is present in up to 90 per cent of patients. Ten per cent of cases appear to be due to new mutations in the *PKD* genes. Ten per cent of patients will have a family history of intracranial bleeds due to berry aneurysms.

The examination findings include:

- bilateral irregular flank masses in the abdomen
- nodular hepatomegaly (from liver cysts) (75 per cent of patients by the seventh decade)

- aortic regurgitation, mitral valve prolapse, or tricuspid regurgitation may be detected due to associated cardiac valve defects
- inguinal and umbilical hernias may also be present.

Relevant investigations include:

- serum chemistry profile – to assess renal function
- full blood count – although anaemia in ADPKD is less common than in other forms of CKD
- urinalysis – this will demonstrate invisible haematuria in 25 per cent and proteinuria in 18 per cent
- ultrasonography – this is the most appropriate imaging modality to identify the renal cysts
- cerebral magnetic resonance angiography – to look for berry aneurysms; it should be reserved for patients with a family history of intracerebral bleeding (10 per cent of families).

Alport's syndrome

Alport's syndrome is an inherited syndrome of haematuria, progressive renal impairment, sensorineural deafness, and eye abnormalities. It has a prevalence of 1:5000 live births, and accounts for 2–3 per cent of patients with end-stage renal disease. An X-linked inheritance pattern is present in 80 per cent of cases, with autosomal recessive and autosomal dominant forms accounting for 15 per cent and 5 per cent of cases, respectively. All forms are caused by mutations in type IV collagen genes (usually the *COL4A5* gene). The presentation can be variable.

- Some patients present with intermittent visible haematuria, often in association with respiratory tract infection.
- Nephrotic syndrome develops in 40 per cent of cases in early adulthood.
- End-stage renal disease and therefore uraemic symptoms usually develop during the third decade.
- Overt deafness becomes apparent during the second decade of life.

On examination, the key abnormalities are:

- hypertension – which is common once renal dysfunction has developed
- anterior lenticonus on formal eye examination – found in 15 per cent of patients, this corre-

lates with the development of progressive renal dysfunction

- asymptomatic perimacular granulations on fundoscopy – found in 30 per cent of patients
- reduced hearing acuity – may be noticeable on bedside testing during the second decade.

Relevant investigations include:

- urinalysis demonstrates invisible haematuria from infancy
- progressive proteinuria develops from the second decade of life
- urea and creatinine become elevated as renal function declines and end-stage renal disease usually develops during the third decade
- renal biopsy is usually required for diagnosis, although audiometry and genetic testing may provide additional information.

Renal stone disease

Renal stone disease has a prevalence of up to 10 per cent in industrialized nations and is higher in some areas such as the Middle East. The modes of presentation are:

- pain – a stone passing through the renal pelvis or ureter induces severe colicky loin pain that radiates to the groin, testis, or labia (ureteral colic)
- urinary symptoms – stones impacted at the vesicoureteric junction may cause urinary frequency and pain in the penile tip or clitoris
- visible haematuria – this may occur during episodes of ureteral colic, or may occur in isolation
- recurrent urinary tract infection
- incidental finding – stones that are confined to the renal pelvis are often asymptomatic and are usually identified in imaging investigations undertaken for other reasons.

Bladder stones may cause haematuria, symptoms due to recurrent urinary sepsis, or frequency and urgency of micturition (stranguary) that can be very distressing. Seek out risk factors for stone disease (Box 10.5).

Examination of a patient with ureteral colic will demonstrate an agitated patient in obvious distress. The skin will be pale and clammy, although there is usually no haemodynamic compromise. Abdominal

---

BOX 10.5 RISK FACTORS FOR RENAL STONE FORMATION

General risk factors:
- age (peak age – third decade of life)
- family history of stone disease
- previous history of stone disease
- previous urinary tract infection
- risk factors for hypercalcaemia (sarcoidosis, hyperparathyroidism, malignancy)
- gastrointestinal disease (e.g. Crohn's disease – increases oxalate absorption)
- gout
- obesity
- diabetes mellitus.

Environmental factors:
- occupation (particularly hot working environments, e.g. foundry workers and bakers)
- inadequate fluid intake
- high animal protein diet
- low urine volume.

Drug-related factors:
- drugs that may form stones directly:
  - triamterene
  - aciclovir
  - indinavir
- drugs that promote stone formation indirectly:
  - loop diuretics
  - calcium and vitamin D supplements
  - glucocorticoids
  - antacids
  - theophylline
  - acetazolamide
  - salicylates
  - probenecid
  - vitamin C.

---

examination usually demonstrates no abnormality apart from mild loin tenderness. Fever and haemodynamic compromise in a patient with stone disease raises the possibility of sepsis from an obstructed kidney (pyonephrosis). Urgent drainage of the affected kidney after resuscitation and appropriate antibiotic treatment is required.

Appropriate investigations include:

- dipstick urinalysis – which will usually demonstrate invisible haematuria

- serum chemistry – for renal function, calcium and uric acid
- non-contrast enhanced spiral CT – currently the preferred option for identifying renal and ureteral stones.

In recurrent stone formers perform a metabolic screen (24-hour urine for calcium, phosphate, oxalate, uric acid, sodium, citrate, and pH) to determine whether there is an underlying metabolic abnormality that requires treatment to prevent further stone formation.

> **IMPORTANT**
> Fever, hypotension and loin tenderness in a patient with stone disease suggests the presence of an infected, obstructed kidney (pyonephrosis). Once resuscitated, urgent imaging and drainage of the kidney is required to prevent irreversible loss of renal function and potentially death.

Urothelial malignancy

The cardinal feature of transitional cell carcinoma of the urinary tract is painless haematuria. This may be visible or invisible. Any patient above the age of 40 years with haematuria requires urological evaluation as a priority.

Bladder tumours may cause irritative symptoms of frequency, urgency, nocturia, and dysuria. Loin pain may indicate the presence of ureteral obstruction. Weight loss and other symptoms of systemic malignancy develop late in the course of disease.

In the history, seek evidence of risk factors for urothelial malignancy. These include:

- cigarette smoking
- occupational exposure to aromatic amines and polyaromatic hydrocarbons
- previous exposure of the bladder to ionizing radiation (for example radiotherapy for cervical or prostate carcinoma)
- previous treatment with cyclophosphamide or phenacetin
- prolonged immunosuppression (for example in organ transplant recipients)
- chronic cystitis, bladder calculi, long-term indwelling catheters, and schistosomiasis all predispose to bladder squamous cell carcinoma.

On examination, signs of urothelial malignancy are uncommon. Advanced disease may be associated with cachexia, the presence of a pelvic mass, and irregular hepatomegaly.

Appropriate investigations include:

- urine cytology
- renal tract imaging with ultrasonography, contrast-enhanced CT or MRI
- cystoscopy and ureteroscopy.

> **IMPORTANT**
> Any patient above the age of 40 years with haematuria (visible or invisible) requires urgent evaluation by a urologist to look for malignant disease of the urinary tract.

Urinary tract infection

Urinary tract infection (UTI) is a very common medical problem with 50–60 per cent of women having at least one UTI during their lifetime. The risk in men is much lower at 5 per 10 000 per year. The classic symptoms are frequency and urgency of micturition, dysuria, and/or suprapubic pain.

Fever is not a feature of lower UTI. Infection of the upper urinary tract is suggested by acute onset flank pain, nausea, vomiting, myalgia and fever. Lower tract symptoms may or may not be present.

Enquire about factors that predispose to UTI, including:

- pregnancy
- recent urinary tract instrumentation
- diabetes mellitus
- immunosuppression
- underlying disease that may predispose to urinary tract obstruction (stones, renal cysts, urinary tract malignancy, urinary diversion procedures e.g. ileal conduit)
- a functionally abnormal urinary tract (e.g. vesico-ureteric reflux, neurogenic bladder)
- renal failure
- renal transplantation
- prostatitis-related infection.

In addition, determine the relationship of UTI symptoms to sexual intercourse and the use of spermicidal agents.

On examination look for fever and assess the circulation to identify evidence of upper urinary tract infection and septic shock. Examine the abdomen. Lower urinary tract infection may be associated with suprapubic tenderness alone. The presence of significant loin tenderness suggests pyelonephritis. In men with UTI, perform a digital rectal exam; prostate tenderness suggests the presence of prostatitis.

The key investigations are:

- dipstick urinalysis – the presence of blood, protein, nitrites and leucocyte esterase strongly suggests UTI
- culture of a clean-catch urine specimen – a bacterial count of $>10^5$ colony-forming units (CFU)/mL is considered significant bacteriuria.

In uncomplicated UTI, no further investigations are necessary. Recurrent or upper tract UTI requires further investigation with imaging (ultrasonography, intravenous urography or CT) to look for evidence of structural or functional urinary tract disease.

SUMMARY

Key features of the history

Presenting symptoms:

- disorders of micturition:
  - frequency of micturition
  - poor urine stream
  - dysuria
- disorders of urine volume:
  - polyuria
  - oliguria
  - anuria
- disorders of urine composition:
  - haematuria
  - proteinuria
  - pneumaturia
  - miscellaneous (e.g. solid material in urine)
- pain
- oedema
- uraemic symptoms (Box 10.2)
- symptoms of systemic disease – infective, inflammatory or malignant disease.

The rest of the history:

- past medical history (Table 10.2)
- gynaecological and obstetric history – menstrual, contraceptive, and pregnancy history
- drug history – including all prescribed, over-the-counter, and herbal remedies
- dietary history – sodium and protein intake
- social history – smoking history, alcohol intake, and socioeconomic status
- occupational history – identify risk of exposure to nephrotoxins and infectious agents
- family history – of renal disease and diseases associated with renal disease
- ethnic and geographical background.

Key features of the examination:

- examination of the kidneys and urinary tract
  - palpation of the kidneys and bladder
  - auscultation for vascular bruits
- blood pressure measurement
- general examination
  - *face* – thickened skin, rash, loss of subcutaneous fat, moon face
  - *eyes* – perilimbal calcification, subconjunctival haemorrhage, lenticonus, retinopathy
  - *skin* – scratch marks, rashes, pigmentation, skin turgor
  - *nails* – dystrophy, leuconychia, Beau's lines, splinter haemorrhages
  - *praecordium* – pericardial rub and cardiac murmurs
  - *chest* – lung crackles, pleural effusions, pleural rubs, respiratory pattern
  - *limbs* – oedema, peripheral neuropathy, peripheral pulses and vascular bruits.

FURTHER READING

Davison A (ed). 2005. *Oxford textbook of clinical nephrology*, 3rd edn. Oxford: Oxford University Press.

11 THE GENITOURINARY SYSTEM

Christine A Bowman

INTRODUCTION

Sexually transmitted infections (STIs) are common and a major cause of morbidity and mortality. Some examples are given below.

- Genital chlamydial infection is the leading cause of pelvic inflammatory disease (PID). Complications include tubal infertility and ectopic pregnancy.
- Disseminated gonococcal infection can cause septic arthritis and endocarditis.
- Sexually acquired reactive arthritis (SARA) may be triggered by an immunological response to chlamydia and gonorrhoea.
- Oncogenic strains of human papilloma virus (HPV) are co-factors for anogenital neoplasia.
- Neonatal herpes following primary genital herpes in late pregnancy can cause neurological damage or death.
- Untreated syphilis may cause significant cardiovascular and central nervous system disease, and in pregnancy it can cause intrauterine death or congenital syphilis.
- Chronic hepatitis B infection can result in cirrhosis and hepatoma.
- Human immunodeficiency virus (HIV) infection, without appropriate therapeutic intervention, will progress to acquired immune deficiency syndrome (AIDS) and death.
- STIs are co-factors in the transmission of HIV.

STIs and HIV infection are also major causes of social, emotional and psychological distress, and are associated with stigma and taboos. They may destabilize sexual relationships and impact on the integrity of the partnership and/or family.

CLINICAL HISTORY

Taking a sexual history

- Details of sexual partners and specific sexual activities direct appropriate investigations and anatomical site swabbing. For example, pharyngeal and rectal swabs are part of routine testing of MSM (men who have sex with men) practising receptive oral and anal sex.
- Some infections are more common in certain higher risk groups or high prevalence geographical areas (e.g. syphilis and hepatitis B are more common in MSM, trichomoniasis is more common in African Caribbeans, and chancroid in individuals who have had sex in tropical countries).
- Timing from sexual contact to testing is important. Incubation periods vary from short (2–10 days) for symptomatic gonorrhoea to long (6–12 weeks for secondary syphilis). Many infections may be asymptomatic for months or years before producing symptoms (e.g. genital herpes and warts).
- Ask the following details about the last sexual contact:
  - When was it?
  - What kind of sexual contact occurred? Heterosexual/homosexual, vaginal, anal, oral sex, insertive or receptive?
  - Was the contact a one-off casual encounter or someone with whom the patient has had sex on a number of occasions over a period of time (a regular sexual contact). Is the contact in a higher risk group for, or actually known to have, STIs or HIV?
  - Did the contact take place locally/in another UK location/abroad (differing prevalence of STIs and antibiotic resistance patterns exist).
- Ask about other sexual contacts in the past 3 months and 12 months. Ask about lifetime exposure to higher risk activities (e.g. commercial sex work or use of commercial sex worker, sex between men, injecting drug use (self or partner), partner from a high infection prevalence area).
- Have condoms been used consistently? Patients often report that condoms split or come off during sex.

- Ask women patients about current contraception current or previous pregnancies and last menstrual period (LMP). Pregnancy can cause symptoms including abdominal pain and altered vaginal discharge.
- Ask about previous urinary or genital symptoms. Is this a recurrent problem such as genital herpes or is it related to a non-STI diagnosis such as a genital dermatosis?
- Are there any other medical conditions which may predispose to genital symptoms, e.g. diabetes, immunosuppressive drug use or chemotherapy (more troublesome candidiasis, herpes and warts)?

Presenting symptoms

This section describes the common presenting symptoms in patients with an STI or other genito-urinary conditions.

Women

Vaginal discharge

Post-pubertal girls and women normally have some physiological vaginal discharge. The amount and consistency varies with age, contraceptive method and menstrual cycle. Puberty, use of the combined oral contraceptive pill and pregnancy are all associated with a hormonally induced increase in vaginal discharge. Ask about the characteristics of the discharge, e.g. a 'fishy' offensive discharge associated with bacterial vaginosis, 'cottage cheese-like'

discharge with candidiasis (associated with itching and soreness), and highly offensive discharge with a retained tampon (Table 11.1).

> **IMPORTANT** *i*
> 'Red flag' list for vaginal discharge
>
> - Chlamydia – common, may be asymptomatic. Complications – pelvic inflammatory disease, chronic pelvic pain, ectopic pregnancy and infertility. Occasionally – reactive arthritis. Can be passed from mother to baby during vaginal delivery.
> - Gonorrhoea – less common than chlamydia but similar complications and maternal transmission risks. May be asymptomatic. Rare but serious complications of disseminated infection including septic arthritis.
> - Herpes simplex virus (HSV) – lesions on cervix may give profuse vaginal discharge. External ulcers may or may not be present. May be misdiagnosed as thrush. Serious risk to baby if first episode occurs during late pregnancy.
> - Foreign object (tampon) – highly offensive discharge. Features of fever, rash and hypotension suggest toxic shock syndrome requiring urgent medical intervention.
> - Cancer – rare but extremely serious.

Vulval itching and/or soreness

If associated with an offensive discharge consider *Trichomonas vaginalis*. Eczema, contact dermatitis,

Table 11.1 Causes of vaginal discharge

Frequency	Cause
Most common	Physiological/hormonal (contraceptive pill, pregnancy) Candida ('thrush') Bacterial vaginosis (BV)
Common	Chlamydia Gonorrhoea Trichomoniasis (TV)
Less common	Genital herpes simplex virus (HSV) Genital warts
Occasional	Foreign object (tampon) Streptococcal infection
Rare	Cancer

Table 11.2 Causes of vulval itching or soreness

Frequency	Cause
Most common	Candida ('thrush') Genital herpes simplex virus Vulval dermatoses, e.g. eczema, contact dermatitis
Common	Genital warts Trichomoniasis Vulval psoriasis
Less common	Lichen sclerosus
Occasional	Other skin diseases including vulval intraepithelial neoplasia Streptococcal infection

psoriasis and lichen sclerosus are other causes of these symptoms (Table 11.2). See also candidiasis (above).

> **IMPORTANT**
>
> 'Red flag' list for vulval itching and/or soreness
>
> - Vulval skin diseases mimic symptoms of thrush.
> - Lichen sclerosus is an intensely itchy skin disease which untreated can lead to loss of or fusion of the labia. It is associated with a small increased risk of vulval cancer.
> - Vulval intraepithelial neoplasia (VIN) is potentially premalignant skin condition which may present as pigmented lesions.
> - Vulval cancer – rare but extremely serious.

Dyspareunia (pain on intercourse)

Superficial dyspareunia (pain or discomfort on initial penetration) is often due to vulval soreness or ulceration. Deep dyspareunia is pain during full penetration, which is felt inside the pelvis and lower abdomen. This may indicate PID. Other causes include endometriosis.

Pelvic and lower abdominal pain

The differential diagnosis includes PID, ectopic pregnancy, endometriosis, urinary tract infections and irritable bowel syndrome.

Irregular bleeding per vagina

This includes intermenstrual and post-coital bleeding. Causes include chlamydial or gonococcal cervicitis and PID.

Table 11.3 Causes of urethral discharge

Frequency	Cause
Most common	Chlamydial non-gonococcal urethritis (NGU) Non-chlamydial NGU
Common	Gonorrhoea
Occasional	Genital herpes simplex virus Trichomoniasis Urinary tract infection Secondary to thrush balanitis
Rare	Foreign object

> **IMPORTANT**
>
> 'Red flag' list for urethral discharge
>
> - Recurrent NGU may occur without reinfection.
> - Chlamydia – common, may be asymptomatic. Complications in men – acute epididymitis, reactive arthritis. Serious complications for female partners.
> - Gonorrhoea – less common than chlamydia but similar complications and maternal transmission risks. May be asymptomatic. Rare but serious complications of disseminated infection including septic arthritis.

Men

Urethral discharge

A profuse, purulent urethral discharge associated with marked dysuria is common in gonorrhoea. Non-gonococcal urethritis (NGU) usually produces milder symptoms. Forty per cent of acute NGU cases are caused by *Chlamydia trachomatis* (Table 11.3).

Dysuria

May occur with or without discharge. Test for urinary tract infections (UTIs) as well as STIs.

Pain and swelling in the testicles/epididymis

Chlamydia and gonorrhoea can both cause acute epididymo-orchitis. Other causes of testicular pain include torsion, underlying malignancy and mumps.

Rectal pain or discharge

Individuals practising receptive anal sex are at risk of proctitis due to gonorrhoea, *Chlamydia trachomatis*, herpes simplex and lymphogranuloma venereum (LGV).

Both sexes

Painful genital ulceration

Painful genital ulceration is commonly due to genital herpes (Table 11.4). Ulceration is often preceded by itch or soreness and associated with dysuria and inguinal lymphadenopathy. Syphilitic ulcers are often painless.

Table 11.4 Causes of genital ulceration

Frequency	Cause
Most common	Genital herpes simplex virus
Common	Excoriation secondary to itching (candidiasis, trichomoniasis or vulval dermatosis)
Less common	Idiopathic genital ulceration Erythema multiforme Syphilis (primary chancres usually painless) Chancroid (usually from foreign contact)
Occasional	Lichen sclerosus Other skin diseases Behçets disease
Rare	Vulval cancer

Table 11.5 Causes of genital skin lumps

Frequency	Cause
Most common	Genital warts (condylomata acuminata)
Common	Molluscum contagiosum Sebaceous cysts/epidermal cysts Coronal papillae in men Vulval papillae in women Skin tags
Less common	Scabies papules
Occasional	Condylomata lata of secondary syphilis Bowenoid papulosis (vulval or prostatic intraepithelial neoplasia)
Rare	Squamous cell cancer Melanoma

> ### *i* IMPORTANT
> 'Red flag' list for genital ulceration
>
> - HSV – lesions on cervix may give profuse vaginal discharge. External ulcers may or may not be present. May be misdiagnosed as thrush. Serious risk of neonatal herpes if primary genital herpes simplex occurs in the mother during late pregnancy.
> - Syphilis ulcers may be painful if superadded bacterial or herpetic infection.
> - HIV seroconversion illness can present with painful genital ulcers.
> - People having sex abroad may pick up tropical genital ulcer infections, e.g. chancroid, granuloma inguinale, LGV.
> - Squamous cell carcinoma – rare but extremely serious.

> ### IMPORTANT *i*
> Genital skin lumps
>
> - Condylomata lata of secondary syphilis can look like genital warts; syphilis serology will be positive in secondary syphilis.
> - Patients often think they have warts when they have noticed normal anatomical features, e.g. vulval papillae in women and coronal papillae in men.
> - Scabies may present with itchy papules on the genitals.

Genital skin lumps

The commonest cause of genital skin lumps is genital warts, which are sometimes itchy (Table 11.5). Molluscum contagiosum in adults appears as smooth, umbilicated, papular lesions in the pubic region, lower abdomen, thighs, scrotum and external genitalia.

Generalized skin rashes

Generalized skin rashes affecting the palms and soles of the feet, and associated with mouth and genital ulceration and generalized lymphadenopathy, are common features of secondary syphilis and HIV seroconversion.

Itchy skin

Pubic itching can be caused by scabies (usually also itch all over body with relative sparing of the head and neck), pediculosis pubis, folliculitis (especially after shaving) and dermatoses (eczema, psoriasis, contact dermatitis, lichen sclerosus).

PHYSICAL EXAMINATION

General examination when indicated

- Are there any systemic signs? For example fever, tachycardia or hypotension could indicate severe gonococcal PID, HIV seroconversion or may point towards a non-STI based diagnosis (e.g. Stevens–Johnson syndrome).

- Look for skin rashes (e.g. generalized rashes including palmar and plantar lesions in secondary syphilis and HIV seroconversion, painful pustular lesions near affected joints in disseminated gonococcal infection (DGI), erythematous plaques on extensor surfaces (psoriasis) or flexural eczema.
- Look inside the mouth for mucous patches of secondary syphilis, pharyngitis of acute HIV seroconversion, oral candida of immunocompromised HIV patients, Wickham's striae associated with lichen planus.
- Examine for generalized lymphadenopathy (secondary syphilis, HIV).

Genital examination

- Look for tender or non-tender lymph nodes in the groins:
  - tender groin nodes are common with genital herpes
  - large rubbery non-tender groin nodes are common with primary syphilis.
- Look for skin rashes/folliculitis in the pubic area, visible pubic lice or their eggs.

In men (Fig. 11.1)

- Examine the penile shaft, glans penis, prepuce, scrotum (Fig. 11.2) and perianal area.
- Look for inflammation and erythema, blisters, ulceration, warts, molluscum contagiosum.
- Look for obvious urethral discharge.

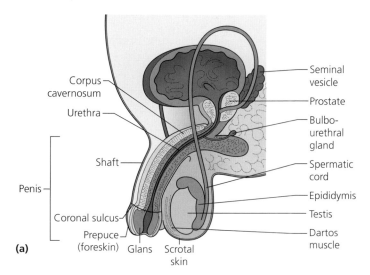

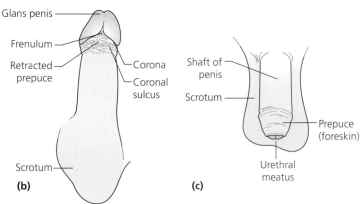

Figure 11.1 Male genital anatomy.

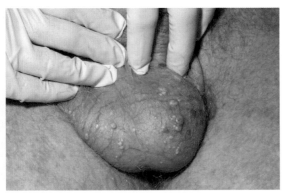

Figure 11.2 Sebaceous epidermal cysts on scrotum.

- Examine the scrotal contents for swelling/pain in testicle or epididymis.
- If there is history of receptive anal intercourse pass a proctoscope to look for inflammation/ulceration/pus/bleeding/warts.
- Collect two urine samples.
  - Send the first-catch urine for chlamydia and gonorrhoea testing by nucleic acid amplification testing (NAAT) (a 'first-catch' sample must include the first few drops of urine produced).
- Dip the second catch urine for protein, blood, nitrites and sugar and send for microscopy, culture and sensitivity if indicated.

In women (Fig. 11.3)

- Examine the vulva, introitus, perineum and perianal area.
- Pass a vaginal speculum.
- Determine the characteristics of any vaginal discharge:
  - smelly (bacterial vaginosis (BV), trichomoniasis (TV), retained tampon)
  - frothy (BV, TV)
  - homogeneous white (BV/normal)
  - cottage cheese and adherent (*Candida*)
  - thick yellow purulent (mucopurulent cervicitis/TV).
- Is mucopurulent cervicitis present with mucopus at cervical os and contact bleeding on swabbing?

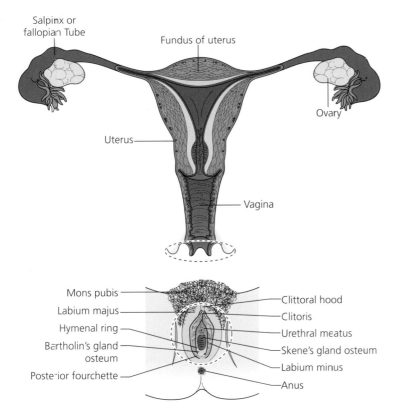

Figure 11.3 Female genital anatomy.

- Do a bimanual per vaginal (PV) examination to look for:
  - tenderness on moving the cervix (cervical excitation)
  - adnexal tenderness and abdominal tenderness (may indicate PID).
- Do a pregnancy test if abdominal pain is present to exclude ectopic pregnancy.

INVESTIGATIONS

All new patients attending genitourinary medicine (GUM) clinics (regardless of their presenting complaint) are encouraged to have testing for:

- *Chlamydia trachomatis* – by NAAT on a first-catch urine in men and a cervical swab in women. Alternatively, non-invasive *Chlamydia* testing can be performed on vaginal swabs and urine samples. However, the sensitivity of these tests is lower than that of cervical testing.
- *Neisseria gonorrhoea* – both by NAAT testing as above and by swabs from urethra plus cervix in women, for microscopy and culture (plus antibiotic sensitivities where isolated).
- Syphilis – by serological testing and by dark ground microscopy if a suspicious ulcerative lesion is found.
- HIV – by blood test (or non-invasive buccal swabbing if the patient has needle phobia).

Even asymptomatic patients are offered screening tests for these four infections as:

- all of the above infections may be detected in patients without any signs or symptoms of infection
- untreated, the patient is at significant risk of serious complications
- the available diagnostic tests are highly sensitive and specific
- therapeutic intervention cures *Chlamydia*, gonorrhoea and syphilis and prevents progression of HIV infection to AIDS and death
- treatment of these infections reduces onward transmission to sexual partners and mother-to-child transmission in pregnant women.

In addition to the four infections discussed above, other tests may be offered dependent on the sexual history, symptoms and signs.

- Sexual contacts of gonorrhoea are offered pharyngeal swabs and rectal swabs for culture.
- MSM including receptive anal intercourse are offered pharyngeal swabs and rectal swabs (via a proctoscope) for *N. gonorrhoeae* culture and swabs for *Chlamydia* testing.
- MSM with proctitis should also have rectal swab testing for LGV and herpes simplex virus detection by polymerase chain reaction (PCR).
- Women with vaginal discharge, itching or soreness should have a loop of discharge dissolved in a drop of saline on a microscopy slide (wet preparation) examined under low-power, dark ground microscope for *Trichomonas vaginalis*, clue cells of BV, hyphae and spores of *Candida*. In addition, vaginal swab material on a dry slide can be used for Gram staining and microscopic examination for evidence of BV or candidiasis.
- Patients with genital ulcers should have swabs taken from the ulcer for detection of herpes simplex by PCR and for dark ground microscopy for the spirochaetes of syphilis if indicated.
- Patients from areas with a high prevalence of hepatitis B, MSM and intravenous drug users and their sexual contacts should have blood tested for hepatitis B and be offered vaccination if non-immune.
- Urine should be sent for microscopy, culture and sensitivity when urinary tract infection is suspected or if there are positive findings on urinalysis.
- Urine should be sent for pregnancy testing in women with abdominal pain.

COMMON DIAGNOSES

Urethral and vaginal discharge

Chlamydia

- *Chlamydia trachomatis* is the commonest bacterial STI.
- Highest prevalence of genital chlamydial infection is in the 16–25-year-old age group.
- The incubation period is 7–21 days.

Chlamydia in women

History:

- 80 per cent of women with uncomplicated chlamydia have no symptoms (see Box 11.1 for complications)
- when present, symptoms include:
  - increased vaginal discharge (may be offensive, mucopurulent or blood-stained)
  - dysuria
  - irregular periods
  - post-coital bleeding
  - lower abdominal pains
  - deep dyspareunia.

Examination:

- is frequently unremarkable
- may find an offensive discharge and mucopurulent cervicitis with contact bleeding and mucopus exuding from the cervical os.

Chlamydia in men

History:

- 50 per cent of men with uncomplicated chlamydia have no symptoms.
- Urethral discharge and dysuria are the most common symptoms of NGU (see Box 11.2).
- *Chlamydia* causes 40–50 per cent of first episode NGU in men.

BOX 11.1 GENITAL TRACT COMPLICATIONS OF CHLAMYDIA IN WOMEN

- **PID**: In around 20 per cent of untreated women, infection may ascend into the uterus and salpinges causing PID. Chlamydial PID is the commonest cause of tubal infertility and ectopic pregnancy in developed countries.
- **Bartholin's abscess**: With vulval pain and tender cystic swelling in the Bartholin's gland.
- **Neonatal chlamydial ophthalmia neonatorum**: Pregnant women with genital chlamydia may pass the infection to their baby during labour.
- Babies with chlamydia may develop sticky eyes 5–14 days after delivery and later suffer with chest and ear infections.

CLINICAL PEARL

In pre-pubertal girls, *Chlamydia* can infect the vulval and vagina epithelium – this is highly suggestive of sexual abuse.

BOX 11.2 TESTING FOR CHLAMYDIA

- NGU in men can be diagnosed on microscopy of Gram-stained urethral discharge and finding >5 pus cells per high power field. Threads seen in first-catch urine indicate anterior urethritis.
- Chlamydia is best detected using NAAT on first-catch urine in men or cervical sample in women (vaginal and urine samples are less sensitive in women).

Examination:

- may be unremarkable
- may find whitish or mucopurulent urethral discharge
- sometimes associated with a circinate balanitis, that is annular lesions with slightly raised borders on the glans penis
- will elicit testicular and epididymal pain and tenderness if the infection ascends to give acute epididymo-orchitis.

Chlamydia at other sites

Chlamydia can infect the pharynx (rarely symptomatic), rectum (usually asymptomatic) and conjunctiva (giving a mild conjunctivitis) in both sexes.

Gonorrhoea

Gonorrhoea is caused by the bacterium *Neisseria gonorrhoeae*. In adults, *N. gonorrhoeae* may infect the columnar epithelial cells of the urethra, cervix, rectum and conjunctiva. In pre-pubertal girls, the vulval and vaginal epithelium are susceptible to gonococcal infection. Isolation of *N. gonorrhoeae* in children is extremely suggestive of sexual abuse. Gonorrhoea is less common than chlamydia and the highest prevalence is in the 16–25-year-old age group. Co-infection with other STIs (e.g. *Chlamydia* (40 per cent) and trichomoniasis) is common.

Gonorrhoea in men

History:

- In men the incubation period is usually short with urethral symptoms occurring 2–10 days after infection, most commonly 5–8 days after exposure.
- Most men (over 80 per cent) with urethral gonorrhoea are symptomatic with a purulent urethral discharge and dysuria (often described as being 'like passing razor blades').
- Rectal infection causes symptoms of proctitis (pain on defecation with discharge per rectum) in around 10 per cent of cases.
- Pharyngeal infection is usually asymptomatic.

Examination:

- Profuse purulent urethral discharge and urethral meatus inflammation is common (Fig. 11.4).
- If infection ascends to produce acute epididymo-orchitis, the epididymis and testicle become tender and swollen.
- Inflamed rectal mucosa with mucus, pus and contact bleeding are seen via the proctoscope in gonococcal proctitis.

Gonorrhoea in women

History:

- frequently asymptomatic in women (50–70 per cent)
- symptoms, if present, commonly develop within 10 days of exposure and include:
  - vaginal discharge
  - dysuria

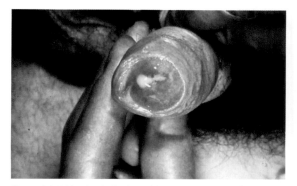

Figure 11.4 Urethral discharge in a man with gonorrhoea.

- lower abdominal pain
- irregular periods
- post-coital bleeding
- dyspareunia.

Examination:

- Offensive discharge and mucopurulent cervicitis with contact bleeding and mucopus exuding from the cervical os.

Genital tract complications

- Gonococcal pelvic inflammatory disease:
  - Untreated infection may spread to pelvic organs causing an acute onset of PID.
  - Admission to gynaecology is indicated for intravenous antibiotics.
  - Complications of gonococcal PID include infertility and ectopic pregnancy.
- Abscesses of paraurethral (Skene's) glands or Bartholin's glands cause painful, tender fluctuant swellings.
- Pregnant women with gonorrhoea can pass this infection to the baby at delivery. The baby may develop a purulent conjunctivitis/sticky eye 2–10 days after delivery. Blindness may result from inadequate treatment.

Investigations for gonorrhoea

- Gram stain of urethral, cervical or rectal discharge for the Gram-negative intracellular diplococcus *N. gonorrhoea*.
- Culture on selective media.
- NAAT testing on a first-catch urine in men and a cervical swab in women and by swabs from urethra plus cervix in women.

Trichomoniasis

Trichomoniasis is an STI caused by the flagellated protozoan *Trichomonas vaginalis*.

In women

Trichomoniasis infects the vagina, ectocervix, vulva, urethra, paraurethral glands and Bartholin's glands. History:

- Vaginal discharge is the commonest symptom. Amount and consistency varies. An offensive vaginal discharge associated with dysuria, vulval soreness and itch is common. Lower abdominal pain occurs in some.

- 10–50 per cent are asymptomatic.
- Symptoms may arise 4–28 days after infection or may develop weeks or months later. Symptoms may be intermittent, fluctuating throughout the menstrual cycle.

Examination:

- Marked vulvo-vaginitis, profuse offensive vaginal discharge (Fig. 11.5) and a 'strawberry cervix'.

Trichomoniasis is not itself a cause of PID, but it may be found in association with other STIs such as chlamydia and gonorrhoea which are.

In men

Trichomoniasis infects the urethra and subpreputial sac. Less commonly found in glans penis, epididymis and prostate gland.

History:

- Trichomoniasis is frequently asymptomatic, most men are seen in GUM as trichomoniasis contacts.
- It may cause dysuria and discharge.

Examination:

- Often there is little to see.
- There may be urethral discharge.
- Balanoposthitis (inflammation of the glans and foreskin), epididymitis and prostatitis are uncommon findings with trichomoniasis.

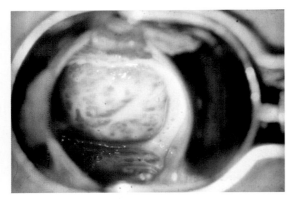

Figure 11.5 Vaginal discharge seen through a speculum in a patient infected with *Trichomonas vaginalis*.

Diagnosis:

- A saline wet preparation using a loop of discharge from the vagina or urethra, viewed under low power dark ground microscopy identifies the motile flagellated protozoans in around 70 per cent of cases for women but has a much lower sensitivity in men.
- Culture using specific media has a higher detection rate.
- PCR tests are in clinical trials.
- Cervical cytological examination may report *Trichomonas* seen on the smear. Cytology smears have poor specificity for *Trichomonas* and false positives may occur.

Candidiasis ('thrush')

Women: vulvo-vaginal candidiasis

Candidiasis is the most common cause of vaginal discharge associated with vulval itch and soreness. *Candida albicans* causes over 85 per cent of cases, *Candida glabrata* up to 15 per cent of cases; other *Candida* species are occasionally causative agents.

History:

- predisposing factors include: inflammation of mucosal epithelium, e.g. from eczema, contact dermatitis, etc., frictional inflammation/micro-abrasions after sexual contact, stress, recent antibiotic treatment, diabetes, obesity, pregnancy, oral steroids or other immunosuppressant drugs, immunosuppression for malignancy and its treatment, HIV infection
- vaginal discharge from candidiasis may range in consistency from watery through to 'cottage cheese'-like
- vulval itch and soreness
- superficial dyspareunia.

Examination:

- inflammation of vulva and vagina, erythema ± excoriations. small satellite lesions may be seen
- vaginal discharge – which may be white and adherent to the vaginal walls – not smelly.

Diagnosis:

- Based on clinical appearance.

- Microscopy is of limited value as hyphae and spores are seen in about 60 per cent of cases only; may, however, exclude other causes of symptoms e.g. *Trichomonas vaginalis.*
- Many women have detectable candidal spores on microscopy of vaginal secretions or *Candida* isolated on vaginal culture without having any symptoms – asymptomatic carriage should not be treated.
- Patients and their doctors frequently misdiagnose thrush – assuming that all vulva itch or itchy vaginal discharge is due to *Candida.*
- If symptoms fail to resolve with antifungals, repeated medication should be discouraged, and proper assessment should include screening for other genital infections and examination to exclude skin conditions such as eczema and lichen sclerosus.

Men: balanoposthitis

Candidiasis may cause balanitis with redness, soreness and itching of the glans penis with or without posthitis (inflammation of the mucosal lining of the foreskin). This is more common in men with tight foreskins, poor hygiene or a predisposing factor, especially diabetes. Balanitis occurring within 24 hours of unprotected vaginal intercourse is likely to be due to a hypersensitivity reaction to the female partner's yeast infection. Treatment with topical antifungal creams or antifungal steroid combinations is usually effective.

Bacterial vaginosis

Bacterial vaginosis is the most common cause of offensive vaginal discharge, and results from an imbalance of commensal bacterial in the vagina. Lactobacilli are relatively decreased and a mixture of *Gardnerella vaginalis*, anaerobic bacteria and other organisms, sometimes including mycoplasmas and *Ureaplasma*, predominates. The anaerobic bacteria produce amines (e.g. putrescine and cadaverine).

History:

- Vaginal discharge with a fishy odour often worse after unprotected sex, as the ejaculate is alkaline and this makes the amines more volatile.
- Mild itch may occur but more significant vulval soreness and itch suggest a different/additional

cause (for example, trichomoniasis or BV plus candidiasis).
- Often there are no symptoms.

Examination:

- thin, homogeneous, whitish, sometimes frothy vaginal discharge that smells of fish.
- inflammation of the vulva, vagina and cervix is minimal.

Diagnosis:

- clinical
- can be confirmed using microscopy. Culture is unhelpful, *G. vaginalis* may be isolated in women without active BV.

Pelvic pain

Pelvic inflammatory disease

This is usually the result of infection ascending from endocervix up through the endometrium and endosalpinges.

Causes

- *Chlamydia trachomatis* (most common)
- *N. gonorrhoeae*
- *Mycoplasma genitalium*

Usually polymicrobial, including anaerobes ± coliforms.

Complications

- Chronic pelvic pain
- Fitz–Hugh–Curtis syndrome: right upper quadrant (RUQ) pain and tenderness due to perihepatitis.
- Tubal blockage and dysfunction of cilia causing ectopic pregnancy and tubal infertility.

Clinical diagnosis

History:

- sexual history
- previous STIs or episodes of PID
- contraceptive usage:
  - recent insertion of intrauterine contraceptive device (IUCD) increases risk of PID
- last menstrual period:
  - exclude ectopic pregnancy

- abdominal pain
  - central or bilateral lower abdominal pain
  - RUQ pain due to perihepatitis occurs in 10–20 per cent PIDs (Fitz–Hugh–Curtis syndrome)
- symptoms related to sex:
  - deep dyspareunia
  - post-coital bleeding
- irregular PV bleeding
- change in vaginal discharge
- urinary symptoms
  - dysuria may be a symptom of chlamydia or gonorrhoea
  - UTIs may give abdominal pain
- bowel symptoms
  - to suggest gastrointestinal cause of symptoms
- systemic symptoms including fevers, sweats.

More common in gonococcal PID ± tubo-ovarian abscess.

Examination:

- Assess the patient's vital signs – is the patient systemically unwell with high temperature, tachycardia, low blood pressure?
  - These patients need admission to assess response to intravenous antibiotics and to arrange further investigations as indicated.

> **IMPORTANT**
>
> The clinical diagnosis of PID is unreliable:
> - PID may be asymptomatic.
> - Clinical signs lack sensitivity and specificity.
> - There is a wide differential diagnosis.
> - Always screen for STIs including tests for *N. gonorrhoeae* and *C. trachomatis* from lower genital tract.
> - C-reactive protein (CRP) may be raised.
> - Always do a pregnancy test to exclude ectopic pregnancy.
> - Laparoscopy is not a first-line investigation but can provide a definite diagnosis and exclude other causes of pelvic pain including endometriosis and ovarian cysts in women who fail to respond to antibiotic treatment.
> - Ultrasound may also help to exclude other causes of pelvic/lower abdominal pain.

- Examine the abdomen:
  - lower abdominal tenderness
  - RUQ tenderness.
- Perform a bimanual examination to look for:
  - adnexal tenderness
  - uterine tenderness
  - cervical excitation (pain on moving the cervix during bimanual examination).
- Pass speculum:
  - Visualize cervix and look for inflammation with contact bleeding, mucopus arising from cervical os (mucopurulent cervicitis).
  - Perform STI screen with Gram stains and cultures for *N. gonorrhoeae* and NAAT testing for *Chlamydia* and *N. gonorrhoeae*.

Differential diagnosis

- Ectopic pregnancy
- Acute appendicitis
- Endometriosis
- Complications of ovarian cyst (e.g. torsion of ovary)
- Urinary tract infections/cystitis
- Bowel problems including irritable bowel syndrome and constipation
- Functional pain.

Urinary tract infections

Urinary tract infections (UTIs) are common in women, but uncommon in men under 50 years old (and recurrent infections in men indicate referral to urology to investigate underlying causes). Older men may get UTIs secondary to bladder outflow obstruction from prostatic hypertrophy, which may also require urological intervention.

Causes of cystitis

- Urinary tract pathogens arising from bowel flora, most commonly *Escherichia coli* and other coliforms, *Staphylococcus saprophyticus*, *Proteus* species.
- Recurrent bacterial cystitis may be triggered by inadequate fluid intake or by sex ('honeymoon cystitis').
- Abacterial cystitis – no organism isolated.
- *Chlamydia trachomatis* can give a painful haemorrhagic cystitis as well as dysuria and lower abdominal pain.

- Interstitial cystitis – not related to infection. Persistent troublesome symptoms often part of a vulva pain syndrome.

History:

- lower abdominal pain, dysuria, frequency, nocturia, strangury and sometimes haematuria
- loin pain and tenderness plus systemic symptoms of fever, malaise, anorexia and vomiting (suggesting ascending infection can cause pyelonephritis).

Men with prostatic hypertrophy may describe poor stream, hesitancy, dribbling after urination and incontinence.

Investigations:

- Send mid-stream urine (MSU) for microscopy, culture and sensitivity.
- If culture is negative or there is a risk of STI send first-catch urine for chlamydia NAAT.
- If recurrent proven UTI arrange renal ultrasound and plain abdominal X-ray to exclude underlying predisposing pathology (e.g. renal calculi). Referral to urology may be indicated.

Testicular pain

Epididymo-orchitis

Causes of epididymo-orchitis:

- sexually transmitted infections, most commonly *Chlamydia* and gonorrhoea (STIs are leading cause in 16–30-year-olds)
- urinary tract infections (more common in men over 40 years)
- viral infections – mumps
- tuberculosis (uncommon).

History:

- gradually increasing pain and tenderness in one or both testicles and or epididymes
- symptoms of associated conditions:
    - urethral discharge and dysuria (NGU)
    - dysuria, nocturia, frequency, strangury and haematuria (UTI)
    - parotid swellings, contact with mumps (mumps)
    - malaise, night sweats, weight loss (TB).

Examination:

- tenderness and swelling of one or both testicles and epididymes
- urethral discharge.

Diagnosis:

- Look for evidence of urethritis by microscopy of Gram-stained urethral smear for pus cells with or without the Gram-negative diplococci of *N. gonorrhoeae*.
- Examine first-catch urine for 'threads'. Screen for STIs.
- Dip test urine for blood, protein and nitrites. Send MSU if present for microscopy, culture and sensitivity.
- If indicated send paired serology for mumps.
- If tuberculosis suspected send three consecutive early morning urine collections for acid fast bacilli smear and tuberculosis culture.

Torsion of testis

- A surgical emergency where torsion of the spermatic cord and testicle cuts off its blood supply leading rapidly to necrosis of the testicle.
- History is of an abrupt onset of pain (often severe) in one testicle.
- More common under 20 years of age but can happen in older men.
- If suspected get urgent surgical/urological opinion.

Testicular tumours

- Usually painless and detected by scrotal examination.
- May give rise to pain in testicle.
- On examination hard or craggy lump felt within the testicle itself.
- If suspected arrange urgent testicular ultrasound.

IMPORTANT   *i*

If ultrasound confirms suspicious testicular lump refer urgently to urology for orchidectomy and then appropriate oncological treatment and follow-up.

Joint pains

Sexually acquired reactive arthritis

Sexually acquired reactive arthritis was previously referred to as part of the triad of Reiter's syndrome – urethritis, arthritis and conjunctivitis. Reactive arthritis is a sterile inflammation of synovial membrane, tendons and fascia triggered by infection at a distant site, usually gastrointestinal or genitourinary. SARA occurs in 0.8–4 per cent of cases of sexually acquired urethritis or cervicitis, is more common in men and in human leucocyte antigen (HLA)-B27-positive patients. The causes are:

- *C. trachomatis* (commonest)
- *N. gonorrhoeae* (<20 per cent)
- *Ureaplasma urealyticum.*

History:

- onset of arthritis usually within 3 months of sex with a new partner
- may be a family history of HLA-B27-related seronegative arthritis
- 80 per cent men give a recent history of urethral discharge with dysuria, sometimes with epididymo-orchitis
- women may complain of vaginal discharge arising from a mucopurulent cervicitis but they often have no genital symptoms or signs
- asymmetrical pain, swelling and stiffness of one or more joints (knees and feet are most commonly affected)
- lower back pain from sacroiliitis
- pain in the feet on walking especially over heels (inflammation of Achilles' tendon insertion and plantar fasciitis)
- red eyes: conjunctivitis or uveitis (pain, photophobia and blurring of vision)
- itchy scaly plaques similar to psoriasis
- systemic symptoms: malaise, fatigue, fever.

Examination:

- asymmetrical joint swelling, tenderness and decreased range of movement
- tenderness and swelling at sites of tendon or fascial attachments and over tendon sheaths
- pain on direct sacral pressure (sacroiliitis)
- red eyes due to conjunctivitis or uveitis (slit-lamp examination essential if pain, photophobia and blurring of vision present)

- psoriasiform rash may occur including pustular psoriasis of soles of feet (keratoderma blennorrhagica)
- nail dystrophy
- stomatitis, oral ulceration and geographical tongue
- genital examination may detect urethral discharge and circinate balanitis in men or vulvitis, vaginal discharge and mucopurulent cervicitis in women.

Less common complications include:

- heart lesions: asymptomatic; tachycardia; rarely pericarditis and aortic valve disease
- renal pathology including proteinuria, microscopic haematuria, aseptic pyuria
- thrombophlebitis of lower limbs, subcutaneous nodules, meningoencephalitis, nerve palsies.

Disease progression:

- usually self-limiting over 4–6 months; 50 per cent have recurrent episodes
- aggressive arthritis more likely if HLA-B27-positive
- around 20 per cent may have chronic symptoms lasting over 12 months
- erosive joint damage may occur
- inadequately treated acute uveitis may lead to blindness.

Diagnosis:

- clinical
- Gram stain of male urethral discharge; culture for *N. gonorrhoeae*, NAAT for *C. trachomatis*, full screen for STIs
- investigation of arthritis: erythrocyte sedimentation rate, C-reactive protein, rheumatoid factor, plasma urate, angiotensin-converting enzyme (ACE) level, full blood count
- urinalysis
- HLA-B27 genotype
- X-rays of affected joints
- synovial fluid analysis
- ophthalmic assessment.

Septic arthritis – gonococcal

Disseminated gonococcal infection (DGI) occurs in 1–3 per cent of cases of gonorrhoea. It is more common in women and MSM in whom asymptomatic mucosal infection is frequent. Most have arthritis or arthralgia as a principal symptom. Septic arthritis may be very joint destructive.

There are two clinical syndromes, which may represent different stages of DGI:

- triad of tenosynovitis, dermatitis and poly-arthralgia:
  - small sterile joint effusions
  - blood cultures only positive if taken within two days of acute onset
- purulent arthritis without associated skin lesions:
  - usually affects one joint, often the knee, ankle or wrist. *N. gonorrhoeae* can be isolated from aspirated effusion
  - blood cultures negative.

Rare complications include endocarditis, meningitis, osteomyelitis.

History:

- sexual history – assess recent risks of exposure to *N. gonorrhoeae*
- genital symptoms – urethral/vaginal discharge
- proctitis – pain on defecation, blood or discharge per rectum
- joint symptoms – which affected, pain, swelling, redness, decreased range of movement
- skin lesions
- systemic symptoms, fever and malaise.

Examination:

- There may be a polyarthralgia (usually affecting knees, wrists, small joints of hand, ankles and elbows) with small sterile effusions or septic arthritis – red, hot, tender joint(s).

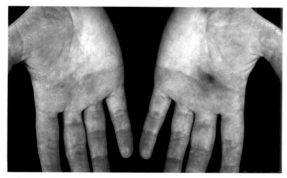

Figure 11.6 Disseminated gonococcal infection lesion on palm.

- Skin lesions start as red macules and become either vesiculopapular then pustular or haemorrhagic then purpuric (especially on palms and soles). Small in number, painful and often close to affected joint, they last 4–5 days but cropping may occur (Fig. 11.6).

Diagnosis:

- All patients should have full STI screen.
- Blood cultures.
- Aspirate joint effusions for microscopy and culture.

Genital ulceration

Genital herpes

Genital herpes is caused by HSV types 1 and 2. Following primary infection, HSV ascends sensory nerves from the site of initial infection and becomes latent in local sensory ganglia. Viral reactivation causes episodes of recurrent herpes or asymptomatic shedding (asymptomatic shedding is common and often the source of onward transmission). Seventy-five per cent of people infected with HSV are not aware that they have genital herpes either because their symptoms are very mild/absent or because the symptoms have been assumed to be due to something else (most commonly thrush).

History:

- sexual history including cold sores in sexual partners and oral sex
- previous similar episodes
- painful genital lesions – blisters or ulcers
- may be preceded by prodromal symptoms of tingling in same area or pain in the back, buttock and back of leg
- itching, soreness, discharge which may mimic candidiasis with vulval/perineal/perianal itch, soreness and vaginal/urethral discharge
- swelling of vulva or prepuce
- tender or swollen groin lymph nodes
- dysuria
- difficulty passing urine – may become intensely painful/acute urinary retention
- systemic symptoms – malaise, fever, headache, myalgia.

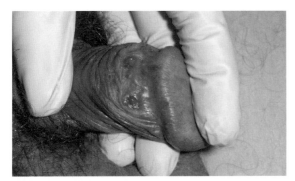

Figure 11 7 Recurrent herpes on penis.

Examination:

- tender, superficial ulceration:
  - women may have extensive involvement of vulva, perineum and cervix associated with labial oedema especially in primary herpes. It may be too painful to pass a speculum during an acute episode
  - men commonly get ulcers on the glans penis, prepuce or penile shaft (Fig. 11.7)
- perianal and intra-anal/rectal lesions can occur
- in recurrent episodes localized small clusters of superficial painful blisters which progress to tender ulcers are common
- tender lymph nodes in groins.

Complications:

- psychological
- adhesions
- secondary infection of lesions
- sacral radiculopathy – leading to urinary retention, constipation
- aseptic meningitis
- erythema multiforme.

Diagnosis:

- Initial provisional diagnosis is based on clinical history and examination.
- Confirmation by HSV culture or PCR on swabs from ulcers/blisters.
- HSV serology is not used routinely in the UK because of the limitations in usefulness and poor predictive value in low prevalence populations. Complement fixation tests (CFTs) are of poor specificity in differentiating between HSV type 1

and type 2. Positive CFTs may simply reflect previous perioral cold sores. IgM antibody response to primary infection may take many weeks to develop. More specific glycoprotein G antibody tests are expensive but better at differentiating between past infections with the two strains. However, 50 per cent of primary genital HSV is due to HSV type 1 infection.

- Dark ground tests if primary syphilis possible.
- Syphilis serology and HIV serology.
- Full STI screen when symptoms allow.

Genital ulcer differential diagnosis:

- genital herpes
- excoriations (e.g. secondary to vulvovaginitis)
- syphilis, primary and secondary
- HIV including seroconversion illness
- herpes zoster
- idiopathic ulceration
- erythema multiforme
- Behçet's disease
- tropical ulcers.

Syphilis

Syphilis is caused by the spirochaete *Treponema pallidum*. The incidence of syphilis in the UK has increased since 2000. There have been recent outbreaks in both heterosexual and MSM sexual networks. Long-term complications occur in 30–40 per cent of untreated individuals and include gummatous disease (a granulomatous nodule with a necrotic centre and fibrous capsule), cardiovascular syphilis and neurosyphilis. Pregnant women with infectious syphilis have a high risk of vertical transmission with fetal intrauterine death or congenital syphilis. Syphilis significantly increases the risk of HIV transmission.

Infectious syphilis (early syphilis)

This occurs in the first 2 years after infection. The infection may be divided into primary, secondary or early latent syphilis on the basis of clinical findings and serology results.

Primary syphilis

History:

- Lesions appear 9–90 days (commonly 2–3 weeks) after exposure: one or more painless chancre(s) develop at the site of inoculation.

Parenchymatous disease (10–20 years after untreated initial infection)

Chronic progressive meningoencephalitis causing cerebral atrophy – dementia and general paralysis of the insane (GPI).

History:

- may come from carers or relatives – poor memory, dulling of intellect, lack of insight and judgement, delusions and confusion, mood swings
- convulsions
- incontinence.

Examination:

- assess mental status
- look for:
  - fine tremor of lips, tongue and hands
  - dysarthria
- examine pupils (Argyll Robertson pupils in about 25 per cent)
- examine tendon reflexes and plantar response (hyperactive tendon reflexes and extensor plantar responses from pyramidal tract lesions)
- spastic paraplegia.

Tabes dorsalis (15–25 years after infection)

History:

- attacks of severe pains
  - acute 'lightning' attacks often affecting the legs
  - acute onset episodes of epigastric pain and vomiting (gastric crisis)
  - symptoms of other tabetic crises due to smooth muscle spasm which can affect rectum, bladder, urethra, kidneys and larynx
- unsteadiness (ataxia)
- incontinence
- impotence.

Examination:

- high-stepping gait
- loss of tendon reflexes and impaired deep pain, vibration and position sense. Positive Romberg's sign (dorsal column degeneration)
- bilateral ptosis
- Argyll Robertson pupils in about 50 per cent
- optic atrophy
- Charcot's joints.

Cardiovascular syphilis

- May develop 10–30 years after infection in about 10 per cent of untreated patients.
- Aortitis:
  - coronary artery ostia stenosis
  - calcification and aneurysm of ascending aorta
  - aortic regurgitation.

History:

- initially asymptomatic
- later symptoms include:
  - dull substernal pain
  - angina
  - paroxysmal nocturnal dyspnoea (left ventricular failure)
  - stridor, cough, dysphagia and Horner's syndrome (pressure symptoms from the aneurysm).

Examination:

- signs of aortic regurgitation.

Diagnosis of late syphilis:

- clinical findings
- syphilis serology – raised VDRL and TPPA
- CSF – raised white cell count, protein and positive VDRL/FTA/TPPA
- chest X-ray.

Congenital syphilis

Untreated early infectious syphilis in a pregnant woman has a 70–100 per cent risk of transmission to the baby resulting in stillbirth in up to a third of cases.

Early congenital syphilis – presenting within 2 years of birth

Signs include snuffles, vesiculo-bullous lesions, condylomata lata, lymphadenopathy and hepatosplenomegaly.

Late congenital syphilis – presenting over 2 years old

- Examine:
  - face – saddle nose, flat face with frontal bossing, linear scars (rhagades) at corners of mouth
  - teeth – Hutchinson's incisors (small, pegged and centrally notched) and Moon's molars (rounded)
  - eyes – choroido-retinitis
  - bones – sabre tibia
  - neurological deficits, e.g. deafness.

Problems with syphilis serology:

- May be negative in early primary infection.
- Low grade positive serology often persists after successful treatment.
- Unable to distinguish syphilis from other treponemal infections, e.g. yaws, endemic syphilis and pinta.
- Acute false-positive VDRL occurs after immunizations and with viral infections.
- Chronic false-positive VDRL occurs with autoimmune diseases (sometimes before they declare themselves) and leprosy.

Chancroid

Chancroid is an STI caused by *Haemophilus ducreyi*. It is uncommon in the UK.

History:

- recent sexual contacts in high prevalence areas e.g. Africa and Asia (incubation period is 3–10 days)
- painful ulcers on genitals or perianally
- tenderness in groins.

Examination:

- One or more painful ulcers at the site of bacterial inoculation. These so called 'soft sores', are not indurated, have a necrotic base, ragged undermined edge, and bleed easily.
- Tender groin lymphadenopathy which progresses to form fluctuant buboes.
- Complications are more common in men who may develop phimosis or partial loss of tissue of the glans penis ('phagedenic ulcer').
- Systemic spread does not occur with chancroid.

Diagnosis:

- Often made on clinical grounds with exclusion of other causes of genital ulceration.
- Culture of *H. ducreyi* is rarely available.
- PCR tests are very sensitive and usually done as part of the multiplex PCR, which also looks for syphilis and HSV types 1 and 2.

Lymphogranuloma venereum

Lymphogranuloma venereum is an STI caused by *C. trachomatis* serovars L1, L2 and L3. It is highly prevalent in parts of Africa, Asia and South America but it is rare in western Europe. Recent outbreaks have been detected in some European cities in MSM (most of whom were also HIV positive). It is a marker of 'unsafe' sex and associated with other STIs, HIV and hepatitis C. LGV may cause unpleasant symptoms and long-term complications. It may be misdiagnosed (e.g. as Crohn's or cancer).

History:

- sexual history and risk factors
- painless erosions/ulcers on genitals, perianal region or in mouth – the primary lesion (appears after incubation for 3–30 days) is transient and may be unnoticed.

Examination:

- A painless papule/pustule/shallow erosion may be seen at site of bacterial inoculation – the primary lesion is transient and may be unnoticed.
- Secondary lesions (usually 10–30 days after primary):
  - Inflamed and swollen regional lymph glands, e.g. in groin (inguinal syndrome)
  - acute haemorrhagic proctitis (anorectal syndrome)
  - periadenitis and bubo formation occurs and may ulcerate, discharging pus and creating chronic fistulas
  - 15–20 per cent develop the 'groove sign': lymph nodes in femoral and inguinal systems separated by inguinal ligament
  - systemic spread is associated with fever, arthritis, pneumonitis, perihepatitis.
- Tertiary phase lesions:
  - proctitis
  - acute proctocolitis
  - fistulae
  - strictures
  - chronic granulomatous disfiguring condition of the vulva ('esthiomene').

Long-term complications:

- lymphoedema of genitals (elephantitis) with persistent suppuration and pyoderma
- association with rectal cancer.

Diagnosis:

- swabs from ulcers/inflamed rectal mucosa for NAAT (PCR) for *Chlamydia*. If positive, reconfirm and send to reference lab for serotyping
- if bubo present aspirate and send for PCR as above
- serology (e.g. CFT, micro-IF).

Donovanosis (granuloma inguinale)

Donovanosis is caused by *Klebsiella granulomatis*. It is not commonly seen in the UK, and it is seen only in patients with sexual contacts in tropical countries.

History:

- sexual history and risk factors
- ano-genital ulcers and enlarged lymph nodes.

Examination:

- painless friable ano-genital ulcers or hypertrophic lesions associated with enlarged regional lymph nodes
- abscesses and pseudo-buboes in tissues overlying the groin lymph nodes
- untreated the lesions may spontaneously resolve or slowly spread causing local tissue destruction and rarely haematogenous spread to bones and viscera.

Diagnosis:

- commonly made by identifying Donovan bodies in smears or tissue biopsies.

Genital lumps

Genital warts

Genital warts are caused by human papilloma virus (HPV). There are over 100 strains of HPV, but only a few (mainly types 6 and 11) cause external genital warts. These HPV types are *not* associated with cervical cancer.

HPV infections are very common. About 80 per cent of the sexually active population will carry HPV in their genital tract at some time. Most infections (90 per cent) do not result in visible warts but are subclinical (they may still be infectious to others). Most infections are self-limiting over time though it may take several months or even years to clear during which the visible warts may recur.

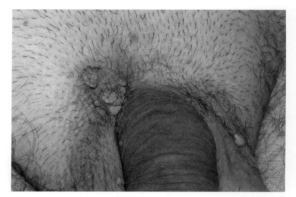

Figure 11.10 Warts at base of penis.

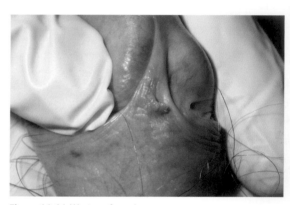

Figure 11.11 Wart on frenulum.

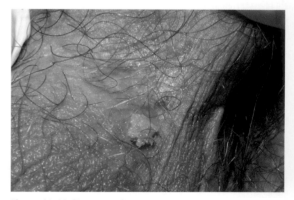

Figure 11.12 Close-up of wart.

History:

- warty lumps on genitals or around anus
- vaginal discharge
- genital itch – may occur with warts especially when the virus is becoming more active prior to warts appearing.

Examination:

- warts may vary in size, number and appearance (Figs 11.10–11.12).
- usually feel 'gritty' to fingertip.

Molluscum contagiosum

Molluscum contagiosum is caused by a pox virus, and is often misdiagnosed as genital warts.

History:

- itchy lumps – in adults these lesions are usually found on the genitals, buttocks, thighs or abdomen.

Examination:

- small, smooth, umbilicated, papular skin lesions.
- in immunocompromised HIV patients, lesions may be found in other sites (e.g. the face).

Molluscum contagiosum occurs in children in non-genital locations (e.g. the arms) resulting from innocent non-sexual contact. The lesions are self-limiting but may cause itch. Scratching the lesions may auto-inoculate the virus into adjacent skin.

Infestations

Pediculosis pubis – pubic lice/'crabs' (Phthirus pubis)

Pubic lice (Fig. 11.13) may be spread by intimate contact with an infested contact or by shared bedding and clothing of a heavily infested person. Sexual contact is not essential.

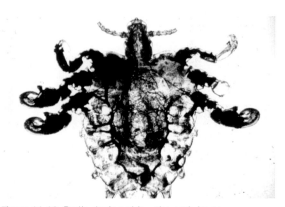

Figure 11.13 *Pediculosis pubis* – the crab louse.

History:

- pubic itch
- sometimes patients notice the lice moving or see the eggs attached in the hairs.

Examination:

- Public lice look like small brown freckles – you may see them move.
- The eggs attached in the hairs.
- Pubic lice may be found in hairs on the legs and abdomen of more hirsute patients and in eyelashes and eyebrows. They do not thrive in the denser hair of the head.

Scabies

Scabies is an infestation caused by the *Sarcoptes scabiei* mite which burrows into skin and then lays its eggs. Transmission is by skin to skin contact as may occur in both sexual and non-sexual contact. Fomite spread may also occur – mites can survive up to 72 hours away from the body. The symptoms may take 4–6 weeks to develop.

History:

- generalized pruritus (often sparing the head and neck) worse at night, caused by a hypersensitivity reaction to the mite's excrement.

Examination:

- Burrows may be seen between the fingers and at the wrists and elbows.
- Lesions in the genital area are often papular or nodular.
- Immunocompromised patients including those with HIV may develop crusted lesions that are highly transmissible (Norwegian scabies).
- Diagnosis is usually made on the basis of clinical appearance but scrapings from burrows examined under light microscopy can confirm the infestation.

Blood-borne viruses

HIV

Primary HIV infection (PHI)/seroconversion illness

History:

- PHI may be asymptomatic.

- Symptoms of PHI usually occur 2–6 weeks after acquiring HIV and vary in severity from mild and transient to acutely debilitating:
  - generalized rash
  - generalized lymphadenopathy, pharyngitis (glandular fever-like symptoms)
  - acute oro-genital ulceration
  - myalgia, arthralgia, fever, headache (flu-like or viral meningitis-like symptoms)
  - acute nausea, anorexia and diarrhoea.

Examination:

- pyrexia
- widespread maculo-papular rash
- superficial ulceration or deeper aphthous ulcers in mouth and ano-genital areas
- pharyngitis
- generalized lymphadenopathy and hepatosplenomegaly
- neck stiffness and photophobia.

Diagnosis:

- Early in seroconversion the HIV antibody test may be negative. Newer fourth generation tests detect HIV earlier by identifying both HIV IgM and p24 antigen. Always specify 'possible seroconverter' on request form. If tests negative repeat after 2 weeks.
- Patients with HIV usually experience several years without any symptoms following recovery from seroconversion. Patients remain infectious during this period and at risk of progression to AIDS and death.
- Since 1996 drug therapy with highly active antiretroviral therapy (HAART) has had a huge impact on life expectancy and quality of life of patients living with HIV.
- With appropriate healthcare HIV-positive patients may now live a near normal lifespan.
- HAART has also reduced the risk of mother-to-child HIV transmission from 20–40 per cent (dependent on mother's health and co-factors for transmission) to less than 1 per cent.
- Undiagnosed and untreated, HIV infection progressively destroys the immune system.

Patients with HIV-related immunodeficiency

History:

- prolonged episodes of herpes simplex
- persistent frequently recurrent candidiasis
- oral candidiasis
- odd-looking mouth lesions, e.g. oral hairy leucoplakia, Kaposi's sarcoma
- recently developed or worsened seborrhoeic dermatitis or psoriasis
- molluscum contagiosum on the face
- unexplained weight loss or night sweats
- persistent diarrhoea
- gradually increasing shortness of breath and dry cough
- recurrent bacterial infections including pneumocystis pneumonia (PCP; Fig. 11.14)
- indicator diseases, e.g. tuberculosis, lymphoma and PCP.

Diagnosis:

- It is important to consider testing for HIV in any patient with symptoms that might suggest HIV-related disease.

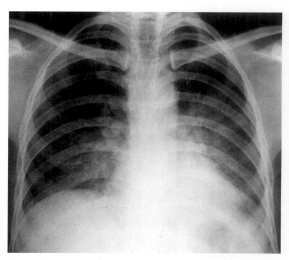

Figure 11.14 Pneumocystis pneumonia in a patient with human immunodeficiency virus infection.

Hepatitis B

- The hepatitis B virus (HBV) is a DNA virus that can be easily transmitted by sexual contact. It is readily transmitted vertically from mother to child at delivery.
- Other routes of transmission include injecting drug use with shared contaminated equipment, needlestick injury, exposure to infected blood products/tissues.
- Sexually acquired HBV is more common among MSM, intravenous drug users, commercial sex workers, patients from high prevalence areas and their sexual contacts.
- High-risk patients are therefore screened for current HBV infection (surface antigen present) and evidence of previous infection and natural immunity (core antibody) or successful previous vaccination (surface antibody). Patients vulnerable to infection are then offered hepatitis B vaccination.
- HBV infection may cause acute hepatitis with jaundice or remain asymptomatic. Patients with chronic hepatitis are at risk of cirrhosis and hepatoma.
- See Viral hepatitis for more details (p. 381).

Hepatitis C

- The hepatitis C virus (HCV) is much more difficult to transmit sexually or vertically than HBV.
- The risk of sexual transmission of HCV is, however, significantly increased in individuals with HIV and in MSM practising high-risk sexual activities e.g. 'fisting' (insertion of a fist into the sexual partner's rectum for sexual gratification), which may traumatize the ano-rectal epithelium.
- More common routes of HCV transmission include injecting drug use with shared contaminated equipment, needle-stick injury, exposure to infected blood products/tissues.
- HCV infection may cause acute hepatitis with jaundice or remain asymptomatic. Patients with chronic hepatitis are at risk of cirrhosis and hepatoma.
- See Viral hepatitis for more details (p. 381).

SUMMARY

History – common presenting symptoms in patients with an STI or other genitourinary condition:

- women
    - vaginal discharge
    - vulval itching and/or soreness
    - dyspareunia (pain on intercourse)
    - pelvic and lower abdominal pain
    - irregular bleeding per vagina
- men
    - urethral discharge
    - dysuria
    - pain and swelling in the testicles/epididymis
- both sexes
    - painful genital ulceration
    - genital warts and other skin lumps
    - skin rashes
    - itchy skin
    - rectal pain or discharge (if receptive anal sex).

Sexual history – ask the following details about the last sexual contact:

- When was it?
- What kind of sex?
- Casual or regular contact?
- In a higher risk group/known to have an STIs or HIV?
- Where? (local/UK/abroad)

Also ask about:

- other sexual contacts in the last 3 and 12 months
- lifetime exposure to higher risk activities
- condom use.

Other important history:

- current contraception, current or previous pregnancies and LMP
- previous urinary or genital symptoms?
- other medical conditions that may predispose to genital symptoms.

Examination – general examination when indicated:

- look for systemic signs
- look for skin rashes
- examine inside mouth
- generalized lymphadenopathy?

Genital examination:

- examine groin for lymph nodes
- ?skin rashes/folliculitis in the pubic area/visible pubic lice or their eggs.

In men:

- examine penis, prepuce, scrotum and perianal area
- look for inflammation and erythema, blisters, ulceration, warts, molluscum contagiosum
- ?urethral discharge
- examine the scrotal contents for swelling/pain
- if history of receptive anal intercourse pass a proctoscope to look for inflammation/ulceration/pus/bleeding/warts.

In women:

- examine the vulva, introitus, perineum and perianal area
- using a vaginal speculum assess vaginal discharge and cervix
- bimanual PV examination
- pregnancy test on urine if abdominal pain.

Investigations – all new patients attending GUM clinics are encouraged to have testing for:

- *C. trachomatis* by NAAT on a first-catch urine in men and a cervical swab in women
- *N. gonorrhoea* both by NAAT and by swabs from urethra, cervix, pharynx and rectum as appropriate for microscopy, culture and sensitivity on selective media
- syphilis – by serological testing or by dark ground microscopy if a suspicious ulcerative lesion is found
- HIV – by blood test
- other tests may be offered on sexual history, symptoms and signs, e.g. herpes PCR, microscopy for BV/trichomoniasis/*Candida*.

FURTHER READING

British Association for Sexual Health and HIV (BASHH) guidelines. Available at: www.bashh.org/guidelines.

Pattman R, Snow M, Handy P, *et al.* (eds). 2005. *Oxford handbook of genitourinary medicine, HIV and AIDS*. Oxford: Oxford University Press.

12 THE NERVOUS SYSTEM

Adrian Wills

INTRODUCTION

In spite of rapid technological advances, the successful diagnosis of neurological disease depends on the ability to take a thorough history from patients, relatives and eyewitnesses. Skilled neurologists often have slightly obsessive personalities and may spend long hours perusing the medical records looking for a previously unrecognized nugget of clinical information which reveals the diagnosis. The three fundamental questions that need answering are always:

- Where is the lesion?
- What is the pathology?
- What is the treatment?

Inexperienced clinicians often order sophisticated (and expensive!) investigations hoping that the diagnosis may be revealed, but sadly this rarely happens. Many investigations are relatively sensitive but not necessarily disease specific: for instance, white matter lesions revealed by magnetic resonance imaging (MRI) of the brain have an entirely different significance in younger and elderly patients.

The neurological examination should be thought of as a form of hypothesis testing, scrutinizing ideas generated by the patient's history. However, students and trainee doctors are often assessed on their ability to perform a competent neurological examination, and in exams such as MRCP PACES, the neurology and cardiology stations are the main pass/fail discriminators in borderline candidates. The examination should be practised by rote so that it becomes almost reflexive in nature. With experience the most relevant components can be cherry-picked but to accomplish this safely may take years of training.

This chapter is confined mainly to the discussion of neurological illness in adults; paediatric neurology is a separate specialty and is covered in Chapter 22.

CLINICAL HISTORY

Headache

Headache is an extremely common symptom and most people experience some form of headache at some stage in their lives. There are numerous headache classification systems but the most practical strategy is to differentiate between acute and chronic syndromes: acute headaches may indicate sinister pathology, chronic headaches rarely do.

Acute headaches may be hyperacute (instantaneous) or evolve over hours to days. Instantaneous headaches may be extremely severe ('worst ever') and associated with loss of consciousness, meningism and focal neurological signs. The most common cause is a subarachnoid haemorrhage (Fig. 12.1) but there are many others (see Box 12.1).

BOX 12.1 CAUSES OF INSTANTANEOUS HEADACHE (LIFE-THREATENING CAUSES IN BOLD)

- **Subarachnoid haemorrhage**
- **Venous sinus thrombosis**
- **Cerebral haemorrhage (especially posterior fossa)**
- **Phaeochromocytoma**
- Low pressure headache
- Thunderclap and ice pick headaches

Headaches that evolve over days to hours may be sinister, particularly in a headache-naïve patient, although it is important to remember that even a first attack of migraine may lead to an urgent hospital admission. Meningism (neck stiffness, photophobia) demands urgent investigation and may be caused by bacterial (including tuberculosis) and viral meningitis or encephalitis (also associated with altered mentation, seizures and focal neurological signs). Migraine (throbbing headache),

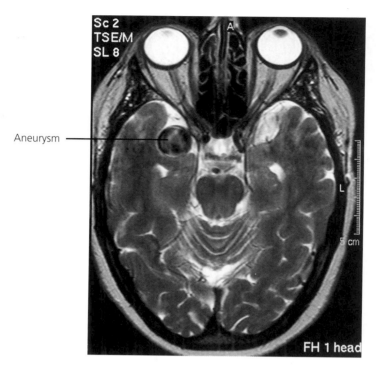

Aneurysm

Figure 12.1 T2-weighted magnetic resonance image showing a large aneurysm in the right temporal lobe.

often lasting several hours, is usually paroxysmal and associated with photophobia, visual symptoms (including scotomas, phosphenes and fortification spectra), phonophobia, nausea and/or vomiting and a desire to lie still or even sleep. This contrasts with other idiopathic paroxysmal headache disorders such as cluster headache, in which the pain is relieved by movement and is associated with autonomic features (see Box 12.2).

BOX 12.2 SYMPTOMS IN AUTONOMIC HEADACHE (INCLUDING CLUSTER)

- Eye watering
- Nasal stuffiness
- Horner's syndrome (paroxysmal)
- Isolated ptosis
- Conjunctival injection

Chronic headaches are usually benign and most often caused by tension headache or chronic daily headache (with or without associated analgesic overuse). The pain may be quite diffuse, nondescript,

maximal over the vertex with no particular exacerbating or relieving factors. 'Red flags' that should prompt further investigation include:

- pain worsened by lying flat, or pain that wakes the patient at night
- focal neurological symptoms/signs
- visual obscurations (transient blurring on standing – may indicate imminent coning)
- jaw claudication, shoulder aching and scalp tenderness (temporal arteritis in elderly patients)
- loss of visual acuity or haloes (glaucoma).

Acute glaucoma may cause marked systemic upset including headache, nausea, vomiting and malaise. Other caused of chronic headache are shown in Box 12.3. Trigeminal neuralgia is a particularly unpleasant lancinating pain (lasting seconds), mainly affecting the cheek and precipitated by speaking or touching the affected area. Low-pressure headaches are relatively common after neurosurgical shunt insertion or lumbar puncture (headache worse on standing up) but can occur 'spontaneously' because of leakage of cerebrospinal fluid (CSF) via the meninges (usually spinal).

BOX 12.3 RARER CAUSES OF CHRONIC HEADACHE
- Chronic carbon monoxide poisoning
- Obstructive sleep apnoea
- Hypercapnia
- Drugs
- Malignant hypertension (including eclampsia)
- Idiopathic intracranial hypertension
- Low pressure headaches
- Venous sinus thrombosis
- Post-traumatic (medico-legal cases)
- Subdural haematoma
- Polycythaemia

BOX 12.4 RARER CAUSES OF LOSS OF CONSCIOUSNESS
- Vertebro-basilar strokes, transient ischaemic attacks (TIAs) and migraine
- Hydrocephalic attacks
- Carotid sinus sensitivity
- Insulinoma
- Poor diabetes control

Loss of consciousness

The most common dilemma in everyday practice is differentiating between:

- seizure disorders
- cardiovascular syncope
- non-epileptic attacks (pseudoseizures).

The comments of an eyewitness are absolutely crucial; without this it is often impossible to make a diagnosis, although this is often revealed with the passage of time (watchful waiting). Table 12.1 shows the main historical discriminators. Other rarer causes are shown in Box 12.4. Syncopal attacks are more likely to be benign in younger patients but note that structural heart disease and arrhythmias are not confined to elderly people.

Patients may use the term 'blackout' and this covers a wide range of symptoms including:

- loss of consciousness
- pre-syncope (may be a white out)
- paroxysmal visual loss
- vertigo or dizziness
- falls.

Drop attacks may be idiopathic (sudden fall due to loss of tone in the legs without loss of consciousness) or precipitated by emotion e.g. laughter (cataplexy) often associated with other features of narcolepsy including vivid dreams and sleep paralysis.

CLINICAL PEARL
- Vertebro-basilar insufficiency and thoracic outlet syndrome are both rare conditions; try to think of alternative common diagnoses when a patient complains of dizziness on head movement or tingling in the hand (e.g. benign positional vertigo and carpal tunnel syndrome).
- Carpal tunnel syndrome can cause symptoms involving the whole arm.
- Isolated vertigo is rarely caused by migraine or epilepsy.

Table 12.1 Distinguishing between epilepsy, syncope and non-epileptic attacks

	Epilepsy	Syncope	Non-epileptic attack disorder
Pallor	–	+	–
Prodrome	–	+	–
Situational	–	+ orthostatic	+ stress
Incontinence	++	+	+
Lateral tongue biting	++	–	–
Jerking	++ prolonged	+ brief	+++ very prolonged
Pelvic thrusting	–	–	+++
Gaze aversion	–	–	+++
Nausea	–	++	–

Weakness

Hyperacute weakness is usually caused by *vascular disease* (stroke) and is most commonly unilateral, reflecting transient or permanent loss of perfusion in the cerebral hemispheres or brainstem. *TIAs* are classically defined as lasting up to 24 hours but in clinical practice are usually of much shorter duration. Bilateral weakness (usually lower limb) or quadriplegia is a marker of *spinal cord disease*.

Acute weakness

Acute weakness (evolving over hours to days) may also be unilateral or paraparetic, reflecting inflammatory or neoplastic disease involving the brain and spinal cord, respectively. Rapidly evolving quadriplegia may be associated with sensory symptoms (Guillain–Barré syndrome/diphtheria) or not (myasthenic crisis, botulism, polymyositis, polio). Most of these conditions can also lead to diaphragmatic involvement and bulbar dysfunction.

Chronic or progressive weakness

Chronic or progressive weakness may be indicative of a range of organic (Table 12.2) and non-organic pathologies (chronic fatigue syndrome/abnormal illness behaviour). Proximal weakness presents with difficulty on stairs, getting out of a chair or combing hair. Distal weakness usually manifests as 'trips' over pavements or uneven surfaces or difficulty doing up buttons, writing, etc. Fatiguability (as a symptom rather than sign) can be a remarkably unhelpful discriminator and is seen in a range of conditions other than myasthenia gravis.

Sensory symptoms

Positive (tingling, dysaesthesia, paraesthesia) and *negative* (numbness) sensory symptoms can reflect pathology anywhere in the sensory pathways. The presence of positive sensory symptoms can be useful in discriminating between *genetic* (Charcot–Marie Tooth, CMT) and *acquired* (chronic inflammatory demyelinating polyneuropathy, CIDP) neuropathies as well as epilepsy/migraine (positive) versus stroke (negative). Neuropathic pain (*cf* diabetes) is often lower limb predominant and described as burning, stinging or throbbing. Allodynia is defined as pain caused by normally non-painful stimuli (e.g. touch), whereas hyperpathia implies a lowered pain threshold.

Bladder symptoms

Urinary urgency, frequency (see Chapter 10) and nocturia are associated with an 'upper motor neurone (UMN)' bladder and characteristic of spinal cord disease, especially demyelination. A 'neuropathic' bladder (cauda equina, rarely caused by neuropathy) causes loss of bladder sensation with dribbling incontinence. Cord transection (usually traumatic) leads to complete loss of voluntary bladder control although automatic reflexive manoeuvres (e.g. stroking the thigh) can be utilized to assist bladder emptying. Frontal lobe disorders may lead to loss of inhibition with urination taking place in socially embarrassing (for the relatives rather than patient) situations.

Autonomic symptoms

A variety of neurological pathologies (Box 12.5) may lead to autonomic dysfunction and consequent symptoms including:

Table 12.2 Causes of chronic progressive weakness (with associated features)

	Distribution	Cranial nerve symptoms	Bladder symptoms	Sensory symptoms
Neuropathy	Distal	Rare	Rare	Common
Myopathy	Proximal	Unusual	Rare	Rare
Neuromuscular junction	Proximal	Common	Rare	Rare
Radiculopathy	Asymmetrical	Rare	Common (lumbosacral)	Common (pain)
Anterior horn	Asymmetrical	Common	Rare	Rare
Spinal cord	Pyramidal	Never	Common	Common
Brainstem	Pyramidal	Common	Rare	Common
Cerebral cortex	Pyramidal	Common	Rare (*cf* frontal)	Common

- sphincter disturbance (bladder and bowels)
- change in sweating pattern (excessive, loss of, gustatory)
- photophobia (pupillary dilatation, e.g. Adie pupil)
- night blindness (Horner's syndrome)
- orthostatic hypotension
- xerostomia (dry mouth, dry eyes)
- erectile and ejaculatory failure
- vomiting (gastroparesis).

BOX 12.5 NEUROLOGICAL CAUSES OF AUTONOMIC DYSFUNCTION

- Diabetic neuropathy
- Guillain–Barré syndrome
- Hereditary sensory and autonomic neuropathy (HSAN)
- Diphtheria
- Lambert–Eaton myasthenic syndrome (LEMS)
- Botulism
- Paraneoplastic disorders
- Autoimmune pandysautonomia
- Morvan's syndrome
- Enzyme deficiencies (e.g. tyrosine hydroxylase)

Cranial nerve symptoms

- *Anosmia* is usually caused by non-neurological pathologies (sinusitis, coryza), but it can be a useful marker following head injury and may occur in idiopathic Parkinson's disease and other rarer syndromes (Refsum's disease – heredopathia atactica polyneuritiformis). Anosmia is usually accompanied by a reduced sense of taste (dysgeusia).
- *Neurological visual loss* is more often bilateral, whereas *retinal pathology* tends to cause unilateral symptoms. Neurological field deficits tend to respect the vertical meridian, whereas retinal disorders respect the horizontal. Monocular loss of vision can be a harbinger of stroke, especially in elderly patients. Patients with homonymous hemianopia can complain of clumsiness (because they may ignore visual cues on the clinically affected side). Bitemporal hemianopias can cause particular difficulties with reading because of loss of fixation.
- *Diplopia* is usually of sudden onset. Sixth nerve palsies cause images to be 'side by side', whereas third and fourth nerve palsies tend to cause vertically related or angulated images. Monocular diplopia either reflects retinal or psychosomatic pathology. Fluctuating diplopia is classically described in myasthenia gravis but can occur in other conditions.
- *Hearing loss* can have a neurological origin: unilateral due to a cerebello-pontine lesion; bilateral due to mitochondrial disease, Sjögren's syndrome and other vasculitides, sarcoid, haemosiderosis. Vertigo is more commonly caused by labyrinthine disease: it worsens on eye closure and is precipitated by head movement. Meniere's disease causes a triad of hearing loss, vertigo and tinnitus.
- *Neurological dysphagia* may affect liquids first (remember to ask about nasal escape) whereas mechanical obstruction (oesophageal stricture) tends to preferentially affect the swallowing mechanism for solids. Neurological causes of dysphagia are shown in Box 12.6.

BOX 12.6 NEUROLOGICAL CAUSES OF DYSPHAGIA

- Stroke
- Brainstem tumours
- Motor neurone disease
- Guillain–Barré syndrome
- Polio and other enteroviruses
- Diphtheria
- Botulism
- Myasthenia gravis and Lambert–Eaton myasthenic syndrome
- Mitochondrial disease
  - Mitochondrial neurogastrointestinal encephalomyopathy (MNGIE) syndrome
- Rare genetic syndromes:
  - Oculopharyngeal muscular dystrophy (OPMD)
  - Fazio–Londe disease (progressive bulbar palsy of childhood)

The symptomatology of speech disorders and cognitive dysfunction will be covered in the examination section.

Disorders of sleep

Daytime somnolence is usually secondary to poor sleep hygiene (shift working, excessive alcohol consumption) but can be a feature of narcolepsy, idiopathic hypersomnolence or, rarely, tumours of the hypothalamic or pineal region. Obstructive sleep apnoea usually affects obese individuals with a history of loud snoring and fragmented sleep and may also present with daytime somnolence.

Abnormal motor activity in sleep is relatively common. Most people experience myoclonic jerks on falling asleep at some stage in their lives but if the myoclonus becomes prolonged or spills over into wakefulness this should be investigated. Abnormal nocturnal motor activity (e.g. sleepwalking, kicking movements) is usually secondary to a non-rapid eye movement (REM) parasomnia but frontal lobe epilepsy also needs to be considered. The acting out of dreams can be dangerous and is seen in REM sleep disorders because of a failure of the mechanisms leading to muscle paralysis; these patients may have features of parkinsonism.

Orthopnoea is usually caused by cardiac or respiratory disease, but ventilatory failure due to diaphragmatic weakness can be a presenting feature of motor neurone disease and some muscular dystrophies. The accessory muscles of respiration tend to be relatively inefficient in the supine posture and this is compounded during REM sleep. Patients with night-time hypoxia can complain of nocturnal enuresis (diuresis induced by overactivity of atrial natriuretic peptide) as well as daytime somnolence and early morning headaches.

EXAMINATION

The neurological examination can be broken down into component parts:

- higher function and speech
- cranial nerves
- limbs
- gait
- special situations.

Every patient should have a general medical examination, paying particular attention to blood pressure, weight, urinalysis, the cardiovascular, respiratory and abdominal systems and the presence of skin lesions. Examination of the back is often forgotten: look for kyphosis and scapular winging. Listen for bruits (spinal arteriovenous fistula).

Higher function and speech

All right-handers (and 40 per cent of left-handers) are left hemisphere dominant; therefore make a record of the patient's handedness. The Mini-mental State Examination (www.minimental.com) is useful but relatively insensitive in frontal lobe disorders. A score of less than 24 may suggest a dementing process but depressive pseudodementia and acute confusional states may cause diagnostic difficulty. The presence or absence of primitive reflexes (Box 12.7) can be useful in differentiating between dementia and pseudodementia.

BOX 12.7 PRIMITIVE REFLEXES
- Palmo-mental – involuntary contraction of mentalis elicited by stimulation of the thenar eminence.
- Grasp – apply distally moving deep pressure over part of the palmar surface.
- Rooting – patient turns mouth towards tactile stimulus on ipsilateral cheek.
- Sucking – place spatula or spoon in patient's mouth.
- Pout reflex – closure of the mouth with pouting of the lips elicited by tapping around the mouth is non-specific and can occur in UMN pathology and may be associated with a prominent jaw jerk.

Speech may be classified as:

- dysphasic
- dysphonic (p. 196)
- dysarthric (p. 196).

Dysphasia (aphasia), defined as impairment in the production of language, usually implies cortical dysfunction. Dysphasia can be divided into receptive and expressive components. *Receptive dysphasia* sounds fluent but nonsensical with poor comprehension (Wernicke's). *Expressive dysphasia* (Broca's) is often agrammatical and hesitant but comprehension is usually preserved. In this situation, asking the patient to follow commands can test comprehension. Repetition can be useful (e.g. say after me 'no ands ifs or buts') and is usually impaired in Broca's, Wernicke's and conduction (lesion in arcuate fasciculus) aphasia.

Tests of *frontal lobe function* performed at the bedside include cognitive estimates (e.g. 'How far is it to Paris?'), but remember to take into account the educational background of the patient. Other tests, which can be applied selectively, include verbal fluency and Luria's three-step sequence: ask the patient to copy you as you make a fist, then put your palm vertical on table, the put palm flat on table – repeat in sequence and, when the patient has mastered the sequence, observe as they continue the sequence alone. Failure to perform the sequence is considered an abnormal response. The examiner holding out a hand and observing that the patient will repetitively attempt to perform a handshake demonstrates perseveration.

Dyspraxia is defined as an inability to perform a complex sequence of movements where a command has been understood and in the absence of significant motor or sensory deficits. Asking the patient to copy certain hand positions or mime an action can test this. Impairment usually implies dysfunction of the contralateral parietal lobe. Dressing and constructional dyspraxias (e.g. copy a clock face) are seen in non-dominant parietal lobe lesions.

Agnosia means non-recognition and may be visual, tactile or auditory. Placing a familiar object in the subject's hand with eyes closed may test for tactile agnosia. The pathology is usually in the contralateral parietal lobe. Visual agnosias include prosopagnosia, which implies an inability to recognize familiar faces. This is commonly associated with bilateral lesions of the parieto-occipital regions. Various classifications of memory are used, including:

- long/short term
- episodic/semantic
- retrograde/anterograde
- visual/verbal.

Digit span is not a test of memory but of alertness (patients with Korsakoff's psychosis often have preserved digit span). To assess digit span, say random numbers (such as 5–7–2–4) and ask the patient to repeat them back. Incrementally increase the list of numbers by one digit each time. A normal adult digit span is 7 ± 2 digits.

THE CRANIAL NERVES

I Olfactory

If smell bottles are unavailable, ask about sense of smell. Anosmia can be a useful sign particularly when gauging the severity of head injuries.

II Optic

Test colour vision with Ishihara charts. When acquired loss of colour vision is associated with loss of visual acuity this implies optic nerve dysfunction. The Snellen and Jensen charts have overlapping functions but the former is more sensitive. Each eye should be tested in turn and a correction for refractive errors documented either using the patient's glasses or a pinhole. In papilloedema (Fig. 12.2) due to raised intracranial pressure visual acuities are preserved until late in the disease process. This contrasts with optic neuritis or infiltration, where acuity is often markedly impaired.

Test the visual fields by sitting opposite the patient (Fig. 12.3). Uncooperative or aphasic patients can have their fields crudely measured by observing their reaction to menace (pretend to poke their eye with your finger!). Test for visual inattention first and then ask the patient to close each eye in

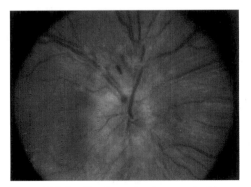

Figure 12.2 Papilloedema due to a cerebral tumour. From: Ogilvie C, Evans CC (eds), *Chamberlain's symptoms and signs in clinical medicine* (12th edition), with permission. © 1997 London: Hodder Arnold.

CLINICAL PEARL

The duration of anterograde amnesia is an extremely useful indicator of the severity of head injury.

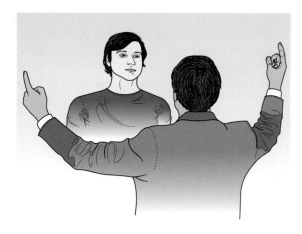

Figure 12.3 Testing visual fields by confrontation. From: Gray D, Toghill P (eds), *An introduction to the symptoms and signs of clinical medicine*, with permission. © 2001 London: Hodder Arnold.

turn, comparing their visual field with yours. Subtle defects can be picked up with a red pin, which is also used to document the blind spots.

In general, monocular defects are usually caused by ocular, retinal or optic nerve pathology. Constricted fields occur in glaucoma or chronic papilloedema. Tunnel vision may arise in association with retinitis pigmentosa and should not be confused with tubular vision in hysterical patients. Central scotomas are usually caused by optic nerve or macular disease (Fig. 12.4). Altitudinal defects (horizontal meridian) indicate retinal vascular pathology or ischaemic optic neuropathy. Defects affecting both eyes may indicate a lesion of or behind the optic chiasm (vertical meridian). The common patterns of field loss are shown in Figure 12.4.

Test the pupillary reactions to light and accommodation. Pupils of different sizes (anisocoria) with accentuation of the difference in dim light suggests a sympathetic defect.

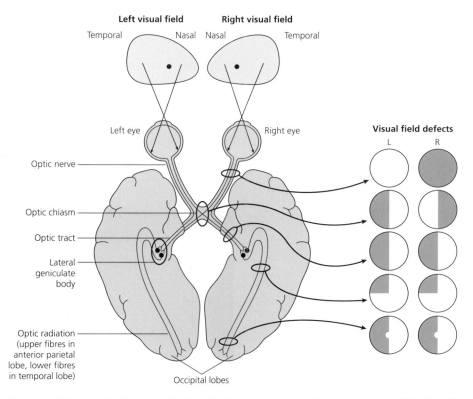

Figure 12.4 Diagram of the visual pathways with visual field defects produced by lesions at specific sites. From: Gray D, Toghill P (eds), *An introduction to the symptoms and signs of clinical medicine*, with permission. © 2001 London: Hodder Arnold.

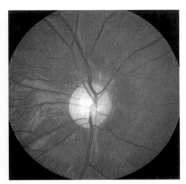

Figure 12.5 Primary optic atrophy. From: Ogilvie C, Evans CC (eds), *Chamberlain's symptoms and signs in clinical medicine* (12th edition), with permission. © 1997 London: Hodder Arnold.

There are four main causes of a unilaterally dilated pupil:

- oculomotor palsy
- tonic (Adie) pupil – the pupil does not react to light but does react to accommodation (light-near dissociation)
- iris damage – the pupil is usually irregular
- administration (which may be surreptitious) of atropine or scopolamine.

The Argyll Robertson pupil (which, like an Adie pupil, shows light-near dissociation) is usually small, irregular and bilateral. Syphilis is the usual cause and the lesion is thought to be in the rostral mid-brain.

Horner's syndrome is caused by interruption of sympathetic fibres. The pupil is small and reacts normally to light and accommodation. The main clinical features are miosis, mild ptosis, upside down ptosis (lower lid elevation), apparent enophthalmos, transient conjunctival hyperaemia and iris heterochromia (more common in congenital Horner's). The causative lesion may be in the brain, spinal cord, brachial plexus or sympathetic chain. Episodic anisocoria may occur in seizures, migraine and cluster headache.

Perform funduscopy, looking at the disc, vessels and retinal background. Beware of diagnosing unilateral optic atrophy (Fig. 12.5) where colour vision is preserved. The swinging flashlight test (Marcu–Gunn pupil or relative afferent papillary defect) is a useful check in this situation. Accommodation should be normal in a relative afferent papillary defect.

III Oculomotor, IV trochlear, VI abducens

All external ocular muscles are supplied by cranial nerve III except the lateral rectus and superior

Right eye

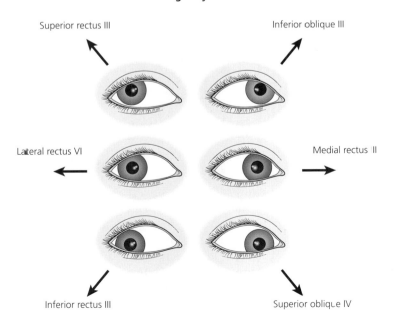

Figure 12.6 A simplified scheme of the action of cranial nerves III, IV and VI and the individual muscles on eye movements. From: Gray D, Toghill P (eds), *An introduction to the symptoms and signs of clinical medicine*, with permission. © 2001 London: Hodder Arnold.

oblique muscles (supplied by VI and IV, respectively). If the patient complains of double vision:

- the false image is always outermost
- the false image disappears when the affected eye is covered
- the diplopia is maximal in the direction of action of the affected muscle.

Oculomotor palsies (Fig. 12.6) are usually accompanied by complete ptosis because of interruption of fibres supplying levator palpebrae superioris. This contrasts with Horner's syndrome, in which the ptosis is subtle, and the pupil is constricted. A pupil-involving oculomotor palsy is usually caused by a surgical lesion, particularly a posterior communicating artery aneurysm. Lateral rectus palsies cause horizontal diplopia whereas superior oblique palsies are worse on looking inferomedially such as when descending stairs or reading. Vertical nystagmus is far more likely to be neurological in origin than horizontal nystagmus, which can also occur in vestibular dysfunction. When testing smooth pursuit movements always look for a jerky quality or saccadic intrusion, which accompanies cerebellar and brainstem disease. Finally, ask the patient to look at alternating targets to demonstrate hypo- or hypermetria (undershooting or overshooting the appropriate position, respectively) and an internu-

clear ophthalmoplegia (an impairment of *adduction* of the affected eye on horizontal gaze).

V Trigeminal

The trigeminal nerve consists of motor and sensory components and supplies the muscles of mastication as well as general sensation to the face via its ophthalmic, maxillary and mandibular divisions (Fig. 12.7). The corneal reflex has a consensual component. This is particularly useful in the presence of an ipsilateral facial nerve palsy leading to facial weakness. On mouth opening the direction of deviation of the jaw is ipsilateral to the lesion. The jaw jerk is tested by tapping the point of the mandible with a tendon hammer; if pathologically brisk this implies pathology above midbrain level (e.g. pseudobulbar palsies).

VII Facial

Lower motor neurone (LMN) palsies tend to cause complete ipsilateral facial weakness, whereas the upper face is relatively preserved in UMN lesions (because of bilateral representation). Ask the patient to shut their eyes tight, raise their eyebrows and smile or purse their lips. The chorda tympani branch accompanies the facial nerve along some of its length and this explains why patients with Bell's palsy (Fig. 12.8) may complain of loss of taste from the anterior two-thirds of the tongue. This can be tested by applying various sweet/bitter/salty solutions. General sensation to the anterior two-thirds of the tongue is supplied by the trigeminal nerve, whereas the glossopharyngeal supplies taste and general sensation to the posterior third.

VIII Auditory

Cranial nerve VIII has auditory and vestibular components. Remember to use an auroscope.

Rinne's test

Whisper into the subject's ear from a distance of 1 m and compare both sides. Patients should hear a 512 Hz vibrating tuning fork more loudly when it is placed in the air (air conduction > bone conduction) adjacent to the pinna compared with resting it on the mastoid process (Rinne test). This is reversed in conductive deafness where bone conduction is better than air conduction.

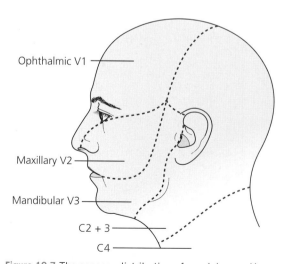

Figure 12.7 The sensory distribution of cranial nerve V. From: Gray D, Toghill P (eds), *An introduction to the symptoms and signs of clinical medicine*, with permission. © 2001 London: Hodder Arnold.

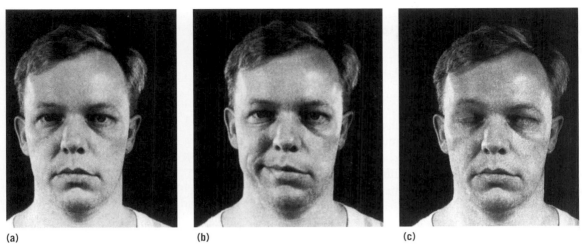

(a)   (b)   (c)

Figure 12.8 Left Bell's palsy. (a) At rest, the nasolabial fold is less prominent and the corner of the mouth droops. (b) On smiling. (c) On attempted closure of the eyes, the left eye rolls upward. From: Gray D, Toghill P (eds), *An introduction to the symptoms and signs of clinical medicine*, with permission. © 2001 London: Hodder Arnold.

Weber s test

Place a vibrating 512 Hz tuning fork in the middle of the patient's forehead. In unilateral *sensorineural* hearing loss the sound is heard louder on the contralateral side. In unilateral *conductive* loss the sound is heard louder on the ipsilateral side. Hallpike's manoeuvre is performed by rapidly lying the patient flat with their head turned to one side. The patient needs to be instructed to report sensations of dizziness while the examiner observes for nystagmus. Latency and fatiguability on repeated manoeuvres suggest a vestibular lesion. Have a vomit bowl handy! Note that Romberg's test (standing the patient upright with eyes closed and noting an increased sway with a tendency to fall) may be positive in vestibular disease.

IX Glossopharyngeal

Cranial nerve IX forms the afferent limb of the gag reflex and can be tested by applying an orange stick to the back of the throat. However, many normal subjects show remarkable tolerance to this manoeuvre. Where dysphagia is a problem the gag reflex is not particularly useful and a much more robust means of assessing the likelihood of aspiration is to ask the patient to swallow a small quantity of water. Doctors can do this just as easily as speech therapists. Clearly in motor disorders such as motor neurone

disease the presence of impaired palatal sensation should lead to a diagnostic reappraisal.

X Vagus

This nerve supplies the palatal musculature. In unilateral lesions the palate is deviated away from the affected side. Ask the patient to say 'aaaah'.

XI Accessory

The accessory nerve supplies the sternocleidomastoid (SCM) and trapezius muscles and you can test it by asking the patient to shrug their shoulders and turn their head to one side. The SCM is controlled by the ipsilateral hemisphere whereas the contralateral hemisphere supplies the trapezius. Knowledge of this anatomical arrangement is useful, particularly in the assessment of functional disorders.

XII Hypoglossal

The hypoglossal nerve supplies the muscles of the tongue. Ask the patient to protrude their tongue and look for deviation from the midline. In LMN lesions the tongue is ipsilaterally wasted and deviates towards the side of the lesion. Test the dexterity of tongue movements by asking the patient to rapidly alternate it from side to side. Slowness of movement without wasting implies spasticity. Fasciculation should be observed with the tongue at rest and inside the mouth.

Dysphonia is usually associated with disorders of the vocal cords and the voice has a hoarse or whispering quality. There may be impairment or alteration of a voluntary cough.

Dysarthria or impaired articulation has many non-neurological causes such as mouth ulcers. Neurological disease affecting the cerebellum, extrapyramidal system or laryngeal musculature (upper or lower motor neurone in nature) may cause various forms of dysarthria. Cerebellar speech is described as staccato in nature and is mimicked by drinking too much alcohol. Bulbar palsies (LMN) cause a nasal twang. Pseudobulbar palsies (UMN) are guttural or growling ('Donald Duck') and often associated with other features such as emotional incontinence and a brisk jaw jerk. Extrapyramidal speech (idiopathic Parkinson's disease (IPD)) is quiet, monotonous and indistinct; there may be an acquired stammer. Chorea may also cause dysarthria and the speech is explosive with repetition of phrases.

CLINICAL PEARL

Asking the patient to say 'p', 't', 'k' tests lip, tongue and palatal dexterity, respectively.

THE LIMBS

Remember to enquire about pain. Look for wasting or fasciculation (irregular vermiform movements or twitching of muscles). Ask the patient to hold their arms outstretched with palms facing the ceiling to observe pronator drift which can be seen in mild pyramidal weakness. Power should be documented using the Medical Research Council (MRC) scale (Box 12.8). Observe for postural tremor.

Motor system examination

It is conventional to start with the motor system (Fig. 12.9). Examine the upper limbs first, and do not forget to inspect the muscles of the shoulder girdle. Describe tone as increased or normal (decreased tone is a term best avoided).

BOX 12.8 MRC SCALE TO GRADE MUSCLE POWER
- Grade 0 = no movement
- Grade 1 = flicker or trace of contraction
- Grade 2 = active movement only if gravity eliminated
- Grade 3 = active movement against gravity
- Grade 4 = active movement against gravity and some resistance
- Grade 5 = normal power

- A spastic (pyramidal) increase in tone is best assessed by rapid flexion/extension movements at the elbow and is described as 'clasp knife', as the limb seems to suddenly give way.

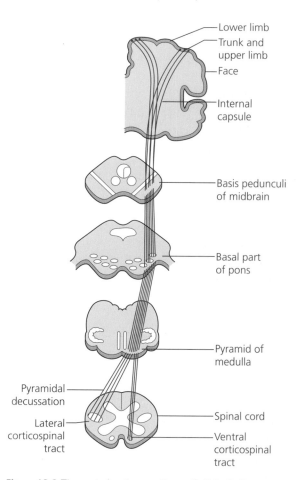

Figure 12.9 The motor pathways. From: Ogilvie C, Evans CC (eds), *Chamberlain's symptoms and signs in clinical medicine* (12th edition), with permission. © 1997 London: Hodder Arnold.

- Extrapyramidal increases in tone can be demonstrated at the wrist by slow flexion/extension movements.
- Cogwheeling has a ratcheting quality whereas in 'lead pipe' rigidity the increased tone is unchanged throughout the range of passive movement.
- 'Gegenhalten', seen in patients with dementing disorders, describes an inability to relax where it feels as though the subject is deliberately trying to frustrate the examiner. Do not take it personally!

The muscles examined will vary according to the clinical scenario, but in the vast majority of cases eight upper limb muscle groups will suffice:

- shoulder abduction (axillary nerve – C5)
- elbow flexion (musculocutaneous nerve – C5, 6)
- elbow extension (radial nerve – C7, 8)
- wrist extension (radial nerve – C7, 8)
- finger extension (radial nerve – C7, 8)
- finger flexion (median and ulnar nerves – C7, 8)
- finger abduction (ulnar nerve – C8, T1)
- a median innervated muscle (usually abductor pollicis brevis – C8, T1).

It is worth learning the root values and nerve supply of the muscles tested.

Examination of the deep tendon reflexes follows next (biceps, triceps and supinator). Finger flexion jerks may indicate an UMN lesion but this can also be observed in anxious patients. If asymmetrical, this latter sign is likely to have added significance (Table 12.3). Hoffman's sign (flicking of the distal thumb leading to flexion of the fingers) may be suggestive of an UMN lesion.

The deep tendon reflexes are graded as:

- 0 – absent
- ± – present with reinforcement
- + – depressed
- ++ – normal
- +++ – increased.

Reinforcement can be obtained by jaw clenching or Jendrassik's manoeuvre (patient links hands and pulls). Deep tendon reflexes may also be inverted whereby the tested reflex is absent but there is spread to a lower level. This indicates an LMN lesion at the level of the reflex but an UMN lesion below.

The main superficial reflexes are the abdominal (upper T8/9, lower T10/11), cremasteric (L1/2) and anal (S4/5). These are absent in some UMN syndromes. The cremasteric reflex can be elicited by stroking the inner aspect of the thigh with consequent ipsilateral testicular elevation.

Assess coordination by asking the subject to perform a hand-tapping task (listen to the rhythm) and the finger–nose test (ask the patient to alternately touch their nose and your finger as quickly as possible). Past pointing or intention tremor is a hallmark of cerebellar disease and, in contrast to other tremulous disorders, the amplitude increases as the finger nears the target. Classical pill-rolling tremor, virtually diagnostic of idiopathic or drug-induced parkinsonism, is a low frequency resting tremor that ameliorates on posture although it can also be

Table 12.3 Main deep tendon reflexes

Reflex	Nerve	Root
Biceps	Musculocutaneous	C5/6
Supinator	Radial	C5/6
Triceps	Radial	C7
Finger flexors	Median/ulnar	C8
Knee	Femoral	L3/4
Ankle	Tibial	S1/2

SMALL PRINT

Brachial neuritis (Parsonage–Turner syndrome) is a rare disease but very satisfying to diagnose as the patient can be reassured that recovery is likely and recurrence rare. The prodrome consists of severe pain in the shoulder (sometimes bilateral) followed by unilateral upper limb symptoms and signs. Occasionally patients can present with ventilatory failure. Nerve conduction studies (sensory action potentials/compound muscle action potentials) are surprisingly normal but electromyographic abnormalities are usually present. Remember to look for scapular winging (long thoracic nerve). Radiation plexopathy can present decades after treatment; pain is unusual, and the lower trunk spared (shielded by clavicle). Malignant plexopathies tend to involve the lower trunk – look for Horner's syndrome.

seen while the patient is walking. Essential and dystonic tremors are prominent on posture (arms outstretched, palms facing floor) and tend to improve when the arm is resting.

Examination of the lower limbs should include assessment of tone by rapid, passive flexion of the subject's hip and knee. The examiner should feel for the spastic 'catch' which accompanies pyramidal disorders. Clonus is best demonstrated by rapid ankle dorsiflexion: sustained clonus of greater than four beats is considered pathological. Observe for wasting/ fasciculations and also for isolated lower limb tremor, which is strong evidence for idiopathic Parkinson's disease. Assessment of power should include hip flexion/ extension, knee flexion/extension and ankle plantar and dorsiflexion. Elicit the knee and ankle reflexes next. Scratching an orange stick along the lateral border of the sole and then turning medially to finish below the first metatarsal elicits the plantar response. An extensor plantar response is always pathological in any patient over the age of 12 months. Finally, assess the gait and perform Romberg's manoeuvre by asking the patient to stand with their feet slightly apart and eyes closed. This should only be recorded as positive if the patient would fall without the intervention of the examiner (be prepared!).

> **CLINICAL PEARL**
> Patients with UMN lesions can present with an isolated foot drop; look for extensor plantar response. A commoner dilemma is sciatic versus common peroneal nerve palsy; in the latter foot inversion is preserved (supplied by posterior tibial branch).

Sensory system examination

The sensory examination follows next (Fig. 12.10). Ideally, one should attempt to map out all the sensory modalities (pinprick, light touch, temperature and joint position/vibration sense) on a chart. In practice, it is better to focus on the important issues:

- spastic paraparesis – find the sensory level with a pin
- functional disorders – complete hemisensory loss with different vibration sense either side of the midline at the sternum.

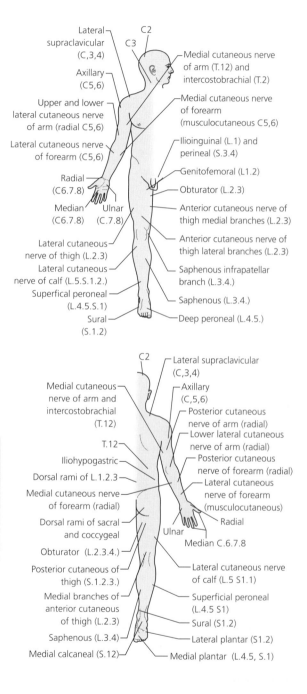

Figure 12.10 Distribution of sensory nerves in the skin. From: Ogilvie C, Evans CC (eds), *Chamberlain's symptoms and signs in clinical medicine* (12th edition), with permission. © 1997 London: Hodder Arnold.

Table 12 4 Abnormal gaits

Type of gait	Description	Common causes
Gait apraxia	Small shuffling steps (*marche a petit pas*)	Small vessel disease, hydrocephalus
Parkinsonian	Shuffling, loss of arm swing	Idiopathic Parkinson's disease
Spastic paraparesis	Stiff ('walking through mud')	Cord lesion, parasagittal lesion
Myopathic	Waddling	Muscular dystrophy
Foot drop	Foot slapping	Neuropathy
Spastic monoplegia	Exaggerated circumduction	Stroke
Cerebellar ataxia	Wide-based ('drunken')	Any cerebellar pathology
Sensory ataxia	Wide-based, foot slapping, deteriorates with eye closure	Subacute combined degeneration of the cord

Remember that loss of joint position sense and vestibular pathology may lead to a positive Romberg's sign, whereas cerebellar pathology does not. Testing two-point discrimination is unlikely to be particularly useful.

The gait

The various gait disturbances encountered in clinical practice are summarized in Table 12.4.

Special situations

The assessment of a patient in coma is shown in Box 12.9 (see also Chapter 24).

BOX 12.9 ASSESSMENT OF COMA
- Glasgow Coma Scale (GCS)
- Pupillary reactions
- Corneal reflexes
- Respiratory effort
- Dolls eye manoeuvre
- Calorics (water in ears)

Patients with ventilatory failure may have diaphragmatic weakness. Abdominal paradox relies on the fact that in normal individuals inspiration when supine causes an outward expansion of the abdominal wall because of the downward movement of the diaphragm. If the diaphragm is weak this movement is reversed and the anterior abdominal wall recedes.

Assessment of sniff is a useful surrogate marker for vital capacity.

INVESTIGATIONS

CT

Computed tomography has been largely superseded by MRI in most situations except acute haemorrhage, head injury (skull fractures) and base of skull lesions. Haemorrhage (Fig. 12.11) shows up immediately on CT imaging (90 per cent sensitivity in subarachnoid haemorrhage if performed within 24 hours). Contraindications include pregnancy (relative), renal failure (contrast agents) and agitation/confusion.

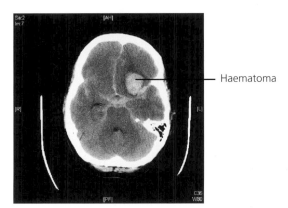
— Haematoma

Figure 12.11 Computed tomography scan showing large subarachnoid haemorrhage. Note blood in fissures and haematoma formation.

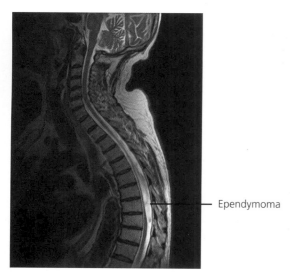

Figure 12.12 T2-weighted magnetic resonance image of cord showing large thoracic intrinsic tumour (ependymoma).

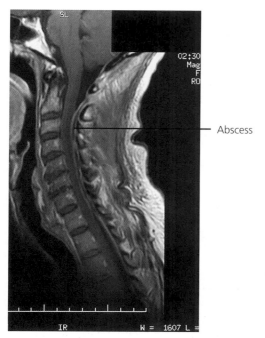

Figure 12.13 T1-weighted magnetic resonance image with contrast showing cervical epidural abscess (note contrast enhancement, indicating pus).

MRI

Magnetic resonance imaging is the investigation of choice in most brain and spinal cord pathologies (Figs 12.12 and 12.13).

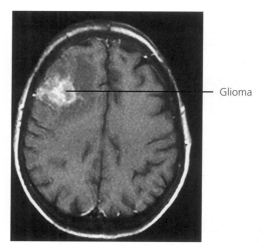

Figure 12.14 T1-weighted magnetic resonance image with contrast showing frontal glioma (note contrast enhancement).

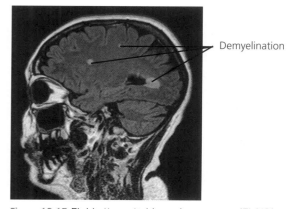

Figure 12.15 Fluid attenuated inversion recovery (FLAIR) magnetic resonance image of brain in a patient with multiple sclerosis. Note demyelinating lesions.

- T1 weighting (CSF looks black) shows up structural pathology, and if contrast is added (usually gadolinium) it may highlight blood–brain barrier breakdown: tumours (Fig. 12.14), acute demyelinating lesions (Figs 12.15 and 12.16).
- T2 weighting (CSF looks white) shows brain and spinal cord inflammation and ischaemia.
- Diffusion weighted imaging (DWI) is useful in acute stroke (lesion looks bright).
- Magnetic resonance angiography now approaches the sensitivity of conventional angiography.

The main drawback of MRI is high sensitivity and low specificity, so applying clinical reasoning is

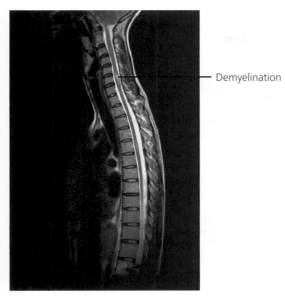
— Demyelination

Figure 12.16 T2-weighted magnetic resonance image of spine showing demyelinating lesions in cervical and thoracic cord.

essential (e.g. subcortical white matter lesions are virtually universal in elderly people and not necessarily pathogenic). Contraindications include pregnancy (risk still unknown but probably low) and ferromagnetic material *in situ* (old aneurysm clips, cardiac pacemakers and defibrillators).

Myelography

Myelography is rarely used now where MRI is available.

Angiography

Angiography is still the 'gold standard' in the detection of aneurysms and other vascular malformations. Its main use is in providing catheter access for interventional neuroradiological techniques.

Electroencephalography

Electroencephalograms (EEGs) are grossly overordered. They should not be used as a diagnostic tool in epilepsy as they are relatively non-specific and non-sensitive. EEG can be useful in classifying epilepsy (e.g. juvenile myoclonic epilepsy and photosensitivity) and may inform therapeutic decision making. Spikes (or spike and wave) and sharp

waves are typical of epileptiform activity. A sleep-deprived EEG has greater sensitivity than non-sleep deprived EEGs (still not foolproof) in the diagnosis of epilepsy.

Other classic EEG patterns are listed in Box 12.10.

BOX 12.10 ABNORMAL EEG RHYTHMS
- Periodic lateralized epileptiform discharges (PLEDS) reflect localized pathology including infection (herpes simplex encephalitis), abscess, metastases.
- Generalized periodic discharges reflect Creutzfeldt–Jacob disease (CJD) and subacute sclerosing panencephalitis (SSPE).
- Pathological slow waves (theta and delta) reflect encephalopathy (including liver failure), hypoxia, dementia, tumour, abscess.

Evoked potentials

Visual evoked potentials (VEPs) are mainly used to detect clinically silent lesions in multiple sclerosis (superseded by MRI). Somatosensory evoked potentials (SSEPs) are used in multiple sclerosis, coma/brain death (utility debatable), intraoperative spinal monitoring, and cortical myoclonus (back averaging). Brainstem-evoked potentials are used in multiple sclerosis and acoustic neuroma (superseded by MRI).

Nerve conduction studies and EMG

Nerve conduction studies can confirm the presence of a sensory neuropathy (low or absent sensory action potentials), motor neuropathy (axonal – low compound muscle action potentials; demyelinating – low conduction velocities, prolonged F waves). They may be normal in small fibre neuropathies (diabetes, hereditary, amyloid). Electromyography should differentiate between neurogenic and myopathic disorders (see specialist textbooks for more information), and confirm the presence of myotonia and neuro-myotonia.

Lumbar puncture

Do not perform lumbar puncture if you suspect raised intracranial pressure or a bleeding/clotting disorder. Lumbar puncture is usually performed at the L4/5 interspace with the patient in a horizontal

CLINICAL PEARL

- Diabetes is the commonest cause of neuropathy in the UK; distal predominantly sensory neuropathy, diabetic amyotrophy (pain and wasting in femoral distribution), nerve entrapments (carpal tunnel syndrome), cranial neuropathy and autonomic neuropathy are relatively common complications.
- If a patient presents with a motor/upper limb-predominant neuropathy consider CIDP.
- Tarsal tunnel syndrome is rare and presents with tingling in the sole of the foot.

lateral decubitus position. Advance the needle at a slight cephalad angle until you feel a 'give' and CSF flows out. Always record the opening pressure using a manometer (normal range 5–20 cm H_2O; can be higher in anxiety or obesity). Perform Queckenstedt's manoeuvre if you suspect a spinal block (pressure on jugular vein leads to transient rise in CSF pressure).

The constituents of the CSF include:

- red cells (from traumatic tap or intracerebral haemorrhage)
- lymphocytes (normal range <4)
- polymorphs (normal range <1)
- protein (normal range <0.6 g/L)
- glucose (normal range >50 per cent of blood glucose, which must be taken concomitantly).

Patterns of CSF abnormality are shown in Table 12.5. If traumatic tap subtract 1 lymphocyte per 500 red cells and 0.01g/L CSF protein per 1000 red cells.

COMMON NEUROLOGICAL DIAGNOSES

Migraine

Migraine is extremely common, especially in females (1-year prevalence: 17.1 per cent females, 5.6 per

Table 12.5 Patterns of cerebrospinal fluid (CSF) abnormality

Condition	CSF findings	Utility
Bacterial meningitis	P>L (unless partially treated or *Listeria*), raised protein +++, low glucose	Aids treatment decisions
Viral meningitis	L>P (unless enterovirus), raised protein +, normal glucose	Aids treatment decisions
Viral encephalitis	L>P (unless enterovirus), raised protein +, normal glucose, PCR (HSV)	Aids treatment decisions
Tuberculous/fungal meningitis	L>P, raised protein +++, low glucose	Aids treatment decisions
Malignant meningitis	L>P, raised protein ++, low glucose	Cytology may confirm origin of primary
Multiple sclerosis	L, OCB (unmatched)	Diagnostic uncertainty, MRI white matter lesions in older patients
CIDP	Raised protein (>1 g/L); diabetes/hypothyroidism cause raised protein also but usually <1 g/L	Differential in CIDP versus CMT and if NCS equivocal (axonal versus demyelinating)
VST/IIH	Normal constituents, raised opening pressure	Diagnostic in IIH, informs decision to order MRV in VST
Creutzfeldt–Jacob disease	Raised 14-3-3 protein	Seen in other neurodegenerative conditions
Intracranial hypotension	Low pressure	In combination with MRI – sagging of brain and gadolinium enhancement +++

CIDP, chronic inflammatory demyelinating polyneuropathy; CMT, Charcot-Marie-Tooth disease; Gd, gadolinium; HSV, herpes simplex virus; IIH, idiopathic intracranial hypertension; L, lymphocytes; MRI, magnetic resonance imaging; MRV, magnetic resonance venogram; NCS, nerve conduction studies; OCB, oligoclonal bands; P, polymorphs; PCR, polymerase chain reaction; VST, venous sinus thrombosis.

cent males). Investigations are not usually required and imaging is invariably normal in typical cases. The main characteristics of migraine are:

- throbbing nature of pain
- patient wants to lie still
- photophobia/phonophobia
- osmophobia
- nausea/vomiting.

Aura may or may not be present and 'positive' symptoms are most common (visual and sensory) though hemiplegia may also occur. The march of migrainous sensory symptoms is usually over minutes and of longer duration than epilepsy and TIA/stroke. Unusual/atypical forms of migraine are listed in Box 12.11.

The main differentials are:

- tension headache (pain like a vice, lack of migrainous features, chronicity)
- medication overuse headache (especially codeine-based products)
- cluster headache (male preponderance, retro-orbital and very severe pain, patient wants to move, autonomic features (unilateral lacrimation, red eye, transient Horner's, nasal stuffiness))
- sinusitis (tender sinuses, seasonal, worse on bending down and coughing).

BOX 12.11 ATYPICAL MIGRAINE VARIANTS

- Vertebrobasilar – diplopia, dysarthria, ataxia, vertigo, loss of consciousness, stuporose state may last for weeks
- Ophthalmoplegic – extraocular paresis during migraine attack, may last for weeks, oculomotor nerve most commonly affected
- Retinal – impaired vision and ipsilateral retro-orbital pain. Ensure that glaucoma has been excluded before making this diagnosis.

Stroke

Stroke is a common cause of hospital admission. In 15 per cent of cases stroke is preceded by TIA, a reversible neurological deficit lasting <24 hours (in practice much shorter duration). TIA offers an opportunity for intervention and can be associated with a high immediate risk of stroke (see Box 12.12).

BOX 12.12 ABCD2 RISK SCORE IN TIA

The ABCD2 risk score is calculated as follows:

- Age 60 years (+1 point)
- Blood pressure at presentation ≥140/90 (+1 point)
- Clinical features
  - Unilateral weakness (+2 points)
  - Speech disturbance without weakness (+1 point)
- Duration of symptoms
  - ≥60 minutes (+2 points)
  - 10–59 minutes (+1 point)
- Diabetes (+1 point)

Thus the risk score attained will be between 0 and 7 points.

An ABCD2 score of ≥4 points indicates a high risk of early stroke and the patient needs to be seen by a specialist and investigated within 24 hours.
Further reading: Johnston SC, Rothwell PM, Nguyen-Huynh MN *et al.* 2007. Validation and refinement of scores to predict very early stroke risk after transient ischaemic attack. *Lancet* **369**: 283–92.

Common risk factors include diabetes, hypertension, atrial fibrillation, hyperlipidaemia, family history, carotid stenosis.

Stroke is of sudden onset (stuttering strokes can occur especially in small vessel disease and cause a stepwise or progressive deterioration) and is associated with loss of function. Rarely positive symptoms may occur (e.g. limb jerking in critical carotid stenosis). Most strokes are thromboembolic (10–20 per cent are haemorrhagic) and anatomical localization is useful (Box 12.13).

- A CT scan should be performed in all stroke patients within 24 hours of onset (sooner if considering thrombolysis) to allow appropriate management (Fig. 12.17).
- Consider carotid ultrasound in total/partial anterior circulation syndrome (TACS/PACS) if endarterectomy is feasible (fit patient) and likely to be of benefit (usually within 6 months of event or sooner and with severe symptomatic stenosis).

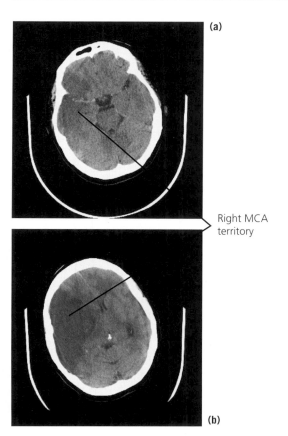

(a)

Right MCA territory

(b)

Figure 12.17 (a) Computed tomography (CT) scan showing hyperdense right middle cerebral artery (MCA) territory in patient with severe left hemiplegia due to stroke. (b) Repeat CT in same patient after 8 hours showing malignant MCA syndrome (note midline shift and sulcal obliteration).

- Full blood count, erythrocyte sedimentation rate (ESR), glucose, lipids, electrolytes and electrocardiography are mandatory in all cases.
- Consider dissection in younger patients.

Admit stroke patients to a specialized unit and consider aspirin (clopidogrel if aspirin-intolerant), angiotensin-converting enzyme inhibitor (do not precipitously lower blood pressure following acute stroke because of risk of hypoperfusion), and statin in all non-haemorrhagic strokes. Mortality is 30 per cent at 1 year.

Parkinson's disease

The prevalence of idiopathic Parkinson's disease (IPD) is 108–164/100 000. The cardinal feature is bradykinesia with or without resting tremor, rigidity and loss of postural reflexes. A true 'pill-rolling' tremor is highly suggestive of IPD or drug-induced parkinsonism (neuroleptics, other dopamine blockers including antiemetics). IPD is usually asymmetrical, reflecting varying degrees of degeneration (dopaminergic loss) of the right and left basal ganglia. All cases of IPD should show an excellent response to levodopa if given in sufficient dosages. Other features include:

- dystonia or dyskinesias (most commonly seen after chronic levodopa therapy)
- bladder symptoms
- hypophonia
- REM-sleep disorders.

Dementia may occur in later stages and is characterized by visual hallucinations, memory impairment and marked fluctuations. In practice the most common cause of diagnostic confusion is essential tremor (ET). *A priori* ET is 10 times as common and tends to cause a postural tremor (if severe it may 'spill over' into rest) and head/voice tremor. Jaw tremor or lower limb tremors are usually caused by IPD. Investigations are rarely needed in IPD or ET. Rarer parkinsonian syndromes are shown in Table 12.6.

SMALL PRINT
Although most textbooks emphasize Wilson's disease it is extremely rare, virtually never presents in the elderly and is not particularly easy to treat.

Table 12.5 Rarer causes of parkinsonism

Condition	Clinical features
Progressive supranuclear palsy	Supranuclear gaze palsy, axial rigidity, early falls, dysarthria/dysphagia, frontal dementia, neck extension (retrocollis)
Multiple systems atrophy	Autonomic failure, cerebellar signs, some response to levodopa, antecollis (extreme forward flexion of neck), preserved intellect, cold extremities, stridor, myoclonus
Corticobasal degeneration	Apraxia, alien limb, dystonia, asymmetry, myoclonus
Vascular Parkinson's	Rare, gait apraxia, pyramidal signs (extensor plantar)
Dementia with Lewy bodies	Early dementia, exquisitely sensitive to neuroleptics (e.g. death)

Epilepsy

The prevalence of epilepsy is 1/200. Peaks of incidence occur in early childhood and in elderly people. Causes in adults include cerebrovascular disease, cerebral tumours, alcohol and following head injury. Cryptogenic epilepsy is relatively common also. Various classifications are used but generalized versus focal is probably the most clinically useful. Generalized epilepsies include absence attacks (rarely presents in adults, brief loss of awareness, three per second spike and wave activity on EEG) and juvenile myoclonic epilepsy (morning jerks, adolescent onset, photosensitive EEG). Most generalized epilepsies cause tonic clonic seizures although atonic and other forms can occur.

Focal epilepsies include partial motor and sensory seizures with or without secondary generalization. Complex partial seizures also have a focal onset but are associated with altered awareness and automatisms including lip smacking, chewing/swallowing movements and stereotypical motor behaviours (picking at clothes etc). Auras may also occur characterized by strong emotions (fear), *déjà/jamais vu*, gustatory and olfactory hallucinations. Sleep deprivation, excessive alcohol consumption and poor compliance/concordance with medication are common triggers. All patients with adult-onset epilepsy should have cerebral imaging (MRI preferable) and an ECG (to exclude long QT interval). An EEG probably has little value in the over-30s as constitutional epilepsy rarely presents beyond the third decade.

Dementia

In practice, dementia implies problems with short-term memory plus one other cognitive domain such as language, praxis, personality and social behaviour. In the 'real world' most patients under 65 who are worried about their memory are anxious or depressed (or both). Many dementia patients are initially relatively unconcerned about their problems and have been dragged to the clinic by a concerned family member or relative. Prevalence of dementia is 1 per cent at age 60. Alzheimer's disease is by far the commonest cause of dementia (70 per cent of cases). Dementia with Lewy bodies, frontotemporal

---

CLINICAL PEARL

The sensory march of symptoms evolves over seconds in epilepsy, minutes in migraine and not at all in stroke/TIA.

BOX 12.14 RARE CAUSES OF DEMENTIA

- Normal pressure hydrocephalus – gait apraxia, fluctuating mental state, urinary symptoms, 'treatable'.
- CADASIL – cerebral autosomal dominant arteriopathy with subcortical infarcts and leucoencephalopathy – range of presentations including migraine, encephalopathy, stroke, dementia. MRI shows prominent temporal lobe involvement (Fig. 12.18). Genetic test available.
- Creutzfeldt–Jacob disease – classical, new variant, iatrogenic and genetic forms. All very rare and usually comprising an ataxic syndrome (apart from classical Creutzfeldt–Jacob disease).
- Limbic encephalitis – paraneoplastic and non-paraneoplastic forms.

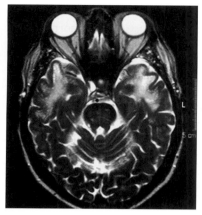

Figure 12.18 T2-weighted magnetic resonance image in a patient with CADASIL showing marked abnormalities in temporal white matter.

dementia and cerebrovascular disease are less common causes. Rare causes of dementia are shown in Box 12.14. All patients with dementia should have cerebral imaging (MRI preferred) plus full blood count, ESR, thyroid-stimulating hormone (TSH), vitamin B_{12} and syphilis serological examination. Consider human immunodeficiency virus (HIV) testing in appropriate clinical setting.

Multiple sclerosis

Prevalence of multiple sclerosis (MS) is about 1/800 in the UK. Most cases are initially relapsing-remitting evolving to secondary progressive. Primary progressive MS is relatively rare (10 per cent and male predominance) and secondary relapsing rarer still. Multiple sclerosis (MS) is thought of as a white matter disease (probably not true!) and the range of clinical presentations reflects this belief: optic neuritis, transverse myelitis, brainstem and cerebellar syndromes. Dementia and epilepsy are rare presentations. The illness is characterized by dissemination in time and place; initially a clinical judgement but more recently, the McDonald criteria (McDonald *et al.*, 2001) allow

CLINICAL PEARL

If a patient says that their symptoms are exacerbated in hot temperatures think of multiple sclerosis.

MRI to act as a paraclinical diagnostic tool. Evoked potentials have been largely supplanted by MRI, but CSF analysis (oligoclonal bands) is still useful in older patients with non-specific MRI features, scan-negative cases or patients with primary progressive disease. The main differentials are shown in Box 12.15.

Motor neurone disease

Motor neurone disease (MND) is known as amyotrophic lateral sclerosis (ALS) in the USA. In the UK ALS is a subtype of MND with mixed upper and lower motor neurone features. Fasciculations are often far more prominent than in other LMN syndromes. Other forms include:

- progressive bulbar palsy
- primary lateral sclerosis (pure UMN features)
- progressive muscular atrophy (pure LMN syndrome).

The incidence of MND is 2/100 000 per year and its prevalence is 7/100 000. About 10 per cent of cases are familial and a minority of these are positive for mutations in superoxide dismutase (*SOD1*). Most patients present with progressive wasting and weakness without sensory symptoms (pain may occur). If the bulbar muscles are involved dysphagia, dysarthria and weight loss are common. Occasionally MND may present with dementia or ventilatory failure. There is often a considerable delay between symptom onset and diagnosis (>1 year).

Myasthenia gravis

Myasthenia gravis (MG) has a prevalence of 5/100 000 and incidence up to 15/1 000 000 per year. Presenting features include:

- diplopia
- ptosis
- dysarthria
- dysphagia
- ventilatory failure
- proximal weakness including 'dropped head syndrome' (also seen in MND).

Reflexes are usually normal (if absent consider Lambert–Eaton myasthenic syndrome). Fatiguability is classical but relatively non-specific and non-sensitive. Most patients with generalized myasthenia have positive acetylcholine receptor antibodies but in ocular myasthenia this test is far less sensitive (50 per cent). Some of these seronegative patients have positive muscle specific tyrosine kinase (MUSK) antibodies. Other diagnostically useful investigations include the Tensilon (edrophonium) test (cardiac monitor and pretreat with atropine), EMG studies (single fibre looking for jitter, repetitive stimulation looking for decrement) and imaging of the thorax (thymoma). Congenital, neonatal and drug-induced (e.g. penicillamine) forms also occur.

Guillain–Barré syndrome

The incidence of Guillain–Barré syndrome is 2/100 000 per year. It is caused by 'molecular mimicry': *Campylobacter* (avian source) is the commonest source of prodromal infection. Patients often complain of quite prominent sensory symptoms (including painful paraesthesiae and back pain) with either ascending or descending weakness. The sensory examination is often remarkably normal. Areflexia is usual but reflexes may still be present early in disease course, particularly in axonal forms. Autonomic involvement is a cause of mortality as is ventilatory failure (25 per cent of cases) and dysphagia. Bladder involvement is unusual and should prompt search for cord or conus pathology.

Perform CSF analysis early to exclude other conditions (CSF is usually acellular in this condition, if not, consider HIV seroconversion, lymphoma, etc.) although the classically described high protein levels may not manifest until second or third week or at all. Nerve conduction studies may also be remarkably normal in the face of a severe clinical phenotype; proximal demyelination usually occurs first (prolonged F waves). There are a number of variants of Guillain–Barré syndrome including Miller Fisher syndrome (ataxia, ophthalmoplegia and areflexia) and the axonal form (common in China, worse prognosis in UK).

Differential diagnosis includes relapsing CIDP (if neuropathy progresses beyond 8 weeks consider this), botulism (descending paralysis, fixed pupils), diphtheria, polymyositis (probably worth checking creatine kinase levels in all acute cases of neuromuscular paralysis), hypokalaemia (check potassium), myasthenia gravis, lead/thallium poisoning (very rare), porphyria (also very rare), acute cord syndrome (reflexes may be depressed due to spinal 'shock'), Lyme disease (radiculopathy) and tick paralysis (not in UK).

CLINICAL PEARL

- Myopathy and chronic respiratory failure: think motor neurone disease, myasthenia, Duchenne/severe Becker's muscular dystrophy, limb girdle muscular dystrophy (LGMD) and acid maltase deficiency
- Cardiomyopathy and neurological disease: consider Becker/Duchenne, LGMD, mitochondrial disease (Kearns–Sayre), Friedreich's ataxia, amyloid, alcohol.

SUMMARY

History

- Migrainous headaches are throbbing, patient prefers to lie still in dark room.
- The comments of an eyewitness are crucial in the assessment of patients with loss of consciousness.
- TIAs usually last for much less than 24 hours.
- An UMN bladder causes frequency, urgency and nocturia.
- Vertigo is usually caused by labyrinthine disease.

- Orthopnoea is usually caused by respiratory or cardiac disease but can be secondary to neuromuscular weakness.

Examination

- Speech can be classified as dysphonic, dysarthric and dysphasic – the latter is almost exclusively caused by neurological disease.
- Standard cognitive tests are not very sensitive in picking up frontal lobe pathology.
- Causes of an LMN facial palsy include Bell's palsy, lesions in the cerebellopontine angle, facial canal and pons, sarcoid, diabetes and Lyme disease.
- Cranial nerves and holes in skull: 12 – hypoglossal canal; 9, 10, 11 – jugular foramen; 7, 8 – stylomastoid foramen; none – foramen lacerum; V3 – foramen ovale; V2 – foramen rotundum; V1 – superior orbital fissure.
- Ensure muscle is at rest when looking for fasciculations, especially tongue.
- Bradykinesia is a *sine qua non* in the diagnosis of IPD.
- Do not forget to examine the gait; in conditions such as gait apraxia (arms normal, cycling movements of legs preserved) and IPD this may be the only abnormal feature of the examination.

FURTHER READING

An interactive online guide to neurological examination. Available at www.neuroexam.com (accessed 1 November 2009).

Brain Journal. 2000. *Aids to the examination of the peripheral nervous system*, 4th edn. Philadelphia: WB Saunders.

Fuller G. 2008. *Neurological examination made easy.* Edinburgh: Churchill Livingstone.

McDonald WI, Compston A, Edan G, *et al.* 2001. Recommended diagnostic criteria for multiple sclerosis: guidelines from the international panel on the diagnosis of multiple sclerosis. *Annals of Neurology* **50**: 121–127.

Neurological examination: an anatomical approach. Available at http://library.med.utah.edu/neurologicexam/html/home_exam.html (accessed 1 November 2009).

13 PSYCHIATRIC ASSESSMENT

Ian H Treasaden and Basant K Puri

INTRODUCTION

At any time up to one in five adults may experience unwanted psychological symptoms such as anxiety, despondency, irritability and insomnia. In the UK, around one in six adults receives treatment each year for primary psychiatric disorders and in a further one in six psychological factors are important contributors to physical illness. Co-morbidity of physical illness and psychiatric disorder is common and often inter-related.

In addition to taking a history and carrying out a physical examination, in the psychiatric assessment of patients you must also carry out a mental state examination to look for signs of mental disorder. In this chapter we explain the key points to look for in the psychiatric history and mental state examination. We then discuss the key routine investigations to carry out. You will then learn about the symptoms and signs of several key psychiatric diagnoses that you can expect to meet in clinical practice.

HISTORY

The key tasks are to:

- understand why this particular patient is presenting in this particular way at this particular time
- be supportive, empathic and non-judgemental.

At least initially, open-ended questions are better than directive, closed questions. For example, it is better to ask 'How are you feeling?', rather than 'Are you feeling low?' In fact, it is usually best to allow the patient time to describe their complaints without interruption for the first 5 minutes or so of the psychiatric interview and then specifically ask if there are any other problems to facilitate the patient talking about matters they may find difficult.

Be aware of potential transcultural issues, including religion, language, illness beliefs and reasons for migration, and emphasize to any official interpreters that they directly translate whatever the patient says and not add comments or their own views.

You must cover the following key areas when you take a psychiatric history.

- Reason for referral.
- Complaints: ask the patient what they see as their main problem, if any. Record verbatim their comments and their explanation of the causes.
- History of presenting illness: record the chronology, nature and development of the symptoms, including precipitating factors and chronic stressors. Many psychiatric disorders have an insidious onset. Be aware that patients, in searching for meaning of their difficulties or in rationalizing them, may incorrectly attribute life events as causes of their mental disorder.
- Family history: detail parental and sibling ages, health, employment and personality. How old was the patient when a close relative died? Is there a history of parental discord or violence? To which parent was the patient closer?
- Family history of psychiatric disorder and criminality: include any family history of suicide. A family tree diagram of ages, relationships and any psychiatric disorder can be useful.
- Personal history:
  - birth – place and date. Was the birth wanted, full-term and was delivery normal? Any obstetric complications?
  - childhood – developmental milestones. History of separations, neurotic traits, bedwetting and of any physical/sexual/emotional abuse or neglect?
  - education – detail primary and secondary schooling, including age of starting and leaving schools. Relationship with other pupils (including any history of bullying or being bullied) and teachers. Difficulties at school, including truancy, exclusion and expulsion. Academic record, including examinations passed. If appropriate, details of higher

education, including college/university, and details of degrees/diplomas.

- work record – establish chronology of occupational history. Did they enjoy their jobs? Longest period of employment in one job. When last worked and its nature. Relationship with workmates. Timekeeping at work. If relevant, reasons for being sacked.
- relationships – sexual orientation. Age of menarche and menstrual history in females. Age at first sexual intercourse and history of sexual relationships. Age on marriage and time known partner before marriage. Age, health (mental and physical), employment and personality of spouse/partner. Who is dominant? Sexual relationship. Contraception. Any discord, including violence, and over what issues.
- children – ages. Whether or not planned/wanted. Any behavioural, mental or physical difficulties. Are more children wanted?
- current social situation – nature of home. Current financial situation. Relationship with neighbours.
- Past medical history:
  - chronology of past significant medical illnesses and operations
  - current medical conditions
  - of particular relevance to psychiatric disorders may be a past history of head injury, brain damage or epilepsy.
- Pre-morbid personality: this relates to how the patient and others would describe the individual before the onset of any mental illness. Any evidence of the following personality traits:
  - introversion/extroversion
  - shyness, introspection or proneness to fantasy
  - over-sensitivity, suspiciousness, paranoid attitude to others
  - over-anxiousness
  - impulsivity
  - obsessionality, rigidity
  - histrionic
  - dominant or submissive
  - low tolerance of stress with liability to temper and/or violence
  - anti-authoritarian attitude
  - characteristic mood

- capacity for enjoyment
- low self-esteem
- immaturity – how old does the patient feel themselves to be?
- ability to sustain interpersonal relationships. Number of friends in whom can confide. Who has been the closest person emotionally for the patient?
- ability to sustain work
- interests/hobbies
- religious beliefs.
- History of alcohol consumption and drug abuse.
  - For alcohol consumption and each drug used, ask:
    - age commenced
    - date since problem
    - amount and type of substance
    - reason for taking, e.g. to counter social anxiety or to blot out experience
    - effects on mental state and behaviour, including liability to violence.
  - Alcohol consumption: does the individual drink on their own or in the mornings? Is there a history of early morning shakes, anorexia, amnesic episodes (memory blackouts), delirium tremens or hallucinosis, epilepsy or fits? History of attempts to abstain, e.g. attendance at Alcoholics Anonymous or at other drug and alcohol services.
  - Does the patient regard alcohol or drug abuse as a problem? Does the patient feel he or she can stop?
- Previous forensic history:
  - age of first conviction, number and type of convictions and sentences received
  - any current law involvement or charges pending?
  - describe circumstances of offences: Were they planned or impulsive? Motivation, e.g. excitement, antisocial attitudes, resentment, anger, for financial gain? Did they follow alcohol or drug abuse? Were there current stresses? Detail offences of violence and whether related to mental disorder.
- Previous psychiatric history: chronology from onset of psychiatric disorder. Dates and places where outpatient or inpatient psychiatric assessment and treatment undertaken. Diagnoses made.

Treatments, including medication, cognitive behavioural therapy (CBT) and electroconvulsive treatment (ECT), received. Include history of self-harm or suicide attempts and when treatment compulsorily given against the patient's will.

- Drug history: current medication treatment and compliance, including non-prescribed medications and alternative complementary medicines. History of adverse reactions or drug allergies.

CLINICAL PEARL

- Always ensure when taking a history that you enquire into any family history of psychiatric disorder, the pre-morbid personality, the previous psychiatric history, and the previous medical history.
- **Life charts**: Summarizing the past family, personal and psychiatric history in a life chart, with the age of the patient and year on the left hand side and significant events on the right hand side, can often illuminate the development of psychiatric difficulties and their relationship to events in the patient's and his or her family's life.

MENTAL STATE EXAMINATION

A psychiatric interview consists of taking a psychiatric history and undertaking a mental state examination; this is analogous to taking a medical history and conducting a physical examination. However, mental state examination does not obviate the need for a relevant physical examination.

---

i **IMPORTANT**

Ideally, mental state examination should be made *throughout an interview* and not merely be considered after taking the history.

A common error in descriptions of mental state examination is to include elements which are part of the history, e.g. the presence or absence of biological symptoms of depressive disorder. The following headings are suggested, though other schemes are also used.

Appearance and behaviour

Appearance

It is useful to note in one sentence what would make the individual immediately recognizable, if possible, to an observer, e.g. the apparent as opposed to actual chronological age, race, sex, accent, posture, prominent physical abnormalities, or abnormal movements, such as tardive dyskinesia or Parkinsonism. Other aspects of appearance include facial expression, self-care, whether the individual looks ill, is underweight, is dirty, or whether the individual is untidy, dishevelled or bizarre.

Manner

This refers to an individual's social and emotional behaviour, in particular their response to others. Is the individual able to establish a good rapport and good eye contact? Does he or she appear friendly, suspicious, reserved, shy, anxious, depressed, hostile, irritable, bewildered, perplexed or withdrawn? The individual may be generally disinhibited in behaviour or appear obviously distracted, e.g. owing to auditory hallucinations (voices).

Mobility

Note the **degree of movement**, such as underactivity and motor retardation (slow, hesitant movements), overactivity and agitation (motor restlessness associated with anxiety but which is also seen in depression) or total lack of movement (stupor). The commonest cause of stupor is no longer schizophrenia but depressive disorder, although such symptoms may also occur in organic states.

Form of movement includes evidence of neurological or drug-induced movement disorders, including tremulousness, tics, parkinsonism, tardive dyskinesia and catatonic features such as posturing. A standard classification is given here.

- Adaptive movements, e.g.:
  - expressive movements such as gesturing
  - mannerisms: abnormal, repetitive, goal-directed movements, e.g. of walk. Most often seen in chronic schizophrenia. Movements appear peculiar and bizarre.

- Non-adaptive movements:
  - habitual non-goal directed spontaneous movements, e.g.:
    - tics (sudden, involuntary, repetitive jerking)
    - chorea (irregular, coarse, jerky, spasmodic)
    - athetosis (slow, writhing, involuntary, affecting extremities)
    - stereotypes (repetitive, non-goal directed, purposeless, e.g. body rocking and foot tapping, seen in chronic schizophrenia, autism and learning disability)
    - orofacial dyskinesia (involuntary, restless movements of face, especially mouth and tongue). This may follow administration of antipsychotic medication but is also seen in the absence of such medication in the elderly
  - abnormal movements induced by interviewer:
    - automatic obedience
    - echopraxia (imitating the interviewer's movements).
- Disorders of posture: waxy flexibility, also called flexibilitas cerea or catalepsy. This catatonic feature is often an awkward, odd, body posture held for a prolonged period by a patient with resistance to an examiner's attempts to alter it, but once altered remains moulded in the new position.

Speech/talk

This refers to the rate, rhythm, fluency, tone, stress and coherence of speech, rather than the underlying thought form or content, for instance:

- Is the rate slow or retarded (seen in depressive disorder), or fast and under pressure (seen in hypomania or manic disorder)?
- There may be *poverty of speech*, both in spontaneous comment and in answer to questions, in schizophrenia.
- Talk may be loud or soft and may be monotonous in tone.
- There may be a normal flow or sudden silences.
- There may be stammering, stuttering, mutism (no speech) or dysarthria (impairment of articulation of speech due to disorder of muscles and the peripheral apparatus of speech).

Affect and mood

Affect usually refers to short-lived emotion (the emotional 'weather') and *mood* to a sustained emotional state (the 'climate'). Affect is also used to refer to the objective, externally observable emotion and mood to a subjective inner experience. The predominant quality of affect/mood should be detailed, e.g. sad, anxious, elated or irritable. Note should be made as to its constancy, e.g. whether it is reactive, whether there is a good or reduced/restricted emotional range, or if the mood is labile (rapidly fluctuating). The appropriateness of mood should also be described. Those with schizophrenia may show emotional blunting/affective flattening, with a reduced emotional range and insensitivity to others' emotions, and/or emotional incongruity, which is the inappropriate presence or absence of mood, e.g. incongruous (inappropriate) smiling and laughter.

Thought

Disorder of thought form

Disorder of thought form is to be distinguished from content of thought as expressed in speech or writing. For example, in mania there may be *flight of ideas* (jumping from one topic to another with a perceptible logical connection) and 'clang' or 'pun' associations. In schizophrenia thinking may be disrupted within a range from loosening of associations between ideas to *frank schizophrenic thought disorder* with illogical associations between ideas, neologisms (invented new nonsensical words) and, in extreme cases, an incomprehensible and incoherent word salad.

Normal individuals may exhibit *circumstantiality* (long winded but goal directed), which should be distinguished from formal schizophrenic thought disorder. *Perseveration*, the illogical and uncontrollable repetition of an idea, phrase or action, may occur in organic mental disorder.

Disorder of thought content

In general, all individuals with a psychiatric disorder will show abnormality of thought content. Within this category the individual's current preoccupations should be described. Enquiry may reveal abnormalities of content such as a preoccupation with grandiose, paranoid or hypochondriacal ideas, guilt feelings, ideas of self-harm or harm to others, phobias (inappropriate situational anxiety with avoidance) and obsessions (non-situational preoccupations), e.g. obsessional thoughts (ruminations). Asking sensitively about suicidal ideas does not increase the risk of suicide. Individuals with schizophrenia may show *poverty of content* (normal in amount but providing little information).

Abnormal beliefs

Over-valued ideas

These are markedly emotionally invested, intense, illogical or false preoccupations or ideas held firmly but not with absolute conviction.

Delusions

Delusions are demonstrably false beliefs out of keeping with the individual's cultural and religious background, often of bizarre and preoccupying content and held with absolute conviction and not amenable to argument. Technically it is the way such beliefs develop and the false basis for them that makes them delusional; the belief itself may coincidentally be factually correct, e.g. delusional jealousy about a spouse who has been unfaithful.

- *Primary delusions* arise spontaneously.
- *Secondary delusions* are understandable in terms of mood state or are secondary to hallucinations.
- *Delusional memory* is a primary delusional recall of a real or false memory.
- *Delusional mood* is where individuals are convinced that there is something odd going on around them which concerns and refers to them, but they do not know exactly what it is. This may precede the occurrence of frank delusions.
- *Passivity phenomena or experiences* are delusions of external control and characteristic of schizophrenia. They may refer to a delusional belief that some external force is making them have particular thoughts, emotions (affect) or actions, or is otherwise affecting their will or giving them bodily sensations (somatic passivity). Such delusions of passivity also include:

- delusions of thought insertion and thought withdrawal – where the individual experiences thoughts being, respectively, put into and removed from his or her mind by some external agency
- thought broadcasting – the delusional belief that one's thoughts are broadcast and can be heard by others. Such delusional beliefs are also referred to as disorders of possession of thought or thought alienation.

The delusion of passive thought broadcast should be contrasted with the paranoid delusion of someone actually reading one's mind which is not a delusion of passivity.

Abnormal experiences/perceptual disorders

Abnormalities in perception of size can occur in temporal lobe epilepsy and parietal lobe lesions, e.g. micropsia or macropsia. Perception of colours may be increased in mania and decreased in depression or distorted by drug abuse, migraine or temporal lobe epilepsy.

- *Depersonalization* is the feeling of being unreal and detached from the outside world and *derealization* the feeling that the outside world is unreal.
- *Illusions* are misperceptions of real objects and are characteristically seen in organic mental disorders such as delirium tremens, e.g. a clock face is seen as a human face. They can occur in normal individuals and are increased by reduced consciousness, reduced sensory input, e.g. in the dark or with sensory deprivation, or in over-anxious individuals.
- *Hallucinations* are false perceptions arising in the absence of external stimuli and may occur in any sensory modality e.g. auditory, visual, olfactory and gustatory. They are classically described as occurring in external space, i.e. outside the head. They should be differentiated from *pseudo-hallucinations*, which are less realistic, usually located in subjective space or internal space inside the head, and are described by patients as often being inside their mind rather than their head and in terms of an 'as if' phenomenon which they know is not real. Such pseudo-hallucinations may occur

particularly in those with a histrionic personality disorder and, indeed, in bereavement reactions where a vision of a loved one may be seen.

- Auditory hallucinations (voices) – when describing these, establish whether one or more voices are present, whether the voice is recognized by the patient, whether the voice is intermittent or continuous, loud or soft and whether the voice or voices occur inside or outside the head. Note should be made of the content of the voices e.g. do they give instructions or directions (command hallucinations)? Do the voices talk in the second person e.g. talking to the patient, or in the third person e.g. two voices talking about the patient in the third person? The latter is a Schneiderian first rank symptom characteristic of schizophrenia, as are auditory hallucinations in which voices repeat or anticipate the subject's thoughts (*echo de la pensé*) or pass running commentaries on the subject's thoughts, feelings or behaviour.
- Visual hallucinations – these may be differentiated into elementary or fully formed complex visions. They are more suggestive of organic mental disorder than auditory hallucinations, e.g. visual hallucinations of insects or animals in delirium tremens.
- Olfactory or gustatory hallucinations – these are seen in temporal lobe epilepsy.
- Tactile hallucinations, e.g. of 'formication' – this is a false perception of insects crawling over or under the skin, and can occur following cocaine abuse.
- Kinaesthetic hallucinations of joint movement – these occur in benzodiazepine withdrawal.

Make a note of any circumstances leading to or precipitating hallucinations. *Hypnagogic hallucinations* can occur even in normal people on going off to sleep, as can *hypnopompic hallucinations* on awakening.

Cognitive function

The following areas should be enquired into in all cases where possible to decide whether a more detailed cognitive assessment is required and as a baseline measure.

Orientation

Enquiries should be made as to whether the patient is orientated in time, e.g. the time of the day, the day, the date, the year and the place, such as the outpatient clinic of a named hospital or, if at home, their home address, and whether they are orientated to important other persons in their life.

Memory

Tests of memory need to be interpreted in the light of the patient's intelligence and general knowledge.

- *Recent memory*: this may be assessed by asking for the patient's age, home address, the current prime minister's name and current events in the news or in the patient's life, e.g. what was eaten at breakfast. It is useful to give a *standard name and address memory test* to new patients. In this subjects are asked to recall a six-part name and address immediately after presentation or 1 minute later, and then after 5 minutes and then at the end of an interview. This is a simple test to apply. While intermediate results are difficult to interpret, extreme results, e.g. no recall or perfect recall after 5 minutes, can be invaluable and the test may be repeated to monitor the patient's mental state at later dates.
- *Distant memory*: this can be tested by asking the patient to give their date of birth, the previous prime minister's or head of state's name and the dates of the world wars.
- *Confabulation*: this is the filling in of memory gaps or deficits with false information should be noted. This is most often seen in Korsakoff's psychosis.

Attention and concentration

Attention refers to a particular point in time. Concentration refers to the ability to sustain attention over time. This is most simply tested by asking the individual to serially subtract 7 from 100 or alternatively by reciting the months of the year in reverse order.

Intelligence

This may be inferred by the individual's vocabulary and reasoning at interview and from consideration of his or her past educational attainments, work record and general knowledge.

Insight

Insight refers to the person's attitudes to their illness and treatment. The patient should be asked for their self-appraisal as to whether they consider that they have a problem and, if so, whether they recognize and regard themselves as ill. If ill, do they consider this physical or mental illness, or 'suffering from nerves'. What does the patient consider as the cause of their illness? For example, is it seen as a reaction to his or her situation or recent events in their life, or due to other people, or did it occur out of the blue? Do they think they need treatment and if so, by what means, e.g. psychological or medication treatment, and whether as an outpatient or inpatient. Ask what they hope will result from an assessment interview, and what they think concerns their relatives and/or friends.

Summary of mental state examination

In conclusion, mental state examination should be:

- systematic
- using appropriate headings
- comprehensive
- accurate.

In different cases particular aspects of mental state examination may need to be given priority and will be of greater clinical relevance. For example:

- cognitive testing in cases of memory impairment
- assessing suicidal risk following an overdose of medication
- attempting to elicit Schneider's first rank symptoms characteristic of schizophrenia in an apparently severely psychotic mentally ill patient.

During mental state examination, attention should be given to the *underlying psychodynamics*, such as the underlying unconscious defence mechanisms characteristically used by the patient, e.g.:

- projection – repressed thoughts or wishes are attributed to other people
- displacement – thoughts and feelings towards one person, e.g. anger, are transferred to others or objects
- denial.

Comment might also usefully be made on the *interviewer's reaction to the patient* – how the interviewer is affected by the patient, including the way the patient made the interviewer feel, i.e. emotions the patient produced in the interviewer. This may reflect the unconscious psychodynamic processes of:

- transference – emotions and attitudes experienced by the patient in the past in relation to others, especially during childhood, are transferred to the therapist
- counter-transference – the professional's emotional reactions and attitudes to the patient
- projective identification – another person is seen as possessing repressed aspects of oneself.

CLINICAL PEARL

Distinguishing dementia from depression: This is an important clinical differential diagnosis. However, up to half of elderly people with depression have cognitive impairment, and a quarter of individuals with Alzheimer's disease and a third with multi-infarct dementia have depressive symptoms. The diagnosis of dementia is favoured by:

- lack of history of depression
- absence of depressed mood on mental state examination
- presence of confabulation, dysphasia and/or perseveration
- poor performance on tests of orientation, general information and sentence repetition, such as the Babcock sentence
- poor recall on a standard name and address memory test after 5 minutes.

Mini-Mental State Examination

The Mini-Mental State Examination (MMSE) (Folstein *et al.*, 1975) is a widely used, brief screening test which assesses cognitive function and language. In particular, it has tests of orientation, registration, attention and calculation, recall and language. The MMSE is copyrighted by Psychological Assessment Resources (PAR), Inc. of Florida – further details can be found at www.minimental.com.

The MMSE does assume a reasonable level of education and, in its absence, a low score may need to be cautiously interpreted. Of a maximum score of 30, unimpaired individuals average a score of 28 while a score of less than 24 is considered abnormal and indicative of cognitive dysfunction. It is more specific than sensitive, i.e. an abnormal score strongly suggests a problem but patients with milder forms of, for instance, dementia may score more than 24 points, especially if they have a high premorbid intelligence and are only in the early stages of dementia. A score of <24/30 suggests organic disorder. A modified MMSE, with a score out of 100, is available to differentiate further those who perform very poorly with easier questions (Teng and Chui, 1987; see Further reading for details).

PHYSICAL EXAMINATION

A full physical examination should be undertaken ideally of all patients presenting for the first time with psychiatric symptoms and for all those admitted to a psychiatric hospital. A full neurological examination is indicated when cognitive impairment is suspected. However, such examinations are all too often omitted or not done thoroughly. This is of special concern as psychiatric patients often have poor physical, including dental, health. Smoking is common among them and many psychotropic medications increase appetite and weight.

Psychiatric disorders can lead to physical symptoms, e.g. alcohol dependency and eating disorders. Individuals with schizophrenia or severe depression may physically neglect themselves, and their mental disorder combined with their medication can lead to obesity, metabolic syndrome, diabetes mellitus and reduced lifespan owing to cardiovascular disease. Psychotropic drugs can also result in other physical side effects, such as extrapyramidal side effects and tardive dyskinesia with antipsychotic medication and hypothyroidism with lithium. Anxiety may conceal unexpressed fear over a developing physical illness such as cancer.

Examination may reveal multiple forearm scars due to self-laceration in those with a borderline personality disorder. In intravenous drug users, needle tracks and injection site abscesses may be evident, as well as an abnormal pupil size in those misusing narcotics. A rapid pulse may be due to anxiety disorder, substance misuse or withdrawal, or undiagnosed hyperthyroidism. A resting tremor may be due to antipsychotic or lithium drug treatment. The interaction between psychiatric and physical illness is summarized below.

Physical examination and assessment also allows documentation of a patient's baseline physical condition. General examination may reveal evidence of anaemia, thyroid disease or liver disease, perhaps due to alcoholism. Examination of pulse, blood pressure and the presence of normal reflexes can usually be easily undertaken in a psychiatric facility.

Interaction between psychiatric and physical illness

- Organic mental disorders – physical illness has direct effect on brain function:
  - delirium/acute confusional state/organic psychosis, e.g. liver failure
  - dementia/chronic organic psychosis
  - postoperative psychosis.
- Maladaptive psychological reactions to physical illness:
  - depression, e.g. after amputation, mastectomy (due to loss)
  - guilt, e.g. fear of burden on relatives
  - anxiety, e.g. before an operation or an unpleasant procedure
  - paranoid reaction, e.g. if deaf, blind
  - anger
  - denial
  - preoccupation with illness
  - prolongation of sick role (fewer responsibilities, more attention).
- Psychosomatic disease – multiple (i.e. biopsychosocial) causes. Life events/stress in physically and emotionally vulnerable individuals leads to changes in nervous, endocrine, and other systems, and to disease. For example, bereavement may precipitate a heart attack, or stress may precipitate asthma, eczema or peptic ulcer.
- Psychiatric conditions presenting with physical complaints:
  - somatic (physical) anxiety symptoms owing to autonomic hyperactivity, e.g. palpitations
  - conversion disorders (via voluntary nervous system), e.g. paralysis
  - depression leading to facial pain, constipation, hypochondriacal complaints, and delusions, e.g. of cancer, venereal disease

- hypochondriacal disorder: excessive concern with health and normal sensations
- somatization disorder
- monosymptomatic hypochondriacal delusions, e.g. delusions of infestation or smell; and other psychotic disorders, e.g. schizophrenia
- Munchausen's (hospital addiction) syndrome
- alcoholism leading to liver disease
- self-neglect.
- Physical conditions presenting with psychiatric complaints:
  - depressive disorder precipitated by cancer, e.g. of pancreas
  - anxiety in hyperthyroidism
  - post-viral depression, e.g. after hepatitis, glandular fever or influenza.
- Medical drugs leading to psychiatric complications
  - antihypertensive drugs leading to depression
  - corticosteroids leading to depression, euphoria
  - antibiotics, e.g. chloramphenicol, streptomycin, cephalosporins, isoniazid, cycloserine, quinolones, may lead to complications such as delirium and psychosis
  - anticancer drugs
  - interferon-α and interferon-β may cause depression and suicide.
- Psychiatric drugs leading to medical complications:
  - overdoses
  - clozapine, leading to neutropenia.

> ### IMPORTANT
> Be aware that those who have been previously physically or sexually abused may be reluctant to be physically examined and will need to be sensitively managed.

FORMULATION

Once the history and the mental state and physical examinations have been undertaken, it is possible to come to an initial formulation of the case, consisting of a summary, differential diagnosis and likely aetiological factors, all of which, in turn, will lead on to further investigations, management and consideration of the prognosis.

Summary

Briefly, this comprises:

- reason for referral, e.g. 'this is a 42-year-old married female shop assistant with two children who presented at the accident and emergency department following an overdose of medication'
- history of current illness, e.g. 'she complains of increasing symptoms over the past 6 months of despondency, anxiety, early morning waking and loss of weight'
- previous psychiatric history, e.g. 'she has had three previous admissions in the past 5 years to a psychiatric hospital with depression, for which she was treated with antidepressants'
- abnormalities on mental state and physical examination, e.g. 'she appears despondent, retarded and has expressed delusions of nihilistic content.'

Differential diagnosis

On the basis of the information available, the *most likely* diagnosis, with reasons for and against, can be made, as well as the most likely *alternative* diagnoses, again with reasons for and against.

Bear in mind a diagnostic hierarchy (see Fig. 13.1), where a given diagnosis takes precedence over those below it, does not exclude co-morbidity, such as substance abuse and other psychiatric disorders.

Aetiology

Co-morbid psychiatric disorders may have differing aetiologies. Aetiological factors are best considered as:

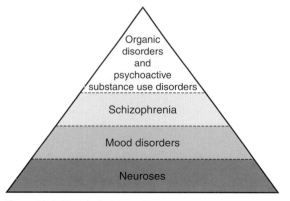

Figure 13.1 Diagnostic hierarchy.

- *predisposing factors* – including a family history of psychiatric disorder, suggesting genetic or family background factors, and pre-morbid personality, e.g. over-anxious personalities may be more prone to depression
- *precipitating factors* – including life events
- *perpetuating factors* – including non-compliance with psychiatric treatment and substance misuse.

Further investigations

These are likely to include gathering further information from independent informants, such as the nearest relative, and the general practitioner, or, indeed, from attending police officers or ambulance crews, and from previous psychiatric and medical hospital records, summaries and reports.

Depending on the differential diagnosis, particular physical investigations may be appropriate, such as:

- blood tests: full blood count (alcohol may produce macrocytosis), C-reactive protein, urea, electrolytes and calcium (may be abnormal in eating disorders), thyroid function tests (dysfunction may be associated particularly with mood disorders), glucose, HbA1c, liver function tests (gamma-glutamyl transferase often abnormal in alcohol-related disease), syphilitic serology, lithium level
- illicit drug screen (urinary or salivary sample): this may be indicated where there is a history of drug abuse or merely positive psychotic symptoms of unknown aetiology
- electroencephalography (EEG): e.g. if epilepsy or lithium toxicity is suspected
- neuropsychological tests: e.g. if dementia or pseudodementia is suspected
- neuroimaging: e.g. to exclude organic brain disorder, tumours, or to check for cortical atrophy in dementia. Magnetic resonance imaging (MRI) gives greater resolution than computed tomography (CT)
- electrocardiography (ECG): this is indicated for patients on specific or high dose antipsychotics. A prolonged QTc interval is associated with risk of a cardiovascular adverse event.

Overall, however, co-morbid physical illness will usually be evident from the history and examination

rather than revealed as an unexpected finding on routine clinical investigations.

Other investigations may be indicated by the presentation, e.g. human immunodeficiency virus (HIV) testing with consent, where there are risk factors or the clinical picture dictates, syphilis screening in dementia, copper levels in suspected Wilson's disease, genetic and chromosomal testing in learning disability, and autoimmune disease screening, e.g. especially for systemic lupus erythematosus. A chest X-ray may be indicated in smokers and those at risk of tuberculosis.

Risk assessment

Risk as a term is now used in preference to dangerousness, as an individual is rarely dangerous to themselves or others all the time but only in certain situations of increased risk.

- Consider the nature and magnitude of risk, e.g. to the physical or mental health of the individual or others, of exploitation, to property, such as fire-raising, or for absconding.
- Is the risk specific, e.g. to children, or general?
- Is it unconditional or conditional, e.g. following drug or alcohol abuse or relapse of mental illness?
- Is the risk immediate, long-term or volatile?

Always ask a patient about current thoughts of harm to themselves or others and any past history of such behaviours. Attempt to corroborate those from informants and past reports and records and document your findings. Consider protective factors. Identifying current mental illness and treating it is often key to the prevention of suicide and violence. A diagnosis of schizophrenia is a poor predictor itself of violence compared to the presence of paranoid delusions or delusions of passivity (threat/control override delusions). A history of previous episodes of parasuicide or apparent unsuccessful suicide attempts still increases the risk of completed suicide.

The Violence Risk Appraisal Guide (VRAG) is an example of an actuarial instrument. It has 12 items. An example of a structured risk assessment tool which looks at both actuarial and dynamic risk assessment factors is the Historical-Clinical-Risk Management-20 (HCR-20), which looks at historical (past and long-term), clinical (present and

CLINICAL PEARL

- Risk assessment takes into account the history, mental state and environment, plus any standard actuarial static or dynamic risk assessment instruments used.
- The assessment should be multidisciplinary and repeated regularly as risk can change.
- It is more accurate in the short term than the long term.
- It should always lead on to an appropriate risk management strategy, which itself is more important than attempting an accurate risk prediction.

short-term) and risk management (future) factors. Risk assessment is incomplete without an appropriate risk management strategy, which itself is more important than attempting an accurate risk prediction. However, risk management does not equate with risk elimination. It is important to consider whether individual and/or situational risk factors have changed.

Management

It is important to consider both the short-term and long-term management and whether this should take place in the community or in an inpatient setting, including if necessary compulsorily under the appropriate mental health legislation. Types of treatment to be considered are:

- *physical*, including pharmacotherapy and electroconvulsive therapy
- *psychological*, including cognitive behavioural therapy, psychodynamic psychotherapy
- *psychosocial*, including modification of environmental factors such as placement in supported supervised accommodation.

Prognosis

This is influenced by the natural history of the disorder itself, as well as individual factors such as compliance with treatment, co-morbid substance abuse and family support. Prognosis can be considered both for the current episode and for the long term.

COMMON PSYCHIATRIC DIAGNOSES

Deliberate self-harm

Deliberate self-harm is a common cause of admission to general and psychiatric hospitals.

- *Suicide* is an intended death by action as decided by a coroner.
- *Non-fatal deliberate self-harm* (parasuicide, attempted suicide) is intentional self poisoning or injury without fatal outcome.

The motivation of deliberate self-harm includes:

- failed suicide attempt in 10 per cent
- cry for help
- emotional relief from situation/distress
- hostility/guilt inducing to influence others
- gamble/ordeal.

Repeated self-mutilation, e.g. repetitive wrist cutting, is characterized by mounting tension relieved by cutting, which may be the result of endorphin

BOX 13.1 ASSESSMENT OF SUICIDAL INTENT AND RISK OF REPETITION

- Never ignore threats. Ask if life is worth living and if suicidal ideas are still present.
- Ask about plans for suicide for the future – both short and long term.
- Hopelessness regarding the future increases risk of repetition.
- Wanted to die?/expected to die/regret survival.
- Previous attempts.
- Social isolation and social problems.
- Life events, e.g. death of spouse, loss of job, criminal charge.
- Psychiatric illness requiring treatment, e.g. depression.
- Enquire also into other factors associated with completed suicide, e.g. alcoholic elderly divorced man living alone.
- Consider need for admission to hospital, including compulsorily.
- 20 per cent of self harms repeat and 1 per cent die in next year. 10 per cent eventually complete suicide.

Table 13.1 Comparison of completed suicide and deliberate self-harm

	Completed suicide	Non-fatal deliberate self-harm
Sex	More males	More females
Age	Late middle age	Late teens/early 20s
Marital status	Widow > divorced > single > married	
Social class	Upper and lower Unemployed and retired	Lower Unemployed
Early childhood	Death of a parent	Broken home
Family history	Depression, suicide, alcoholism	Similar episodes
Physical health	Handicapped, terminal illness	–
Personality	–	Antisocial, borderline, histrionic
Season	Spring	–
Diagnosis	Depression (70 per cent) Alcoholism (15 per cent) Schizophrenia	'Mental distress' Personality disorder 'Reactive' depression
Precipitants	Guilt Hopelessness	Situational crisis
Setting	Planned Alone Suicide note	Impulsive Others present

After Puri BK, Treasaden IH. 2008. *Emergencies in psychiatry*. Oxford: Oxford University Press.

Table 13.2 Hierarchical classification of suicide risk factors and their prognostic utility

Psychiatric		
Current axis I major mental disorder Previous suicide attempt/current suicidal thoughts Co-morbid personality disorder Family history of suicide	} High risk	} Very high risk
Psychosocial		
Adverse childhood experiences Permanent adverse life situations Acute psychosocial stressors	} Low risk	
Demographic		
Male		
Adolescent male or older male or female		

After Puri BK, Treasaden IH. 2008. *Emergencies in psychiatry*. Oxford: Oxford University Press.

release. Tables 13.1 and 13.2 give further details of the differences between completed suicide and non-fatal deliberate self-harm and their associated risk factors, and Box 13.1 details the assessment of suicidal intent and risk of repetition.

Schizophrenia

Schizophrenia is characteristically a chronic relapsing severe psychotic mental illness, usually presenting with acute symptoms which may progress to a chronic syndrome with disintegration of personality and deterioration in social functioning. Schizophrenia may cover a diversity of conditions of uncertain biological origin, but including genetic predisposition. The incidence is 1 in 100, and the typical onset is in adolescence or early adulthood.

Schizophrenia is defined by its symptomatology:

- *Positive symptoms*: delusions, hallucinations, thought disorder, inappropriate affect
- *Negative symptoms*: lack of motivation, social withdrawal, poverty of speech, blunted or flat affect.

Table 13.3 details the different syndromes of schizophrenia (which may co-exist).

Schneider's first rank symptoms are characteristic of schizophrenia and can be summarized under three headings:

- *Passivity experiences* – which include:
  - thought insertion or thought withdrawal. The closely related phenomenon of thought broadcasting is often associated with or regarded as a variant of thought withdrawal
  - feelings of thoughts, impulses (drives) or actions being controlled by an external

agency. These, like thought insertion, are regarded as 'ego-boundary' disorders
  - haptic, kinaesthetic or thermal hallucinations seemingly imposed by an external agency (somatic passivity).
- *Delusional perception* – this occurs when abnormal significance, usually of self reference, is attached to a normal perception without any understandable logical or emotional justification.
- *Auditory hallucinations* – in this voices repeat or anticipate the patient's thoughts (*echo de la pensé*), or talk about them in the third person; this includes the passing of running commentaries on their thoughts, feelings or behaviour.

Duration of symptoms for diagnosis of schizophrenia:

- According to the *International classification of diseases* (ICD)-10, symptom duration must be 1 month or more
- According to *Diagnostic and statistical manual of mental disorders* (DSM)-IV, third revision, symptom duration must be 6 months or more.

Types of schizophrenia

- Paranoid
- Hebephrenic (early onset, negative symptoms, flattening of affect, emotional incongruity, e.g. inappropriate smiling and laughter)
- Catatonic
- Residual
- Simple (slowly progressive negative symptoms)

The types often overlap and can reflect the stage seen.

Course

The course is varied with only around 20 per cent recovering completely, as shown in Figure 13.2. Prognostic indicators are listed in Table 13.4 and the types of non-affective psychoses, including schizophrenia, are listed in Box 13.2.

Mood (affective) disorders

In mood (affective) disorders, the primary disturbance is of affect or mood, and other symptoms derive from this. The term is restricted in use to

Table 13.3 Syndromes of schizophrenia

Syndromes of schizophrenia	Symptom
Psychomotor poverty (= negative symptoms)	Poverty of speech Flatness of affect Decreased spontaneous movement
Disorganization	Inappropriate affect Thought disorder
Reality distortion	Delusions Hallucinations

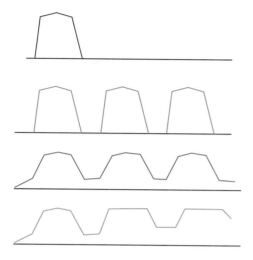

One episode
22%

Several episodes
35%

No return to normality after first episode
8%

Increasing impairment with each episode
35%

Figure 13.2 Course of schizophrenia. After Shepherd M, Watt D, Falloon I *et al.* 1989. The natural history of schizophrenia: a five-year follow-up study of outcome and prediction in a representative sample of schizophrenics. *Psychological medicine. Monograph supplement* **15**: 1–46.

Table 13.4 Prognostic indicators in schizophrenia

Good	Bad
No family history	Family history
Good premorbid personality	Shy, solitary
Functioning in occupational spheres	Poor work record
Precipitating cause	No precipitant
Acute onset	Gradual onset
Prominent affective symptoms	Blunt affect
Prompt treatment	Delayed treatment

moods of sadness (depression) and elation (mania) and not other moods such as anxiety or anger. These disorders tend to be periodic or recurrent with often full recovery in between episodes, unlike schizophrenia.

The term depression can refer to:

- Unhappiness within normal range and not persistent, e.g. grief.
- A symptom of, and secondary to, another psychiatric disorder, such as schizophrenia or alcohol or drug dependency or a physical illness.
- A primary affective depressive psychiatric syndrome, where the primary disorder is of depressive affect, but other symptoms such as anxiety are often present.

If depression is a primary mood (affective) disorder, it is then important to distinguish whether it is:

- *Unipolar* (a depressive episode or a recurrent depressive disorder)
- *Bipolar* (recurrent episodes of depression with at least one past hypomanic or manic episode).

BOX 13.2 TYPES OF NON-AFFECTIVE PSYCHOSES
Delusional disorders: persistent delusion or delusional system; not bizarre. These include:

- paranoia
  - single delusion (mono-delusional)
  - sometimes develops from paranoid personality disorder
  - morbid delusional jealousy (Othello syndrome)
  - erotomania (de Clérambault's syndrome)
  - Capgras' syndrome (delusional double)
  - Fregoli's syndrome (delusion that a familiar person takes on a different appearance).
- Paraphrenia, e.g. in elderly: delusions and hallucinations.
- Paranoid schizophrenia: delusions and hallucinations, with affective and personality deterioration.

Schizoaffective disorder: both definite schizophrenic and affective (depressed, manic or mixed) symptoms are prominent simultaneously.

Other classifications of depression include:

- reactive vs. endogenous depression (with diurnal variation of mood, loss of weight and early morning waking)
- neurotic vs. psychotic depression (with delusions and/or hallucinations)
- major depression vs. dysthymia (less severe and chronic).

Depression

- Core symptoms:
  - low mood
  - loss of interest and enjoyment (anhedonia)
  - reduced energy leading to increased fatigability and diminished activity.
- Cognitive symptoms:
  - suicidal thoughts
  - guilt
  - poor concentration and attention
  - low self-esteem and self-confidence leading to feelings of unworthiness and worthlessness
  - pessimism and hopelessness
  - helplessness.
- Somatic syndrome (biological or vegetative symptoms):
  - appetite disturbance, usually loss of appetite
  - weight loss
  - constipation
  - low sexual libido
  - amenorrhoea in females
  - sleep disturbance.
- Other symptoms:
  - anxiety
  - paranoid symptoms
  - hypochondriacal symptoms.
- Psychotic symptoms:
  - delusions: these are characteristically mood congruent, e.g.
    - hypochondriacal, e.g. of cancer, appearance
    - poverty
    - nihilistic, e.g. 'I'm dead', 'I've no blood'
    - evil, e.g. 'I'm evil', 'I'm the devil'.
  - hallucinations: these are usually auditory and perceived to be outside the head, e.g. accusing voices, the voice of the devil.

Hypomanic and manic states

The core symptom is elevated mood (elation and excitement).

- Hypomania (ICD-10)/hypomanic episode (DSM-IV-TR) – this is when the condition is of less severity and there are no psychotic symptoms.
- Mania (ICD-10)/manic episode (DSM-IV-TR) – this is when the condition is of greater severity and associated with marked impairment in social or occupational functioning or hospitalization.
- Mania/manic episodes may be without or with psychotic symptoms (ICD-10) or psychotic features (DSM-IV-TR).
- Patients with a history of hypomania or mania by definition have bipolar affective disorder (ICD-10)/bipolar disorder (DSM-IV-TR), even if they have had only one such episode.
- A mixed episode (mixed affective psychosis) may occur in which the criteria are met simultaneously for both a manic episode and a major depressive episode.

The bipolar spectrum

DSM-IV-TR also divides bipolar disorder into:

- bipolar 1 disorder – characterized by a history of one or more manic or mixed episodes and usually major depressive episodes
- bipolar II disorder – characterized by one or more major depressive episodes accompanied by at least one hypomanic episode.

Clinical features of hypomania and mania

- persistent elevation of mood, but also fleeting sadness/tearfulness (micro-depressions)
- irritability
- disinhibition
- increased energy and drive
- increased sexual libido and sexually disinhibited behaviour
- thoughts racing
- pressure of talk
- flight of ideas (jumping from one topic to another but with a logical connection) and clang associations and punning

- over-activity
- decreased sleep
- weight loss
- increase in self-esteem and grandiosity, e.g. spends money excessively.

In mania alone:

- grandiose and religious delusions, e.g. 'I am God'
- hallucinations – these are usually mood congruent and auditory, e.g. hearing the voices of angels, and tend to be transitory.

Rapid cycling bipolar affective disorder

This refers to individuals with bipolar affective disorder who have four or more episodes of depression or hypomania/mania within a year, or two or more complete cycles, switching between depression and hypomania/mania, which have been continuous without remission. Most are resistant to lithium treatment. A syndrome of ultra-rapid cycling within a period as short as 24 hours has also been described.

Organic mental disorders

Primary organic disorders are those where aetiology is primarily due to disorders, injuries or insults affecting the brain directly or with predilection, e.g. Alzheimer's disease, or is secondary due to systemic disorders affecting the brain as one among other organs or body systems affected, e.g. hypothyroidism. Table 13.5 indicates the clinical differences between acute and chronic confusional states/organic disorders/psychoses.

Alcohol and drug abuse

- *Drug abuse*: the excessive inappropriate non-medical use of drugs to the detriment of health and social functioning.
- *Drug dependence*: the compulsion to take the drug to experience psychic effects and/or avoid discomfort or its absence.
- *Psychological dependence*: the drug is taken to produce pleasure or relieve distress (situational), e.g. cannabis.
- *Physical dependence (addiction)*: occurs if there is drug withdrawal (withdrawal symptoms) associated with tolerance, i.e. with time less response to same dose and/or need for larger dose for same effect, e.g. opioids.

Alcohol dependence

Edwards and Gross (1976) classically described features of alcohol dependence that follow chronic heavy drinking:

- a narrowing in the repertoire of drinking behaviour
- salience of drink-seeking behaviour
- increased tolerance to alcohol
- repeated withdrawal symptoms:
  - within 12 hours after the last alcoholic drink, there is tremor, insomnia, nausea, increased sweating, anorexia and anxiety symptoms
  - 10–60 hours after the last drink: generalized withdrawal fits may occur
  - after 72 hours: delirium tremens

Table 13.5 Clinical differences between acute and chronic confusional states/organic disorders/psychoses

Acute confusional state/organic disorder/psychosis	Chronic confusional state/organic disorder/psychosis
Acute onset	Insidious onset
Disorientation, bewilderment, anxiety, poor attention	
Clouding or impaired consciousness, e.g. drowsy	Clear consciousness
Perceptual abnormalities (illusions, hallucinations)	Global impairment of cerebral functions, e.g. recent memory, intellectual impairment, and personality deterioration with secondary behaviour abnormalities
Paranoid ideas/delusions	
If delusions and/or hallucinations, termed delirium	
Fluctuating course with lucid intervals	Progressive course in dementia Static course in head injury and brain damage
Reversible causes, e.g. infective, metabolic, toxic, traumatic, degenerative, vascular, alcohol/barbiturate withdrawal	Irreversible

- repeated relief or avoidance of withdrawal symptoms by further drinking
- subjective awareness of a compulsion to drink
- reinstatement of the syndrome after abstinence.

Alcohol withdrawal may cause fits in hospitalized patients, including postoperative fits in surgical wards.

Assessment

- History: establish the pattern of drinking, including the average number of units of alcohol drunk each week, and any evidence of alcohol dependence, such as withdrawal symptoms. The CAGE questionnaire (Table 13.6) can be used routinely to screen for alcohol problems; two or more positive answers to the four questions indicate problem drinking.
- Mental state examination: this may show evidence of low mood, confabulation and pathological delusional jealousy, all related to alcohol abuse.
- Physical examination: particular attention should be paid to the presence of (Puri *et al.*, 2003):
  - withdrawal signs – such as tremor, flushing
  - hepatic disease – such as liver palms, spider naevi, hepatomegaly
  - evidence of accidents or fighting – such as haematomas, cuts, broken ribs
  - concomitant illicit drug abuse – such as venepuncture marks.
- Investigations: the following laboratory investigations may be useful:
  - mean cell volume (MCV) showing macrocytosin
  - gamma-glutamyl transpeptidase (GGT)
  - aspartate aminotransferase (AST)
  - blood alcohol concentration
  - plasma uric acid.

Table 13.6 The CAGE questionnaire

C	Have you ever felt you should **C**ut down on your drinking?
A	Have people **A**nnoyed you by criticizing your drinking?
G	Have you ever felt **G**uilty about your drinking?
E	Have you ever had a drink first thing in the morning (an **E**ye-opener) to steady your nerves or get rid of a hangover?

An important distinction to be made is that between *alcohol dependence* and *alcohol abuse*. Alcohol abuse, including alcohol intoxication, is a far greater cause than alcohol dependence of attendance at accident and emergency departments. Alcohol abuse is also associated with increased risk of morbidity and death from accidents, self-harm and suicide and in the UK is present in half those convicted of violent offences, including homicide, and also in around 60 per cent of those who are victims of assault.

A level of alcohol consumption above 21 units of alcohol a week in men and 14 units a week in women is associated with increased physical and psychiatric complications. (One unit of alcohol contains 8–10 g of ethanol and is equivalent to one standard measure of spirits, a standard glass of sherry or table wine, or half a pint of beer or lager of standard strength.)

Neurotic and stress-related disorders

Concepts of neurosis

- Neurosis is a general term for a group of mental illnesses in which anxiety, phobic, obsessional, and hypochondriacal symptoms predominate. The dominant symptom determines the formal diagnosis, but several commonly co-exist.
- Neurotic symptoms differ from normal symptoms such as anxiety only by their intensity, not qualitatively.
- Neuroses are abnormal psychogenic (psychologically caused) reactions.
- Most neuroses are precipitated by normal life stressors and are often associated with a vulnerable personality disorder, especially dependent and anankastic (obsessional) personality disorders.
- Neurosis is twice as common in women compared to men and also among the homeless and prisoners.

Anxiety disorders

- Anxiety is a normal mood and, like pain, a warning.
- Anxiety is accompanied by bodily (somatic) symptoms (Fig. 13.3, Table 13.7) because of Cannon's (adrenergic) fight or flight reaction.
- Primary generalized anxiety disorder is rare compared with mixed anxiety and depressive

Table 13.7 Psychological features of generalized anxiety disorder

Symptoms	Characteristics
Psychic	Feelings of threat and foreboding Difficulty in concentrating or 'mind going blank' Distractible Feeling keyed up, on edge, tense or unable to relax Early insomnia and nightmares Irritability Noise intolerance (e.g. of children or music)
Panic attacks	Unexpected severe acute exacerbations of psychic and somatic anxiety symptoms with intense fear or discomfort Not triggered by situations Individuals cannot 'sit out' the attack
Other features	Lability of mood Depersonalization (dream-like sensation of unreality of self or part of self) Hypnagogic and hypnopompic hallucinations (when, respectively, going off to or waking from sleep) Perceptual distortion (e.g. distortion of walls or the sound of other people talking)

IMPORTANT

Benzodiazepines should not be prescribed as hypnotics for more than 10 nights, or as anxiolytics for 4 weeks, owing to the risk of dependency.

disorder. Most psychiatric disorders and some physical disorders, e.g. epilepsy, thyrotoxicosis and phaeochromocytoma, can present with symptoms of anxiety.

- Anxiety is more often associated with other psychiatric disorders, such as depression, than primary generalized anxiety disorder, especially when the onset is after the age of 35 years.
- Cognitive therapy and anxiety management techniques are effective treatments for generalized anxiety disorder.

Panic disorder

- Panic attacks are discrete periods of intense fear or discomfort caused by acute psychic and somatic anxiety symptoms, which are unexpected and not triggered by situations.

- Panic disorder is effectively treated by CBT.
- Antidepressants, especially selective serotonin re-uptake inhibitors (SSRIs) and clomipramine, are also beneficial in panic disorder.

Mixed anxiety and depressive disorder

This is diagnosed when symptoms of both anxiety and depression are present, but neither condition is severe enough to justify a separate diagnosis.

The term *neurosis*, now much less often used, has latterly not been considered to include depression if this is the predominant symptom, whereupon it should instead be classified under mood (affective) disorders as a depressive episode.

Phobic disorders

- Fear is a normal prudent situational anxiety.
- A phobia is an inappropriate situational anxiety with avoidance.
- Specific (isolated) phobia, such as of animals, is the most common, but agoraphobia, a fear not only of open spaces but of crowds and difficulty in making an easy escape, is most often seen by psychiatrists.
- In social phobia there is a fear of formal social occasions in which one feels under scrutiny from others, e.g. eating in public, talking in small groups.
- Exposure techniques are the psychological treatment of choice and may involve homework assignments.

Obsessive-compulsive disorder

This is a non-situational preoccupation with subjective compulsion despite conscious resistance. Symptoms can include thoughts (ruminations/obsessions) and/or acts (rituals/compulsions) e.g. checking, washing. Insight is generally maintained and patients will refer to their complaints in terms of 'it's silly but I can't stop it'. Individuals do recognize the thoughts or images as their own. Obsessional symptoms are common in depressive disorder which may be the primary diagnosis requiring treatment.

Post-traumatic stress disorder

This is a reaction of normal individuals to major trauma. It is characterized by intrusive recollec-

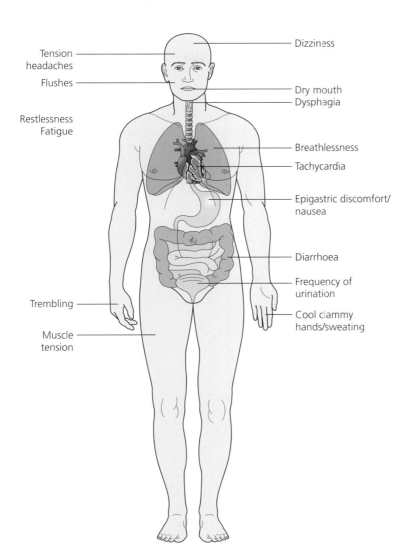

Tension headaches

Flushes

Restlessness
Fatigue

Trembling

Muscle tension

Dizziness

Dry mouth
Dysphagia

Breathlessness

Tachycardia

Epigastric discomfort/ nausea

Diarrhoea

Frequency of urination

Cool clammy hands/sweating

Figure 13.3 Somatic clinical features of generalized anxiety disorder. After Puri BK, Laking PJ, Treasaden IH. 2003. *Textbook of psychiatry*, 2nd edn. Edinburgh: Churchill Livingstone.

tions (flashbacks), recurrent distressing dreams of the event, emotional numbing, increased autonomic arousal, hypervigilance and avoidance of thoughts, places, people and activities that arouse recollections of the trauma. The onset is generally within 6 months of the event (as opposed to *acute stress reactions*, which occur immediately following the trauma) and symptoms persist for at least 1 month.

Dissociative (conversion) disorders

These are characterized by a psychogenic (psychologically caused) alteration in an individual's state of consciousness or personal identity, such as amnesia or fugue (unexpected journeying with amnesia). In conversion disorders there is a loss or change in bodily function, usually affecting the voluntary nervous system, such as paralysis or anaesthesia. Dissociative and conversion disorders classically have an unconscious motivation to resolve intrapsychic conflict and may show the following features:

- primary gain (to resolve conflict or reduce anxiety)
- secondary gain (e.g. the attention of others)
- symptom choice may be symbolic of the conflict and reflect modelling of symptoms either the individual or others have experienced
- *la belle indifférence* (calm acceptance of symptoms).

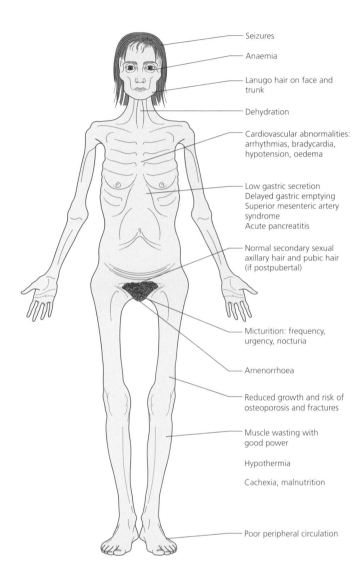

Seizures

Anaemia

Lanugo hair on face and trunk

Dehydration

Cardiovascular abnormalities: arrhythmias, bradycardia, hypotension, oedema

Low gastric secretion
Delayed gastric emptying
Superior mesenteric artery syndrome
Acute pancreatitis

Normal secondary sexual axillary hair and pubic hair (if postpubertal)

Micturition: frequency, urgency, nocturia

Amenorrhoea

Reduced growth and risk of osteoporosis and fractures

Muscle wasting with good power

Hypothermia

Cachexia, malnutrition

Poor peripheral circulation

Figure 13.4 Physical features associated with anorexia nervosa. After Puri BK, Laking PJ, Treasaden IH. 2003. *Textbook of psychiatry*, 2nd edn. Edinburgh: Churchill Livingstone.

Eating disorders

These include anorexia nervosa, bulimia nervosa, binge eating disorder and obesity. Although there is a degree of overlap between anorexia and bulimia nervosa, both being common in young females, those with anorexia nervosa are significantly underweight and have associated characteristic physical and psychological concomitants, most notably amenorrhoea and low mood, whereas patients with bulimia nervosa have normal or slightly above average weight. In both conditions, however, there is a morbid dread of fatness. Bingeing and vomiting are

dangerous activities because of their effect on the body electrolytes.

Anorexia nervosa

This is characterized by (Fig. 13.4):

- body weight maintained 15 per cent below expected for age and height
- weight loss self-induced by restriction of intake, self-induced vomiting, self-induced purging, excessive exercise, use of appetite suppressants and/or diuretics
- morbid dread of fatness (over-valued idea)

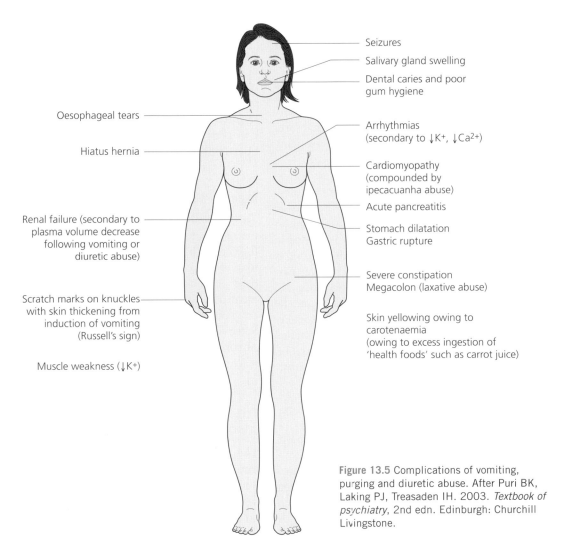

Seizures

Salivary gland swelling

Dental caries and poor gum hygiene

Oesophageal tears

Hiatus hernia

Arrhythmias
(secondary to $\downarrow K^+$, $\downarrow Ca^{2+}$)

Cardiomyopathy
(compounded by
ipecacuanha abuse)

Acute pancreatitis

Stomach dilatation
Gastric rupture

Renal failure (secondary to
plasma volume decrease
following vomiting or
diuretic abuse)

Severe constipation
Megacolon (laxative abuse)

Skin yellowing owing to
carotenaemia
(owing to excess ingestion of
'health foods' such as carrot juice)

Scratch marks on knuckles
with skin thickening from
induction of vomiting
(Russell's sign)

Muscle weakness ($\downarrow K^+$)

Figure 13.5 Complications of vomiting, purging and diuretic abuse. After Puri BK, Laking PJ, Treasaden IH. 2003. *Textbook of psychiatry*, 2nd edn. Edinburgh: Churchill Livingstone.

- self-set low weight threshold
- disturbance of endocrine function to produce amenorrhoea in women and loss of sexual interest and potency in men (in pre-pubertal onset there is a delay in puberty and growth restriction). Note that taking oral contraception may mask the development of amenorrhoea.

Bulimia nervosa

This is characterized by (Fig. 13.5):

- bingeing
- preoccupation with and craving for food

- attempts to counteract excessive calorie intake by:
  - self-induced vomiting – the use of fingers for this can lead to thickening of the skin of the knuckles (Russell's sign)
  - self-induced purging
  - alternating periods of starvation
  - use of appetite suppressants, diuretics, thyroid preparations or, in diabetes, deliberately not complying correctly with insulin treatment
- morbid dread of fatness
- self-set low weight threshold
- possible history of anorexia nervosa or atypical anorexia nervosa.

Personality disorder

Personality can be defined as the lifelong persistent and enduring characteristics and attitudes of an individual, including that person's way of thinking (cognition), feeling (affectivity) and behaving (impulse control and ways of relating to others). Personality consists of *character*, those aspects acquired over time, and *temperament*, those aspects of personality that are hereditary or congenital.

Personality disorder can be defined as an abnormal, extreme and persistent variation from the normal (statistical) range of one or more personality attributes (traits), causing the individual and/or his or her family and/or society to suffer. Care is needed in making a diagnosis of personality disorder during an episode of another psychiatric disorder. However, personality traits are continuous from adolescence and before, while symptoms of behaviour due to mental illness are discontinuous and episodic. Personality disorder not only increases vulnerability to mental illness (pathogenic) but may colour its presentation (pathoplastic) and also worsen the course and treatment response, including by non-compliance.

Personality disorders tend to cluster into four groups:

- withdrawn (odd and eccentric) – including paranoid and schizoid personality disorders
- dependent (anxious and fearful) – including anxious (avoidant) and dependent personality disorders
- inhibited – including anankastic (obsessive-compulsive) personality disorder
- antisocial (dramatic, flamboyant and erratic) – including histrionic, impulsive, borderline and dissocial (including psychopathic) personality disorders. Psychopathy is characterized by affectionlessness, impulsivity, egocentricity, lack of empathy and guilt and failure to learn from experience, including punishment.

Autism

This is a pervasive developmental disorder and is manifested before the age of 3 years. It is characterized by abnormalities in functioning in the areas of social interaction and communication, and by restricted repetitive behaviour. It occurs three to four times more often in boys than girls. Twin stud-

ies suggest that genetic factors are of importance. The disorder can lead to gaze avoidance and inability to relate to others. Other signs include disorders of speech and language and non-verbal communication, resistance to change, mannerisms and other odd behaviours, emotional lability, distractibility, overactivity, poor sleep, enuresis (bed-wetting) and encopresis (soiling), as well as seizures in about a quarter of the cases by the time of adolescence.

Asperger's syndrome

This is characterized by the same kind of abnormalities of reciprocal social interaction that typify autism together with a restricted stereotyped repetitive repertoire of interests and activities, but there is no general delay or retardation in language or cognitive development. Most individuals are of normal intelligence but are clumsy. Boys outnumber girls in a ratio of 8:1. Some cases probably represent mild varieties of autism. Abnormalities persist into adolescence and adult life when psychotic episodes may occasionally occur.

Attention-deficit hyperactivity disorder/hyperkinetic disorder

The characteristic features are of impaired attention, impulsivity and overactivity, occurring in more than one environment, i.e. not just at home or school, of early onset under 6 years of age, and of long duration.

Associated clinical features include extreme restlessness, poor attention with difficulties learning resulting, impulsivity, accident proneness and recklessness, disobedience, temper tantrums and aggression, all of which exhaust the parents and predispose the individual, including through resulting poor school adjustment, to conduct disorder. The overactivity generally lessens as the child grows older but it may persist into adult life.

The boundary between normal overactivity and hyperkinetic disorder is an area of dispute, given that up to a third of children may be perceived by their parents as overactive and a fifth similarly described by their schoolteachers. The controversy is compounded by treatment with stimulant drugs such as methylphenidate, which paradoxically reduce overactivity in such cases.

Learning disability

Learning disability, or mental retardation (deficiency or subnormality), is intellectual deficit from birth or an early age. Learning, short-term memory, use of abstract concepts and problem-solving are impaired with specific functions sometimes being affected more than others. Clinical features vary with the degree of learning disability/mental retardation, which is usually subdivided into mild, moderate, severe and profound learning disability based on IQ, though the diagnosis may be made on the basis of social performance, especially as formal intellectual testing may not be possible when individuals are of severe or profound learning disability.

- Mild learning disability (IQ 50–70): this represents 80 per cent of people with learning disability. Specific causes are uncommon. Such individuals may need practical help and special education but are able to sustain themselves independently.
- Moderate learning disability (IQ 35–49): this group accounts for about 12 per cent of those with learning disability. They do require special education and supervision but can manage some independent activities.
- Severe learning disability (IQ 20–34): specific aetiological causes are usual. This group accounts for 7 per cent of those with learning disability. They require close supervision and much practical help.
- Profound learning disability (IQ below 20): again, specific aetiological causes are usual. This accounts for 1 per cent of those with learning disability. They may require assistance with basic self-care and co-morbid physical problems are common.

Postpartum psychiatric disorders

Maternity blues

Up to two-thirds of women have a short-lived disturbance of emotions, including weeping and depression, commencing between 3 and 5 days after delivery and lasting for 1–2 days, but not beyond 10 days.

Puerperal psychosis

There is usually a lucid interval of 2–3 days following parturition, followed by a prodromal period of insomnia, restlessness and confusion, and then by a rapidly fluctuating clinical picture until the nature of the psychosis becomes clear. Affective psychosis occurs in 70 per cent and schizophrenia in 25 per cent. Always assess the risk of the patient harming her child or herself in such cases.

Postnatal depression

The onset is usually after that for postpartum maternity blues and puerperal psychosis, characteristically in or after the third week postpartum. There is a slow progression of symptoms of fatigue, anxiety, insomnia, irritability, restlessness and loss of libido. Feelings of inadequacy about caring for the baby are common. Depressive symptoms may be masked and early recognition is important. Aetiological factors include ambivalence towards the baby, previous history of termination, lack of social support, and chronic marital and social difficulties.

SUMMARY

Aim of psychiatric assessment: to understand why this particular patient is presenting in this particular way at this particular time.

History:

- reason for referral
- presenting complaints
- history of presenting illness
- family history
- family history of psychiatric disorder
- personal history
- previous medical history
- previous personality
- history of alcohol consumption and psychoactive substance abuse
- previous forensic history
- previous psychiatric history
- drug (medication) history.

Mental state examination:

- appearance and behaviour
  - appearance
  - manner

- - motility
  - speech/talk
- affect and mood
- thought
  - form
  - content
- abnormal beliefs, e.g. delusions
- abnormal experiences/perceptual disorders, e.g. hallucinations, illusions
- cognitive function
  - orientation
  - memory
  - attention and concentration
  - intelligence
- insight.

FURTHER READING

Edwards G, Gross MM. 1976. Alcohol dependence: provisional description of a clinical syndrome. *British Medical Journal* **i**: 1058–1061.

Folstein MF, Folstein SE, McHugh PR. 1975. 'Mini-mental state'. A practical method for grading the cognitive state of patients for the clinician. *Journal of Psychiatric Research* **12**: 189–198.

Puri BK, Laking PJ, Treasaden IH. In press. *Textbook of Psychiatry*, 3rd edn. Edinburgh: Churchill Livingstone.

Teng EL, Chui HC. 1987. The Modified Mini Mental State (3MS) Examination. *Journal of Clinical Psychiatry* **48**: 314–318.

14 THE MUSCULOSKELETAL SYSTEM

Alan J Hakim

INTRODUCTION

Disorders of the musculoskeletal system make up 20–25 per cent of a general practitioner's workload and account for significant disability in the general population. The symptoms and signs range from focal to widespread and can be associated with a number of systemic pathologies typically affecting the skin, eyes, lungs, kidneys, bowel, endocrine and nervous systems. These disorders are primarily the realm of the rheumatologist, orthopaedic surgeon, neurologist, and pain specialist; equally many disorders may present to allied healthcare professionals such as physiotherapists, osteopaths and chiropractors dealing with musculoskeletal pain and dysfunction.

It is common to find that musculoskeletal assessment is either omitted in medical notes or the term 'arthritis' or 'rheumatism' appears in the history without further elaboration. Rather than becoming overwhelmed with making a diagnosis from over 200 forms of 'arthritis', it is clinically more useful to describe the distribution and nature of the symptoms and signs, together with the impact on function, and be able to undertake a focused history and examination of other systems when a systemic disorder is suspected.

CLINICAL HISTORY

At the end of the history taking you should be able to determine:

- whether the condition is most likely mechanical or inflammatory
- whether it is acute or chronic, and persistent or intermittent
- the distribution of joints/soft tissues/nerves/muscles involved
- functional and psychosocial impact
- treatments tried and their effectiveness

- presence of associated end-organ/systemic pathology.

The chief symptoms to identify in the musculoskeletal assessment are:

- pain
- stiffness
- swelling
- impaired function
- constitutional.

Pain

Record the site, radiation, nature and relieving and aggravating factors.

Site and radiation

It may be possible to localize pain to specific sites. Pain may be focal (e.g. along a bone, tendon, or muscle), or it may be diffuse over or within a joint. Pain may radiate giving symptoms away from the site of the pathology. For example:

- a trapped nerve due to mechanical damage of vertebral bodies (cervical or lumbar spondylosis) or a prolapsed disc may cause pain along the nerve affected; in sciatica pain may be felt from the buttock down the outside of the leg to the foot. Nerve entrapment in the neck may be felt in the shoulder and hand
- hip pain (normally felt in the groin) may radiate to the knee and vice versa.

The ability to describe which joints are involved is fundamental. First, classify the condition according to whether it is:

- *monoarticular* – one joint involved
- *pauciarticular* – up to four joints involved
- *polyarticular* – more than four joints involved
- *axial* – affecting the spine.

Second, consider the symmetry and distribution. Symmetry (involvement of the same joints on

Table 14.1 Common associations between musculoskeletal disorders and other diseases

Musculoskeletal disorder	End-organ/systemic associations
Inflammatory	
Autoimmune rheumatic disease	
Rheumatoid arthritis, Sjögren's syndrome, Systemic lupus erythematosus (SLE), Scleroderma, Polymyositis	Dry eyes/mouth. Cornea and scleral damage Skin – nodules, vasculitis Renal – glomerulonephritis Lung – fibrosing alveolitis, effusions Cardiovascular – accelerated ischaemia, thrombosis, pericarditis, pulmonary hypertension Nervous system – mononeuritis, cerebral vasculitis Blood – pancytopenia, lymphoma
Seronegative spondyloarthropathies	
Ankylosing spondylitis	Eye – uveitis Lung – fibrosis Cardiovascular – aortic valve prolapse
Psoriatic arthritis	Skin – rashes, nail pitting/ridging/onycholysis
Enteropathic arthropathy	Bowel – inflammatory bowel disease
Reactive arthritis	Genitourinary – infection
Crystal arthropathies	
Gout	Diabetes Hypertension Hypercholesterolaemia (metabolic syndrome) Chronic renal impairment
Vasculitides	
Giant cell arteritis	Scalp/facial pain Visual disturbance/blindness
Wegener's granulomatosis, Polyangiitis	Lung – vasculitis Renal – glomerulonephritis
Churg–Strauss	Asthma Eosinophilia
Small vessel vasculitis	Malignancy Hepatitis Human immunodeficiency virus (HIV)
Mechanical	
Osteoarthritis	Co-morbidities of ageing
Tendinopathy, spondylosis/spondylolisthesis	Collagen connective tissue disorders (Marfan's or Ehlers–Danlos syndrome) and joint hypermobility syndrome (mitral valve disease, lens dislocation, easy bruising/bleeding, hernias, pelvic floor prolapse)
Nerve entrapment	Carpal tunnel syndrome (diabetes, thyroid disease, acromegaly)
Pain	
Focal bone pain	Fracture Primary or secondary bone tumour
Chronic widespread	Anxiety Depression

Continued

Table 14.1 *Continued*

Musculoskeletal disorder	End-organ/systemic associations
Metabolic bone disease	
Osteoporosis, Osteomalacia	Dietary 'fads' Eating disorders Malabsorption syndromes Hepatic disease Renal disease Widespread skin disease Myeloma-induced osteoporosis Fractures
Osteogenesis imperfecta	Fractures, dental decay, hearing loss
Paget's disease of bone, chondromalacias	Osteosarcoma Deformity Nerve entrapment Fractures

either side of the body) is typical of the inflammatory autoimmune rheumatic diseases (ARDs) (Table 14.1). Look for common patterns.

- In rheumatoid arthritis (RA) the metacarpophalangeal (MCP) and proximal interphalangeal (PIP) joints are usually symmetrically involved with sparing of the distal interphalangeal (DIP) joints.
- Asymmetry is more typical of conditions such as osteoarthritis (OA), gout, and psoriatic arthritis (PsA); the PIP and DIP joints are often involved.
- Axial disease affecting the spine and sacroiliac joints is typical of ankylosing spondylitis (AS).

Chronic widespread pain (CWP) – generalized pain for more than 3 months – is common. Up to 10 per cent of the general population describes having CWP. It may be a consequence of:

- multiple joint problems or a myopathy
- fibromyalgia – multiple tender points in muscles and tendon insertions
- joint hypermobility syndrome
- polymyalgia rheumatica – pain in the shoulder girdle (neck, shoulder, upper arm) and/or pelvic girdle (lower back, hips and thighs).

Nature

Pain is described in many different ways. Given its variability, a description of the pain may be of limited value. It is more helpful to understand the patient's loss of function as a consequence. However, some characteristics are important:

- paraesthesia or weakness in the distribution of a nerve root, e.g. nerve entrapment or inflammation (mononeuritis)
- focal, constant pain, waking the patient. This may be a bone lesion such as a malignancy or infection
- sudden acute pain in the absence of trauma. In the spine this may be an acute vertebral fracture, perhaps from osteoporosis or malignancy. It may be a sign of an inflamed disc. In a large joint think about a cartilage tear, septic arthritis, spontaneous haemarthrosis or tendon rupture.

Relieving and aggravating factors

As a rule mechanical disorders (e.g. OA, spondylosis, and tendinopathies) are worsened by activity and relieved by rest. In severe degenerative disease the pain may, however, be present at rest and disturb sleep. Inflammatory disorders tend to be painful both at rest and during activity and are associated with worsened stiffness after periods of prolonged rest. The patient may note that stiffness is relieved somewhat by movement. Both mechanical and inflammatory disorders may be worsened by excessive movement.

> **CLINICAL PEARL**
> Some patients can identify relieving factors such as hot/cold compress, straps/supports, acupuncture, massage and physiotherapy, etc. It is helpful to know what relieves their pain and to what degree.

The majority of patients will have taken pain killers. Find out:

- which ones they have taken – know your pharmacology; patients may have tried non-steroidal anti-inflammatory drugs (NSAIDs), paracetamol, opioids, neuroleptic agents, anti-depressant agents, or topical gels/creams
- why did the patient stop taking the painkiller? Did it not work at all? Were there side effects and if so what? Were they worried about becoming dependent on a drug and therefore didn't take it?

Before abandoning analgesia as unhelpful find out:

- the frequency and maximum dose tried
- whether there was any relief that then wore off.

A number of patients say their painkiller did not work but on further questioning it may become clear that either they did not take enough, frequently enough, or the drug worked for a few hours and then wore off. Converting the painkiller to a long-acting slow-release formula may reduce the 'on–off' effect; one example is the use of a 12-hour slow release formula in the evening giving relief of early morning stiffness and pain.

Stiffness

A patient may not be able to differentiate 'stiffness' from pain and swelling. Difficulty moving a joint may be a combination of all three symptoms. However, many patients will recognize the phenomenon of worsened joint stiffness after a period of rest. Prolonged stiffness is associated with inflammatory arthritis; typically it lasts 1–2 hours and eases with heat and movement. The duration may be a guide to inflammatory disease activity.

Short periods of *generalized stiffness* (up to 30 minutes) are not meaningful. *Localized joint stiffness* of short duration may be a feature of mechanical disorders. These short episodes tend to be intermittent and occur throughout the day after any period of rest.

Stiffness may also occur in a normal joint. Some people 'crack' or 'click' their joints to relieve themselves of the symptom. This and the clicking are usually benign and not associated with long-term risk of joint damage. If however a clicking joint or tendon also hurts at the time of the click this would suggest a mechanical problem that needs assessment.

Finally, stiffness may be the result of a *tendon nodule or fibrosis*. At its extreme the tendon mechanism may get stuck; this is termed 'triggering' and is most often seen in the flexor tendons of the fingers.

Swelling

Joint swelling is indicative of an inflammatory condition, infection (septic arthritis) or trauma and may be due to soft tissue inflammation, thickening of the synovial membrane or an excess of synovial fluid causing an effusion.

Consider the possibility that swelling may be a consequence of peripheral oedema, cellulitis, deep vein thrombosis or varicose veins. Trauma may lead to the rapid development of an effusion. This may be synovial fluid or blood (haemarthrosis). Occasionally, and in the absence of trauma, an effusion may be very rapid in onset and so painful that the patient cannot move the joint. In these circumstances a septic arthritis should be considered.

> **CLINICAL PEARL**
> Swelling does not always imply the presence of an inflammatory arthritis. In particular swelling can often be seen in OA; in the hands this is usually due to bone nodules. Occasionally in OA cartilage debris and calcium crystals within the joint may induce an effusion. Typical joints affected in this way include the knee, hip and shoulder.

Impaired function

Difficulty with specific movements may occur as a consequence of pain, tissue damage, fibrosis (contractures), fusion (bone ankylosis), or neuropathy. Functional impairment may have a profound impact on mood and sleep leading to anxiety, depression, and fatigue.

Every patient is different in their perception of the problem, coping strategies for activities of daily living (hygiene, cooking, and dressing), and integration (relationships and sexual activity, social interactions, work, and exercise). Take a social and treatment history to identify the impact on these aspects of well-being. As well as use of medications, identify coping strategies and modifications to the environment that support activity, e.g. occupational therapy advice and home adjustments (hand rails, gadgets, downstairs wash facilities, ramps instead of steps, etc.).

Constitutional symptoms

Patients with arthritis may describe symptoms of fatigue, fever, sweating and weight loss. A number of other diseases and disorders may manifest as or have complications of a musculoskeletal origin. Table 14.1 describes some of the 'extra-articular manifestations' or associations seen in arthritic conditions (although the list is not exhaustive).

SIGNS

General screen

At the end of a 'screening' inspection of the musculoskeletal system it should be possible to identify which sites are affected and to what degree. A more detailed examination of the sites involved is then required. There are four parts to the physical assessment: inspection, palpation, movement and function.

Inspection

Look for swelling, deformities, nodules, asymmetry, muscle wasting, scars, skin pathology (Table 14.2, Figs 14.1–14.3).

Perform the gait, arms, legs, spine screen (Doherty et al., 1992). This is a rapid screening of joint movement designed to identify affected areas (Table 14.3, p. 240, Fig. 14.4, p. 242).

Palpation

Be gentle, avoiding excessive pressure or sudden movement that may cause unnecessary pain. If a joint, muscle, or tendon is swollen, painful, or there

Table 14.2 Physical examination – general inspection: standing the patient in the anatomical position, look at them from the front, rear and side. At all times think about symmetry. The numbering in the table aligns with that in Figure 14.1

Position	Observation
Front	
1. Neck	Abnormal flexion (torticollis)
2. Shoulder	Muscle bulk across the chest
3. Elbow	Full (or hyper) extension
4. Pelvis	Level – tilted lower on one side may be leg length difference or spinal curvature (scoliosis)
5. Quadriceps	Muscle bulk
6. Knee	Alignment – bow-legged (varus deformity) or knock-kneed (valgus deformity) Swelling Operation scars
7. Midfoot	Loss of midfoot arch – flat feet
Rear	
8. Shoulder	Muscle bulk across deltoid, trapezius, and scapular muscles
9. Spine alignment	Scoliosis (curvature to side, Fig. 14.2) Operation scars (including neck)
10. Gluteal	Muscle bulk
11. Knee	Swelling
12. Calf	Muscle bulk, swelling
13. Hindfoot	Out-turning (eversion) of the heel associated with flat foot Achilles tendon swelling
Side	
14. Spine alignment	Cervical – normal lordosis Dorsal/thoracic – normal kyphosis (Fig. 14.3) Lumbar – normal lordosis
15. Knee	Excessive extension – hypermobility

is a reduced range of movement then feel for warmth of inflammation using the back of the fingers. Gently squeeze individual joints and palpate soft tissues for tenderness.

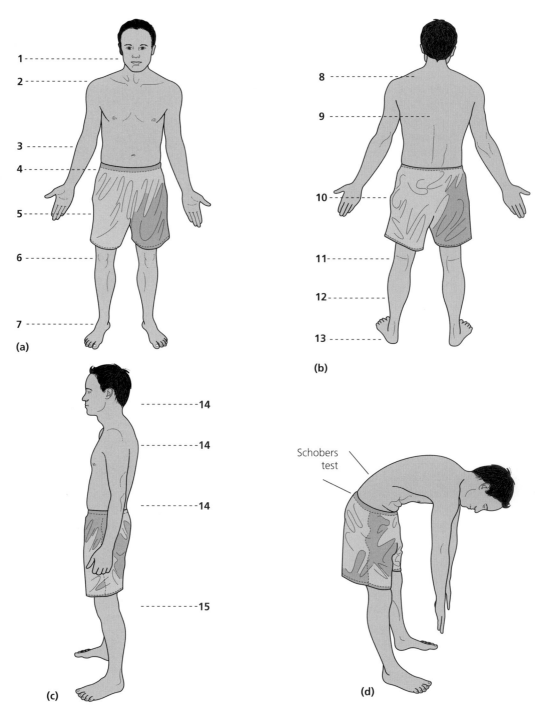

Figure 14.1 Physical examination – general inspection. Measure lumbar flexion using Schöbers' test. With the patient standing upright make a horizontal mark across the sacral dimples and a second mark over the spine 10 cm above. The patient then bends forward as far as possible. Re-measure the distance between the marks. It should increase from 10 cm to >15 cm; less suggests restriction. (Note: just looking at ability to bend forwards and not at lumbar expansion is inadequate; the individual may have good range of hip movement giving false impression of lumbar mobility.)

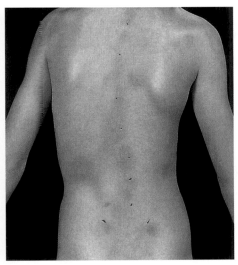

Figure 14.2 Scoliosis. From: Gray D, Toghill P (eds), *An introduction to the symptoms and signs of clinical medicine*, with permission. © 2001 London: Hodder Arnold.

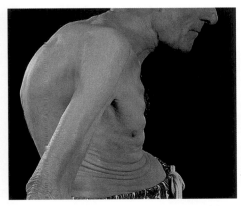

Figure 14.3 Severe kyphosis as the result of the collapse of multiple vertebrae due to myeloma. From: Gray D, Toghill P (eds), *An introduction to the symptoms and signs of clinical medicine*, with permission. © 2001 London: Hodder Arnold.

Ask whether any areas of the body are numb or weak and be prepared to perform a sensory or motor neurological examination, respectively, after the screening assessment.

Movement

Regional examination of the musculoskeletal system (Coady *et al.*, 2004) is beyond the scope of this chapter. For now, focus on being able to perform the screen, but we would encourage you to learn regional examination during the course of an attachment to a musculoskeletal firm and to read the *Arthritis research campaign handbook* and DVD giving a detailed demonstration of joint and soft tissue examination (Coady, 2005).

At any one site, there are three assessments of movement:

- *Active movement* – the patient doing it themselves
- *Active movement against a resisting force* – the patient holds a position while the assessor places a gentle force against it. If pain is induced it may indicate tendon pathology
- *Passive movement* – the assessor moves the joint. This may be necessary if a patient cannot move because of weakness or pain. Always perform passive movement slowly and gently in order to ascertain the extent of range of movement without causing undue pain. Full range on passive movement but limited or no range on active movement suggests the problem is neurological or muscle/tendon rather than articular.

Range of movement on each side of the body should be compared. Look for excessive movement (hypermobility). Note a painful hypermobile joint may still move in what seems to be a normal range for the general population.

Function

Loss of movement leads to loss of function. Patients often learn to compensate. Consider what the joint does thus focusing attention on what the issues might be. For example:

- unable to rotate the shoulder to place hand behind back – how does this person manage washing, or doing up a brassiere?
- cannot bend knee – how do they sit or climb stairs?

Regional examination of the hips and knees

- Ask the patient to lie on the couch after completing the general screen. Perform the *log-rolling test* of the hips by placing the legs in extension and gently rolling the entire limb back and forth

Table 14.3 Physical examination screening tool – gait, arms, legs and spine

Position	Observation	Command
Standing	*Gait:* Smooth movement Arm swing Pelvic tilt Normal stride length Ability to turn quickly	'Walk to the end of the room, turn, and walk back to me'
	Lumbar spine: Lumbar expansion (Fig. 14.1) Lumbar lateral flexion	'Bend forward and touch your toes' 'Place your hands by your side; bend to the side running your hand down the outside of your leg toward your knee…'
	Hip: The Trendelenburg test – if the opposite side of the pelvis drops below the horizontal level this suggests weakness of the hip abductors on the weight-bearing leg	'Stand on one leg… now the other' *Note: Patient may not be able to do this if frail, has a neurological problem, unstable hypermobility, or a knee or ankle problem*
Sitting facing you: Neck and thoracic spine (Fig. 14.4)	*Neck:* Smooth movement, no pain/stiffness Forward flexion Side flexion Extension Rotation *Thoracic spine:* Smooth movement, no pain/stiffness Lateral chest expansion Rotation	'Bend forward chin to chest' 'Bend sideways ear to shoulder' 'Tilt head back' 'Turn head to the …, chin to shoulder … other side' See respiratory examination for technique 'Fold your arms, turn body to the…'
Sitting facing you: Hands, wrists, elbows and shoulders (Fig. 14.4)	*Hand:* Hand, wrist, finger swelling deformity Hand pronation Observe palms and grip function – gently squeeze the metacarpophalangeal joints by compressing the row of joints together Assess for pain Feel for warmth Look for operation scars Wrist extension and flexion *Elbows:* Look for nodules, rash *Shoulders:* Abduction to 180° Rotation	'Place both hands out in front, palms down and fingers straight' 'Turn the hands over, palms up' – 'make a fist' 'Place palms of hands together as if to pray, with elbows out to the side', 'with the elbows in the same position place the hands back to back with the fingers pointing down' 'Bend your elbows bringing your hands to your shoulders' 'Raise arms out sideways, hands above your head' 'Touch the small of your back'

Continued

Table 14.3 *Continued*

Position	Observation	Command
Sitting facing you: Hips, knees and ankles (Fig. 14.4)	*Hips:* Gently turn inward and outward looking for symmetry, restriction, pain *Knees:* Flex and extend, feeling the patella with palm of hand for 'crepitus' (grinding), and back of hand for warmth Feel back of the knee, calf and Achilles tendon for pain and swelling *Ankles and feet:* Gently squeeze the metatarsophalangeal joints of the toes by compressing the row of joints together Assess for pain Feel for warmth	'Turn your ankles in a circular motion' 'now up and down' 'Wiggle your toes'

looking for pain in the groin and limitation of internal or external rotation, comparing left and right sides.

- *Thomas' test* is used to identify hip flexion deformity. It is only useful if there is no flexion deformity of the ipsilateral knee. With the patient lying flat, fully flex the opposite hip and knee; this flattens lumbar lordosis. Look at the knee on the involved side. It should remain flat on the couch. If it is now elevated off the couch and cannot be flattened there is an ipsilateral hip flexion deformity present that may be due to arthritis or tight hip flexors.
- Assess the knee for an effusion by eliciting the bulge sign and ballotting the patella.
  - The *bulge sign test* is helpful in identifying a small effusion. It is performed with the knee fully extended and the muscles relaxed. Displace the effusion by stroking the thumb down the medial side of the knee below the patella margin. This creates a recess or dimple and the lateral side of the knee may fill. Now stroke the lateral side of the knee and observe the medial recess refill.
  - *Ballottement* is useful if a large knee effusion is present. In the same position as above, use the index finger to push the patella straight down. Release quickly and repeat the motion. In the presence of an effusion you can feel the patella knocking against the femur below.

INVESTIGATING MUSCULOSKELETAL DISORDERS

Having identified the distribution, symmetry, and possible associated extra-articular manifestations of disease, it should now be possible to determine whether the condition is regional or generalized, and mechanical or inflammatory. Laboratory and radiological investigations are used to support a diagnosis, assess severity, and may be of prognostic value.

Laboratory tests

Screening tests for inflammation and autoimmune rheumatic diseases

- Erythrocyte sedimentation rate (ESR).
- C-reactive protein (CRP): unlike the ESR, it is unaffected by anaemia or hyperglobulinaemia, both of which may be present in ARDs.
- Full blood count: anaemia of chronic disease, leucopenia, lymphopenia, and thrombocytopenia may be present in ARDs. Though they may be directly associated with disease, they may be the consequence of drug therapies, in particular disease modifying anti-rheumatic drugs (DMARDS) such as methotrexate and azathioprine, and biological therapies. NSAIDs, by inducing peptic ulcer disease and gastrointestinal blood loss, might cause anaemia.

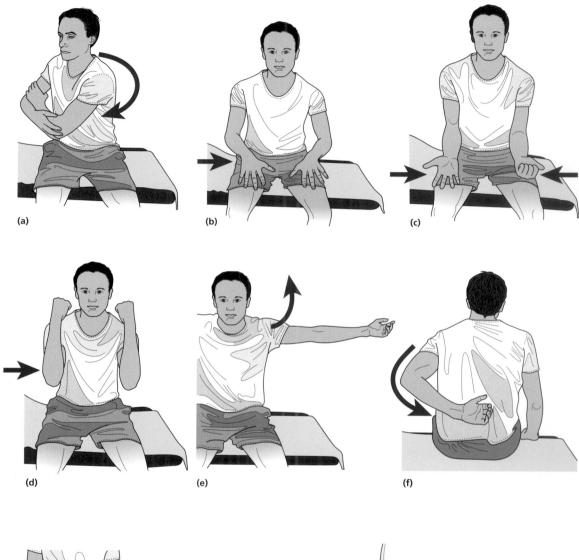

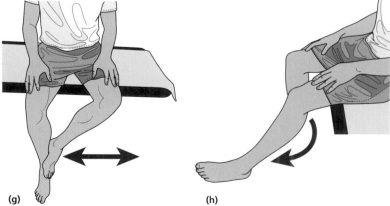

Figure 14.4 Physical examination screening (see Table 14.3 for commands).

- Urea and electrolytes, and serum uric acid: renal impairment may be a manifestation of an ARD. Equally it may be a result of drug treatment (e.g. NSAIDs, ciclosporin), or other co-morbidity e.g. diabetes or hypertension. Chronic renal impairment may result in high serum uric acid levels and low vitamin D levels, leading to gout and osteomalacia respectively.
- Urinalysis: protein and blood in the urine may indicate glomerulonephritis or infection. Detailed microscopy for inflammatory casts and culture is warranted.
- Liver function tests: abnormalities may be drug-induced or a manifestation of autoimmune hepatitis. Infections such as hepatitis B and C are also associated with inflammatory arthritis. Note that a raised alkaline phosphatase (ALP) might be from bone and alanine transferase (ALT) from muscle rather than liver.
- There are many causes for a raised creatine kinase (CK). In the context of diffuse muscle pain (myalgia) and inflammation a raised CK suggests myositis.
- Rheumatoid factor (RF) is of value in establishing the diagnosis of RA. However, up to 5 per cent of the population may be positive for RF with no consequence. Equally, only 70–80 per cent of patients with RA are RF positive.
- Rheumatoid factor may be positive in other rheumatic diseases such as Sjögren's syndrome and SLE, chronic infections such as subacute bacterial endocarditis and hepatitis C, and chronic lung and liver disease.
- Anticyclic citrullinated peptide (anti-CCP) antibody is a marker for diagnosis and prognosis in RA. Anti-CCP antibody is detected in 50–60 per cent of patients with early RA. It is a marker of erosive disease and predicts development of RA in patients with non-specific inflammatory symptoms. The test is therefore valuable when the history suggests RA but the clinical signs are minimal and the RF is low or negative.
- Anti-nuclear antibody (ANA) is often positive in the ARDs (Table 14.1). Over 95 per cent of patients with SLE have a positive ANA. The test, however, is not specific and may be positive in other end-organ diseases such as thyroiditis and hepatitis.

Screening tests for focal bone pain or diffuse myalgia and fatigue

- Check for an abnormal ESR, CRP, and FBC that might suggest the presence of a malignancy.
- A raised calcium suggests either hyperparathyroidism, malignancy involving bone, or sarcoidosis.
- Focal bone pain with a raised ALP but normal calcium may suggest Paget's disease, a bone cyst or tumour, fracture or osteomalacia.
- Diffuse myalgia may be due to polymyalgia rheumatica (raised ESR but normal CK), polymyositis (raised ESR and CK), endocrinopathies (hypo- and hyperthyroidism) or vitamin D deficiency.
- Laboratory investigations should be normal in CWP due to fibromyalgia and joint hypermobility syndrome.

Other specific laboratory tests

- Extractable nuclear antigens (ENA) are helpful in separating out the ARDs and identifying risk for specific pathologies such as renal disease. The common ENAs are:
  - anti-Ro and anti-La – found in Sjögren's syndrome, SLE, and RA
  - anti-SM and RNP – found in SLE
  - anti-centromere and Scl-70 – in systemic sclerosis
  - anti-Jo-1 – in polymyositis.
- Antiphospholipid and anticardiolipin antibodies are associated with arterial and venous thrombosis, spontaneous abortion, and acute cerebral vasculopathy. They are found primarily in antiphospholipid syndrome and SLE.
- Antineutrophil cytoplasmic antibody (ANCA); cANCA and pANCA are associated with the vasculitides (Table 14.1).
- Infections: tests to consider include blood cultures, synovial fluid culture if there is an effusion, antistreptolysin O titre (ASO titre), hepatitis B and C serology, parvovirus B19 IgG and IgM, and a human immunodeficiency virus (HIV) test.

Radiological tests

Plain radiographs are a simple and helpful tool (Fig. 14.5). Radiological changes due to inflammatory conditions such as RA, gout and psoriatic arthropathy include:

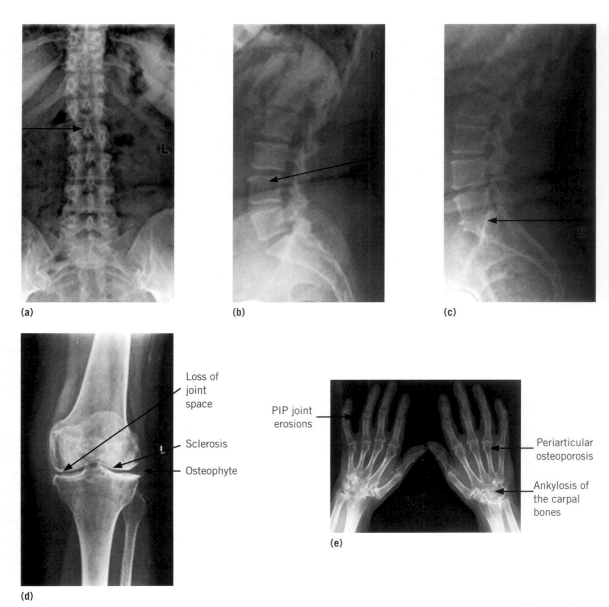

Figure 14.5 Radiographic examples of common musculoskeletal pathologies. (**a**) Anteroposterior (AP) view of a normal lumbar spine. Follow the transverse processes to assess alignment. (**b**) Lateral view of the lumbar spine. Normal alignment but note anterior osteophytes on the upper margin of L3 and L4. (**c**) Degenerative disc L5/S1 with anterior osteophytes. (**d**) AP view of the left knee – osteoarthritis. (**e**) Erosions of small joints of the hands and wrists – rheumatoid arthritis. PIP, proximal interphalangeal.

- soft tissue swelling
- periarticular bone demineralization
- diffuse loss of joint space
- erosions – seen at the far margins of the joint where the cartilage no longer covers bone

- gross joint destruction in advanced erosive disease. This may lead to joint dislocation, subluxation, or ankylosis (fusion of the joint surfaces).

Mechanical or degenerative conditions such as OA manifest radiologically as:

- bony nodules – osteophytes at joint margins
- bone cysts along the joint line
- sclerosis along the joint line
- focal or diffuse loss of joint space
- chondrocalcinosis – pyrophosphate crystal deposition in the fibrocartilage
- loose bodies – bone debris in the joint space.

Other imaging techniques include the following.

- Ultrasound – this can assess soft tissue injuries, including the deep tendon structures, and is an aid to local corticosteroid injections. Ultrasound can also be used to identify early erosions.
- Isotope bone scanning – this is valuable in identifying areas of high bone turnover. Isotope uptake is increased at sites of bone metastases, fractures, Paget's disease, infection (osteomyelitis), and inflammation (e.g. sacroiliac joints in AS).
- Magnetic resonance imaging (MRI) – this provides highly detailed information on the anatomy and pathology of soft tissues and joints. It is particularly valuable in assessing the presence of erosions in the hands and feet, inflammatory and mechanical disorders of the spine and spinal cord, and tendon, ligament, and cartilage abnormalities of the shoulder, hip, and knee.

COMMON MUSCULOSKELETAL DIAGNOSES

Neck pain

About 10 per cent of the adult population experiences neck pain at any one time, although many people do not seek medical help. About 1 per cent of adults with neck pain develop neurological deficit. Most neck pain occurs at the level of C5–C6 and is mechanical in nature due to disc degeneration.

Nerve root (radicular) pain is usually sharp with paraesthesia radiating into the arms or hands. Common causes for radicular pain are compression by an intervertebral disc or an osteophyte encroaching on the nerve root exit foramen.

> **IMPORTANT**
> Indicators of serious pathology in lumbar pain:
> 'red flags' of serious pathology that requires further investigation with blood tests and plain radiographs are:
> - presenting under age 20 and over age 55 years
> - prolonged stiffness (>6 weeks)
> - sudden onset of severe pain
> - pain that disturbs sleep (>6 weeks)
> - thoracic pain
> - nerve root symptoms – including spinal claudication (pain on walking resolved by rest), saddle numbness, and loss of bladder or bowel control
> - chronic persistent pain (>12 weeks)
> - weight loss
> - history of carcinoma.

Lumbar pain

The lifetime incidence of lower back pain is about 60 per cent and the greatest prevalence is between ages 45 and 65 years. Over 90 per cent of low back pain is mechanical and self-limiting. Low back pain can arise from disc degeneration (spondylosis) or inflammation of the thoracic or lumbar spine and sacroiliac joints. Pain may be referred from the retroperitoneum or pelvic viscera, e.g. renal pain.

It is important to ensure there is no evidence of a vertebral fracture, bone metastases, sequestered prolapsed disc, discitis, infection, or onset of an inflammatory condition such as AS. Vertebral fractures appear on radiographs as either flattening of the whole vertebra ('compression' fracture) or, more commonly, with loss of height on the anterior border of the vertebra ('wedge' fracture).

A motor and sensory neurological examination of the arms and legs is essential in suspected cases of nerve root entrapment, cord compression, or spinal stenosis at the neck. Similarly an examination of the legs is essential if pathology is suspected in the lower spine.

The management options for chronic low back pain due to degenerative disease and in the absence of serious pathology include:

- exercise advice
- manipulation
- analgesia
- transcutaneous nerve stimulation (TENS)
- 'back schools' – education.

Chronic widespread pain

Chronic widespread pain is present in 5–10 per cent of the general population. In the absence of diffuse degenerative or inflammatory rheumatic disease the two most common conditions found in association with CWP are fibromyalgia and joint hypermobility syndrome.

In addition to diffuse tenderness at discrete anatomical sites patients with fibromyalgia experience a range of symptoms including fatigue, mood and sleep disturbance. Fibromyalgia is also found in up to 25 per cent of patients with RA, AS, SLE, and joint hypermobility syndrome. Fibromyalgia and joint hypermobility syndrome also overlap symptomatically with chronic fatigue syndrome in many ways. Care must therefore be taken to avoid misdiagnosing fibromyalgia as the only cause for pain. If joint hypermobility syndrome is suspected, look for generalized hypermobility, particularly in the fingers, elbows, lumbar spine, knees, and feet (flat feet), easy scarring and bruising, and evidence of soft tissue elasticity, such as hernias and pelvic floor prolapse. Other metabolic causes of fatigue should always be excluded, e.g. hypothyroidism, hypoadrenalism, hypo/hyperglycaemia, and anaemia.

Fibromyalgia is considered when *all* of the following are present:

- pain in the left and right side of the body
- pain above and below the waist
- axial skeletal pain
- pain present for at least 3 months.

Tenderness should be elicited over 11 or more of 18 sites (Fig. 14.6) by palpation using the thumb with a pressure sufficient to make the nail blanch. The nine sites (repeated each side) are:

- occiput at the paraspinal muscle insertions of the neck
- lower cervical spine at the inter-transverse spaces at the level C6–7
- trapezius, mid-way along the upper border

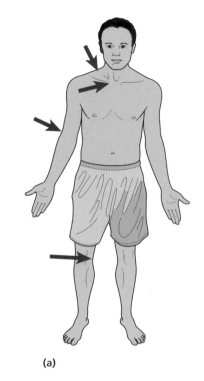

(a)

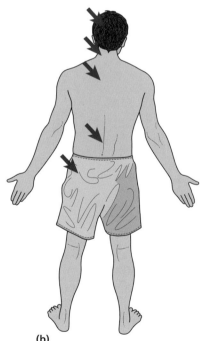

(b)

Figure 14.6 Trigger points in fibromyalgia. There are nine sites repeated on both sides to give a maximum score of 18.

- origin of supraspinatus, just above the spine of the scapula at its medial border
- second rib at the costochondral junction
- lateral humeral epicondyle, 2 cm distal from the epicondyles
- lower lumbar spine
- gluteal, in the upper inner quadrant
- knee, medial fat pad proximal to the joint line.

The emphasis in management is an explanation and reassurance that there is no serious underlying inflammatory/systemic condition or damage to the joints and muscles. Although exercise may cause a short-term increase in pain, a prolonged aerobic exercise programme may help. Pacing daily activities is also important, avoiding patterns of overactivity when well, followed by inactivity due to pain and fatigue. Pacing is a key component of cognitive behavioural therapy, a chronic pain programme that, alongside aerobic rehabilitation, may be of significant benefit to patients with fibromyalgia, CWP and joint hypermobility syndrome. NSAIDs and opioid analgesics usually do not work. Tricyclic antidepressants (such as amitriptyline) and neuroleptic agents (such as gabapentin and pregabalin) may be helpful.

Osteoarthritis

Osteoarthritis is a chronic degenerative and mechanical disorder characterized by cartilage loss. It is the most common form of arthritis, estimated to affect 15 per cent of the population of the UK over the age of 55 years. It is second only to cardiovascular disease as a cause of disability. Weight-bearing joints are chiefly involved (e.g. facets in the spine, hip and knee). However, OA can be generalized with a 'nodal' form that typically affects the PIP and DIP joints of the hands (Fig. 14.7).

Risk factors for OA that should be considered in the history include:

- obesity
- family history (particularly the 'nodal generalized' form)
- high bone density such as osteopetrosis ('marble bone syndrome')
- fractures through the joint line
- abnormal bone/joint formation – dysplasias
- neurological or muscular disease leading to weakness and abnormal mechanical forces on a joint.

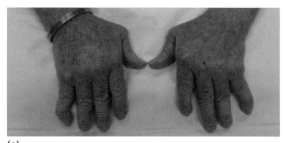
(a)

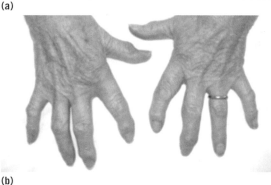
(b)

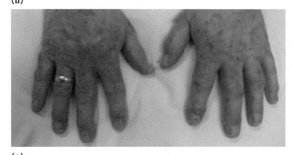
(c)

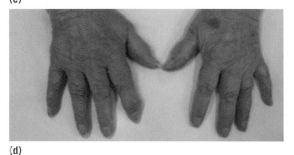
(d)

Figure 14.7 Common arthropathies affecting the hands. (a) Rheumatoid arthritis – symmetrical metacarpophangeal swelling and ulnar drift. Thumb 'Z' and proximal interphalangeal (PIP) joint 'swan neck' deformities. (b) Osteoarthritis – distal interphalangeal (DIP) 'Heberden's' and PIP 'Bouchard's' nodes. (c) Symmetrical PIP and DIP swelling, psoriatic rash, nail pitting and onycholysis. (d) Asymmetrical thumb and DIP swelling. Gouty nodules on both thumbs and right second DIP joints in particular.

There is little evidence to link OA with repetitive injury from occupation, except perhaps knee bending in men. Dockers and miners have a higher incidence of knee OA.

Interventions for OA include exercise to build muscle strength, encourage weight loss, and improve endurance and joint proprioception (position sense). NSAIDs, paracetamol and opioid analgesics are effective. Intra-articular injections of long-acting anaesthetic may help pain. Occasionally an OA joint may be inflamed due to debris in the joint; here corticosteroid joint injections are useful. Intra-articular injection of hyaluronic acid derivatives (viscosupplementation) may also reduce pain and swelling for 2–6 months in mild-moderate cases. Glucosamine and chondroitin sulphate supplements may have an analgesic effect in mild-moderate OA of the knee; there is little evidence for their use in OA at other sites. There is some evidence that avocado/soya bean supplementation, evening primrose oil, and omega-3 fish oils improve pain. Management should also include ways to reduce the impact of disability. Options include occupational therapy and physiotherapy. Surgery may be required when conservative therapy is unsuccessful.

Rheumatoid arthritis

Rheumatoid arthritis (Fig. 14.8) is the most common ARD and is characterized by the presence of a symmetrical destructive polyarthritis with a predisposition for the small joints of the hands, wrists and feet. It is more common in women than men and may present at any age though most often in the third to fourth decade. Criteria for the diagnosis of RA are shown in Table 14.4. It is important to remember

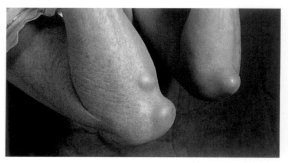

Figure 14.8 Rheumatoid nodules over the elbows and forearms. From: Ogilvie C, Evans CC (eds), *Chamberlain's symptoms and signs in clinical medicine* (12th edition), with permission. © 1997 London: Hodder Arnold.

Table 14.4 The 1987 American College of Rheumatology criteria for the diagnosis of rheumatoid arthritis: at least four criteria must be fulfilled

Criterion	Comments
Morning stiffness	Duration at least 1 hour lasting >6 weeks
Arthritis of at least three joints	Soft tissue swelling[1] lasting >6 weeks
Arthritis of hand joints	Wrists, metacarpophalangeal or proximal interphalangeal joints, lasting >6 weeks
Symmetrical arthritis	At least one area, lasting >6 weeks
Rheumatoid nodules (Fig. 14.8)	
Positive rheumatoid factor	
Radiographic changes	Erosions, particularly wrists, hands, and feet

[1]Common sites: metacarpophalangeal joints, proximal interphalangeal joints, wrist, elbow, knee, ankle, metatarsophalangeal joints.

that there are a number of 'extra-articular' manifestations to the disease (Table 14.5).

Onset is typically insidious and progressive pain, stiffness and symmetrical swelling of small joints occurs. Up to a third of patients may have a subacute onset with symptoms of fatigue, malaise, weight loss, myalgia, morning stiffness and joint pain without overt signs of swelling. A mono- or bilateral arthropathy of the shoulder or wrist may account for up to 30–40 per cent of initial presentations, and the knee 5 per cent. Any synovial joint can become involved.

Spontaneous rupture of tendons and ligaments is uncommon, but typically occurs at the wrist, hand and rotator cuff in the shoulder. More often, tenosynovitis (tendon inflammation) and weakening of ligaments lead to joint instability and subluxation.

The management of RA requires a multidisciplinary approach. Details of drug therapy are beyond the scope of this chapter but patients may require a combination of analgesics, DMARDs and sometimes steroids. A proportion of patients do not respond to DMARDs and require biological therapies (antitumour necrosis factor (TNF) α, B cell depletion, or IL-6 inhibition). Regular liaison with physiotherapists, occupational therapists, podiatrists, social services and surgeons is important in managing complex cases.

Ankylosing spondylitis

Ankylosing spondylitis is one of the seronegative inflammatory arthropathies. The ESR or CRP may be raised but the ANA, RF and ENAs are negative. Included in this group of conditions are psoriatic arthritis (PsA), enteropathic arthritis and reactive arthritis. They are characterized by axial involvement of the skeleton with sacroiliitis.

Patients are typically below 40 years of age with a male to female ratio of approximately 3:1. The condition occurs more frequently in Caucasian populations. The criteria for the diagnosis of AS are shown in Box 14.1.

There is often an insidious onset of low back pain and morning stiffness that tends to improve with exercise. Large joints (hips and knees) may be involved and in PsA small joint disease may mimic RA. Patients may also have insertional tendonitis at several sites outside the spine including the Achilles tendon, intercostal muscles, plantar fascia and a dactylitis (sausage-shaped swelling) of the fingers and toes.

Table 14.5 Organ disease associated with rheumatoid arthritis

Organ	Manifestation	Frequency (per cent)
Lymph nodes	Enlargement	50
Spleen	Enlargement	20
Lungs	Pleurisy	30
Heart	Pericarditis	10
Muscle	Atrophy Myositis	Very common 1, rare
Bone	Osteoporosis	Common
Skin	Nodules	20
Eyes	Sicca syndrome (dry eyes, dry mouth)	10
Nervous system	Nerve entrapment Mononeuritis multiplex Cord compression due to cervical disease	Common Uncommon Rare

BOX 14.1 DIAGNOSTIC CRITERIA FOR ANKYLOSING SPONDYLITIS (MODIFIED NEW YORK CRITERIA)

Clinical criteria:
- low back pain and stiffness for >6 months improving with exercise but not relieved by rest
- limitation of lumbar spine movements in lateral and forward flexion
- limitation of chest expansion relative to normal values for age and sex.

Radiological criteria:
- greater than or equal to Grade II bilateral sacroiliitis
- grade III or IV unilateral sacroiliitis.

Combined diagnostic criteria:
- definite AS if one radiological and one clinical criterion
- probable AS if three clinical criteria or a radiological criterion without signs or symptoms satisfying the clinical criteria.

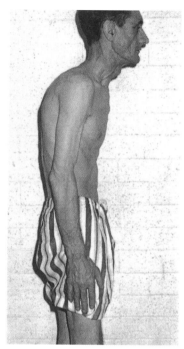

Figure 14.9 Characteristic 'question mark' posture in ankylosing spondylitis. From: Ogilvie C, Evans CC (eds), *Chamberlain's symptoms and signs in clinical medicine* (12th edition), with permission. © 1997 London: Hodder Arnold.

Later in the disease the spine may become fused with a loss of lumbar lordosis and an increase in thoracic kyphosis – the so-called 'question-mark' posture (Fig. 14.9). In order to be able to look ahead the AS patient adopts a hyperextension at the neck, increasing cervical lordosis.

The extra-articular manifestations in AS include:

- constitutional features of fatigue, weight loss, low-grade fever, and anaemia
- iritis – this occurs in up to 40 per cent of cases but has little correlation with disease activity in the spine
- upper lobe or bilateral pulmonary fibrosis. Pleuritis can occur as a consequence of insertional tendonitis of the costosternal and costovertebral muscles. Fusion of the thoracic wall leads to rigidity and reduction in chest expansion
- aortic valve prolapse.

Radiological evaluation is the most helpful form of investigation. The classical findings include sacro-iliac joint sclerosis and erosions, syndesmophytes (calcific thickening of spinal ligaments) and squaring of vertebrae. Isotope bone scanning can highlight inflammation at the sacroiliac joints. MRI may show joint erosions, and oedema and fatty change in the bone marrow induced by inflammation.

General principles for therapy include:

- patient education
- exercise, physiotherapy and hydrotherapy
- avoid smoking
- NSAIDs
- anti-TNF α therapy.

Psoriatic arthritis

Psoriasis affects 1–2 per cent of the population and 10 per cent of these develop arthritis. Psoriatic arthritis may affect any peripheral joint as well as the axial skeleton and sacroiliac joints. Nail lesions occur in up to 90 per cent of patients with PsA. These lesions include pitting, ridging, and onycholysis (see Fig. 14.7, p. 247).

There are five clinical patterns of psoriatic arthritis:

- distal, involving the distal interphalangeal joints
- asymmetrical oligoarthritis
- symmetrical polyarthritis, indistinguishable from RA
- arthritis mutilans
- spondyloarthropathy.

The radiological features associated with PsA that help to differentiate it from RA include:

- asymmetry
- DIP joint disease
- osteolysis of terminal phalanges with 'pencil-in-cup' deformities
- cervical and lumbar spondylitis
- ankylosis
- periostitis (inflammation of periosteum).

Also, unlike RA, periarticular osteopenia is uncommon.

The treatment of PsA is like that of RA with NSAIDs, DMARDs (particularly methotrexate and leflunomide), and biological therapies. Systemic corticosteroids should be avoided as they may worsen the skin disease. Intra-articular steroids may be helpful.

Gout and hyperuricaemia

Gout is a group of conditions characterized by hyperuricaemia and uric acid crystal deposition in the joints, skin and renal tract leading to an inflammatory arthritis, tophaceous gout, nephrolithiasis and nephropathy respectively. Table 14.6 outlines the risk factors for developing gout.

The condition is more common in men than women and tends to occur from the fourth decade on. The most common symptom is an acute, self-limiting, monoarthritis; up to 60–70 per cent of attacks first occur in the big toe. Other frequently involved joints include the ankle, foot, knee, wrist, elbow (olecranon bursa), and the small joints of the hands. Gout can mimic RA and septic arthritis.

Tophi are subcutaneous deposits of urate. The classic sites are the pinna of the ear, bursa of the elbow and knee, Achilles tendon, and the dorsal surface of the small joints of the hands (see Fig. 14.7, p. 247). Tophi are usually painless, though the overlying skin may ulcerate and become infected. Those most at risk of tophi are patients with prolonged severe hyperuric-aemia, polyarticular gout, and elderly patients with primary nodal OA who are on diuretics.

Synovial fluid analysis should be undertaken, looking for negatively birefringent needle shaped crystals with polarized light microscopy; the absence of crystals, however, does not rule out the diagnosis. The serum uric acid level may be normal during an acute attack. Uric acid levels are nevertheless of value when monitoring the effectiveness of therapies that lower serum urate. Late features on radiographs may be tophi near joints, tissue swelling, joint erosions, periosteal new bone formation, and joint deformity.

Public health improvement measures to prevent gout are yet to be proven. However avoiding excess weight gain and alcohol, controlling hypertension, and exposure to diuretics, may have some effect on reducing risk of gout. Otherwise, there are two phases to therapy: treatment of the acute attack, and treatment of chronic disease. Acute attacks should be managed with a combination of NSAIDs, colchicine and corticosteroids. In the longer term, agents that reduce serum urate should be used, the most common of these being allopurinol.

Table 14.6 Common causes of hyperuricaemia and gout

Primary gout 'metabolic syndrome'	Male sex Age >40 years Obesity Family history Renal impairment Hypertension
Overproduction of uric acid	Excess alcohol and purine rich foods intake Cell lysis – tumour lysis syndrome Myeloproliferative disease Haemolytic anaemia Psoriasis Drugs – cytotoxics, warfarin
Underexcretion of uric acid	Renal failure Drugs – salicylates, diuretics, laxatives, ciclosporin, levodopa, ethambutol, pyrazinamide
Inherited syndromes	X-linked HPRT deficiency (Lesch–Nyhan syndrome) X-linked raised PRPP synthetase activity

HPRT, hypoxanthine guanine phosphoribosyl transferase; PRPP, phosphoribosylpyrophosphate synthetase.

Osteoporosis

This remains a significant cause of morbidity and mortality. Peak bone mass is usually achieved in the third decade and is determined by both genetic and environmental factors. After the age of 35 the amount of bone laid down is less than that reabsorbed during each remodelling cycle. The net effect is age-related loss of bone mass. Up to 15 per cent of bone mass can also be lost over the 5-year period immediately post menopause. Symptomless reduction in bone mass and strength results in an increased risk of fracture; it is the resulting fractures that lead to pain and morbidity.

Major risk factors to be considered in osteoporosis are:

- race (white or Asian > African Caribbean)
- age
- gender
- family history of maternal hip fracture
- previous low trauma fracture (low trauma defined as no greater than falling from standing height)
- long-term use of corticosteroids

- malabsorption disorders
- endocrinopathies – hyperparathyroidism, hyperthyroidism, low vitamin D
- inflammatory arthritis e.g. RA, AS, SLE.

Other risk factors include:

- low body mass index (BMI <16 kg/m^2)
- late menarche and early menopause
- nulliparity
- reduced physical activity
- low intake of calcium (below 240 mg daily)
- excess alcohol intake
- smoking
- malignancy (multiple myeloma).

Plain radiographs are insensitive for assessing bone mass. The standard technique for measuring bone mineral density (BMD) is dual energy X-ray absorptiometry (DEXA). This gives two readings, the 'T' and 'Z' scores:

- 'T' score is the individual's bone mineral density compared with the mean bone mineral density achieved at peak bone mass (i.e. around age 35) for the same sex and race. Most analyses and studies have focused on the T score
- 'Z' score is the individual's bone mineral density compared with that for someone of the same age, sex and race.

One standard deviation below the mean is equal to a twofold increase in the risk of fracture. This means that an individual with a BMD three standard deviations below the mean has an eightfold increased risk of fracture, compared with a 'normal' individual of the same age.

Calcium, phosphate and ALP levels are normal in osteoporosis. Investigation should include a screen for malignancy and biochemical abnormalities of bone (i.e. ESR, urea and electrolytes, liver function test, serum immunoglobulins, calcium and phosphate).

Management focuses on reducing the risks, falls assessment, and adequate daily calcium (1 g) and vitamin D (800 IU) intake. Specific therapies such as bisphosphonates and strontium ranelate may prevent further bone loss and reduce fracture risk after the menopause.

Osteomalacia

Osteomalacia results either from deficiency of vitamin D (poor intake, lack of sunlight exposure, malabsorption, liver or renal disease) or rare abnormalities of phosphate metabolism (renal tubular acidosis, hypophosphatasia).

A decrease in the ratio of mineral to matrix leads to softening of bone. Symptoms include bone pain, bone deformity, fractures, and proximal muscle weakness with a 'waddling gait'. Plasma levels of calcium and phosphate are usually reduced and ALP raised. Hypocalcaemia may give rise to paraesthesia and tetany; rarely, it can cause cardiac dysrhythmia, convulsions, or psychosis.

The classical radiographic change is the pseudo-fracture (Looser's zone), found most often at the ribs and clavicles, outer border of the scapulae, pubic rami, femoral neck, and metatarsals. They appear as incomplete, radiolucent fracture lines perpendicular to the cortex, with poor callus formation.

Management requires treatment of the underlying cause and adequate vitamin D replacement. Many bony deformities persist despite treatment (unless due to simple dietary deficiency and treated in childhood) and may require surgery, e.g. tibial/fibular osteotomy to correct lower limb alignment.

Infection and arthritis

Infection may give rise to systemic inflammatory arthritis or vasculitis. The condition 'reactive arthritis' is also recognized. The disorder is characterized by conjunctivitis, urethritis or colitis, skin lesions in the palms and soles, and either a pauci- or polyarthritis. It is usually triggered by sexually transmitted infection such as with *Chlamydia trachomatis*. The acute inflammatory reaction is treated with NSAIDs and corticosteroids and often 'burns out' after 6–18 months. It may leave lasting joint damage.

IMPORTANT *i*

Septic arthritis constitutes an acute emergency. The presentation is usually one of a rapid onset of severe pain in a hot swollen joint, the pain so severe that the patient cannot bear for it to be touched or moved.

Septic arthritis is an acute mono- or pauci-articular pathology. Staphylococcal, gonococcal, pneumococcal, *Escherichia coli*, and *Mycobacterium tuberculosis* infection are among the more common causes. Diagnosis is made by culture of synovial fluid and treatment involves high dose antimicrobial therapy for up to 6 weeks (or 9 months if tuberculosis).

Neoplasia and bone pain

Focal pain, swelling, or a low trauma fracture in the spine or long bones should alert suspicion. Primary tumours of bone include the benign (but often very painful) osteoid-osteoma, chondromas, and malignant osteosarcoma. Metastatic carcinoma may be secondary to a primary lesion in the lung, breast, prostate, kidney or thyroid. Haematological malignancies including lymphomas and leukaemias may also lead to diffuse bone involvement. Multiple myeloma, a neoplasia of plasma cells, is an important example; it is associated with widespread bone destruction, hypercalcaemia, and renal impairment.

SUMMARY

Key features of the presenting history are:

- pain
    - site and radiation
    - nature
    - relieving and aggravating factors
- stiffness
- swelling
- impaired function
- constitutional symptoms.

Include the following in your physical examination:

- inspection:
    - swelling
    - deformities
    - nodules
    - asymmetry
    - muscle wasting
    - scars
    - skin pathology
    - perform the gait, arms, legs, spine screen

- palpation:
    - feel for warmth of inflammation
    - gently squeeze individual joints and palpate soft tissues for tenderness
- ask whether any areas of the body are numb or weak – be prepared to perform a sensory or motor neurological examination
- movement:
    - active movement
    - active movement against a resisting force
    - passive movement
    - compare range of movement on each side of the body
    - look for excessive movement (hypermobility)
- function:
    - loss of movement leads to loss of function
    - consider what the joint does
- regional examination of the hips and knees:
    - log-rolling test of the hips
    - Thomas' test to identify hip flexion deformity
    - assess the knee for an effusion: bulge sign test; ballottement.

FURTHER READING

Coady D, Walker D, Kay L. 2004. Regional examination of the musculoskeletal system (REMS): a core set of clinical skills for medical students. *Rheumatology* **43**: 633–9.

Coady D. 2005. *Regional examination of the musculoskeletal system – A handbook for medical students*. York: Arthritis Research Campaign Trading Ltd.

Doherty M, Dacre J, Dieppe P, *et al.* 1992. The 'GALS' locomotor screen. *Annals of the Rheumatic Diseases* **51**: 1165–1169.

Hakim AJ, Clunie G, Haq I. 2006. *The Oxford handbook of rheumatology*. Oxford: Oxford University Press.

15 THE ENDOCRINE SYSTEM

Peter Mansell

INTRODUCTION

Diabetes mellitus is becoming a major public health problem. This is particularly true for type 2 diabetes, the prevalence of which is increasing rapidly due to the association with obesity and physical inactivity. Much of the morbidity, and cost, of diabetes care is due to the associated complications, rather than directly to hyperglycaemia and its management.

Thyroid disease and polycystic ovarian syndrome are also prevalent conditions. Most other endocrine disorders are uncommon, although of considerable clinical interest and often associated with a wide range of symptoms and signs. The increasing sophistication and availability of biochemical testing means that the final diagnosis and management of endocrine disorders is now almost entirely dependent on the measurement of the concentrations of either hormones themselves, or metabolites influenced by those hormones. As biochemical testing has become progressively more reliable and straightforward, an increasing number of patients with endocrine or metabolic disorders are now diagnosed at an early, often pre-symptomatic stage, e.g. early type 2 diabetes, subclinical thyroid dysfunction and mild hypercalcaemia due to hyperparathyroidism.

DIABETES MELLITUS

Symptoms

The classic triad of symptoms associated with diabetes mellitus consists of:

- thirst
- polyuria (often nocturia)
- weight loss.

Many patients will also experience pruritus or balanitis, fatigue and blurred vision. Some people, particularly those with newly presenting *type 1 diabetes mellitus* (T1DM) or with marked hyperglycaemia in *type 2 diabetes mellitus* (T2DM), may have a 'full house' of symptoms, in which case it is generally not difficult to suspect the diagnosis. However, other patients, particularly those with only modestly elevated blood glucose concentrations in T2DM, will have fewer, milder symptoms, and some may be entirely asymptomatic. Note that symptoms potentially suggestive of diabetes may have alternative causes, particularly in elderly people, for example, frequency and nocturia in an older man may be due to bladder outflow obstruction, and many medical disorders are associated with weight loss.

The symptom complex of thirst, polydipsia and polyuria most commonly suggests a diagnosis of uncontrolled diabetes mellitus but can occur in other settings. Some patients taking diuretics will experience similar symptoms. A dry mouth, perhaps associated with drug usage (e.g. tricyclic antidepressants) or certain medical conditions (e.g. Sjögren's syndrome), may lead to increased fluid intake in an attempt at symptom relief. In addition, there are other metabolic disorders which can interfere with the concentrating ability of the renal medulla and hence cause increased urine output with compensatory thirst. Such conditions include diabetes insipidus, hypercalcaemia, hypokalaemia and (on occasions) renal failure.

Weight loss is a symptom that always requires further evaluation as this may have a serious underlying cause. Some patients do not appear to notice or to report weight change, and it can be helpful to obtain objective evidence from prior weights recorded in hospital or their general practitioner's (GP's) notes. In some patients with weight loss, particularly those who are elderly, it can be difficult to be certain whether their diabetes has been sufficiently uncontrolled to account for this, or whether the weight loss may be due to a second diagnosis. A pragmatic trial of improved diabetes management may be required to see if the weight loss resolves.

The rest of the history

When seeing a patient presenting with symptoms of possible diabetes, or where this is being re-evaluated, you should also ask relevant questions to try to establish the following.

1. If the patient already has complications of diabetes

> **i   IMPORTANT**
> 30–50 per cent of patients with newly diagnosed T2DM will already have tissue complications at diagnosis due to the prolonged period of antecedent moderate and asymptomatic hyperglycaemia.

Complications will not be present in patients with new and recently diagnosed T1DM, but may occur in all others. The complications of diabetes are broadly divided into:

- microvascular complications (often diabetes specific)
- macrovascular complications.

The most important microvascular complications are retinopathy, nephropathy and neuropathy. When taking a history, you should therefore ask about these complications and specifically about any changes to vision and about neuropathic symptoms.

The most common form of a diabetic neuropathy is a '*glove and stocking*' distal sensory (or sensorimotor) neuropathy, although in practice the hands are rarely affected. Such a sensory neuropathy may be painless, but note that numbness is sometimes not noticed or reported by the patient and is first identified on examination. Some patients experience a symptomatic painful neuropathy with added sensations such as burning, shooting pains or paraesthesiae, characteristically worse at rest and particularly at night.

Other forms of neuropathy can occur in diabetes including a mononeuropathy (e.g. an isolated cranial or individual peripheral nerve palsy), and an autonomic neuropathy, most commonly manifest as impotence in men, but more rarely causing postural hypotension or a gastrointestinal motility disorder with vomiting and a disturbed bowel habit.

Your evaluation of a patient with diabetes is not complete without obtaining a history of hypertension and symptomatic macrovascular disease (Fig. 15.1):

- cardiovascular disease (angina, myocardial infarction, heart failure, revascularization procedures)
- cerebrovascular disease (transient ischaemic attack or stroke)
- peripheral vascular disease (claudication, foot ulceration or amputation).

As a corollary to the above, when you see a patient presenting with clinical problems which may possibly be associated with diabetes, you should determine whether that patient has diabetes or not. For example, all patients with newly diagnosed cardio-, cerebro- or peripheral vascular disease should be assessed for diabetes.

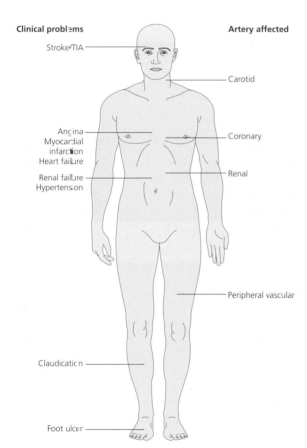

Clinical problems — Artery affected
Stroke/TIA
Carotid
Angina
Myocardial infarction
Heart failure
Coronary
Renal failure
Hypertension
Renal
Peripheral vascular
Claudication
Foot ulcer

Figure 15.1 Macrovascular disease in diabetes and associated clinical problems.

2. The type and cause of diabetes (see later; this will include full past medical, drug and family histories)

3. The effect of diabetes, and of its management and complications, in the social history

Ask the patient how they look after their diabetes and how this affects their daily life. Diabetes management may affect functioning or occupation – patients on insulin in particular may have problems with hypoglycaemia, or adapting to shift working, and are restricted from certain occupations and holding a vocational driving licence. Complications such as reduced vision or foot ulceration will affect daily activities and quality of life.

Physical examination

Patients with established diabetes should have an annual review. This consists of:

- measurement of blood pressure
- funduscopy or retinal photography for retinopathy
- assessment of visual acuity
- a check of the integrity of foot pulses and sensation
- a urine test for (micro-) albuminuria, the hallmark of diabetic nephropathy.

When examining the eye, check visual acuity first. Then dilate the pupils with tropicamide (or equivalent) eye drops as it is generally much easier to look for signs of retinal disease using an ophthalmoscope through a dilated rather than an undilated pupil. Ophthalmoscopy takes a lot of practice to become competent.

First look for lens opacities. Then focus on the optic disc. Subsequently follow each of the superior and inferior temporal and nasal vascular arcades out to the periphery and back again to the disc. Finally, inspect the macula by asking the patient to look directly into the ophthalmoscope; if the patient finds the light painfully bright, reduce its intensity.

The signs and classification of retinopathy depend on the stage of the disease (Table 15.1, Fig. 15.2). *Maculopathy* is defined as any changes occurring within one optic disc diameter of the fovea. You

may also see signs of previous laser therapy for retinopathy (Fig. 15.3).

Examine the foot, first looking for signs of ulceration, infection or deformity (Figs 15.4 and 15.5). Any deformity such as a prominent bunion or metatarsal

Table 15.1 Stages of diabetic retinopathy

Stage of retinopathy	Signs
Background	Microaneurysms (dots), blot haemorrhages, hard exudates
Pre-proliferative	Soft exudates, venous irregularities, IRMA
Proliferative	New vessels on the disc or elsewhere
Advanced	Scarring, fibrosis
Maculopathy	Any retinopathy close to the fovea

IRMA, intraretinal microvascular abnormalities.

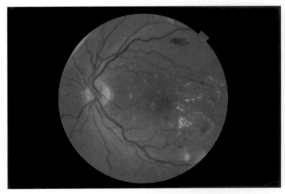

Figure 15.2 Pre-proliferative diabetic retinopathy.

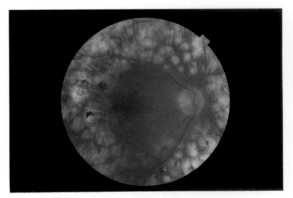

Figure 15.3 Laser scars from photocoagulation in diabetic retinopathy.

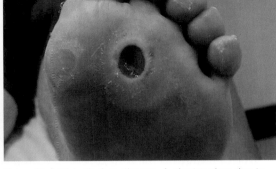

Figure 15.4 Diabetic foot disease. A plantar ulcer due to neuropathy.

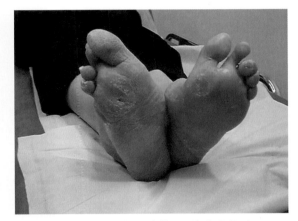

Figure 15.5 Bilateral deformed Charcot's feet due to diabetic neuropathy.

heads, claw toes, a prior minor amputation or Charcot's foot is a risk factor for subsequent ulceration. Thick callus can accumulate at pressure points and erode the underlying healthy skin.

Next, assess for peripheral vascular disease by palpating for the dorsalis pedis and tibialis anterior foot pulses – if these are absent or difficult to find, check for the popliteal and femoral pulses and listen for a femoral bruit.

Finally check for neuropathy by testing sensation and the ankle reflex. Look in particular for a 'sock' distribution of sensory loss; if there is loss of sensation in the feet, examine the hands as well.

There are frequently no abnormalities on physical examination in patients with T1DM, particularly those who are younger or who do not have long-standing disease. Those who have had T1DM for more than a few years and all of those with T2DM (even from first diagnosis) may have tissue complications of diabetes identified at annual review, and there may therefore be additional signs of cardiovascular or cerebrovascular disease.

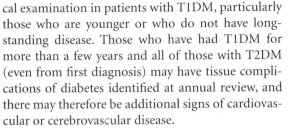

> **IMPORTANT**
> Patients with a new diagnosis of what is apparently T2DM should have a full general examination as, occasionally, the diabetes may be the presenting feature of (but secondary to) another disorder e.g. acromegaly, haemochromatosis or Cushing's syndrome.

Investigations

The diagnosis of diabetes mellitus rests solely on laboratory blood glucose concentrations (see below). Further investigations may be required in occasional patients in whom it is thought that the diabetes may be secondary to another medical disorder. Tests essential in the further evaluation and longer-term assessment of patients with diabetes are:

- HbA1c – as a marker of longer-term glycaemic control
- serum lipid profile
- urea, electrolytes and creatinine – as indicators of renal function (now generally converted to estimated glomerular filtration rate, eGFR)
- liver function tests – in view of the association with non-alcoholic fatty liver disease (NAFLD).

Diagnosis and classification of diabetes mellitus

Diabetes mellitus is formally diagnosed solely using laboratory blood glucose tests. The presence of glycosuria, a raised HbA1c and elevated capillary blood glucose meter readings raise the possibility of diabetes but are insufficient for diagnosis.

In the great majority of patients, diabetes is diagnosed on the basis of symptoms and a random venous

> **_i_ IMPORTANT**
> Blood glucose meters are accurate enough for
> _monitoring_ but should never be relied upon
> without laboratory back-up either for _diagnosis_
> or for evaluating patients who are unwell with
> decompensated diabetes (ketoacidosis or
> hyperosmolar state), or with reduced consciousness
> due to possible hypoglycaemia.

> **CLINICAL PEARL**
> The blood glucose concentration at diagnosis is
> not useful as a guide to whether an individual
> patient has T1DM or T2DM. Patients with T1DM
> can be in severe ketoacidosis with a blood glucose
> less than 20 mmol/L, and even below 10 mmol/L
> on occasions, whereas T2DM can present with a
> hyperosmolar state with blood glucose levels over
> 50 mmol/L.

plasma glucose concentration above 11.1 mmol/L. Other patients may require a fasting blood glucose or a 75 g _oral glucose tolerance test_ (OGTT), which is performed the morning after an overnight fast of 8–14 hours (water is permitted). After a baseline blood sample is taken for a venous plasma glucose level, an adult patient is given 75 g glucose in 300 mL water to drink over 5 minutes. A further blood sample is taken after 2 hours. Table 15.2 provides guidance on interpretation of the results of an OGTT.

Just one abnormal blood test is needed to make the diagnosis in patients with typical symptoms of diabetes, with two abnormal results required in those who are asymptomatic. The categories _impaired glucose tolerance_ (IGT) and _impaired fasting glycaemia_ (IFG) are defined as there is a significant rate of progression to T2DM. Impaired glucose tolerance in particular is associated with a considerably increased risk of macrovascular disease, almost to the degree seen in T2DM. The scheme for diagnosing diabetes is not entirely intuitive. It is, for instance, possible to have both IFG _and_ IGT. In addition, a fasting plasma glucose consistent with IFG or even in the normal range does not fully exclude a possible diagnosis of diabetes.

Diabetes mellitus is not a single disorder. In the UK, 85–90 per cent of patients will have T2DM (formerly non-insulin-dependent diabetes, NIDDM) and the majority of the remainder will have T1DM (formerly insulin-dependent diabetes, IDDM). It is important to make this distinction, as initial management from diagnosis is so different. Table 15.3 lists clinical features that are useful in distinguishing T1DM from T2DM, and many patients will clearly fit one or other pattern. In a small number of patients,

Table 15.2 Venous plasma glucose concentrations (mmol/L) and diagnostic criteria for diabetes in a 75 g oral glucose tolerance test

	Fasting plasma glucose	Plasma glucose at 2 hours
Normal	≤6.0	<7.8
Impaired fasting glycaemia	6.1–6.9	
Impaired glucose tolerance		7.8–11.1
Diabetes	≥7.0	>11.1

Table 15.3 Clinical features helpful in discriminating between type 1 and type 2 diabetes at initial presentation

Clinical feature	Type 1 diabetes	Type 2 diabetes
Diabetic ketoacidosis	Prone	Very rare
Ketonuria (dipstick +++)	Common	Rare
Symptoms	Severe, acute	Mild, chronic
Obesity	Uncommon	Very common
Weight loss	Moderate/severe	Nil/moderate
Age	Any but often <30	Any but often >30
Complications at diagnosis	Never	Common
Affected first-degree relative	Uncommon (5 per cent)	Common
Other OSAID*	Common	Uncommon
Islet cell antibodies	Usual (80 per cent+)	Absent

*OSAID, organ-specific autoimmune disease e.g. autoimmune thyroid disease, Addison's disease, pernicious anaemia, vitiligo.

it is not always possible to be certain whether they have T1DM or T2DM at the time of diagnosis. In particular, although age is a pointer to diabetes type, it is far from an absolute discriminator, as T2DM is now prevalent in obese younger people, even teenagers, and T1DM can occur in elderly people.

In addition to T1DM and T2DM, there is a small number of patients in whom diabetes can be monogenic, part of another disease or syndrome, secondary to another condition, drug-induced or due to primary disease of the exocrine pancreas. The classification of diabetes is summarized in Table 15.4 (note: only selected, more common 'other' causes of diabetes are given).

Hypoglycaemia

In normal physiology, a fall in blood glucose concentration below normal causes a reduction in endogenous insulin production and a counter-regulatory response with the release of glucagon, adrenaline, cortisol and growth hormone. There is also autonomic activation which, together with the increase in circulating adrenaline induces a variety of symptoms including:

- anxiety
- palpitations
- tremor
- sweating
- hunger.

Many patients with diabetes recognize these symptoms as a 'warning' and know that they need to take additional carbohydrate to restore their blood glucose concentration. If warning symptoms are delayed, absent, not recognized or not acted on, progressive hypoglycaemia will lead to *neuroglycopenia*, with a variety of symptoms such as blurred or double vision, loss of concentration and difficulty word finding. A further fall in blood glucose will cause a reduction in conscious level and eventually fitting and/or coma.

It is generally not difficult to suspect an episode of hypoglycaemia in patients who are known to have diabetes, particularly if they are being treated with insulin or sulphonylureas. Significant hypoglycaemia not associated with diabetes is much more difficult to recognize. Hypoglycaemia should be considered in all patients who present with symptoms suggestive of intermittent sympatho-adrenal activation and/or neuroglycopenia (as described above) whether or not they are known to have diabetes.

Table 15.4 Classification of diabetes mellitus (very rare causes have been omitted)

Type	Causes
Type 1	Pancreatic islet B cell deficiency Autoimmune or idiopathic
Type 2	Defective insulin action or secretion
Others	Genetic defects of B cell function: • MODY (autosomal dominant), mitochondrial disorders Diseases of the exocrine pancreas: • chronic pancreatitis • pancreatectomy • carcinoma • cystic fibrosis • haemochromatosis Endocrinopathies: • acromegaly • Cushing's syndrome Drug or chemical induced: • corticosteroids Gestational diabetes

SMALL PRINT

Spontaneous hypoglycaemia, although clinically very significant, is rare.

Summary

Diabetes mellitus is much more than a disorder of glucose metabolism. The complications of diabetes can affect many of the organ systems leading to associated cardiac, vascular, renal, retinal, neurological and other disorders. The satisfactory evaluation and management of a patient with diabetes requires knowledge of the wider manifestations of the condition and an understanding of its impact on the individual as a whole.

THYROID DISEASE

Thyroid disease generally presents either as an endocrine disorder and/or as a thyroid swelling (nodule or goitre).

Thyroid dysfunction

There are two serum thyroid hormones. Both the total and free (non-protein bound) concentrations of thyroxine (T4) are higher than those of the more biologically active tri-iodothyronine (T3). The serum thyroid hormone concentrations determine the rate of metabolism. Thyroid-stimulating hormone (TSH) derives from the pituitary gland and, due to negative feedback, is generally suppressed in thyroid overactivity and increased in underactivity. In normal health, the serum levels of TSH, T4 and T3 show little diurnal or seasonal variation.

- *Thyrotoxicosis* denotes any excess of thyroid hormones, whereas *hyperthyroidism* refers more specifically to overactivity of the thyroid gland per se.
- *Hypothyroidism* denotes thyroid underactivity, and the term *myxoedema* is generally only used to describe clinically severe hypothyroidism.

The clinical features associated with thyroid over- and underactivity are fairly predictable and opposite.

Presenting symptoms

The principal and contrasting presenting symptoms of hyper- and hypothyroidism are given in Table 15.5.

Some patients with marked thyroid dysfunction will present with a 'full house' of clinical symptoms. However many patients will have only some, or less severe, symptoms. In addition, others may have some symptoms that are apparently paradoxical; in particular, on occasions, patients with thyroid overactivity can present with weight gain, rather than weight loss, if the increase in appetite is greater than that in the metabolic rate. Conversely, some elderly patients may have so-called 'apathetic' thyrotoxicosis, superficially more resembling hypothyroidism. Hypothyroidism, particularly if prolonged or severe,

Table 15.5 Contrasting symptoms in hyper- and hypothyroidism

Symptom	Hyperthyroidism	Hypothyroidism
Palpitations	Present	Absent
Tremor	Present	Absent
Weight change	Weight loss	Weight gain
Appetite	Increased	Decreased
Bowel frequency	Increased	Decreased
Temperature (subjective)	Hot/sweaty	Cold/dry skin
Mood	Hyperactive	Depressed
Exercise tolerance	Decreased	Decreased
Periods (women)	Light/infrequent	Heavy

can on occasions cause additional clinical features. Nerve entrapment can result in carpal tunnel syndrome and pleural or pericardial effusions occasionally occur.

There is naturally a degree of correlation between the severity of symptoms in thyroid dysfunction and the degree of biochemical disturbance. However, some patients can become quite unwell with relatively minor changes in biochemistry, whereas others with gross biochemical disturbance may be relatively asymptomatic.

The descriptions hyper- and hypothyroidism do not provide a full diagnosis. Thyrotoxicosis, in particular, has several potential causes, the most common being:

- autoimmune Graves' disease
- toxic multinodular goitre
- thyroid adenoma
- viral thyroiditis
- post-partum thyroiditis
- drug-associated – such as amiodarone.

> **SMALL PRINT**
> Rarely, severe prolonged hypothyroidism can result in *myxoedema coma* presenting with inanition (lack of energy), hypothermia and a reduced conscious level due to a grossly suppressed metabolism.

i IMPORTANT
Try to establish the aetiology of thyrotoxicosis, as this determines the natural history of the condition and also influences clinical management.

When undertaking an evaluation of a patient with thyroid disease, you should therefore not only elicit symptoms and signs directly related to thyroid dysfunction, but also seek for pointers towards the underlying cause (see Table 15.6). It is often helpful to ask about the duration of symptoms. The clinical severity of Graves' disease in particular often changes with time and, in retrospect, patients may recall episodes months or even years previously where they had transient symptoms. By contrast, nodular thyroid disease is often fairly mild and more stable over time.

Remainder of the history

Thyrotoxicosis associated with a *painful goitre* strongly suggests a diagnosis of viral (de Quervain's) thyroiditis. Graves' disease is autoimmune in origin, and so if you suspect Graves' disease, find out whether the patient has any associated autoimmune disease or whether any close relative is affected.

Hyper- or hypothyroidism first occurring within about 6 months of pregnancy is suggestive of *postpartum thyroiditis*, which is often self-limiting. A few drugs can cause thyroid dysfunction, most notably amiodarone (both hyper- and hypothyroidism) and lithium, which causes hypothyroidism.

Table 15.6 Clinical features which may be of value in determining the cause of thyroid dysfunction

Physical sign	Cause of thyroid dysfunction
Lid retraction/lid lag	Any thyrotoxicosis
Thyroid-associated ophthalmopathy	Graves' disease
Smooth, symmetrical goitre	Graves' disease, thyroiditis
Irregular goitre	Nodular disease
Painful/tender symmetrical goitre	Viral thyroiditis
Pre-tibial myxoedema/acropachy	Graves' disease

Some patients with Graves' disease develop an associated eye problem variously described as thyroid eye disease (TED), Graves' ophthalmopathy, or thyroid associated ophthalmopathy (TAO). Patients may describe a discomfort in their eyes, a bulging or prominent appearance, puffiness or swelling around the eyes, double vision or, very rarely, visual loss.

CLINICAL PEARL
The severity of thyroid dysfunction and of thyroid-associated ophthalmopathy (TAO) may not follow a parallel course. TAO can first occur some time after thyrotoxicosis appears or be the initial feature of Graves' disease occurring with normal thyroid function tests or even hypothyroidism.

Physical examination

Patients with thyrotoxicosis from any cause will often have signs compatible with the symptoms described above including:

- tachycardia (irregular pulse if in atrial fibrillation) with increased pulse volume
- finger tremor
- warm and sweaty skin
- brisk tendon reflexes
- weight loss.

Rarely, patients with severe thyroid overactivity may be in heart failure. By contrast, those with hypothyroidism may have:

- bradycardia with cool dry skin
- slowly relaxing tendon reflexes
- weight gain.

However, there may be no significant physical signs, particularly if the biochemical derangement is mild.

All patients with thyroid dysfunction, and also those presenting with a neck swelling in the region of the thyroid, should be examined for the presence of a goitre or nodule. Examine the thyroid by standing behind the seated patient (Fig. 15.6). Place your thumbs behind the patient's neck and rest the tips of your ring fingers on the ends of the patient's clavicles. Use the index and middle fingers of each hand to palpate the thyroid.

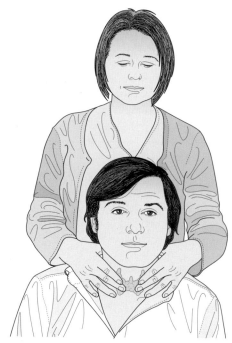

Figure 15.6 Clinical examination of the thyroid gland.

- If a goitre is present, note whether the gland is generally enlarged (both lobes and isthmus).
- Is the gland tender (uncommon) and does it appear smooth or nodular?
- Is there an abnormal consistency – is this hard (rare) or rubbery, suggestive of Hashimoto's disease in hypothyroidism?
- Ask the patient to swallow some water. A normal gland moves upwards on swallowing, but if tethered to surrounding structures, suspect a malignancy.
- Assuming the gland does move up on swallowing, feel for the trachea in the suprasternal notch below it – if this is impalpable, the gland has a retrosternal extension and may cause tracheal compression.
- Are the cervical lymph nodes enlarged?
- Finally, in a thyrotoxic patient listen with a stethoscope over the goitre for a bruit, which is virtually diagnostic of Graves' disease.

Common causes of a thyroid swelling and their clinical characteristics are given in Table 15.7.

Table 15.7 Causes of thyroid enlargement and their characteristics

Aetiology	Type of thyroid enlargement	Other features
Graves' disease	Diffuse	Bruit, TAO
Hashimoto's	Diffuse	Rubbery
Acute viral	Diffuse	Tender
Iodine deficiency	Diffuse	
Single nodule	Nodule	
Malignant	Nodule or diffuse	May be fixed. Nodes
Cyst	Discrete	
Multinodular	Multiple nodules	

TAO, thyroid associated ophthalmopathy.

Patients with thyrotoxicosis of any cause may have lid retraction and/or lid lag. The thyroid overactivity causes contraction of the levator palpebrae superioris, which has some sympathetic innervation, The upper lid may therefore retract sufficiently to expose an arc of white cornea above the upper border of the iris, producing a 'staring' appearance. This effect may be further demonstrated by eliciting 'lid lag'. Gently hold the patient's chin to keep the head steady, place your other hand above the eyeline so that the patient needs to look upwards. Then ask the patient to follow your hand, using their eyes only, as you lower this below the horizontal over a period of 3 seconds or so. In thyroid overactivity, movement of the upper lid may lag behind that of the eye, transiently exposing the cornea above the upper border of the iris.

Only patients with Graves' disease develop additional symptoms and signs of TAO. Unequivocal changes of TAO, if present, are therefore diagnostic of Graves' disease. TAO can result a variety of signs, which should be determined. The most common sign, which can be difficult to ascertain clinically, is *proptosis*, where the eyeball is pushed forward by retro-orbital inflammatory tissue. Patients with proptosis will have a staring appearance, but this should not be confused with simple lid retraction. Forward protrusion of the eye in proptosis may lead to exposure of the cornea *below* the lower arc of the iris, as well as above the upper border. True proptosis may also be recognized by prominence of the eyeballs when looking down from above the patient's head.

The patient may also have periorbital oedema (see below) and abnormalities of movement of extra-ocular muscles which patients may describe as 'double vision'; look for disconjugate gaze on examining eye movements (see examination of cranial nerves, Chapter 12). Rarely, TAO can lead to loss of vision through compression of the optic nerve, so check visual acuity. In severe proptosis, corneal exposure can lead to scarring – check that patients can voluntarily close their eyes fully.

It is important to assess for *all* features of TAO. Some patients have:

- marked periorbital oedema, which causes a striking change in facial appearance and considerable distress, but is not medically serious
- visual loss due to optic nerve compression without other apparent signs of TAO
- changes which may be asymmetrical and occasionally even unilateral.

Full evaluation of TAO can be difficult and should be left to the expert, once it has been identified.

> **SMALL PRINT**
> Occasional patients with Graves' disease and TAO may have a thickening of the skin over the shin (pretibial myxoedema) and other areas and, very rarely, thyroid acropachy, with clubbing and pain and swelling in the hands and wrists due to periosteal new bone formation.

ADRENAL DISEASE

Adrenal cortex

Cushing's syndrome

The term Cushing's syndrome refers to the clinical state associated with excess endogenous cortisol production from any cause. Cushing's disease refers specifically to cortisol overproduction secondary to excessive adrenocorticotropic hormone (ACTH) release from a pituitary adenoma, and excludes the other causes of Cushing's syndrome, namely ectopic ACTH production and autonomous adrenocortical overactivity. The term 'cushingoid' variously refers to patients with clinical features resembling Cushing's syndrome, either resulting from chronic exogenous corticosteroid use or spontaneously without biochemical disturbance.

The major clinical features of Cushing's syndrome include:

- increased and redistributed adiposity with loss of muscle bulk (myopathy), leading to a typical general appearance with central obesity, thin limbs (a 'lemon on matchstick' appearance), a moon face and a 'buffalo' hump due to expansion of the interscapular fat deposits. The myopathy may cause considerable weakness, such that the patient cannot easily get out of a low chair or a bath, and not be able to rise from a squatting position – a useful, simple clinical test for a proximal myopathy
- loss of subcutaneous connective tissue leading to thin skin and easy bruising, and also to abdominal striae, which are typically purple
- hyperandrogenism, which in women may lead to acne, hirsutes, frontal balding and amenorrhoea
- systemic effects including hypertension and glucose intolerance
- psychological effects (common) such as mood changes and depression.
- Cushing's syndrome can be difficult to recognize and diagnose because some of the associated clinical features are very common but the syndrome itself is rare. Hypertension, obesity, T2DM and hirsutes occur frequently, individually and collectively; it would be almost impossible to screen patients with these features alone for steroid overproduction as very few will have Cushing's syndrome.

> **CLINICAL PEARL**
> Select patients for screening for possible Cushing's syndrome on the basis of more discriminatory clinical features including osteoporosis, myopathy, purple abdominal striae, thin skin and easy bruising.

Patients thought likely to have Cushing's syndrome on clinical grounds should first be investigated with biochemical screening tests. The two tests most commonly used are:

- overnight dexamethasone test – serum cortisol taken at 9am will not be suppressed by dexamethasone
- 24-hour urinary collection for free cortisol.

Patients who have abnormal results on screening tests should be referred to a specialist endocrinologist for further confirmatory tests and investigation of the cause of the Cushing's syndrome because the interpretation of these tests is fraught with difficulties and pitfalls.

Addison's disease

Underproduction of corticosteroids can occur either as a result of failure of the adrenal glands (primary adrenocortical insufficiency, Addison's disease), or secondary to pituitary failure.

Addison's disease is rare, and the diagnosis is often delayed. Patients with marked primary adrenocortical insufficiency may have a classic collection of clinical features including:

- weight loss
- fatigue
- weakness
- dizziness on standing (due to postural hypotension)
- brown skin pigmentation.

Pigmentation extends to areas not exposed to the sun and is often particularly marked in natural skin creases, established scars and inside the cheeks. Patients may also present with or describe episodes of extreme lethargy, abdominal pain, vomiting and hypotension, a so-called 'addisonian crisis', which can be fatal if not recognized and appropriately treated.

Patients with severe Addison's disease, and particularly those in a crisis, will typically have hyponatraemia, hyperkalaemia and a raised serum urea due to dehydration, although electrolytes can be normal in early or mild disease. The short synacthen test, showing a subnormal stimulated serum cortisol concentration, is the 'gold standard' diagnostic investigation.

Other adrenal cortex disorders

- *Conn's syndrome* results from primary overproduction of aldosterone. It is an uncommon cause of hypertension, often in association with hypokalaemia, although the latter is generally not severe enough to cause symptomatic muscular weakness.
- Excess androgen production – see hirsutes (p. 267).

Adrenal medulla

Phaeochromocytoma

Phaeochromocytoma is a disorder of the adrenal medulla or the sympathetic chain where there is overproduction and release of excess catecholamines. It is a cause of secondary hypertension, and may be suspected when there are additional associated features resulting from the variable catecholamine release, including:

- fluctuating and sometimes severe hypertension
- headache
- fainting (from postural hypotension)
- sweating
- anxiety.

PITUITARY DISEASE

The commonest cause of pituitary gland dysfunction is an adenoma in the anterior part of the gland, but other disorders in adjacent structures (parapituitary lesions) can lead to a similar presentation. Pituitary disease is generally manifest as clinical problems associated with one or more of:

- pituitary hormone overproduction
- pituitary underfunction (hypopituitarism)
- pressure effects from a large adenoma on other local structures.

Pituitary hormone overproduction

Prolactinoma

In premenopausal women, an increase in serum prolactin causes oligo- or amenorrhoea, infertility and galactorrhoea. An elevated serum prolactin concentration is most commonly due to a prolactinoma, but there are other causes, including pregnancy, breastfeeding, primary hypothyroidism and certain drugs. In men, a raised serum prolactin may or may not cause symptoms associated with hypogonadism, and there are usually no endocrine effects in older women. Prolactinomas in men and older women therefore usually present with pituitary gland failure or with local pressure effects from a large pituitary adenoma rather than with the endocrine manifestations of hyperprolactinaemia.

Acromegaly

Acromegaly (literally 'large extremities') is due to excess growth hormone production from a pituitary adenoma. This results in a striking clinical syndrome with numerous manifestations. The most obvious changes are an alteration in appearance with enlarged supra-orbital ridges, deepened nasolabial folds, a prominent jaw and a 'coarse' facies (Fig. 15.7). The teeth become wide-spaced and there may be mandibular prognathism with the teeth in the lower jaw protruding in front of those in the upper jaw, leading to problems with occlusion, with either natural or artificial teeth. The hands and feet are broad, the former being described as 'spade-like' (Fig. 15.8), and patients may describe a change in ring or shoe size. The skin is thick and greasy. Patients also variously develop arthopathies, entrapment neuropathies (e.g. carpal tunnel syndrome), hypertension, glucose intolerance or diabetes and heart failure.

The change in appearance, although often eventually quite striking, is very gradual in onset, and it

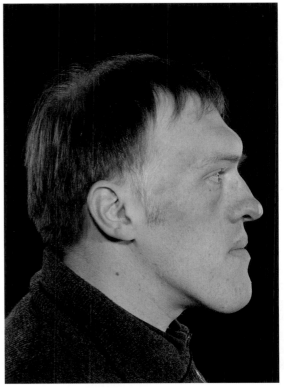

Figure 15.7 The face in acromegaly.

is not unusual for the diagnosis to be first suspected by a new GP, dentist or even medical student meeting the patient for the first time. Some people have constitutional physical features resembling acromegaly, for whom the term 'acromegaloid' is sometimes

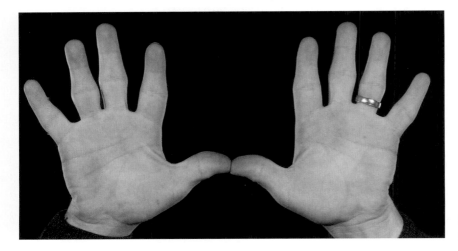

Figure 15.8 The hands in acromegaly.

used. Biochemical confirmation of the diagnosis of acromegaly is made where there is failure of near-complete suppression of serum growth hormone levels during a glucose tolerance test.

Cushing's disease

See p. 263.

Pituitary underfunction (hypopituitarism)

Anterior pituitary gland failure leads to clinical features resulting from a combination of one or more of secondary adrenocortical, thyroid and gonadal dysfunction. Growth hormone deficiency may also occur and is the probable cause of the characteristically associated finely wrinkled skin. It is not difficult to identify patients with pituitary gland failure when they present with gonadal dysfunction (e.g. amenorrhoea, infertility or impotence) as, on testing, the relevant sex hormone (oestradiol or testosterone) concentration is reduced with low or inappropriately normal gonadotrophin (luteinizing hormone (LH) and follicle-stimulating hormone (FSH)) concentrations. However, other patients may present more insidiously with less definite symptoms such as fatigue, weakness, weight loss and faintness, and there may be little in the way of physical signs other than pale skin, conjunctival pallor due to anaemia and, in men, reduced facial and body hair growth. The diagnosis of hypopituitarism is consequently often delayed.

Pressure effects

A large pituitary adenoma or other para-pituitary lesion can cause and sometimes present with pressure effects on local structures with or without endocrine effects. The classic presentation is with a *bitemporal hemianopia* (loss of the temporal visual field in both eyes; Fig. 15.9), as a pituitary adenoma extends upwards to compress the optic chiasm. The visual field loss can be minor or extensive and, at a late stage, there can be loss of visual acuity or even blindness. Lateral extension of a pituitary or para-pituitary lesion may cause pressure on one or more of the oculomotor nerves (cranial nerves III, IV, VI), and so patients may describe *diplopia*, and there may be abnormalities of eye movements on clinical testing.

All patients with known or suspected pituitary disease should have a clinical assessment of visual acuity, visual fields by confrontation, and of eye movements. These clinical tests should be backed up with a formal visual field test and with magnetic resonance imaging (preferred) or computed tomography.

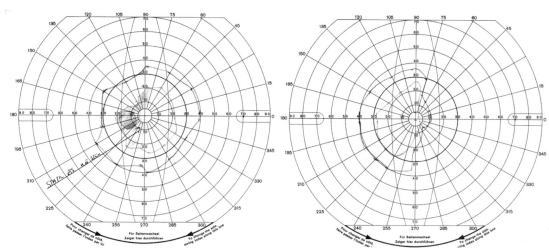

Figure 15.9 Restricted visual fields with a pituitary adenoma. There is complete temporal hemianopia on the right and partial temporal field loss on the left side.

Diabetes insipidus

Diabetes insipidus results from a deficiency in anti-diuretic hormone (ADH) produced in the posterior lobe of the pituitary gland. It can occur either as an isolated condition or in association with, generally severe, anterior pituitary or para-pituitary disease. Classic presenting symptoms are thirst and poly-uria (cf diabetes mellitus). The diagnosis is made by documenting a high urine volume output (generally exceeding 3 L/day), then excluding other potential causes for this, and finally establishing an inappro-priately low urine concentration (osmolality) in the presence of a high serum osmolality during a water deprivation test.

OTHER SYMPTOMS AND ENDOCRINE DISORDERS

Increased availability of hormone testing means that many patients are referred to endocrinologists with the diagnosis already made or suspected. Other patients are sometimes referred with one or more of a series of symptoms for evaluation which may or may not have an endocrine cause, such as those described below.

Fatigue

As a solitary complaint in the absence of other symp-toms, weight change or abnormalities on physical examination, it is unusual to find a definite organic cause for fatigue. However, consider anaemia, thy-roid dysfunction, Addison's disease and hypo-pituitarism. A diagnosis of chronic fatigue syndrome should only be considered after reasonably excluding other possible medical conditions.

Hypoglycaemia

It is not uncommon for patients to self-diagnose 'hypoglycaemia' on the basis of intermittent symp-toms of, for example, fatigue, weakness or tremor, particularly if the complaints appear to improve after ingesting carbohydrate. Home capillary blood glucose meter readings can be misleading and are not sufficiently accurate or reliable enough to diag-nose spontaneous hypoglycaemia. Genuine fasting hypoglycaemia therefore needs to be established by laboratory testing but is rare. Endocrine causes include insulinoma, Addison's disease and hypo-pituitarism, and also consider liver failure.

Sweating

It is unusual to find a definite underlying medical cause in the absence of other symptoms and signs. Sweating can occur as a side effect of medication and also obesity. Endocrine causes include thyrotoxico-sis, acromegaly and phaeochromocytoma.

Collapse/altered consciousness/funny turns

Such symptoms are much more likely to be due to cardiovascular or neurological disorders than endo-crine disease, but consider hypoglycaemia, Addison's disease, hypopituitarism and phaeochromocytoma.

Hypertension

Endocrine disorders are well recognized as impor-tant causes of secondary hypertension. Consider Conn's syndrome (hypokalaemia), Cushing's syn-drome (somatic features) and phaeochromocytoma (additional symptoms – see above).

Hirsutes

Excess hair growth in women is a common present-ing complaint. Look for other evidence of hyper-androgenism such as acne and frontal balding, and also signs of virilization, which suggests the presence of grossly elevated androgen levels. Polycystic ovar-ian syndrome is very common, and is also associated with amenorrhoea/oligomenorrhoea and infertil-ity. Congenital adrenal hyperplasia, Cushing's syn-drome and adrenal and ovarian androgen secreting tumours are all rarer causes of hirsutes. In many women, there is no clear underlying pathology – so-called 'idiopathic' hirsutes.

Obesity

Weight gain and obesity rarely have a definable and treatable underlying endocrine disorder. Hypothy-roidism is associated with weight gain, but this is often relatively modest. There will generally be additional clinical features in weight gain due to Cushing's syndrome.

SUMMARY

- The diagnosis of diabetes mellitus can only be made on the basis of laboratory blood glucose measurements.
- In most patients, diabetes mellitus is diagnosed with a random blood glucose concentration exceeding 11.1 mmol/L in the presence of typical symptoms, but pre-symptomatic diabetes is also common.
- It is usually (but not invariably) possible to distinguish between T1DM and T2DM on initial presentation.
- There is a high prevalence of vascular disease in patients with diabetes mellitus.
- All patients with diabetes mellitus should have an annual review including screening for associated retinal, renal and foot complications.

- Thyrotoxicosis is not an adequate diagnosis – try to establish the aetiology.
- The clinical severity of thyroid dysfunction and associated ophthalmopathy often do not run in parallel in Graves' disease.
- Diabetes, hypertension, obesity and hirsutes are common – use more discriminatory clinical features to select patients for biochemical screening for Cushing's syndrome.
- Hypopituitarism can present insidiously.
- Obesity and fatigue, as isolated symptoms, rarely have an endocrine cause.

FURTHER READING

Turner HE, Wass JAH (eds). 2002. *Oxford handbook of endocrinology and diabetes*. Oxford: Oxford University Press.

16 THE BREAST

Oleg Eremin and Jennifer Eremin

INTRODUCTION

The primary biological function of the human female breast is to provide essential nutrition and protective antibodies for the newborn infant. It is also a very important aesthetic and sexual embodiment of the female form and a woman's perception of her body image.

The female breast arises from within the subcutaneous compartment of the chest wall and when fully developed, extends from the second to the sixth ribs, and from the lateral margin of the sternum to the mid-axillary line. In the young female, the nipple is at the level of the fourth intercostal space. However, its position varies depending on pregnancies, lactational status and age. The breast lies on the fascia covering the pectoralis major, part of serratus anterior, and the upper part of the rectus sheath. The superolateral aspect of the breast may extend into the axilla, through the deep fascia of the axillary floor, to lie in contact with the upper and medial wall of the axilla. The breast is a mixture of fat, stromal elements and glandular structures (Fig. 16.1). Distribution of these various components is influenced by age, pregnancy and lactation, and menopausal status.

The glandular component is made up of 15–20 lobes. Each lobe consists of 20–40 lobules connected together by ducts, areolar and fibrous tissue (Fig. 16.2). The lobules consist of clusters of alveoli (50–100), which drain into the terminal lobular ductules. The ductules join up to form ducts, which become prominent and are referred to as lactiferous ducts in the nipple and areolar area (Fig. 16.1). The areola consists of pigmented, rugose skin with subcutaneous smooth muscle fibres arranged concentrically and radially. The epithelium contains sweat glands, sebaceous glands and accessory mammary glandular tissue. The nipple protrudes from the areola and is covered by thick, corrugated pigmented skin. It

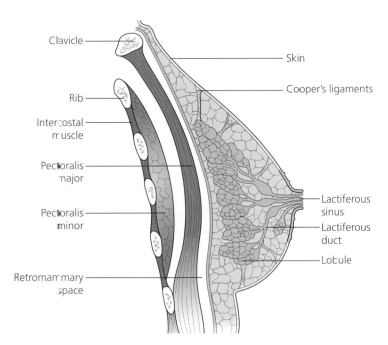

Labels: Clavicle, Rib, Intercostal muscle, Pectoralis major, Pectoralis minor, Retromammary space, Skin, Cooper's ligaments, Lactiferous sinus, Lactiferous duct, Lobule

Figure 16.1 Cross-sectional macroscopic architecture of the female breast. Reproduced from Fig. 14.1, Cross-sectional area of the female breast, p 498, Chapter 14, Heys SD, Eremin JM, Eremin O. Breast. In: Eremin O (ed.), *The scientific and clinical basis of surgical practice*, Oxford University Press, with permission © 2001.

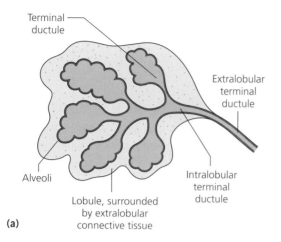

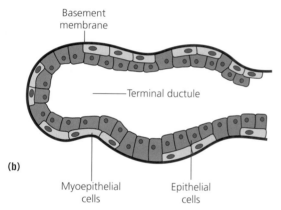

Figure 16.2 Microscopic architecture of the terminal lobular unit of the female breast. Reproduced from Fig. 14.2 Terminal lobular unit: microanatomy, p 498, Chapter 14, Heys SD, Eremin JM, Eremin O. Breast. In: Eremin O (ed.), *The scientific and clinical basis of surgical practice*, Oxford University Press, with permission © 2001.

contains erectile smooth muscle fibres arranged in a concentric and spiral manner.

The breast is subject to changes, induced by the woman's hormonal milieu, pregnancy and post-partum lactation. It is also an organ that develops a range of benign and malignant conditions resulting in a variety of clinical manifestations (as well as occult lesions), usually readily observed and evaluated by examination, imaging and needle biopsy.

This chapter sets out the essential information that the clinician requires to ensure that an accurate diagnosis is established and appropriate management pathways formulated.

CLINICAL HISTORY

Pain

Pain is one of the commonest presenting disorders in the female breast, occurring in both pre-and post-menopausal women. It may vary in intensity, duration and frequency, be present in multiple quadrants and in both breasts, radiate into the nipple–areolar area and/or axilla and be associated with diffuse or focal tenderness. In most women, there is no obvious or serious underlying breast pathology present; the pain can be a feature of benign fibrocystic changes, and rarely cancer. In males, pain is not uncommon in gynaecomastia (swelling of male breast).

Lump

A discrete lump, nodularity or thickening is the next most common mode of presentation. Size may vary (frequently 'pea-sized'), but can be large. Onset may be acute (several days) or longstanding (several months). Fluctuation with the menstrual cycle is common in young women. Pain and tenderness are features of cysts, less common with fibroadenomas (unless rapidly growing or phylloides tumours), uncommon with cancer, except with rapidly expanding, aggressive (grade 3) and inflammatory tumours. The commonest lump in women below 30 years is a fibroadenoma; in women 30–45 years, a cyst and those over 45 years, cancer.

> **SMALL PRINT**
> Rarely, non-breast cancers (e.g. lymphomas) can present as lumps in the breast.

Nipple discharge

Discharge is the next most common presentation, occurring from a single or multiple ducts, one or both breasts, and is clear, coloured or bloody. Physiological discharge is usually bilateral, from multiple ducts and in premenopausal women often following pregnancy and lactation. Profuse and prolonged discharge, with high levels of serum prolactin, is due to a pituitary microadenoma – a rare disorder. Pathological discharge is usually unilateral, involves

Table 16.1 Nipple discharge: causes and prediction based on pertinent clinical features associated with the discharge

Cause	Clinical features
Postpartum galactorrhoea	Copious, frequent, milky discharge, multiple ducts (bilateral), long duration; reproduced clinically but no other relevant findings on examination
Mammary dysplasia (premenopausal)	Minimal, occasional, coloured, clear or bloodstained discharge, single or multiple ducts; difficult to reproduce but breast nodularity or tenderness may be present
Periductal mastitis (premenopausal)	Recurrent, purulent or bloodstained discharge, single or several ducts; may be reproduced clinically, areolar induration, inflammation, tenderness, and nipple retraction (variable degree) may be present
Duct ectasia (peri- and postmenopausal)	Copious, frequent, coloured (green, brown, black) or bloodstained discharge, multiple ducts (bilateral), long duration, reproduced clinically, areolar tenderness and nipple retraction (variable degree) may be present
Papilloma, single	Minimal, clear, serous or bloodstained discharge, single often localizable duct, short duration; occasionally tender areolar swelling, pressure on latter or isolated duct may reproduce discharge
Papilloma, multiple	Prominent, serous or bloodstained discharge, multiple ducts, not infrequently; may be reproduced clinically, but with no breast masses felt
Ductal carcinoma: *in situ*, invasive	Variable, serous or bloodstained discharge, short duration, single or multiple ducts; may be reproduced clinically, but with no breast masses felt; a palpable retroareolar mass or Paget's disease of nipple may be present
Drugs (contraceptive pill, antidepressants etc.)	Minimal, intermittent, clear, milky discharge, several ducts, long duration, difficult to reproduce clinically, no relevant findings
Endocrine tumours (pituitary adenoma, Chiari–Frommel syndrome, etc.)	Copious, frequent, clear, milky discharge, multiple ducts (bilateral), long duration; may be reproduced clinically, no other relevant findings, abnormal serum levels (on repeated testing) of prolactin

Modified from Table 14.2 (Nipple discharge: aetiological factors and clinical features) in Eremin O (ed.), *The scientific and clinical basis of surgical practice*. Oxford: Oxford University Press, with permission © 2001.

a single or a few ducts, is serous (positive for blood on testing) or overtly bloody, with or without palpable lesions and occurs in pre- and postmenopausal women. Intraduct papilloma is the commonest cause. Ductal carcinoma *in situ* is a less common cause (Table 16.1).

Nipple changes

Retraction (intermittent, partial or chronic) is often a concern to women. It can be idiopathic or associated with malignancy in the retroareolar region, but usually is seen in the postmenopausal breast and is secondary to glandular atrophy and replacement by fibrosis and major duct ectasia. Congenital absence is very rare, whereas accessory nipples are seen in 2 per cent of women. Alterations of size and shape are seen with prominent duct polyps or malignant growths. Inflammatory changes, with induration of the nipple, with or without purulent discharge, are seen with periductal inflammation. Paget's disease (nipple ulceration, eczematous changes) is associated with ductal carcinoma, often occult. This is an uncommon presentation in contrast with eczema of skin and/or areola of the breast, which occurs in all age groups.

Axillary symptoms

Axillary symptoms and signs may be local or associated with breast disturbances. Mastalgia frequently radiates into the axilla with associated axillary or breast tenderness. Not infrequently, patients (both sexes) present with a swelling in the axilla. Lymphadenopathy is the commonest cause with confirmation of nodal size, architecture and histopathology by ultrasonography and core cut biopsy. Lymphoma, metastatic nodal disease (occult breast cancer, melanoma, others) are also possible likely diagnoses. In younger patients, reactive (non malignant) changes may occur with viral infections or trauma/inflammation of the skin of upper limbs and body. Lipomas or infected adnexal glands in the skin are other common lesions found in the axilla.

PHYSICAL EXAMINATION

Inspection

Prior to carrying out a physical examination of the patient, perform an inspection (in the presence of a female chaperone) with the patient sitting on the edge of the couch, with her arms by her side, followed by elevation of the arms above her head and finally with her arms tensed (to fix the pectoral muscles) on her hips. This rapid visual inspection may reveal a range of features which could provide a clue

Table 16.2 Clinical features which may be detected on inspection

Area inspected	Clinical features detected on inspection
Breast as a whole	Changes/discrepancies in size, shape or contour
Breast skin	Puckering and/or tethering Oedema (*peau d'orange*) Features of inflammation (swelling, redness) Skin nodules, mass with or without ulceration
Nipple areolar complex	Swelling Retraction Eczematous changes or ulceration Nipple discharge: • single or bilateral • single or multiple ducts • fluid being clear, serous, greenish, whitish or bloody
Lymph draining areas	Axilla: diffuse swelling or discrete lump(s) Supraclavicular fossa: diffuse swelling or discrete lump(s) – lymphadenopathy (benign or malignant – secondary or primary); lipoma

as to the possible underlying disease process (Table 16.2). In the case of breast cancer it may suggest the likely TNM staging.

Palpation

Palpation of the breasts

Examine the patient (in the presence of a female chaperone) lying on the examination couch in a comfortable position on her back, with the arms raised above her head, preferably with the back of the head lying on her interlocked palms. The examination is carried out from either side (right side – author's preference). If necessary, the patient can also be examined sitting on the edge of the couch and facing the clinician. This position may be of help in examining the axilla, especially in an obese patient and when ascertaining fixity of breast lesions to the chest wall (pectoral muscles being put on tension intermittently). The supraclavicular fossae can be examined lying or sitting, preferably sitting, with the clinician standing behind the patient.

The examination should commence with the normal (asymptomatic) breast, if the breast symptoms/complaints are unilateral. The breasts are examined first with the patient's head lying on her hands, followed by the axillae and finally the supraclavicular fossae, and any other anatomical site, if deemed appropriate (e.g. spine or abdomen, if there is suspicion of metastatic spread to those areas). Examine the breast with the fingers (extended or slightly flexed) of both hands in a gentle manner, but graded pressure may be necessary to define more precisely localized or focal clinical features. Using the fingertips of both hands may help to better establish the basis of the breast lesion. Before commencing the examination, ask the patient to point out or localize with her own fingers the site and extent of her concern.

The examination follows a clockwise sequential process as depicted in Figure 16.3. For example, commencing in the upper outer quadrant (1) of the left breast (standing on the patient's right hand side), followed by the lower outer (2), lower inner (3) and upper inner (4) quadrants of the left breast. The nipple and areolar complex (5) examination is next carried out with the extended fingers of both hands. The nipple may be gently squeezed (with the patient's approval) to reproduce the discharge and

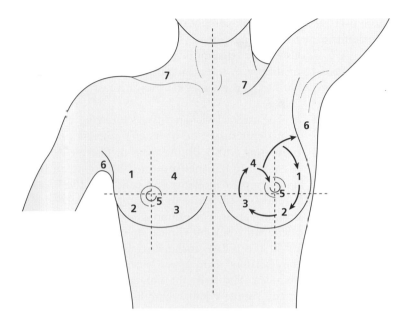

Figure 16.3 Diagram of the female breast showing areas of clinical interest (1–7) to be examined. Stand on the patient's right hand side, with the patient's left arm elevated and hand placed behind her head, and systematically examine the left breast with both hands (→ 1–5) (see text for details). The procedure is repeated for the right breast. Stand on the patient's right hand side and hold her abducted right upper arm and flexed forearm with your right hand. Systematically examine the right axilla with your left hand (→ 6) (see text for details). The procedure is repeated for the left axilla but using the right hand. If deemed appropriate the supraclavicular (7) and cervical areas are also examined (see text for details).

for testing for blood, as well as making smears (fixed, air-dried) for cytological assessment. The contralateral breast (right) can be examined from either the same (right) or opposite side of the patient; in both instances the same sequential approach is used. Palpation should incorporate examination of the axillary tail of the breast, which can be prominent (e.g. in pregnancy) and felt behind the lateral border of the pectoralis major muscle. Particular attention is given to the area of the patient's concern and to any focal abnormality detected on palpation. There may be variable pain/tenderness elicited on examination and you need to not only document this, but to ensure that the patient is willing for the examination to continue, modifying the degree of pressure applied.

The breast examination should ascertain the segment or quadrant (see Fig. 16.3) of the breast involved, whether or not the lesion is in the breast substance, and if there is involvement of the overlying skin and/or underlying muscles. In the former case, skin puckering or tethering suggests possible involvement by cancer spicules of the dermis and associated inward skin retraction. A lump with overlying skin oedema (*peau d'orange*) is indicative of blockage of dermal lymphatics and advanced tumour stage (T_4). Similarly, adherence or fixity to the pectoral muscles is a feature of a T_4 cancer.

CLINICAL PEARL

Careful assessment of a lump can indicate whether the breast lesion is benign or malignant:

- if it is rounded, smooth, mobile, tense and tender it is most likely to be a cyst (30 to 45 years of age)
- if it is rounded, smooth, mobile, firm and non-tender it is most likely to be a fibroadenoma (under 30 years of age)
- malignant lumps are rare in women under 30 years and uncommon under 40 years (4 per cent of breast cancers). Cancers are usually irregular, firm or hard, with variable involvement of overlying skin or deeper structures.

All lumps should be carefully measured using skin calipers and the findings recorded in the notes. In modern practice, many patients are referred with a short history (<2 weeks), and poorly defined features (intermittent lump with fluctuations in size, vague thickening/nodularity). Where clinical assessment fails to establish any underlying disease or basis for the presenting complaint, young patients (<30 years) can be reassured and discharged. Selective use of imaging may be necessary to define the possible underlying cause (e.g. a suspected fibroadenoma) in some of these young women, and in those over 30 years of age, where both benign and malignant conditions are more likely to occur.

Inflammatory changes (pain, redness and associated swelling – abscess) can be a presenting complaint. If localized to the skin (but not involving the breast) it is usually an infected sebaceous cyst or skin follicle. Infection is seen in the postpartum period shortly after commencing breastfeeding and can involve any breast segment. Involvement of the nipple–areolar complex (pain, swelling, nipple discharge) in non-pregnant women can occur due to periductal mastitis, often in women who smoke. Examination may reveal a firm or hard, regular or irregular mass, all features suggestive of cancer.

Nipple discharges are tested for blood and smears made for cytology (fixed and air dried) if adequate samples can be produced, either by the clinician or patient.

Palpation of the lymph draining areas

Following examination of the breast, the lymph draining areas (axilla, supraclavicular fossa) on each side are carefully examined. The axilla is usually palpated with the patient lying supine, the examiner using the tips of her/his fingers (left hand, right axilla), standing on the patient's right side, and the right hand for the left axilla. If need be, the axilla can be examined with the patient sitting on the side of the couch and facing the clinician. When examining the axilla, the arm is brought down and held at chest level by the non-examining hand (Fig. 16.3).

The examination of the axilla should be systematic with the four walls of the pyramidal axilla palpated:

- medial – serratus anterior
- lateral – inner aspect of upper arm
- posterior – subscapularis
- anterior – inner aspect of pectoralis major.

Also palpate the central contents. If examination of the lateral wall is found to be awkward with this approach, the hands may be reversed. In obese women, the fat in the axilla can readily mask underlying pathology and axillary ultrasonography may be required to define more precisely any suspected lymphadenopathy. A diffuse swelling (excess normal fat accumulation) is not infrequent; lipomas can also occur and can be either relatively well-defined or diffuse. A recent, rapid increase in size (>3 cm) with tenderness may be indicative of sarcomatous change.

The supraclavicular fossa should be examined in patients suspected of having a breast cancer or presenting with a diffuse mass or discrete lump in the fossa. In patients suspected of having a malignant lymphadenopathy (no cancer in the breast), careful assessment needs to be made of the regional draining areas. For example, with axillary lymphadenopathy and no clinical or imaging abnormality in the breast, malignant cutaneous lesions of the ipsilateral arm, upper back, and chest must be excluded. Similarly, the cutaneous draining areas of the supraclavicular lymph glands (scalp, neck, face) need to be assessed. In the latter case, evidence of other suspicious lymph nodes in the neck area may suggest an occult/associated malignancy of the oro- or nasopharynx. In both lymph draining areas, lymphadenopathy of recent onset may be a presenting feature of a lymphoma. If such a diagnosis is suspected then lymphadenopathy in other lymphoid compartments (contralateral axilla and neck, inguinal areas and abdomen) needs to be confirmed or refuted. More definitive confirmation of a generalized abnormal lymphadenopathy will be obtained with computed tomography (CT).

Enlarged axillary nodes are relatively common and are a cause of worry for patients. One of the commonest causes is a benign systemic viral infection (e.g. glandular fever in young women) and may persist for some months after apparent resolution of the viral infection. A not infrequent cause of unilateral axillary lymphadenopathy of acute onset is a cutaneous injury of the ipsilateral arm, for example, due to a laceration, or skin abrasion as a result of gardening, or a scratch by an animal (e.g. cat).

In a small number of women with a prominent and persistent lymphadenopathy an ultrasound-guided core biopsy or fine needle aspiration is performed to establish a more definite diagnosis. Where a lymphoma is suspected, the whole node needs to be removed to establish a reliable histopathological diagnosis.

COMMON DIAGNOSES

Benign breast disease

Mastalgia

Mastalgia is one of the commonest breast disorders experienced by women and is a common symptom in women presenting to their general practitioner. An underlying fear of breast cancer induces many women to seek medical help. After significant disease is excluded, in the majority of patients (80 per cent) the symptoms respond to simple reassurance and supportive measures. Others (20 per cent) require more definitive treatment. Of this latter group, the majority of women with cyclical mastalgia (CM), and two-thirds of women with non-cyclical mastalgia (NCM), obtain good relief with appropriate use of available therapies.

There are three main types of mastalgia: CM (commonest), NCM and extra-mammary (EM) (uncommon); the pertinent clinical features of these are summarized in Boxes 16.1–16.3.

BOX 16.1 CYCLICAL MASTALGIA

Clinical profile:
- commonest (60 per cent) cause of mastalgia
- pain intensity >4.0 cm on a 10 cm visual analogue scale described as dull ache, heaviness
- pain duration >5–7 days per month (10 per cent of women); usually latter half of cycle
- frequently in upper/outer quadrant, radiating into upper arm/axilla; diffuse, bilateral, one breast usually predominates
- interferes with sleep (10 per cent), work and/or social activity (10 per cent), physical activity (30 per cent) and sexual activity (45 per cent)
- third to fourth decade, persists and recurs; 15 per cent undergo spontaneous remission, 45 per cent resolve at menopause.

Aetiological profile:
- no correlation with fibrocystic changes in breast
- no consistent hormonal abnormalities, either systemically or locally in the breast
- increased breast volume, but body water not increased (diuretics not recommended)
- dietary fat and caffeine are proposed factors – no benefit in reduced intake
- enhanced by anxiety, depression and stress, but patients no more neurotic than controls
- association of CM and breast cancer documented, but the risk is very low; no precautions required.

BOX 16.2 NON-CYCLICAL MASTALGIA

Clinical profile:
- occurs in 35 per cent of women with mastalgia
- pain is constant or intermittent, unilateral or bilateral, can be sharp and short-lived
- within a breast quadrant; can be diffuse and radiate into the axilla
- fourth to sixth decade, mainly postmenopausal; subsides spontaneously but may persist.

Aetiological profile:
- benign pathology – infective mastitis in premenopausal women, duct ectasia, large cysts, enlarging fibroadenomas
- trauma – external, post surgery
- hormones – hormone replacement therapy (HRT), contraceptive pill
- breast cancer – (2.5 per cent) presenting with pain as primary symptom
- medication. The following may cause NCM:
  - antidepressants, antipsychotics and anxiolytics
  - antihypertensive/cardiac drugs (spironolactone, methyldopa, digoxin)
  - antimicrobial agents (ketoconazole, metronidazole)
  - others – cimetidine, domperidone, ciclosporin
- idiopathic – in many women there is no obvious cause.

BOX 16.3 EXTRA-MAMMARY MASTALGIA

Clinical profile:
- responsible for 5 per cent of cases of mastalgia
- costochondritis or Tietze's disease (second to third costal cartilages + swelling)
- herpes zoster infection
- pain referred from painful shoulder
- mastalgia mimics – ischaemic heart disease, reflux oesophagitis, gallbladder diseases, pulmonary emboli.

Breast cysts

Five to 10 per cent of women will, at some stage, present with a macrocyst. Microcysts are more common but tend to be occult. Breast cysts are commonest between the ages of 35 and 50, but can occur outside this age range, particularly in women who have been taking HRT.

Cysts arise from breast lobules, with two types being identified. The first is lined by flattened epithelium and the second by apocrine, secretory epithelium. Cysts with flattened epithelium have high sodium and low potassium concentrations, with a sodium:potassium ratio of >4. Cysts with apocrine-type epithelium have low sodium and high potassium concentrations, with a sodium:potassium ratio of <4. Breast cyst fluid has been shown to contain hormones (androgens, prolactin and calcitonin), enzymes, growth factors and immunoglobulins.

Patients present with a palpable lump or nodularity. When acute and large, the lump can be tender and the patient complains of pain. Typically cysts are well-circumscribed, smooth, mobile and, on occasion, tender lumps. More than one may be palpable within either one or both breasts. On mammography, in breasts that are not dense, a well-defined opacity may be seen (Fig. 16.4). Ultrasound confirms the cystic nature of the lesion (Fig. 16.5). The cyst can be aspirated if causing symptoms and/or the patient wishes to have the fluid removed. The fluid may be straw-coloured, bluish-green or brown. If it is blood-stained, an intracystic papilloma or cancer is a possibility and the fluid should be sent for cytological examination. If an intracystic lesion is visualized, a core cut biopsy or fine needle aspiration cytology (FNAC) may be carried out. Under ultrasound guidance the cyst may be aspirated to dryness with complete resolution. The cyst may recur and require further aspiration. As a general rule, patients are not reviewed after having the cyst aspirated. If the cyst recurs on a regular basis, with or without blood, it is best to excise it. In some patients who have recurrent and multiple cysts, a 6-month course of danazol may reduce the number and subsequent rate of cyst formation. If the cysts are multiple, frequent, requiring numerous aspirations, there may possibly be an increased risk of cancer.

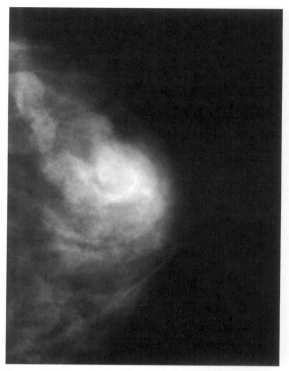

Figure 16.4 Mammogram showing a well-defined, dense, oval opacity suggesting a benign lesion, possibly a cyst. Reproduced with permission from Lincoln Breast Unit.

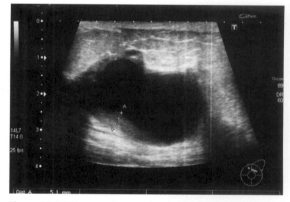

Figure 16.5 Ultrasound scan of a cyst in the breast: typical well-defined border with hypoechoic contents. Reproduced with permission from Lincoln Breast Unit.

A galactocoele is a single, smooth swelling, typically in the subareolar area. It develops in the breast during late pregnancy or during lactation. Aspiration reveals milky fluid, but in longstanding cases the contents may be inspissated and difficult to aspirate.

Solid lumps

Benign lumps in the breast are common, may be discrete, well-circumscribed (fibroadenoma) or diffuse (nodularity, linear thickening, asymmetry). In the latter there may be fluctuations in size over time and over the menstrual cycle. The lumps are frequently painless, but can be associated with localized or diffuse breast pain or tenderness.

Fibroadenoma

Fibroadenomas are well-circumscribed, smooth, firm and mobile lumps and can be multiple. They are usually seen in premenopausal females, particularly those under the age of 35. The microarchitecture and histological features of fibroadenomas suggest that they arise from a single lobule. Diagnosis is confirmed by imaging with ultrasound in young women, or ultrasound and mammography in those aged 35 years and older. It can be picked up as an incidental finding, often calcified, in the screening population. In women under the age of 25 a core cut biopsy is not done unless there are worrying features on ultrasonography. Core cut biopsies are recommended in women over the age of 25, as occasionally a fibroadenoma may turn out to be a malignant lesion in women in their late 20s or early 30s. If the lesion clinically is small (<2 cm) and the patient does not wish to have surgery, then it can be left *in situ* and excision carried out if and when the lesion begins to increase in size. If the lesion is causing significant symptoms and/or is increasing in size, the patient is advised to have it removed. Occasionally, in young women a large lesion (>5 cm) may occur. These giant fibroadenomas are best removed as they may lead to cosmetic deformity if removed late. Even with large fibroadenomas, the cosmetic results of surgery are good.

Mammary dysplasia

A number of benign breast lesions arise as a result of abnormal or exaggerated alterations of the normal physiological and morphological changes within the breast. These aberrations of normal development and involution (ANDI) form the basis for a variety of pathophysiological entities and include:

- adenosis – increase in acini and glandular tissue
- fibrosis or sclerosis – increased deposition of dense fibrous tissue, with loss of elastic tissue and fat
- cystic changes – numerous cysts (macro or micro)
- epitheliosis – hyperplasia of epithelium lining terminal ducts/ductules and acini, which can be typical, atypical or florid leading to papillomatous growths.

Sclerosing adenosis (radial scars)

These lesions in the breast can mimic cancer, both clinically and mammographically. Histologically, the extensive localized fibrosis results in distortion of the normal lobular architecture resulting in dense, spiculated strands. Complex sclerosing lesions are variants, associated with prominent epithelial hyperplasia. They tend to be asymptomatic and detected during breast screening. Breast cancer can be associated with radial scars which should undergo surgical removal or be adequately assessed by mammotomy.

Breast abscesses

These may occur in lactating and non-lactating breasts. The former occur in the puerperium, during lactation and on weaning and are usually caused by staphylococcal or streptococcal organisms. They can occur in any part of the breast and present with typical clinical features of inflammation and a variable systemic inflammatory response. There may be cellulitis with no or minimal pus. When established, a multiloculated breast abscess (confirmed by ultrasonography) is present, and pus can be aspirated. If recurrent aspirations and appropriate antibiotics do not lead to resolution, surgical evacuation is required, particularly if the abscess is multiloculated. The residual cavity is packed with antiseptic-soaked or absorbent dressing. Healing is rapid by secondary intention or by delayed primary closure. Milk is expressed from the breast either manually or by a breast pump. The infant can be fed from the uninvolved breast provided a suitable antibiotic has been prescribed. Non-lactating breast abscesses are usually due to periductal mastitis, occur in the periareolar area, frequently recur, and may result in a mammary duct fistula. There is a strong association with smoking.

CLINICAL PEARL

If the patient is weaning or does not wish to breastfeed, lactation can be suppressed with bromocriptine.

Phylloides tumour

This is an uncommon lesion, present in 1 per cent of all breast neoplasms, usually seen in women between 30 and 45 years. The tumour is characterized macroscopically by the presence of cystic cavities within which fronds of tissue project. Histologically, there is a benign epithelial component and a hypercellular stroma, which comprises most of the tumour. Phylloides tumours may resemble an intracanalicular fibroadenoma or an aggressive sarcoma; the tumour may behave either as a benign (85 per cent) or malignant (15 per cent) lesion. The number of mitoses per 10 high power microscopic fields is an important feature: 0–4 mitoses being benign; 5–9 potentially malignant; and 10 or more malignant.

The tumour can be treated by wide local excision with a surrounding margin of normal tissue. If sarcomatous and aggressive, the patient needs radical surgery to achieve local control of the disease. It spreads by the haematogenous route, therefore axillary lymphadenectomy is not carried out. Radiotherapy and chemotherapy have no beneficial effects.

Miscellaneous lesions

- *Trauma*: this can produce a haematoma which may be slow to resolve; may also lead to fat necrosis, which clinically and mammographically can mimic carcinoma. Ultrasound-guided core cut biopsy will confirm the diagnosis.
- *Mondor's disease*: thrombophlebitis of superficial breast veins, (cause unknown) results in the production of taut, firm, subcutaneous bands with skin dimpling.
- *Skin lesions*: various skin lesions may give rise to lumps – sebaceous cysts, adnexal tumours and blocked blind-ending ducts of areola (Montgomery tubercles).

Duct disturbances

Nipple discharge

Nipple discharge in premenopausal women is likely to be associated with, or be due to, benign disease. It is the predominant clinical feature in up to 10 per cent of women presenting with breast cancer. Nipple discharge is characterized by its appearance.

- Purulent and coloured discharges are usually indicative of benign disease (infection and fibrocystic disease, respectively).
- Spontaneous bilateral milky discharge (multiple ducts) most commonly occurs in women of reproductive age and is called galactorrhoea. It is seen after pregnancy and lactation, sometimes lasting for several years. Rarely, it is due to increased production of prolactin, but in most cases no endocrine abnormality is found. It can be induced by hormones (contraceptive pill) and drugs (tricyclic antidepressants and phenothiazines).
- Clear, serous or bloodstained discharges are not infrequently associated with neoplastic disease (intraduct papilloma(s), intraduct and invasive cancers). Papillomas have little predilection for malignant change, though multiple papillomas have an increased tendency for breast cancer.

Investigations in premenopausal women usually do not demonstrate any abnormality, either by imaging or cytology. If cytology of the discharge reveals epithelial or atypical cells, or is positive for blood, and if localized to one duct, microdochectomy should be carried out. In many women the discharge will stop spontaneously, be minimal or intermittent. In postmenopausal women where the duct cannot be localized, the discharge is bloody or epithelialcells are seen on cytology, a subareolar duct excision is performed. The major ducts and adjacent cone of breast tissue are excised. Table 16.1 summarizes the various likely causes of nipple discharge (see p. 271).

Nipple retraction

This is not an uncommon clinical feature, and can be either congenital or acquired. It may be intermittent or become progressively worse as the patient ages. The most common cause is mammary duct ectasia, frequently seen in postmenopausal women. The majority of women, with no abnormality clinically or by imaging, are reassured.

Mammary duct ectasia and periductal mastitis

These are variations of periductal inflammation leading to duct dilatation and ectasia. Periductal inflammation affects women under the age of 50, is characterized by subareolar or periareolar inflammation, can lead to abscess formation and subsequently a fistula, occurring spontaneously or following surgical intervention. Chronic inflammation can lead to nipple discharge, areolar induration and eventually nipple retraction. The aetiology is unknown, but cigarette smoking, oestrogen deficiency, and infection have all been implicated. The chronic inflammatory process may result in fibrosis and obliteration of the ducts, and nipple retraction.

Duct ectasia affects women over the age of 50 and presents as nipple discharge, affecting several ducts. The discharge varies from clear to black, and blood may be present microscopically or macroscopically. It can cause nipple retraction. Chronic periductal inflammation leads to loss of ductal supporting tissue, with resultant ectasia and retention of secretions.

Malignant breast disease

Carcinoma of the breast is one of the most common cancers (23 per cent of all female malignancies in the developed world), and there are 44 000 new cases per annum in the UK. One in 10 women develops breast cancer during her lifetime. The incidence is increasing worldwide, even in young women, due to undefined factors (diet, pollutants, lifestyle changes). Breast cancer is very rare in women under the age of 25. About 4 per cent occur under the age of 40. There is a plateau in incidence between the ages of 45 and 55, and beyond 55 years it continues to increase steadily into the 80s.

Breast cancer is responsible for 16 000 deaths per annum in the UK. The results of breast cancer treatment are steadily improving, with significantly enhanced survival over the past three decades. Certain risk factors have been established for the development of breast cancer, and these are discussed below. Table 16.3 outlines various risk factors documented for the development of breast cancers, including particular benign breast lesions and their associated risks for breast cancer.

Hormones

Epidemiological studies demonstrate that prolonged exposure to oestrogens, especially if unopposed by progesterones, increases the risk of developing breast cancer. Hormone replacement therapy, given for more than 10 years after the age of the natural menopause, increases the risk of breast cancer. Bilateral oophorectomy before 35 years of age reduces the risk.

Table 16.3 Risk factors for the development of breast cancer

Factor	Enhanced risk of cancer development
Genetic factors	Breast cancer (*BRCA1* and *BRCA2*) gene mutations Familial predisposition (first-degree relatives, bilateral disease, age of presentation <40 years) Familial history of ovarian cancer
Menstrual history	Early menarche and/or late menopause Hormone replacement therapy for >10 years following onset of menopause
Reproductive history	Nulliparity, lack of breastfeeding Late childbearing (first pregnancy >28 years)
Ionizing radiation	Exposure of breast at early age (e.g. patients with Hodgkin's disease receiving mantle radiotherapy before 35 years of age)
Social class	High socioeconomic class
Dietary	High and prolonged intake of saturated fats, alcohol intake above recommended daily amount (1 unit per day)
Benign breast disease	Epithelial hyperplasia (florid) – twofold increase in risk Atypical lobular or ductular hyperplasia – fourfold increase in risk
Mammographic findings	Dense breasts on mammography (particularly in postmenopausal women)

Genetic aspects

Approximately 10 per cent of patients with breast cancer have a family history and 2 per cent a genetically transmitted type of breast cancer. One rare form of inherited breast cancer has a mutation or loss or heterozygosity of the p53 tumour-suppressor gene on the short arm of chromosome 17. This type of breast cancer is seen in the Li–Fraumeni syndrome, with soft tissue sarcomas and other epithelial tumours occurring in members of the family. Another more common type of genetic breast cancer is the Lynch type II syndrome, (autosomal dominant with high penetrance), with a high familial incidence of breast and ovarian cancers. These genetically transmitted cancers have mutations of the *BRCA1* and *BRCA2* tumour suppressor proteins.

> **Box 16.4 Developing breast cancer based on family history, age of onset, bilaterality and association with ovarian cancer**
>
> Low risk:
> - 1 close relative with breast cancer >40 years
> - 2 close relatives with an average age of breast cancer >50 years.
>
> Moderate risk:
> - 1 close relative with breast cancer <40 years or with bilateral breast cancers <60 years
> - 2 close relatives with an average age of breast cancer <50 years
> - 1 close relative with breast cancer <50 years and another relative with ovarian cancer at any age
> - Father and/or brother with male breast cancer at any age.
>
> High risk:
> - 2 close relatives with an average age of breast cancer <40 years
> - 2 close relatives with ovarian cancer
> - mother and/or a sister with both breast and ovarian cancer
> - 3 close relatives with an average age of breast cancer <50 years
> - 3 close relatives with breast or ovarian cancer including at least 1 with ovarian cancer
> - 4 or more relatives with breast or ovarian cancer at any age.

The family history can be defined as shown in Box 16.4:

- low risk (<2 × population lifetime risk of breast cancer)
- moderate risk (2–3 × population lifetime risk of breast cancer)
- high risk (>3 × population lifetime risk of breast cancer).

Those at moderate and high risk should be referred to a secondary/tertiary care centre for further risk evaluation and management.

Pathology of carcinoma of breast

Invasive cancer

- **Invasive ductal carcinoma** (no special type): this is the most common type (75 per cent). Micro-scopically, malignant cells are arranged in various microarchitectural forms, including glandular structures. Many tumours have a prominent connective tissue stromal component (scirrhous). Biological behaviour is variable, ranging from good to poor prognosis. Tumour grading (1–3) systems have been established based on:
  - the degree of tumour differentiation, as assessed by the formation of tubules
  - the variation in size, shape and staining of the nuclei
  - the frequency of mitoses.
- **Invasive lobular cancer**: this is the next most common type (10 per cent). Microscopically, monomorphic tumour cells are arranged in file, alveolar or targetoid patterns. It is frequently multifocal and may be bilateral. It is not associated with microcalcification, and can be difficult to detect by mammography or ultrasonography. Magnetic resonance mammography is recommended to evaluate this type of cancer.
- **Tubular carcinoma**: this forms 5 per cent of all breast malignancies and is increasingly being detected through screening. These are usually small, stellate tumours, and histologically have well-formed glands separated by fibrous stroma. The malignant cells have cytoplasmic projections ('snouts'), extending from the apex of the cell into the duct lumen. Tubular cancer tends to remain localized and it virtually never metastasizes to the regional lymph nodes. The 5-year survival rates approach 95 per cent.
- **Inflammatory breast cancer**: 3 per cent of all breast malignancies seen. Microscopically, these cancers may have features of infiltrating ductal, lobular or medullary cancers, with dermal invasion of the lymphatics by malignant cells, tissue oedema, and a variable degree of infiltration by inflammatory cells. The cancers tend to occur in younger, premenopausal women, and are biologically aggressive with a poor clinical outcome.

Carcinoma in situ

In situ carcinoma arises from the terminal ductular–lobular unit with ductal carcinoma *in situ* (DCIS) limited to ducts/ductules, and lobular carcinoma *in situ* (LCIS) to lobules. Prior to breast screening the incidence of DCIS was 1–3 per cent of excised specimens and 3–6 per cent of all breast cancers. Since the introduction of screening, DCIS has been documented in 15–20 per cent of all breast cancers excised, and in 20–40 per cent of all occult (impalpable) breast cancers excised. The frequency of LCIS has also increased in biopsy/excision specimens. LCIS is classified as lobular neoplasia.

In DCIS there is proliferation of the inner cuboidal cell layer into the lumen and disappearance of the outer layer of myoepithelial cells, but the basement membrane is intact. Histologically the ducts are lined by malignant cells which may have the following patterns:

- comedo – the most common type, characterized by central necrosis and calcification
- non-comedo – cribriform or micropapillary. If the DCIS is <2.5 cm, <15 per cent of such cases will have multifocal disease. If the DCIS is >2.5 cm then more than 40 per cent will have multifocal disease. Approximately 2 per cent of patients with DCIS will develop invasive cancer annually, a 40 per cent risk after 10 years. Microinvasion in DCIS is rare, with only 1 per cent of patients having invasion of regional lymph nodes, presumably due to an occult invasive component.

Comedo carcinoma is biologically the most aggressive type.

Paget's disease of the nipple presents as an eczematous lesion of the nipple with an underlying usually non-palpable carcinoma of the breast. Less frequently there is a serous or bloodstained nipple discharge. A mass is present in up to 40 per cent of cases, either DCIS or invasive ductal carcinoma. Histologically, malignant cells have a characteristic morphological appearance. Paget's cells (95 per cent) found within the epidermis of the nipple are large and rounded, with vacuolated cytoplasm and pleomorphic hyperchromatic nuclei. Removal of the nipple and areolar complex is appropriate treatment in the first instance; mastectomy may be required if the disease is extensive.

Clinical manifestations of breast cancer

Presenting complaint

The most common (70 per cent) presentation is a palpable lump, nodularity or thickening in the breast,

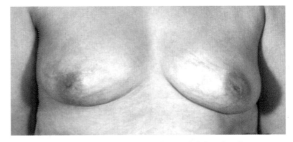

Figure 16.6 Patient presenting with a thickening in upper outer quadrant of left breast. Examination reveals overlying skin tethering, a poorly defined mass and some attachment to the pectoral fascia.

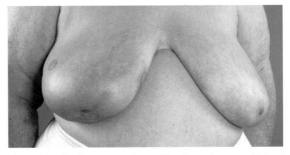

Figure 16.7 Patient presenting with a large lump and bloody nipple discharge. Examination reveals a large mass (T_3) with an inverted nipple.

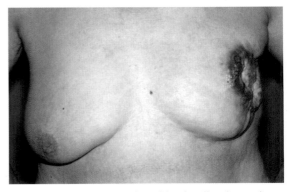

Figure 16.8 Patient presenting with a locally advanced cancer in the left breast (T_4, N_2), present for many months.

usually detected by the patient. Typically the lump is firm or hard, well defined, with an irregular surface. There may be tethering of the overlying skin, with or without attachment to the pectoral fascia (Fig. 16.6). Cancers are situated in the upper outer quadrant of the breast in two-thirds of cases; the remaining

PATIENT:				REFERRING PRACTITIONER:
Surname: First Name: Address: Date of Birth dd/mm/yyyy: Telephone no (home): Telephone no (daytime): NHS number: Date decision to refer:	Mr ☐ Mrs ☐ Miss ☐ Ms ☐ Post Code: Age: Mobile tel no: E-mail: Hospital no: Date of referral:			GP Name: Address: GP telephone no: Safe haven fax no:

REFERRAL DETAILS* (please tick the correct box)

2ww	Yes	No	Routine	Yes	No
Discrete, hard lump ± fixation, ± skin tethering	☐	☐	Women aged younger than 30 years with a lump with benign features (well defined, smooth, mobile)	☐	☐
Female, aged 30 years and older with a discrete lump that persists after her next period, or presents after menopause	☐	☐	Patients with breast pain and no palpable abnormality, when initial treatment (change of bra, simple analgesics (paracetamol)) fails and/or with unexplained persistent symptoms (see protocol for mastalgia)	☐	☐
Female, aged younger than 30 years: with a lump that enlarges with a lump that has features of cancer (see first bullet point) in whom there are other reasons for concern, such as family history (see protocol)	☐ ☐	☐ ☐	Asymmetrical nodularity or thickening that persists at review after menstruation	☐	☐
Female of any age, with previous breast cancer, who presents with a further lump or suspicious symptoms	☐	☐	Infection or inflammation that fails to respond to antibiotics	☐	☐
With unilateral eczematous skin of areola or nipple that does not respond to topical treatment	☐	☐	Nipple discharge: <50 years – bilateral, stains clothes and/or blood stained >50 years – any nipple discharge	☐ ☐	☐ ☐
With nipple retraction or distortion of recent onset (<3 months onset)	☐	☐			
With spontaneous unilateral bloody nipple discharge or which stains clothes	☐	☐			
Male, aged 50 years and older with a unilateral, firm subareolar mass with or without nipple distortion or associated skin changes	☐	☐			

Figure 16.9 Referral guidelines produced for general practitioners to 'fast track' patients suspected of having breast cancer (based on national and local guidelines). Reproduced with permission from the United Lincolnshire Hospitals NHS Trust.

one-third is evenly distributed between the other quadrants and behind the nipple and areola. The next most common presentation is with nipple problems (bleeding, eczematous changes and retraction, Fig. 16.7, p. 281). Pain is uncommon, but is present in a small percentage of patients. Rarely, a patient may present with a large, painful and tender axillary lymph node without any obvious breast abnormality.

Inflammatory breast cancer presents with an enlarged firm breast, oedema and redness of the overlying skin and varying degrees of tenderness on palpation. There may be no clearly defined mass in the breast. About 25 per cent of women in the UK present with large primary tumours (>3 cm T_2, T_3, Fig. 16.7, p. 281), or locally advanced breast cancers (T_4, N_2) (Fig. 16.8, p. 281). In some cases, particularly elderly patients, the tumour may have been present for some time, but hidden by the patient from her relatives due to fear and anxiety (Fig. 16.8). Occasionally patients may even deny the presence of a tumour as a psychological coping strategy. Patients may also present with metastatic disease, for example, pathological bone fractures, malignant pleural effusions, ascites and hepatic metastases, or brain dysfunction with cerebral metastases. To speed up patient referral and establish an early diagnosis, guidelines have been produced for GPs to use (Fig. 16.9).

Diagnosis and staging of breast cancer

Diagnosis

The diagnosis is made on clinical features (Figs 16.6–16.8, p. 281), from various imaging modalities (Figs 16.10 and 16.11), and cytological/histological assessment. In approximately 75 per cent of patients, a diagnosis of cancer can be made clinically. Triple assessment is used: clinical examination, imaging (mammography, ultrasonography), core cut biopsy (usually ultrasound guided), and occasionally fine needle aspiration cytology in the hospital's breast unit. Using this approach, more than 95 per cent of cancers can be diagnosed with a sensitivity of 95 per cent, a specificity of >96 per cent, and a predictive value of >97 per cent. This approach is used in the authors' Rapid Result Clinic.

Staging

Various staging investigations are carried out.

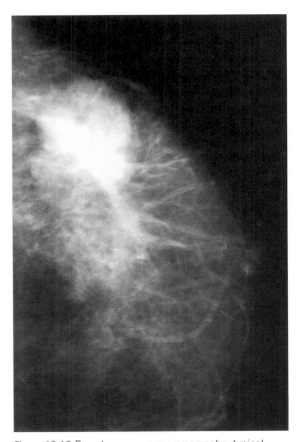

Figure 16.10 Breast cancer on mammography: typical irregular density with architectural distortion and invading projections. Reproduced with permission from Lincoln Breast Unit.

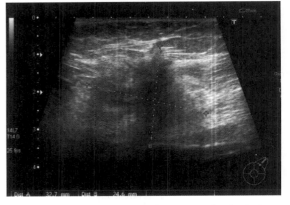

Figure 16.11 Breast cancer on ultrasonography: typical hypoechoic mass with irregular margins and acoustic shadowing. Reproduced with permission from Lincoln Breast Unit.

- Blood tests:
  - full blood count
  - urea and electrolytes
  - liver function
  - serum calcium
  - tumour markers.
- Imaging investigations:
  - chest radiograph and radiographs of any symptomatic areas of the skeleton
  - ultrasound examination of the abdomen is carried out in patients with locally advanced or large tumours
  - computed tomography may be performed, particularly if there are abnormal liver function tests or clinical features suggestive of hepatic metastases and a normal result from abdominal ultrasonography
  - isotope bone scans are not routinely performed for small tumours, but are done where the tumours are >3 cm, or locally advanced cancers (T_3, T_4 and N_2) as there is a likelihood of disseminated disease and tumour deposits in skeletal tissues.

Breast screening

Through screening, many impalpable lesions are now being detected. These include mammographic densities, lesions with clearly defined margins suggestive of benign conditions, areas of microcalcification – linear branching patterns suggestive of comedo DCIS, and aggregates of focal, granular and irregular deposits of calcium. Approximately 75 per cent of malignant microcalcifications are due to DCIS and 25 per cent to invasive cancer. The calcification in DCIS occurs in the debris and secretions of duct lumens, or within the epithelium of ductal malignant cells. In benign conditions, it tends to be present in the stroma. DCIS represents 10–20 per cent of screen detected (mammography) breast cancers. Diagnosis of impalpable lesions is carried out by stereotactic core cut biopsy, or by ultrasound-guided core cut biopsy if it can be seen on the corresponding ultrasound scan. The lesions are then removed by either stereotactic or ultrasound wire-guided localization and excision. The specimen is X-rayed after removal while the patient is anaesthetized to ensure that the opacity or microcalcification has been removed.

Special considerations

Bilateral breast cancers

These can be either synchronous or metachronous, (occurring at least 3 months after diagnosis of the first lesion). Synchronous tumours occur in 1 per cent of patients with breast cancer. Metachronous tumours occur in 4 per cent with a diagnosis of breast cancer. Women with synchronous or metachronous cancers do not necessarily have a poor prognosis. Patients with a genetic predisposition and strong family history are at very high risk of developing bilateral breast cancers, but do not necessarily have a worse prognosis. Such patients, on developing a breast cancer, often express a wish for and undergo bilateral mastectomies.

Breast cancer during pregnancy

Breast cancer is the most common malignant condition occurring during pregnancy. The incidence is approximately 1 in 2500 pregnancies, and poses many medical and psychological problems, both for the woman and her relatives. Breast cancer in pregnancy should be treated using the same management criteria as for the general population. Termination of pregnancy does not alter the prognosis, but may be indicated, especially in the first trimester, if the patient needs to undergo chemotherapy or radiotherapy, because of the risk of significant damage to the fetus. This is a complex issue requiring a multidisciplinary approach and taking into account the various oncological, ethical and psychological issues. There is no evidence that a subsequent pregnancy has any deleterious effects on recurrence of disease or survival, in particular if the cancer was oestrogen receptor negative (ER –ve). In general, women should be advised to wait at least 2 years following treatment before embarking on further pregnancies, as recurrence within this time period carries a bad prognosis.

Male breast cancer

Breast cancer in males is less common than in females (1 in 150 breast cancers). The age group and presentation are not dissimilar to women – lump, ulceration, discharge. Management guidelines are similar to those used for females.

SUMMARY

Key features of the presenting history are:

- Pain
- Lump
- Nipple discharge
- Nipple changes
- Axillary symptoms.

Include the following in your physical examination:

- Inspection
    - breast as a whole: changes/discrepancies in size, shape or contour
    - breast skin: puckering and/or tethering; oedema (peau d'orange); features of inflammation (swelling, redness); skin nodules, mass with or without ulceration
    - nipple–areolar complex: swelling; retraction; eczematous changes or ulceration; nipple discharge
    - lymph draining areas: axilla; supraclavicular fossa
- Palpation – for each breast palpate the:
    - upper outer quadrant
    - lower outer quadrant
    - lower inner quadrant
    - upper inner quadrant
    - nipple and areolar complex
    - axillary tail of the breast
- Palpation – of the lymph draining areas: axilla
    - medial: serratus anterior
    - lateral: inner aspect of upper arm
    - posterior: subscapularis
    - anterior: inner aspect of pectoralis major
    - central: axillary contents
- Palpation – of the lymph draining areas: supraclavicular fossa.

FURTHER READING

Heys SD, Eremin JM, Eremin O. 2001. Breast. In: Eremin O (ed). *The scientific and clinical basis of surgical practice*. Oxford: Oxford University Press.

17 THE HAEMATOLOGICAL SYSTEM

Martin R Howard

INTRODUCTION

Diseases of the blood and associated tissues are common both in community and hospital practice. They produce a remarkably diverse range of symptoms and signs. This heterogeneity is explained by the large number of different ways in which blood may malfunction and result in disease. Most simply, an individual may have a shortage of normal blood cells. The commonest of all haematological syndromes, anaemia, arises from a lack of normal circulating red cells. Underproduction or excessive destruction of white cells (leucopenia) or platelets (thrombocytopenia) also causes distinctive groups of symptoms and physical findings. Conversely, pathological overproduction of cells occurs in the myeloproliferative disorders.

Well-regulated haemostasis is crucial for health and both inadequate coagulation, such as in the inherited disorder haemophilia, and excessive coagulation, as occurs in thrombophilia, can have drastic consequences such as haemorrhage and thrombosis. Much of the clinical haematologist's time is spent in managing malignant diseases of the bone marrow and lymphoid system, and these cancers have their own features. Leukaemias tend to lead to symptoms and signs because of the shortage of normal blood cells whereas lymphomas more often present with the consequences of direct tissue invasion, most commonly enlarged lymph nodes (lymphadenopathy). Both symptoms and signs may be produced by indirect mechanisms. In the malignant disease of plasma cells, myeloma, bone pain and fractures occur because of the secretion of tissue-damaging cytokines by the tumour cells.

A patient may have an isolated blood abnormality causing a predictable clinical presentation but, equally, they may have complex combinations of mechanisms. Patients with certain subtypes of acute myeloid leukaemia often have a shortage of all normal blood cells (pancytopenia) and a failure of haemostasis. Many patients with lymphoma have bone marrow infiltration by the tumour cells causing the symptoms and signs of blood cytopenia in addition to lymphadenopathy. It is important to understand not only the basic connection between blood abnormalities and clinical symptoms and signs (e.g. for anaemia) but also the characteristic clinical patterns of the major diseases of the blood (e.g. anaemia and bone pain in myeloma or anaemia and neurological signs in severe vitamin B_{12} deficiency).

The 'haematological system' can also become deranged in a very large number of non-blood disorders: an appreciation of this fact is important to properly interpret the symptoms and signs that result. The patient with iron deficiency anaemia may well present only with the symptoms of anaemia. Here, the diagnosis of anaemia is only the start, as a search for the underlying cause is crucial. If iron deficiency is confirmed with an appropriate laboratory test, then an exhaustive systemic enquiry and clinical examination is essential to elicit an occult site of bleeding. In this context, even the absence of clinical symptoms and signs of gastrointestinal pathology may not avoid the need for invasive investigation such as endoscopy. This scenario is a reminder that an understanding of the clinical presentation of the common abnormalities of the blood is necessary for general practice and is not confined to the management of rare blood diseases. The clinician who has grasped the significance of the symptoms and signs of iron deficiency anaemia is more likely to make the early diagnosis of otherwise asymptomatic colonic cancer.

One of the rewards of the practice of clinical haematology is the merging of the consulting room and the laboratory. Blood abnormalities first suspected during history taking and examination can be promptly confirmed with a relevant blood test, perhaps a full blood count or a coagulation screen. This chapter addresses the proper interviewing and physical examination of the patient but the role of careful selection of laboratory tests based on accurate clinical findings cannot be underestimated.

CLINICAL HISTORY

Presenting complaint

Anaemia

Anaemia is simply defined as a haemoglobin level below the accepted normal range. It is the commonest of all clinically significant blood abnormalities and has a large number of possible causes (Fig. 17.1). Symptoms result from the blood's reduced oxygen carrying capacity leading to tissue hypoxia and the body's attempts to compensate for this. Patients complain of *fatigue* and *shortness of breath on exertion*; the latter symptom may be ascribed to incipient cardiorespiratory failure. Cardiac overactivity causes *palpitations* and some also complain of *tinnitus*, *dizziness* and *faintness*. Other features include feelings of irritability, restlessness and insomnia. Severe anaemia will eventually lead to alarming symptoms such as dyspnoea at rest, syncope and visual disturbances.

In practice, the severity of symptoms is not only determined by the haemoglobin level. The rapid onset of anaemia will cause more profound upset than its insidious development where the affected person has more time to compensate physiologically and to adjust their lifestyle. Patients who are elderly or frail or who have co-existent heart disease are more vulnerable to the effects of anaemia. The exacerbation of angina is a concerning development.

Leucopenia

There are five different types of white cell in the blood but in clinical practice, the two most significant forms of leucopenia are neutropenia and lymphopenia. These may be isolated or they may co-exist.

Neutrophils are phagocytes: they engulf and destroy foreign material and damaged cells. A shortage of neutrophils (neutropenia) may arise from underproduction or excess destruction. Whatever the mechanism, patients are at risk of infection and other insults. The likelihood of infection can be predicted by the degree of fall in the neutrophil count. Significant bacterial infections are commonly caused by Gram-positive cocci and also Gram-negative bacilli such as *Pseudomonas aeruginosa*, *Escherichia coli*, *Klebsiella* and *Proteus*. Patients may present with fulminant life-threatening infection but early symptoms of neutropenic sepsis can be surprisingly subtle.

Lymphocytes are also essential for normal immunity:

- B lymphocytes produce antibodies against a particular antigen (humoral immunity)
- T lymphocytes interact with antigen-presenting cells in the genesis of the 'cell-mediated response'.

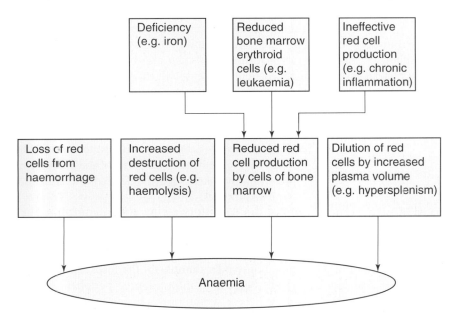

Figure 17.1 Causes of anaemia.

IMPORTANT

In patients known to be at risk of neutropenia – this would include those on drugs known to be associated with agranulocytosis – complaints of general malaise or a persistent sore throat or mouth ulceration should prompt urgent investigation.

A shortage of lymphocytes (lymphopenia) can occur in various malignancies (e.g. lymphoma), in immune deficiency disorders (e.g. human immuno-deficiency virus (HIV) infection) or associated with drug treatment or trauma. Patients with reduced humoral immunity, which can be quantitated by measuring immunoglobulin levels, often present with bacterial infections of the respiratory system, skin and urinary tract. Severe T cell depletion potentially leads to numerous unusual opportunistic infections, including those cause by viruses, fungi and *Pneumocystis*. Rather as with neutropenia, patients with lymphopenia may present with alarming symptoms of fulminant infection or with surprisingly low grade features. Vigilance is needed: in a patient with abnormal cell-mediated immunity, exertional dyspnoea may be the first sign of life-threatening *Pneumocystis* or cytomegalovirus-associated pneumonia.

Thrombocytopenia

Platelets are vital for normal haemostasis. Where there is either a reduced number of platelets (thrombocytopenia) or abnormal platelet function, there is the possibility of a haemorrhagic tendency. Characteristic symptoms include easy bruising and bleeding. There may be heavy periods (menorrhagia), nose bleeds (epistaxes), gum bleeding and excessive blood loss following dental extractions or other surgery. Bleeding from the gastrointestinal or urinary tract may occur but, even in severe thrombocytopenia, this is unusual in the absence of other pathology. Thankfully, cerebral haemorrhage is also a rare event but it must be considered in patients with low platelets who complain of headache or other neurological symptoms. The pattern of bleeding in platelet disorders is distinct from that seen in 'coagulation disorders' (see p. 294).

Failure of coagulation

Formation of a normal clot depends not only on platelets but also on a coagulation component in which a fibrin scaffold (thrombus) is constructed around the platelet plug. Any deficiency in the 'coagulation cascade' – for instance, the deficiency of a single vital coagulation factor, as occurs in haemophilia – will lead to a tendency to bleed. Unlike thrombocytopenia, where oozing into skin and mucous membranes is the predominant problem, patients with abnormal coagulation are more likely to bleed spontaneously into joints (to form a *haemarthrosis*) and into muscles. They complain of local pain and loss of function. In some inherited or acquired bleeding disorders (e.g. von Willebrand's disease or severe liver disease) there are deficiencies of both platelets and the coagulation cascade, and so there is a full range of haemorrhagic symptoms.

Thrombophilia

The clinical term 'thrombophilia' means a predisposition to thrombosis because of an enhanced coagulation mechanism. Many forms of the disease are inherited (e.g. factor V Leiden mutation) and venous thrombosis is the major risk. Affected people have an increased chance of deep vein thrombosis with the typical complaints of lower limb swelling and pain or associated pulmonary embolus. Thrombus may form in unusual sites: unilateral arm swelling suggests axillary vein occlusion. In acquired thrombophilia (e.g. antiphospholipid antibody syndrome) arterial thrombosis can also be a significant factor and patients present with the protean symptoms of myocardial or cerebral infarction.

Haematological malignancy

Haematological malignancy can lead to a very wide range of disease symptoms. Some of the commoner presenting symptoms may be divided into *local* and *systemic* subtypes.

Local symptoms

Patients with lymphoma often present with enlarging, non-tender lumps in the neck, axillae and groins because of infiltration of peripheral lymph nodes. Less commonly, bulky mediastinal or intra-abdominal nodes lead to local compression and respiratory and gastrointestinal symptoms. Oddly, pain is a relatively late manifestation of lymphoma. Similar symptoms may be experienced in chronic lymphocytic leukaemia. A large spleen, seen in both lymphoproliferative and myeloproliferative disorders, leads to a dragging uncomfortable sensation in the left abdomen and, if there is peri-capsular inflammation, a sharp localized pain exacerbated by movement and inspiration.

The characteristic presentation of myeloma is bone pain. This is often in the back – its relentless nature helps to differentiate it from the much more common pain of spinal degenerative disease. Rib pain is another clue. Symptoms such as paraesthesiae and loss of lower limb and bladder function are likely to herald spinal cord compression. Acute leukaemias present more with symptoms of bone marrow failure, those attributable to anaemia, leucopenia and thrombocytopenia, than with symptoms of local infiltration; however, sometimes, particularly in acute lymphoblastic leukaemia, patients experience pain. Neurological symptoms, also more common in the lymphoblastic form, are frequently a sign of central nervous system dissemination.

Systemic symptoms

Lymphomas that are disseminated at presentation are frequently associated with 'systemic symptoms' such as weight loss, night sweats and pyrexia. These have prognostic significance and, once properly documented, are included in the staging system as 'B symptoms'. Their severity is highly variable. Patients with advanced Hodgkin's lymphoma are prone to night sweats, which may be severe enough to drench the nightclothes and sheets. Fatigue and pruritus may also occur. These malignant disorders are themselves forms of acquired immunodeficiency and recurrent infection is a common finding.

Chemotherapy may limit the disease but will tend to further compromise the immune response. In myeloma and Waldenstrom's macroglobulinaemia high levels of serum monoclonal proteins secreted by the malignant cells (paraproteins) can potentially lead to 'hyperviscosity syndrome', with confusion and neurological symptoms.

THE REST OF THE HISTORY

Duration of symptoms

In general, those who have symptoms of recent onset are likely to have acquired disorders whereas a life-long history suggests the possibility of an inherited disorder. This is especially pertinent in patients with a history of easy bruising or bleeding. An inherited disease such as haemophilia is far more likely to cause symptoms from the first year of life than an acquired bleeding tendency such as immune thrombocytopenia (ITP).

History of surgery or trauma

Diagnostic clues may be derived from the patient's response to surgery or trauma. A past history of surgery with a quick recovery suggests a more recent onset of a significant blood abnormality or haematological disorder. In contrast, repeated excessive bleeding following dental extractions or other surgery is consistent with a lifelong bleeding disorder, possibly an inherited disease.

Drug history

It is difficult to exaggerate the importance of a thorough drug history in patients with suspected haematological disease. Many drugs are implicated in abnormalities of the blood such as:

- autoimmune haemolytic anaemia – e.g. cephalosporins, penicillins
- neutropenia – agranulocytosis, e.g. phenothiazines, sulphonamides
- thrombocytopenia – e.g. quinine, thiazide diuretics.

Bone marrow failure with pancytopenia may occur idiosyncratically (e.g. chloramphenicol) or predictably following cytotoxic chemotherapy. Often the situation is complicated as the patient is on multiple agents, several of which may be causative. Here it is helpful to take an exhaustive history of the temporal relationship of the medication to the blood abnormality – if a low platelet count preceded the commencement of a thiazide diuretic then the drug is unlikely to be the culprit.

IMPORTANT

It is vital to spot a drug-related blood abnormality as prompt cessation of the offending agent usually leads to complete resolution of the symptoms, whereas a failure to make the connection and continuation of the drug may have serious consequences (e.g. septicaemia arising from agranulocytosis).

> **BOX 17.1** SELECTED INHERITED BLOOD DISORDERS
>
> Red cell disorders:
> - disorders of the membrane – hereditary spherocytosis and elliptocytosis
> - disorders of haemoglobin – sickle cell anaemia and thalassaemia
> - disorders of metabolism – pyruvate kinase and glucose 6-phosphate deficiencies.
>
> Coagulation disorders:
> - factor deficiency – haemophilia A and B
> - combined factor and platelet deficiency – von Willebrand's disease
> - platelet dysfunction – Bernard-Soulier syndrome (rare)
>
> White cell disorders: rare functional disorders such as chronic granulomatous disease.

It is also obligatory to take a history of drug allergies. Patients with a complex haematological disorder such as leukaemia or lymphoma will inevitably become exposed to many drugs. Whenever there is doubt as to a patient's medication, it is well worth retaking the history with the tablets to hand. Confused, elderly patients are unlikely to be able to spontaneously recall an elaborate list of 10–20 different drugs.

Family history

Many types of blood disorders are inherited and a family history is a key part of the diagnostic process. The presence of the disease in other family members may be elicited by a simple question but to gain a clear understanding the family tree must be documented to gain an appreciation of the likely mode of inheritance of the disorder. A few of the commoner inherited disorders in haematological practice are listed in Box 17.1.

β-**Thalassaemia** is an inherited disorder of red cells. It is an autosomal recessive disorder characterized by reduced or absent production of β haemoglobin chains; the heterozygous (trait or minor) form is usually symptomless whilst the homozygous form leads to the clinically significant disease 'β-thalassaemia major', in which the patient develops symptoms of anaemia early in life. It is not always so straightforward.

In **hereditary spherocytosis** an abnormal red cell membrane leads to haemolysis and possible anaemia. There are many possible causative gene mutations and, accordingly, a variable mode of inheritance. It is important to appreciate this heterogeneity when taking the family history in an affected patient.

A number of coagulation disorders are also inherited. In **haemophilia A and B** (caused by a short-age of clotting factors VIII and IX, respectively) the inheritance is X-linked recessive. Briefly:

- all males with the abnormal gene have haemophilia
- all sons of haemophiliac fathers are unaffected
- all daughters are obligatory carriers
- daughters of female carriers have a 50 per cent chance of being themselves carriers.

The commonest inherited coagulation disorder, **von Willebrand's disease**, is more complicated, with most but not all forms having autosomal dominant inheritance.

The few examples described above emphasize that a well-taken family history requires not only a methodical approach but also a thorough understanding of the genetics of the implicated disease. Note also that ethnic origin and geography are relevant factors. A child from an African Caribbean background is much more likely to present with sickle cell anaemia than a Caucasian child, whereas the converse is true of iron deficiency caused by coeliac disease. Disorders such as thalassaemia are much more common in particular parts of the world.

Lifestyle and social history

A social history is important to understand the causation of blood abnormalities or disease and to allow the optimal management of the patient. Some blood changes are directly related to the patient's lifestyle. Heavy smoking may contribute to polycythaemia, poor diet can cause anaemia because of deficiency of iron or folate, and excess alcohol consumption leads to myriad blood abnormalities including macrocytosis, thrombocytopenia and disordered coagulation.

People with chronic and serious blood diseases want to lead as normal a life as possible. A proper history should lead to an understanding of the individual's support structure and situation outside the hospital clinic and ward. Children with inherited disease such as thalassaemia can easily fall behind at school. The whole family is likely to be under strain; adults may suffer unemployment, financial difficulties and social isolation.

> **CLINICAL PEARL**
>
> An appreciation of all issues surrounding a patient, including their social history, allows a more holistic view of the person's medical care and maximizes their chance of a timely return to normality.

Occupational history

Occupational exposure to benzene or other solvents leads to an increased risk of leukaemia. Similarly, studies have suggested links between various occupations such as agricultural work (and presumed exposure to pesticides) or hairdressing (with exposure to chemical dyes) and lymphoma. In practice, connections of this kind are nearly always conjectural and it is difficult to prove a causative effect in individual people.

Travel history

Symptoms caused by an enlarged spleen will carry an entirely different differential diagnosis if the patient has recently returned from an area where malaria and other tropical infectious diseases are commonplace. The incidence of HIV infection, a disease often associated with blood abnormalities, also fluctuates widely around the world. Patients may not think to offer travel information spontaneously so the question must be asked.

Systems review

This is vital as diseases of non-haematopoietic organs may contribute to blood abnormalities and complicate the investigation and treatment of primary blood diseases. Much time can be wasted searching for a haematological cause of anaemia if previously ignored symptoms of chronic gastrointestinal bleeding are not discovered as part of the systems review. In patients with haematological malignancies such as lymphoma, the presence of unexpected symptoms such as headache or loss of peripheral sensation may reflect extranodal infiltration by disease or side effects of chemotherapy drugs (e.g. neuropathy caused by vincristine). A systematic check for cardiorespiratory symptoms is obligatory to detect significant heart or lung disease which might be exacerbated

Table 17.1 Eastern Cooperative Oncology Group (ECOG) performance status scale

Grade	ECOG
0	Fully active, able to carry on all pre-disease performance without restriction
1	Restricted in physically strenuous activity but ambulatory and able to carry out work of a light or sedentary nature, e.g. light housework, office work
2	Ambulatory and capable of all self-care but unable to carry out any work activities. Up and about more than 50 per cent of waking hours
3	Capable of only limited self-care, confined to bed or chair more than 50 per cent of waking hours
4	Completely disabled. Cannot carry on any self-care. Totally confined to bed or chair
5	Dead

Modified from: Oken MM, Creech RH, Tormey DC et al. 1982. Toxicity and response criteria of the Eastern Cooperative Oncology Group. American Journal of Clinical Oncology 5: 649–55. Credited to the Eastern Cooperative Oncology Group, Robert Comis, MD, Group Chair.

Table 17.2 Karnofsky's performance status scale

Definition	Per cent	Criteria
Able to carry on normal activity and to work. No special care is needed	100 90 80	Normal; no complaints; no evidence of disease Able to carry on normal activity; minor signs or symptoms of disease Normal activity with effort; some signs or symptoms of disease
Unable to work. Able to live at home, care for most personal needs. A varying amount of assistance is needed	70 60 50	Cares for self. Unable to carry on normal activity or to do active work Requires occasional assistance, but is able to care for most of his needs Requires considerable assistance and frequent medical care
Unable to care for self. Requires equivalent of institutional or hospital care. Disease may be progressing rapidly	40 30 20 10 0	Disabled; requires special care and assistance Severely disabled; hospitalization is indicated although death not imminent Very sick; hospitalization necessary; active supportive treatment necessary Moribund; fatal processes progressing rapidly Dead

From: CANCER, Vol. 1, No. 4, 1948, 634–56, © 1948 American Cancer Society. This material is reproduced with permission of Wiley-Liss, Inc., a subsidiary of John Wiley & Sons, Inc.

by intensive chemotherapy treatment. In people presenting with a high haematocrit (polycythaemia) or a high platelet count (thrombocytosis) a systemic enquiry is necessary to exclude secondary causes such as hypoxia and infection before a diagnosis of a myeloproliferative disorder is seriously considered. Where the patient is debilitated it is helpful to formally record this using an accepted scoring system such as the Eastern Cooperative Oncology Group (ECOG) system (Table 17.1) or Karnofsky's (Table 17.2) scales. Document the score, together with other objective measures such as height and weight, and use this to monitor general state or to assess suitability for chemotherapy or other treatments.

PHYSICAL EXAMINATION

Before describing the signs associated with particular haematological syndromes, the importance of initial careful inspection of the patient must be stressed. Many key signs are readily detectable on observation alone and the inexperienced or over-eager examiner can all too easily miss them in his or her enthusiasm to palpate and percuss.

Anaemia

The examination findings can be divided into those potentially found in all patients with significant anaemia ('general') and those connected with particular aetiologies ('specific').

General findings

The most well known sign of anaemia is pallor of the skin. This is not caused by 'thinning' of the blood but by reduced peripheral blood flow. This pallor may be better appreciated by close inspection of the conjunctivae, nail beds, and palmar creases. It is an insensitive sign.

As anaemia becomes more marked, the clinical findings can be explained in terms of a variable degree of cardiopulmonary compensation. Patients are usually comfortable at rest but may become visibly dyspnoeic on minimal exertion. The 'hyperkinetic' circulatory response leads to tachycardia, increased arterial pulsation and cardiac flow murmurs.

In severe anaemia there may be frank cardiac failure with the characteristic cardiomegaly, basal inspiratory crepitations in the lungs, and lower limb oedema. Very low haemoglobin levels can be

---

CLINICAL PEARL

More severe anaemia may cause a systolic flow murmur. This functional murmur must be differentiated from the systolic murmurs of valvular heart disease.

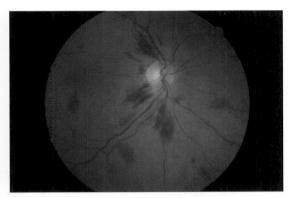

Figure 17.2 Retinal haemorrhages in severe anaemia.

associated with papilloedema and retinal haemorrhages (Fig. 17.2). Anaemia may cause a fever but in practice this is more often a feature of an underlying cause (e.g. malignancy) or a co-existent disorder.

Specific findings

An initial careful inspection of the skin, nails and mouth often reveals diagnostic clues. In severe iron deficiency, the general signs of anaemia may be accompanied by glossitis and angular stomatitis. Because of thinning of the epithelium the tongue can appear dark red in contrast to the facial pallor. If iron deficiency is prolonged it may become smooth and shrunken. The painful red fissures of angular stomatitis appear at the corners of the mouth which may be generally sore. A highly characteristic, but rare, feature of longstanding iron deficiency is koilonychia, in which the nails become concave or 'spooned'. More commonly, and less dramatically, the nails are brittle and ridged.

As epithelial abnormalities also occur in megaloblastic anaemia, simple inspection also reaps rewards in this disorder. In vitamin B$_{12}$ deficiency due to pernicious anaemia, the tongue is typically red, smooth and shiny. More profound epithelial dysfunction leads to the neurological signs of subacute combined degeneration of the cord (see also later) whereas the presence of vitiligo is a reminder of the autoimmune nature of the disease.

Haemolytic anaemias may present with jaundice rather than pallor. The accelerated catabolism of haemoglobin releases increased amounts of bilirubin into the plasma. Where the spleen is the site of red cell destruction, it may be palpable. If there is chronic haemolysis in childhood, for instance in the haemoglobinopathies, then expansion of the marrow cavity leads to skeletal abnormalities including frontal bossing of the skull.

Numerous further examples could be quoted – the anaemia of chronic disease may be associated with any of the signs of the innumerable systemic diseases which cause it – but the core message is that careful examination of the anaemic patient can elucidate not only the signs of anaemia itself but also of the underlying cause.

Leucopenia

Perhaps the most important sign associated with **neutropenia** is pyrexia. In the context of severe neutropenia, it usually has to be assumed that the pyrexia is due to infection and not other aetiologies such as malignancy or a drug reaction. A raised temperature is often the only outward sign of a potentially fulminant infection.

Many people with life-threatening neutropenic sepsis have no signs to indicate the primary focus. Because of the lack of normal neutrophils, classical signs of inflammation are frequently absent, making the diagnosis of infection more difficult than usual. Pneumonia may not be accompanied by the classic signs of consolidation and cellulitis may not lead to the usual degree of tenderness and pain. A thorough systemic examination is obligatory as signs are easily overlooked. Extensively search the skin, including the perineal and perianal regions.

> **CLINICAL PEARL**
> Skin infections cause heterogeneous clinical signs; when in doubt seek an expert dermatological opinion.

The mouth is a common focus of infection in neutropenia. Common findings are the mucosal atrophy and plaques of *Candida*, and ulcers. Neutropenic ulcers are typically yellowish in appearance with regular margins. They may be single or multiple, are not easily removed from the mucosa, and are often painful. Experience is required to reliably differentiate them from other common causes of mouth ulcers in immunosuppressed patients (drug-induced mucositis, aphthous ulcers, herpetic ulcers).

Examination of the neutropenic patient is completed with a careful review of all other systems in turn, with particular reference to the possibility of infection. In this situation, regular examination for new signs is vital; the appearance of a previously unheard murmur may be the only clue to the presence of endocarditis.

In **lymphopenia**, many of the same considerations apply. Undertake examination with knowledge of the likely complicating infections and their characteristic signs. Again, these signs can be surprisingly subtle. In patients presenting with impaired cell-mediated immunity and life-threatening *Pneumocystis jirovecii* (*carinii*) pneumonia, up to half will have no abnormal signs on auscultation of the lungs. The development of marked tachypnoea (and hypoxia) on minimal exertion is usually the main diagnostic feature.

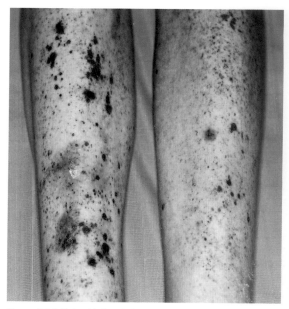

Figure 17.3 Petechial rash in severe thrombocytopenia.

Thrombocytopenia

Minor reductions in platelet count frequently cause no clinical signs but more significant falls (e.g. to less than $50 \times 10^9/L$) usually present as bleeding into the skin (purpura). In general, signs (and symptoms) are more pronounced at any given platelet count where there is reduced platelet production (e.g. in leukaemia) than where there is excessive platelet destruction (e.g. in immune thrombocytopenia).

Thrombocytopenia is a cause of an increase in bruising (ecchymoses). Ecchymoses are easily recognized on routine examination and inspection is usefully accompanied by an enquiry as to the degree of trauma (if any) that produced them. Ecchymoses can be quite persistent and usually undergo a series of colour changes from blue to green and then to yellow and brown as the extravasated blood is degraded. It is sometimes difficult to be certain when bruising is pathological – a scattering of small bruises may be normal in an active child or an athletic adult.

If platelet counts are at very low levels, *petechiae* appear. These are small reddish blue spots (1–3 mm in diameter) which often occur suddenly in the skin in crops (Fig. 17.3). They may arise anywhere on the body but are often found on dependent areas, par-

ticularly the shins. Petechiae are usually less persistent than ecchymoses, tending to disappear within a few days. Because they are composed of extravasated blood they do not fade on pressure. Where these skin signs suggest thrombocytopenia, a careful inspection of the mouth, conjunctivae, and retinas is essential to detect mucosal haemorrhage. In very severe thrombocytopenia, bleeding can be profound leading to haemorrhagic bullae in the skin, blood blisters in the mouth and extensive retinal haemorrhage with reduced visual acuity. The presence of neurological signs is ominous as it suggests a significant intracerebral bleed.

Coagulation failure

The signs associated with a pure failure of coagulation (e.g. a deficiency of coagulation factor(s)) are best understood by describing the findings in severe haemophilia. Here, patients have a pattern of bleeding quite different from that described in thrombocytopenia. Bruising may be increased but the chief characteristics of the disease are acute bleeds into joints and muscles with lifelong sequelae. Fortunately, in the modern era, patients receive optimal prophylactic factor replacement regimens and bleeds are much less frequent and severe chronic

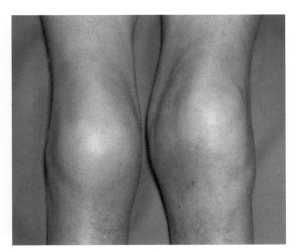

Figure 17.4 Joint swelling and deformity in severe haemophilia.

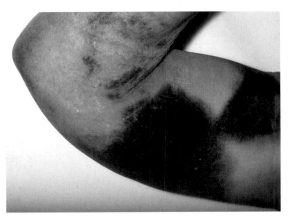

Figure 17.5 Ecchymoses in acquired haemophilia.

joint disease is rare. An acute joint bleed (haemarthrosis) presents as a swollen, tender joint with restriction of movement. The skin is warm to the touch The knees are most often affected, followed by the elbows, ankles, shoulders, wrists and hips. In the absence of optimal treatment, the affected joints of haemophiliac patients become irretrievably damaged with permanent swelling, fixed deformities and associated muscle wasting (Fig. 17.4).

Bleeding into muscles causes both local pain and swelling with eventual discoloration of the skin as the blood drains to the surface. If bleeds into large muscles remain untreated, the compression of adjacent nerves, blood vessels and lymphatics may result. For instance, a bleed into the iliopsoas muscle can compress the femoral nerve, leading to fixed flexion at the hip and sensory loss on the outside of the thigh. In extreme cases, there is wasting of the quadriceps muscle. Chronic muscle bleeding, now rare in developed countries, is a cause of 'pseudotumours', which have the potential to track through surrounding tissues including the skin.

Cerebral bleeding is also rare but the finding of papilloedema or other unexplained neurological signs should alert you to this possibility. The related disorder 'acquired haemophilia' is caused by an acquired antibody against a coagulation factor (generally factor VIII) and is usually seen in the last decades of life. The diagnosis should especially be considered where very extensive bruising develops for no apparent reason in the presence of a normal platelet count (Fig. 17.5).

The signs relating to thrombocytopenia and coagulation failure have been discussed separately for convenience but patients may have a more general failure of normal haemostasis with features of both platelet lack or loss of function and also coagulation deficiency (e.g. in severe von Willebrand's disease, following massive transfusion, or in liver failure).

Thrombophilia

Thrombophilia is a haematological disorder whose physical signs commonly arise from a prothrombotic tendency (i.e. the associated deep vein thrombosis or pulmonary embolism). Patients with thrombophilia may have thrombosis at unusual sites.

Malignancy

Haematological malignancies lead to a protean range of clinical signs and these will be discussed in the disease-orientated section later. At this stage, we will review the examination findings in three specific situations that are 'haematological emergencies'.

Superior vena cava obstruction

Hodgkin's and non-Hodgkin's lymphomas are second only to lung cancer as a cause of superior vena cava obstruction as bulky mediastinal lymphadenopathy is common in these disorders. The mediastinal mass compresses the superior vena cava and the characteristic examination findings, all arising from obstruction of venous return, include plethora and oedema of the face and upper extremities, increased jugular venous pressure and visible dilatation of the collateral veins of the upper thorax and neck. The patient may have a hoarse voice or even stridor.

Spinal cord compression

Myeloma is commonly complicated by spinal cord compression either secondary to vertebral destruction or because of a localized tumour of plasma cells (plasmacytoma). Once suggestive symptoms (e.g. lower limb paraesthesia, urinary difficulty) are reported, an urgent examination will reveal the diagnostic signs. Definitive signs usually appear within a week or so of the symptoms and include loss of sensation below the neurological lesion (sensory level), upper motor neurone weakness in the legs (spastic paraparesis) and loss of sphincter control.

Hyperviscosity syndrome

This may complicate myeloma or, more commonly the IgM-secreting indolent lymphoma termed Waldenström's macroglobulinaemia. High serum monoclonal protein (paraprotein) levels significantly increase blood viscosity which in turn may lead to visual disturbance, heart failure and neurological symptoms. The classic signs of hyperviscosity are

> **BOX 17.2** COMMON CAUSES OF LYMPHADENOPATHY
> Localized:
> - local infection
> - lymphoma
> - metastatic malignancy.
>
> Generalized:
> - systemic infection
> - lymphoma
> - disseminated malignancy
> - other haematological malignancies (e.g. leukaemia)
> - inflammatory disorders (e.g. sarcoidosis, connective tissue disorders).

found in the fundus (distended veins, exudates, haemorrhages and blurring of the optic disc) highlighting the need for routine retinal inspection in patients with haematological disease.

Particular examination skills

Examination of the lymph nodes

Enlargement of lymph nodes is referred to as lymphadenopathy or just adenopathy. A wide range of haematological and systemic disorders may lead to

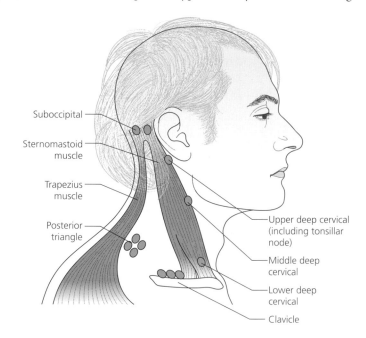

Suboccipital

Sternomastoid muscle

Trapezius muscle

Posterior triangle

Upper deep cervical (including tonsillar node)

Middle deep cervical

Lower deep cervical

Clavicle

Figure 17.6 Normal cervical lymph nodes.

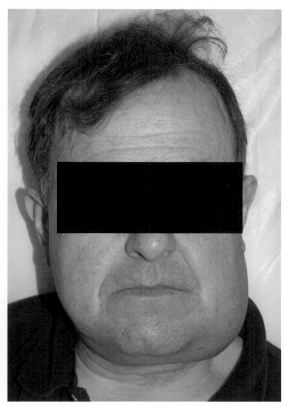

Figure 17.7 Cervical lymphadenopathy in non-Hodgkin's lymphoma.

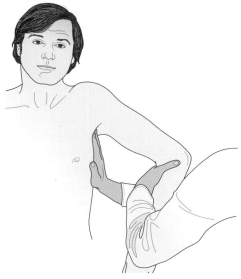

Figure 17.8 Technique for examination of the axillary nodes.

- location
- size (two dimensions)
- shape
- consistency
- presence/absence of tenderness.

lymphadenopathy (Box. 17.2). In clinical practice, examination is usually limited to the peripheral nodes in the cervical, axillary and inguinal regions although, on occasions, bulky intra-abdominal lymphadenopathy may be palpated as an abdominal mass. Optimal examination requires knowledge both of the possible causes of adenopathy and the normal anatomy and drainage of lymph glands.

Examination of the cervical nodes (Fig. 17.6) is most easily performed standing behind the seated patient. After initial inspection – bulky nodes may be visible (Fig. 17.7) – each of the anatomical groups is methodically examined on each side. This systematic approach is necessary as it is easy to miss a solitary enlarged node, particularly the supraclavicular nodes lodged behind the clavicle. It is important for the patient to be entirely comfortable to relax the surrounding muscles.

Where an enlarged node is discovered, document its nature in terms of:

Reactive nodes (e.g. enlarged secondary to infection) are often tender whereas lymphoma infiltrated nodes are classically rubbery and carcinoma infiltrated nodes stony hard but these findings are not consistent.

The detection of cervical lymphadenopathy should lead on to a careful examination of potential drainage sites. A head and neck examination may be usefully supplemented by a specialist ENT referral. A solitary enlarged supraclavicular node can be a sinister sign of metastatic spread from a lung or gastric carcinoma.

The best technique for examining the axillary nodes is illustrated in Figure 17.8. Lie the patient on a couch and support the flexed arm while gently but firmly examining the right axilla with your left hand and the left axilla with your right hand. The nodes are divided into medial, lateral, posterior, central and apical groups. The same methodical approach is adopted as described for the cervical nodes. Inguinal nodes are best examined as part of the abdominal review. The differential diagnosis of a lump in the groin includes hernias and it is helpful to appreciate their features (described elsewhere) as they may be confused with a nodal mass.

The finding of a palpable node or nodes in any of these areas does not necessarily indicate disease. A few small nodes (e.g. up to 0.5 cm) may be felt in a normal neck, particularly in children and younger adults. The tonsillar node at the angle of the mandible may be a little larger. Small incidental nodes in the axillae and inguinal regions are also commonplace. There is no substitute for experience in differentiating small harmless nodes from pathological adenopathy but, in practice, this may be difficult even for the most seasoned examiner. Where there is doubt, a short period of observation may be in order, but if the nodes persist or enlarge then a surgical biopsy is likely to be required.

Examination of the spleen

The spleen is frequently enlarged in blood disorders and in certain systemic diseases (Box 17.3). A normal spleen is not palpable. Examination of the spleen is often performed badly and it is easy to miss both slight splenomegaly and massive enlargement of the organ where it extends across the abdomen into the right iliac fossa. Careful and informed examination will avoid such mistakes.

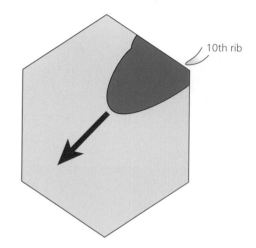

Figure 17.9 Mode of enlargement of the spleen.

10th rib

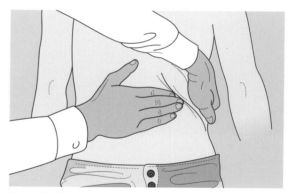

Figure 17.10 Technique for examination of the spleen.

BOX 17.3 COMMON CAUSES OF SPLENOMEGALY
- Acute and chronic infections (e.g. septicaemia, tuberculosis)
- Haemolytic anaemia
- Infectious mononucleosis
- Portal hypertension
- Myelofibrosis[1]
- Chronic myeloid leukaemia[1]
- Polycythaemia vera[1]
- Lymphoma[1]
- Malaria[1]
- Leishmaniasis[1]

[1]May be massive enlargement.

It is essential for the patient to be warm and comfortable and to have confidence in the examiner. First, inspect the abdomen for masses and then enquire regarding the presence of tenderness. Kneel by the bed and, with your forearm horizontal to the abdomen, palpate each sector prior to examination of the major organs. The abnormal spleen enlarges from behind the tenth rib in a line running diagonally across the abdomen through the umbilicus (Fig. 17.9). Commence palpation in the right iliac fossa to avoid missing massive enlargement and gradually move your hand in stages towards the tenth rib while the patient takes deep breaths.

An enlarged spleen will be felt by the tips of the fingers during deep inspiration. The organ has a notch but, in practice, this is rarely detected. If splenomegaly is suspected but the spleen is not palpable using this technique then it is worth rolling the patient half onto their right side with your left hand supporting the left lower ribs – in this position, a slightly enlarged spleen may be moved forward so the tip becomes just palpable ('tippable': Fig. 17.10). Some examiners find it helpful to hold their left hand under the left lower ribs during routine examination.

An enlarged spleen is most likely to be confused with an enlarged left kidney. The spleen has a number of characteristics which should allow it to be definitively identified:

- the spleen has a distinctive shape
- it is impossible to get above the spleen
- the spleen moves with respiration
- the spleen is dull to percussion
- the spleen cannot be felt bimanually or ballotted.

The enlarged left kidney, in contrast, is not dull to percussion (it is covered by the colon) and it can be felt bimanually and can be ballotted. It is worth auscultating an enlarged spleen as there may be a 'splenic rub' signifying inflammation of the capsule. It is not usually possible to diagnose the cause of splenomegaly by simple examination of the organ, although the degree of enlargement does give a clue, particularly where this is massive.

INVESTIGATIONS

A thorough history and careful physical examination allied to logical selection and interpretation of laboratory tests are essential for the accurate diagnosis of blood disorders. Radiological procedures also play a vital role but, in the interests of space, only laboratory investigations will be considered.

Basic techniques for examination of the blood and bone marrow

Most blood disorders are characterized by an abnormality in the blood count (or full blood count). This test is performed on a small sample of venous blood anticoagulated in ethylenediaminetetraacetic acid. A typical blood count report contains a large amount of numerical information and it is therefore useful to adopt a systematic approach to interpretation.

The three most important measurements are the:

- haemoglobin level
- total white cell count
- platelet count.

Further numerical data pertain to red cell number, size, and haemoglobinization (all useful in the diagnosis of anaemia) and a differential white cell count

(relative numbers of neutrophils, lymphocytes, etc.). The latter information is used in the diagnosis of primary disorders of white cells (e.g. leukaemia) and also in systemic disorders where numerical abnormalities of white cells (e.g. neutrophil leucocytosis) are common.

The blood count is generated by an automated analyser; where significant abnormalities are detected, a blood film may be microscopically examined by a trained observer. Blood film morphology has its own complex nomenclature – when a report is obscure, it is worth contacting the laboratory to discuss the findings. Laboratory equipment is not faultless and aberrant results are relatively common. For instance, if a very low platelet count is not associated with typical symptoms and signs then it is worth repeating the sample and asking for a blood film to exclude either a clot in the original sample or 'clumping' of platelets in the anticoagulant.

When the cause of a blood abnormality remains unclear then the bone marrow may be examined. A bone marrow aspirate and trephine biopsy are obtained from the posterior iliac crest by a trained operator. The two samples are complementary. The liquid aspirate sample is better for the assessment of individual cell morphology while the solid biopsy allows assessment of marrow architecture and the detection of low level infiltration by malignant disease.

The start point in the investigation of bleeding disorders is the coagulation screen. This usually consists of the prothrombin time (PT), activated partial thromboplastin time (APTT), and quantitation of plasma fibrinogen. Some common causes of an abnormal screen are shown in Table 17.3.

Table 17.3 Common causes of an abnormal coagulation screen

Prolonged PT	Prolonged APTT	Low fibrinogen
Warfarin	Heparin	DIC
Liver disease	Haemophilia	Liver disease
Vitamin K deficiency	vWD	
DIC	Liver disease	
	Lupus anticoagulant	
	DIC	

APTT, activated partial thromboplastin time; DIC, disseminated intravascular coagulation; PT, prothrombin time; vWD, von Willebrand's disease.

Assessment of the *acute phase response* is a very useful diagnostic tool in general medicine and in patients with blood disorders. Commonly performed measurements are the erythrocyte sedimentation rate (ESR), C-reactive protein (CRP) and plasma viscosity – all have their advantages and drawbacks.

Other tests useful in non-malignant disease

- *Haemoglobin electrophoresis*: this is useful particularly for the diagnosis of haemoglobinopathies.
- *Reticulocyte count*: this is useful in the diagnosis of haemolysis where is it is usually raised.
- *Direct Coombs' (or antiglobulin) test*: this is useful in the diagnosis of autoimmune haemolysis.
- Estimation of *iron (ferritin), vitamin B$_{12}$ and folate* levels: useful in the diagnosis of anaemia.
- *Thrombophilia screen*: useful for investigation of a prothrombotic tendency.

Other tests useful in haematological malignancy

- *Immunophenotyping (flow cytometry), cytogenetics, and molecular biology*: these are all routinely used in the diagnosis, subclassification and monitoring of haematological malignancy (e.g. leukaemia, lymphoma). Blood and bone marrow samples are routinely examined. Molecular biology techniques (e.g. gene microarrays) are gradually moving from the research laboratory to mainstream clinical practice.
- *Serum and urine electrophoresis*: used to detect the monoclonal immunoglobulins and light chains found in myeloma.

COMMON DIAGNOSES

Anaemia

Iron deficiency anaemia

In addition to the general symptoms and signs of anaemia there may be more specific symptoms and signs of endothelial cell dysfunction and, more importantly, the underlying cause of deficiency. Iron is required by many different tissues. Chronic deficiency can lead to a sore mouth, glossitis and angular stomatitis. The nails may become brittle, ridged, flattened and even spooned (koilonychia). Dysphagia may result from an oesophageal web (Plummer–Vinson syndrome). Many patients manifest none of these endothelial problems. In children, iron deficiency is a cause of failure to thrive and behavioural problems.

> ### IMPORTANT   *i*
> It is crucial to understand the cause of iron deficiency. This may be straightforward (e.g. menorrhagia in an otherwise well young woman) but particularly in men and postmenopausal women there is the possibility of occult gastrointestinal bleeding and a serious pathology such as a colonic tumour. A thorough history of gastrointestinal symptoms and examination of the abdomen, including rectal examination, is necessary.

Megaloblastic anaemia

This is essentially caused by deficiency of vitamin B$_{12}$ and/or folate. The most distinctive vitamin B$_{12}$ deficiency syndrome is **pernicious anaemia**, a familial autoimmune disorder where the basic abnormalities are gastric parietal cell atrophy, general epithelial cell atrophy and megaloblastic anaemia. Patients typically (but not always) have premature greying and blue eyes. Co-existent autoimmune disorders include the skin disorder vitiligo. Because of the combination of pallor and jaundice (due to low grade haemolysis) the skin may have a lemon yellow tint.

Epithelial changes include glossitis – this is typically painful – and the neurological syndrome 'subacute combined degeneration of the cord'. The latter arises from demyelination of the dorsal and lateral columns. Common early complaints are of numbness and paraesthesiae in the feet. The clinical signs are of posterior column loss (vibration and position senses with possible Rombergism) and of an upper motor neurone lesion with peripheral neuropathy. Chronic vitamin B$_{12}$ deficiency is also a cause of dementia and optic atrophy. In modern medical practice, vitamin B$_{12}$ deficiency is often detected at an early stage and these neurological complications are now rarely seen.

haemolytic syndromes the red cell destruction is extravascular (in the spleen and/or liver) but on occasion it is intravascular with the dramatic appearance of haemoglobinuria (Fig. 17.11). Specific inherited and acquired haemolytic disorders have their own particular clinical features (e.g. acrocyanosis in cold autoimmune haemolytic anaemia).

Sickle cell anaemia

Sickle cell syndromes are inherited disorders in which there is an abnormal haemoglobin β-chain: red cells 'sickle', becoming misshaped with reduced deformability. Sickle cell trait (Hb AS) causes no clinical problems but sickle cell anaemia (Hb SS) is a serious disorder affecting predominantly the African Caribbean population. Anaemia (due to haemolysis) often causes surprisingly few symptoms as HbS releases oxygen more easily than normal HbA.

In vaso-occlusive crises, patients complain of musculoskeletal pain of variable severity often located around the hips, shoulders and spine. The degree of pain may warrant hospital admission and opiate analgesia. Complications are too numerous to detail here but include cerebral infarction and sequestration syndromes – these should be diagnosed and managed by clinicians with experience of the disease. Other possible signs are lower limb ulceration, proliferative retinopathy and glaucoma. Palpable splenomegaly is not usually a feature as the organ is often infarcted.

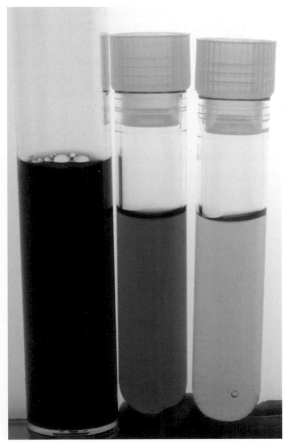

Figure 17.11 Haemoglobinuria (left tube) in intravascular haemolysis.

Haemolytic anaemia

Haemolytic anaemia is caused by increased destruction of red cells. There is either a disorder of the red cell itself (usually an inherited disorder, e.g. hereditary spherocytosis) or an abnormality extrinsic to the red cells (usually acquired, e.g. autoimmune haemolytic anaemia). Significant haemolysis is characterized both by the symptoms and signs of anaemia and features attributable to the accelerated catabolism of haemoglobin. The latter leads to the release of increased amounts of bilirubin into the plasma and the clinical sign of jaundice.

Consequences of chronic haemolysis include palpable splenomegaly and bilirubin gallstones with possible clinical features of cholelithiasis. In most

Thalassaemia

The thalassaemias are a highly variable group of inherited disorders of haemoglobin synthesis. As for the sickle cell syndromes, there are minor forms ('traits') of little clinical significance but also major clinical syndromes. This section will refer only to β-**thalassaemia major**. Anaemia is due to a combination of ineffective red cell formation and haemolysis. Symptoms appear at around 3–6 months of life as the production of fetal haemoglobin falls away. Children fail to thrive and develop the characteristic signs of skull bossing and maxillary enlargement due to compensatory expansion of the marrow space. If not properly managed, the disease can also lead to repeated infections, bone fractures, and leg ulcers.

Regular transfusion is often necessary; the resultant iron overload can damage the liver, endocrine organs and heart.

Disorders of normal haemostasis

Immune thrombocytopenia (ITP)

ITP is a disease in which there is immune destruction of platelets. The symptoms and signs are those described for thrombocytopenia. Many patients have only modest reductions in platelet count and are asymptomatic. There are two distinct forms of the disease (although with some overlap). The acute form is most common in childhood. There is acute onset of haemorrhagic symptoms and signs but the syndrome is self-limiting and serious complications (e.g. cerebral haemorrhage) are very rare. The chronic form is more often seen in adult life but again serious complications are infrequent and many patients only develop significant symptoms of excess bruising and bleeding at very low platelet counts (e.g. less than 10×10^9/L).

Haemophilia

This is an inherited disorder of coagulation. The most common subtypes are the X-linked disorders haemophilia A (deficiency of coagulation factor VIII) and haemophilia B (deficiency of IX). Both types are divisible into mild, moderate and severe forms dependent on the relevant factor level. The joint and muscle bleeds described in the coagulation failure section only affect men with severe disease (factor level less than 2 per cent of normal). Symptoms often first appear when the affected child begins to crawl; the disorder may be confused with non-accidental injury.

von Willebrand's disease

von Willebrand's disease (vWD) is the most common inherited bleeding disorder. The inheritance is more complex than for haemophilia with numerous subtypes. von Willebrand factor (vWF) is an adhesive glycoprotein that both promotes platelet adhesion to damaged endothelium and transports and stabilizes factor VIII. In vWD there is a deficiency of normal vWF and, in more serious cases, there are symptoms and signs of both platelet dysfunction and coagulation deficiency. In practice, the most common complaints are of epistaxes, gum bleeding, menorrhagia, and easy bruising. Milder cases may only experience excess bleeding following surgery or trauma. Haemarthroses and muscle bleeds are rare.

Myeloproliferative disorders

Polycythaemia vera and myelofibrosis

Polycythaemia vera must be distinguished from other causes of a raised haematocrit (e.g. secondary polycythaemia); the recent discovery of the *JAK2* mutation, found in almost all cases of polycythaemia vera, has greatly facilitated the diagnosis. Affected patients often present with symptoms secondary to the raised red cell mass and total blood volume and associated hyperviscosity, such as:

- lethargy
- excess sweating
- dizziness
- pruritus (particularly after a hot bath).

There is an increased incidence of arterial and venous thrombosis and, more rarely, a bleeding tendency due to platelet dysfunction. The classic clinical sign is facial plethora (Fig. 17.12) sometimes accompanied by rosacea. The spleen is palpable in a minority of cases.

The essential features of **myelofibrosis** are bone marrow fibrosis and splenomegaly. The spleen is palpable in almost all cases and massive in around 10 per cent. Hepatomegaly is seen in two-thirds of cases.

Haematological malignancies

Acute leukaemia

Many of the symptoms of acute leukaemia can be explained in terms of the pancytopenia (i.e. anaemia, leucopenia and thrombocytopenia) caused by the infiltration of the bone marrow by leukaemic cells. Specific subtypes of the disease do have additional particular characteristics which will be noted here.

In **acute myeloid leukaemia** (AML), the acute promyelocytic subtype (FAB M3, t(15;17)) is associated with a life-threatening coagulopathy. Neurological

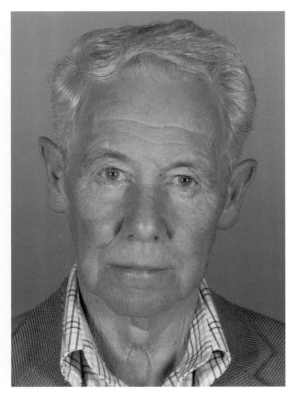

Figure 17.12 Plethoric appearance in polycythaemia vera.

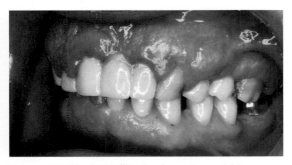

Figure 17.13 Gingival infiltration in acute myeloid leukaemia.

symptoms or signs often indicate intracerebral bleeding. Tissue infiltration (e.g. splenomegaly, skin and gingival infiltration, Fig. 17.13) tends to be more common where there is monocytic morphology (e.g. FAB M5).

In **acute lymphoblastic leukaemia** (ALL), there is a higher risk of central nervous system involvement than in AML. There may be symptoms and signs of raised intracranial pressure (e.g. headache, vomiting, and papilloedema) or cranial nerve palsies (particularly VI and VIII). The T-ALL subtype is a cause of mediastinal lymphadenopathy and pleural effusion. In males, routinely examine the testes.

Chronic leukaemia

The two types of chronic leukaemia are conveniently discussed together but their biology and clinical features are very different.

In **chronic myeloid leukaemia** (CML), patients often present in the chronic phase of the disease with symptoms of anaemia accompanied by anorexia and weight loss. Splenomegaly is the most consistent physical finding; this may be massive causing discomfort, bloating and satiety. Very high white cell counts can lead to the symptoms and signs of hyperviscosity syndrome. The chronic phase may transform to 'blast crisis' where the features are those of acute leukaemia.

In **chronic lymphocytic leukaemia** (CLL), the characteristic symptoms are of anaemia, recurrent infections, and weight loss. Lymphadenopathy and hepatosplenomegaly occur but the spleen is rarely massively enlarged. In advanced disease, other tissues such as the gastrointestinal tract and the lungs may become affected. Fortunately, many patients have early stage disease and diagnosis of CLL is often made from a routine blood count in an asymptomatic patient. The same is increasingly true of CML.

Lymphoma

The clinical presentation of lymphoma is heterogeneous as the disease may involve any organ in the body containing lymphoid tissue; however, we can make some generalizations.

In classical **Hodgkin's lymphoma**, patients usually present with asymmetrical, painless lymphadenopathy. This is most often cervical and, in the nodular sclerosing histological subtype, is frequently associated with a mediastinal nodal mass (a potential cause of superior vena cava obstruction). Nodes may fluctuate in size. Hepatosplenomegaly is common but rarely massive. Systemic symptoms are important in staging and include fever, night sweats and weight loss. The fever may have a cyclical nature (Pel–Ebstein fever).

Non-Hodgkin's lymphoma is divisible into many subtypes but, in broadest terms, there are aggressive potentially curable forms (e.g. diffuse large B-cell lymphoma) and more indolent forms which are less curable (e.g. follicular lymphoma). Lymphadenopathy is a prominent finding (see Fig. 17.7) but the presentation is more varied than in Hodgkin's lymphoma with a greater chance of extra-nodal disease (e.g. central nervous system, gastrointestinal tract, skin). Systemic symptoms are often surprisingly absent until advanced disease.

Myeloma

This is a malignant disorder in which there is an uncontrolled proliferation of plasma cells in the bone marrow. Secretion of proteins by the malignant clone leads to organ dysfunction and destruction. Most patients have bone pain at presentation. This often manifests as back pain and is all too easily dismissed. With time, the pain becomes persistent and severe and may be associated with evidence of bone destruction such as pathological fractures or vertebral collapse leading to scoliosis and loss of height. There is a risk of spinal cord compression.

Infiltration of the bone marrow causes the symptoms and signs of pancytopenia. As normal immunoglobulin levels are low, there is a tendency to recurrent bacterial infection. Renal failure, hypercalcaemia, and amyloidosis will all lead to the recognized symptoms and signs (see other chapters). Hyperviscosity syndrome can arise where there is a very high serum paraprotein level but this is more common in the related disorder, *Waldenström's macroglobulinaemia*.

SUMMARY

- Benign and malignant disorders of the blood are associated with diverse symptoms and signs.
- Abnormalities of normal blood cells and normal coagulation lead to largely predictable symptoms and signs.
- Anaemia typically causes symptoms and signs arising from the blood's reduced oxygen carrying capacity leading in turn to tissue hypoxia and the body's attempts to compensate. These include:
  - fatigue
  - dyspnoea
  - palpitations
  - faintness
  - pallor
  - tachycardia.
- Leucopenia leads to a predisposition to frequent and/or severe infection. Neutropenia classically leads to fulminant bacterial or fungal infection whereas lymphopenia leads to compromised humoral and/or cell-mediated immunity and a wide range of opportunistic infections including bacteria, viruses, fungi and *Pneumocystis*.
- Thrombocytopenia (or abnormal platelet function) causes a haemorrhagic tendency characterized by easy bruising, skin petechiae, and bleeding occurring either spontaneously or excessively after surgery or trauma.
- Coagulation failure, classically seen in the inherited disorder 'haemophilia', commonly presents as bleeding into joints and muscles and excessive bleeding following surgery or trauma.
- Thrombophilia is a clinical disorder of the blood characterized by a predisposition to venous or (less commonly) arterial thrombosis because of abnormally enhanced coagulation.
- Successful history taking in patients with blood disorders requires knowledge of their common features including symptoms and signs, modes of inheritance and aetiological factors (e.g. drugs).
- Clinical examination of the lymph nodes and spleen should be methodical and be performed with an understanding of normal anatomy and the causes of lymphadenopathy and splenomegaly.
- An understanding of the signs and symptoms of 'haematological emergencies' is vital. Examples are: superior vena cava obstruction in lymphoma, spinal cord compression in myeloma and hyperviscosity syndrome in Waldenström's macroglobulinaemia.
- Laboratory tests, including morphological examination of the blood and bone marrow, are crucial in the diagnosis and classification of blood diseases and must be carefully selected.

FURTHER READING

Howard MR, Hamilton PJ. 2007. *Haematology: an illustrated colour text*, 3rd edn. Edinburgh: Churchill Livingstone. A basic haematology text including short sections on history taking, examination, and laboratory tests.

Provan D, Singer CRJ, Baglin T, Dokal I. 2009. *Oxford handbook of clinical haematology*, 3rd edn. Oxford: Oxford University Press. A reference guide with a section on 'The Clinical Approach' to the patient with a blood disorder.

18

SKIN, NAILS AND HAIR

Stuart N Cohen and John S C English

INTRODUCTION

The skin is a highly specialized organ that covers the entire external surface of the body. Its various roles include protecting the body from trauma, infection and ultraviolet radiation. It provides waterproofing and is important for fluid and temperature regulation. It is essential for the detection of some sensory stimuli. Another vital function is the role of the skin in social activity.

A sound understanding of dermatological disease will stand doctors in many specialties in good stead. Skin problems are extremely common and are responsible for 10–15 per cent of all consultations in general practice. Extensive loss of skin function or 'skin failure', e.g. due to widespread burns or erythroderma (Fig. 18.1), can be catastrophic and potentially lethal. Incidental detection of a melanoma during an examination of another system can be life saving. Aside from the multitude of primary cutaneous diseases, the skin can also function as a 'window' into the general health of a patient, with various internal conditions producing specific or non-specific cutaneous changes. Recognition of these can lead to earlier diagnosis of the underlying condition and reduce levels of morbidity. Finally, unlike most internal disease, skin abnormalities are not easily hidden: it is important to recognize that even apparently trivial problems can carry an enormous psychosocial burden.

In this chapter, we outline the specifics of taking a dermatological history, examining the skin and how to describe or document the findings. After a short summary of investigative options, specific diseases of the skin, including inflammatory dermatoses, drug reactions, infections, skin lesions and conditions which may be related to underlying internal disease are detailed. Given that there are around 2000 dermatological conditions described, only common and important conditions, including some that might be especially relevant in the examination setting, can be covered here.

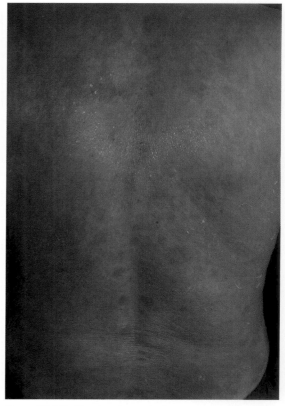

Figure 18.1 Erythrodermic psoriasis.

CLINICAL HISTORY

Fundamentally, a dermatological history is no different from any other.

- Basic information to ascertain includes the duration of symptoms and the sites affected.
- It is useful to know whether the problem is persistent, intermittent, or waxing and waning.
- Any evolution should be noted (e.g. is a lesion growing or is the rash spreading? If so, how fast?).
- The level of itching (pruritus) is important. Box 18.1 provides a list of some conditions that are characteristically very itchy.

BOX 18.1 COMMON CONDITIONS THAT ARE VERY ITCHY

- Eczema
- Scabies
- Lichen planus
- Urticaria
- Nodular prurigo

Pay particular attention to any treatments that have already been tried – some may affect the clinical appearance (such as steroid cream applied to a fungal infection); treatment failure may give useful diagnostic clues (for example, steroid cream applied to actinic keratosis), as well as guiding further intervention. Past medical or skin problems may have an important bearing on the differential diagnosis. For inflammatory conditions, a personal or family history of atopy should be established. Psoriasis is also often familial. Information on occupation may be helpful: an outdoor occupation increases the risk of skin cancer; contact dermatitis might be suspected if chemicals are used at work or if workmates have been similarly affected; and affected household contacts may suggest an infection. An accurate drug history, including any over-the-counter preparations, is essential. Drug eruptions are common and may mimic many other pathologies. It is important to delineate the duration for which a particular drug has been taken. The time course can be instrumental in identifying a culprit drug or at least narrowing down the suspects.

The psychosocial impact of the skin condition should be explored. Patients often do not reveal their distress about a skin problem unless asked directly. There may be embarrassment, poor self-image, social phobia, sexual dysfunction, sleep disturbance due to itching, even frank depression and many other ill effects. Skin disease with associated high levels of psychological morbidity may justify more aggressive intervention. It is also vital to understand the ideas and expectations that the patient has brought to the consultation. Many people hold beliefs about the causes of skin disease, its treatment and the chances of cure. Where these are inaccurate, they can be a major barrier to a successful therapeutic relationship.

PHYSICAL EXAMINATION

A good skin examination requires good lighting and a thorough approach. It can help to be thinking of the differential diagnosis while examining, so that corroborating features can be sought, at specific skin sites, or in the nails or mucous membranes. A logical system of examination can ensure that clues are not overlooked. It is important to palpate the skin, as well as to inspect it.

Examining and describing an eruption

A useful scheme for describing a widespread rash is *DCM* – distribution, configuration, morphology (Box 18.2). Distribution refers to the particular sites affected, whether the changes are bilateral/symmetrical and whether there is a specific pattern to the areas involved, such as flexor or extensor surfaces. Configuration relates to how the individual components making up the rash relate positionally to one another. For example, are they arranged in a line (linear configuration), in a ring (annular) or in clusters? Often, there will not be a specific configuration. However, looking specifically for one is advisable to avoid missing important information and diagnostic clues. Lastly comes morphology, the description of the components of the rash.

BOX 18.2 DCM SCHEME FOR DESCRIBING A WIDESPREAD RASH

- *Distribution*: what are the affected sites? Is the eruption symmetrical?
- *Configuration*: what is the pattern (if any) in which individual component parts of the eruption are arranged?
- *Morphology*: describe the actual features of the component parts of the eruption, e.g. macules, papules, plaques, etc.

There are many specific terms used in dermatology (Table 18.1). Bear in mind that even among dermatologists, there are differences of opinion over usage of some of these terms: exactly what

Table 18.1 A dermatological glossary

Morphological types of lesion	
Macule	A flat (impalpable) circumscribed area of skin discoloration (Fig. 18.2). Some dermatologists restrict the size of a macule, using the term 'patch' for larger lesions – this is unnecessary
Papule	A small, solid, rounded swelling (Fig. 18.3). In the UK, papules must be less than 5 mm in diameter. In the USA, they can be up to 1 cm
Nodule	A solid, usually rounded swelling with a diameter of greater than 5 mm (or 1 cm in the USA) (Fig. 18.4). Nodules may be superficial, as in acne, or deep, even subcutaneous, as in lipoma
Plaque	A lesion that is raised from the surrounding normal skin (i.e. palpable), but flat on top (Fig. 18.5)
Pustule	A relatively small lesion containing visible pus. Most are raised and palpable (Fig. 18.6)
Vesicle	A blister of less than 5 mm in diameter (blister implies a split in the skin below or within the epidermis; blisters are often filled with serous fluid) (Fig. 18.7)
Bulla	A blister of greater than 5 mm (Fig. 18.7)
Weal	A dermal swelling (i.e. a visibly elevated lesion without scaling, usually indicative of urticaria) (Fig. 18.5)
Purpura	Red or purple macules or papules that do not blanch on pressure (Fig. 18.8). This implies that there is extravasation of red blood cells. Small purpura are also known as petechiae and larger ones as ecchymoses
Other common terms	
Eruption	Rash
Erythema	Redness, hence erythematous is red
Excoriation	Broken skin due to scratching. Fresh lesions may be bleeding, older ones are often scabbed
Scale	Partially detached keratin on the skin surface
Crust	Dried exudate, typically golden coloured
Atrophy	Loss of usual thickness of epidermis and/or dermis
Lichenification	Thickening of the skin with increased skin markings, due to chronic rubbing or scratching, usually in the context of eczema (Fig. 18.9)
Hyperkeratosis	Thickened skin due to abnormal keratin production. Often the colour is yellowish
Hypopigmented	Lighter in colour than the individual's normal skin; may occur as a post-inflammatory phenomenon especially in psoriasis
Hyperpigmented	Darker in colour than the individual's normal skin; a very common post-inflammatory phenomenon
Depigmented	Lacking any pigmentation, as in vitiligo
Pruritus	Itch
Xerosis	Dryness

constitutes a small plaque versus a nodule? Is there a size limitation on a macule? These issues are not worth losing sleep over!

As part of *morphology*, consider the colour of the rash – many are erythematous (red), but others can be purple (violaceous), brown (hyperpigmented) or white (hypo- or depigmented). If there are erythematous lesions, do they blanch with pressure? Are the changes well or poorly demarcated? Alongside the morphological characteristics, remember to look for excoriation (breaks in the skin from scratching), xerosis (dryness), scaling and crust.

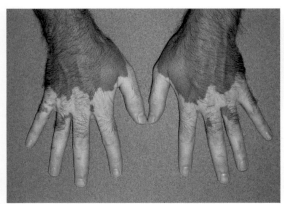

Figure 18.2 Macular eruption of vitiligo.

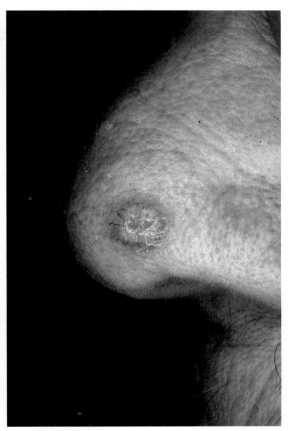

Figure 18.4 Nodulocystic basal cell carcinoma.

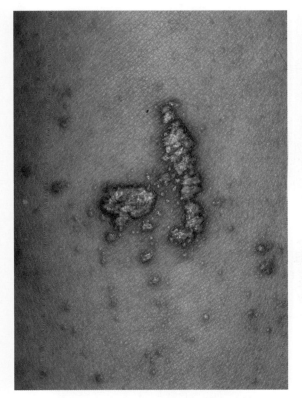

Figure 18.3 Lichen planus demonstrating lichenoid papules, coalescing into plaques, with Wickham's striae on the surface.

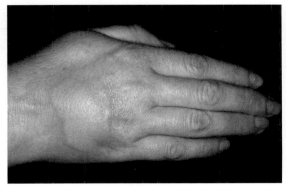

Figure 18.5 A plaque of cold-induced urticaria.

When describing a rash in an examination, try to progress through DCM logically. For example:

'This is a widespread, symmetrical eruption affecting large areas of the trunk. On the limbs it is predominantly over the extensor surfaces. Parts of the scalp are involved, though some areas are completely spared. There is no specific configuration. It consists of clearly demarcated erythematous plaques, with overlying silvery

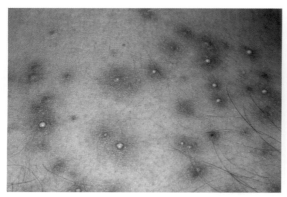

Figure 18.6 Inflamed pustules representing folliculitis.

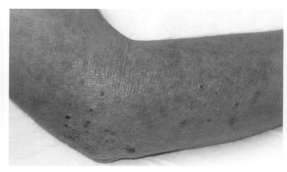

Figure 18.9 A diffuse plaque of eczema on the arm showing lichenification and excoriation (compare this with a plaque of psoriasis on the elbow in Fig. 18.19, p. 315).

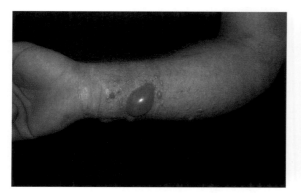

Figure 18.7 Vesiculo-bullous eruption on the forearm.

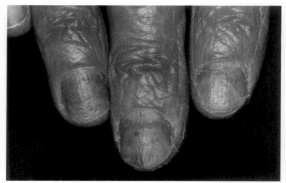

Figure 18.10 Psoriatic nail dystrophy including pitting and onycholysis.

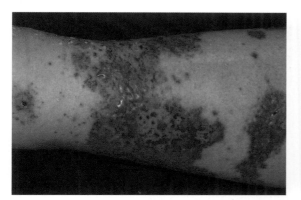

Figure 18.8 Vesiculo-bullous purpuric eruption of the lower leg (leucocytoclastic vasculitis).

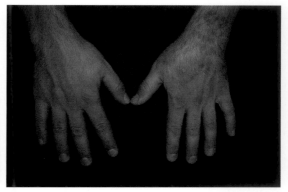

Figure 18.11 Tinea incognito resulting from inappropriate treatment with topical steroid following misdiagnosis.

scale. There is pitting in several fingernails and thickening of the toenails. The diagnosis is chronic plaque psoriasis (Figs 18.10 and 18.19). I would like to examine the joints for evidence of psoriatic arthropathy.'

CLINICAL PEARL

Most inflammatory rashes are bilateral. If you see a unilateral rash, suspect an exogenous cause such as infection (Fig. 18.11).

so well for all lesions. If examining non-melanocytic lesions, consider E as standing for 'everything else'. For example, if you are faced with a basal cell carcinoma, this might be symmetrical, with a well-defined, regular border, skin coloured, 1 cm in diameter and elevated. The key features, however, would be better encapsulated by (Fig. 18.4, p. 309):

> 'This is a skin-coloured pearly nodule, with a rolled edge, central crust and surface telangiectasia'.

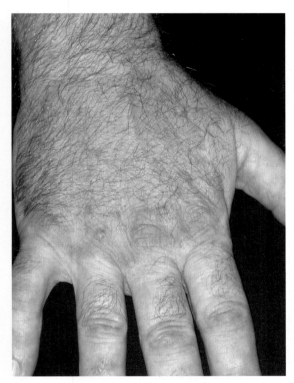

Figure 18.12 Granuloma annulare on the back of the hand.

Describing a lesion

Start by commenting on whether the lesion is solitary or multiple, and then indicate the body site. It is important to think about size, shape, border, surface, colour and elevation. The level of the lesion in the skin may be apparent. For example, actinic keratosis, a superficial abnormality affecting only the epidermis, shows no induration (thickening). Dermatofibromata lie in the dermis – the lesion feels deeper, but still within the skin. The skin overlying a lipoma can be moved over the nodule, indicating that the lesion lies in the subcutis. In general, scaling indicates epidermal involvement, as in eczema; dermal pathology (such as granuloma annulare (Fig. 18.12) or urticaria (Fig. 18.5, p. 309)) tends to cause more induration and elevation.

When describing melanocytic lesions (i.e. moles or suspected melanoma), the ABCDE scheme is useful (Box 18.3). The aim is to differentiate potentially dangerous lesions from those which are harmless (though this should be considered in the context of the history). Note that this mnemonic does not work

---

BOX 18.3 ABCDE SCHEME FOR DESCRIBING MELANOCYTIC LESIONS

- **Asymmetry**: is the lesion asymmetrical in shape or colour?
- **Border**: does the lesion have an irregular border?
- **Colour**: is all or part of the lesion very dark or are there multiple colours?
- **Diameter**: is the diameter greater than 6 mm?
- **Elevation**: has the lesion become elevated when it was once flat?

Malignancy is more likely if one or more of ABCDE is present in a melanocytic lesion (Fig. 18.13). Examination findings should be considered in the context of the history: a mole that is changing rapidly is suspicious even if it lacks all of these features. Check for lymphadenopathy if you suspect a squamous cell carcinoma or melanoma.

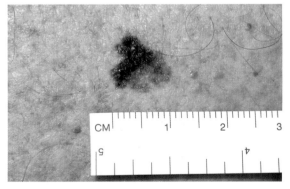

Figure 18.13 Superficial malignant melanoma. It is asymmetrical with an irregular border and colour variation, is greater than 5 mm in diameter and elevated.

Describing a leg ulcer

Ulcers are a somewhat special case. The things to look for in the examination are those that help to identify the underlying cause. Consider:

- site
- size
- border
- surface
- depth
- surrounding skin.

Venous disease is the commonest cause of leg ulceration. Venous ulcers occur in the gaiter area. They are usually superficial and may be large and have a slop-

---

BOX 18.4 SIGNS OF CHRONIC VENOUS DISEASE

- *Oedema*.
- *Ulceration*.
- *Varicose veins*.
- *Haemosiderin deposition*: red-brown macular discoloration originating from blood cells that are extravasated due to raised venous pressure.
- *Lipodermatosclerosis*: thickening of the skin with brownish pigmentation and loss of subcutaneous fat, giving rise to an abnormal contour of the leg, sometimes called the 'inverted champagne bottle appearance'.
- *Venous flare*: tiny purple or red superficial blood vessels.
- *Atrophie blanche*: white scar-like changes.
- *Gravitational eczema*: also known as venous, varicose or stasis eczema/dermatitis.

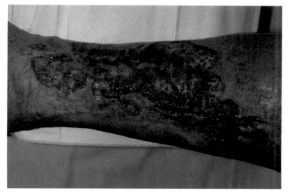

Figure 18.14 A large, irregular venous ulcer with co-existing signs of chronic venous insufficiency.

---

ing edge. They often have a wet surface with granulation tissue, indicating an attempt at healing. Many clues pointing to underlying venous disease may be found in the surrounding skin (Box 18.4, Fig. 18.14).

Arterial ulcers occur over bony prominences, usually the malleoli, or in regions with little or no collateral circulation, especially the toes. They are typically small and 'punched out', implying steep sides, and quite deep. They lack granulation tissue and are usually dry. There may be other signs of arterial compromise such as poor capillary refill times, weak foot pulses and hairless legs. Ask about pain and claudication.

There are many other causes of leg ulceration. Look for purpura around the edge as a sign of vasculitis. Pyoderma gangrenosum (associated with myeloproliferative disorders and inflammatory bowel disease) has a violaceous or gun-metal coloured border (Fig. 18.15).

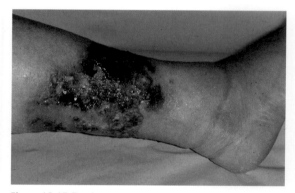

Figure 18.15 Pyoderma gangrenosum on the leg.

IMPORTANT   *i*

'Red flag' findings: some skin cancers present as ulcers – beware an ulcer that is indurated or has a rolled edge (see Fig. 18.33).

Examining alopecia

Key features in delineating the cause of alopecia are whether:

- hair loss is localized, diffuse or patterned
- there is a scarring process.

Scarring is indicated by loss of the follicular openings. The affected area is usually smooth, pink and shiny. Once follicles have been lost, there is no potential for regrowth of hair. In non-scarring alo-

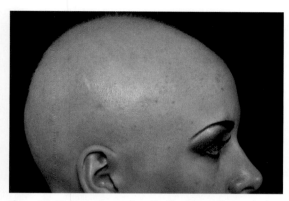

Figure 18.16 Alopecia areata affecting the entire scalp is known as alopecia totalis; this patient has also lost her eyebrows and lashes.

pecia, the affected area usually demonstrates normal skin texture.

The commonest cause of localized non-scarring alopecia is alopecia areata (Fig. 18.16). Think of tinea capitis if there is inflammation or scaling, especially in children. Diffuse non-scarring alopecia may be due to telogen effluvium (occurring a few months after pregnancy, major illness or stress) or iron deficiency. Alopecia arising in a distinct pattern is usually 'age-related', although age of onset is highly variable. Male pattern hair loss starts with temporal recession, followed by frontal recession and loss of hair over the scalp vertex. Female pattern hair loss is characterized by thinning over the crown and vertex, but there is preservation of the frontotemporal hairline.

Scarring alopecia is uncommon and usually localized. It may result from severe tinea capitis or inflammatory conditions such as discoid lupus or a form of lichen planus.

INVESTIGATIONS

Dermatologists often use dermoscopy to visualize changes in the skin. This involves magnification with a handheld device, but considerable experience is required to interpret the findings. It is particularly useful when assessing melanocytic lesions.

If *bacterial infection* is suspected, it is always wise to take a swab for microscopy, culture and sensitivity testing. Viral swabs should be obtained to confirm *herpes simplex or varicella zoster infection*. Note that the carrier medium is different for viral studies.

Where there are blisters or pustules, it is best to swab the contents. This may involve pricking the surface with a needle to gain access.

For *fungal infection*, a skin scraping should be taken. This involves brisk strokes of a scalpel blade across the edge of the affected area, which will typically be scaly. The scale is collected for microscopy and culture. For fungal infection of the scalp (tinea capitis), hair often precludes taking a scraping. Here, brushings can be taken if a suitable implement (similar to a disposable toothbrush with its own sheath) is available; otherwise, hair pluckings should be obtained. Nail clippings should be obtained if fungal infection of the nail is suspected.

Skin biopsy is often helpful to confirm the diagnosis of rashes or lesions. This is carried out under local anaesthesia. A punch biopsy involves harvesting a small circle of skin (3–8 mm in diameter); an incisional biopsy yields a larger ellipse specimen and is useful for deeper pathology such as panniculitis (inflammation of the subcutaneous fat). Excision biopsy removes an entire lesion. Many skin abnormalities can present with non-specific features clinically and histologically, so clinico-pathological correlation and a good relationship between dermatologist and pathologist is essential.

For suspected *contact allergy* perform patch tests. Here, various chemicals are applied under patches on to the patient's back. A standard series is always applied, plus other series or specific substances as indicated. These are left for 48 hours, then removed and the patient is assessed for reactions after another 48 hours. Considerable skill is required for their accurate interpretation, as false-positive irritant reactions are common.

Blood tests are frequently requested in dermatology. These may be to screen for systemic disease in association with skin involvement, or for therapeutic monitoring – immunosuppressives are often required, as well as other potentially toxic drugs.

COMMON DIAGNOSES

Inflammatory dermatoses

Eczema

Eczema presents with dry, red, scaly skin and associated itching. Morphologically, eczema is characterized by ill-defined, scaly erythematous plaques with prominent xerosis (dryness) and excoriations (Fig. 18.9, p. 310). Chronic rubbing or scratching leads to lichenification. Palmoplantar eczema often becomes hyperkeratotic – this in combination with xerosis leads to painful fissures. Acute eczema gives rise to vesicles, which are often incredibly itchy.

There are a number of variants of eczema.

- *Atopic eczema* (or atopic dermatitis) is common in childhood; most cases settle by the mid-teens. In babies, the rash often appears on the face, before localizing to the flexures. In more severe cases, it may become much more widespread. It is often associated with asthma and hay fever, either in the patient or their family. The cause is unknown, but it is associated with altered skin barrier function. The psychosocial effects of severe eczema may be devastating and include low self-esteem, social phobia, bullying, disturbed sleep and poor performance at school or work.
- *Gravitational eczema* (also known as venous, varicose or stasis eczema) is a result of chronic venous disease. It affects the gaiter area of the legs and is usually bilateral. Look for corroborating signs of venous disease (see 'Describing a leg ulcer', p. 312).
- *Seborrhoeic dermatitis* is caused by overgrowth of the commensal yeast *Pityrosporum ovale*. It tends to cause dandruff or thicker scaling on the scalp, as well as a low grade eczematous eruption on the forehead and in the nasolabial folds. Unlike in other forms of eczema, topical antifungals are helpful.
- *Discoid eczema*, unlike most eczema, gives rise to well-defined lesions which are often multiple. These are often intensely itchy and superadded bacterial infection is common (Fig. 18.17).
- *Contact dermatitis* may be either irritant or allergic. The former is caused by direct action of chemicals on the skin, or frequent wetting or hand washing leading to loss of protective oils. The latter involves a type IV hypersensitivity reaction.
  - Irritant contact dermatitis usually affects the hands. It is common in those whose occupations involve wet work or frequent hand washing. Usually dryness is more prominent than inflammation.

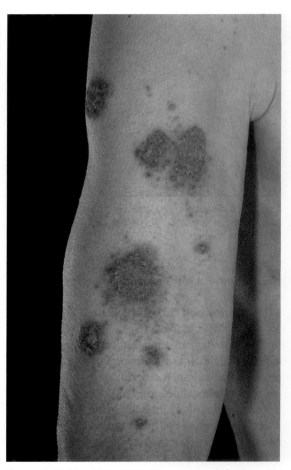

Figure 18.17 Discoid eczema with secondary infection.

- Allergic contact dermatitis (ACD) can result from a vast number of different chemicals. It may be occupational (such as chromate allergy from cement, or rubber allergy) or arise from everyday exposure (such as nickel allergy from jewellery or fragrance allergy from cosmetics). The distribution is often helpful to identify the likely cause. For example, ACD in the axillae is likely to be due to allergy to an ingredient of antiperspirant; rubber allergy from gloves affects mainly the back of the hands and has a relatively clear cut-off at the wrist where the exposure stops. However, if ACD is suspected, patch testing should be performed to confirm allergies definitively, so the patient can be advised accurately on avoidance measures.

Probably related to eczema is a condition known as *nodular prurigo*. This gives rise to intensely itchy nodules which are often excoriated. There is often accompanying xerosis (dry skin). It is very difficult to treat.

> **CLINICAL PEARL**
>
> The mainstay of treatment for all types of eczema is emollients (moisturizers) and topical steroids. Severe cases may require phototherapy or systemic immunosuppression.

Eczema commonly becomes superinfected with *Staphylococcus aureus*. This produces erosions and weeping in the affected area. If the exudate dries, it produces a golden crust. This is known as impetiginized eczema (Fig. 18.17).

Herpes simplex virus (HSV) can also superinfect eczema. The history is usually of sudden (over a few hours), severe deterioration in the skin. Early on, the eruption is made up of monomorphic papules or vesicles. These subsequently break down into small punctate ulcers and then crusts (Fig. 18.18). Depending on the extent and level of viraemia, patients can become severely unwell. Untreated, there is a significant mortality. Treatment is with systemic aciclovir: intravenous therapy is preferred if the patient is very unwell. Topical steroids to treat the eczema may be used in conjunction with aciclovir, but if applied alone may exacerbate the viral infection.

Psoriasis

Psoriasis is a chronic inflammatory condition of unknown cause affecting around 2 per cent of the population. It may be very localized but can affect the entire body surface area. It can produce nail changes and joint disease. Increasingly, it is recognized that it is associated with the metabolic syndrome and a worse cardiovascular risk profile. Psoriasis can carry a huge psychosocial burden. The impact on health-related quality of life is estimated to be similar to that of arthritis, chronic lung disease and myocardial infarction.

- *Chronic plaque psoriasis* is the commonest form. Typically this is a symmetrical eruption of well-

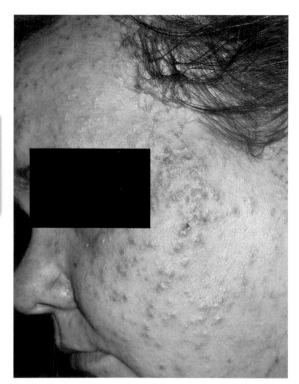

Figure 18.18 Widespread herpes simplex (eczema herpeticum).

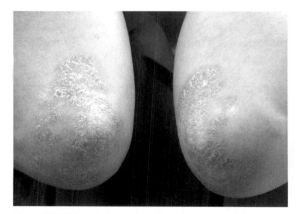

Figure 18.19 Psoriasis on the elbow (compare with eczema on the arm Fig. 18.9, p. 310).

demarcated plaques which may be pink, red or even purple, with overlying scale. These have a predilection for extensor surfaces, notably elbows (Fig. 18.19), knees and sacrum. Other frequently affected sites are the shins, natal cleft and scalp.

It is worth checking for signs in the umbilicus and just behind the ears, as a rash here is highly suggestive of the condition. Look for evidence of Koebner's phenomenon – the rash appearing in previously unaffected sites of trauma. Psoriasis can be exacerbated by stress and certain drugs (e.g. β-blockers, lithium, antimalarials). Sudden withdrawal of oral corticosteroids can lead to dramatic rebound.

- *Guttate psoriasis* (i.e. like rain drops) is characterized by numerous tiny plaques, usually mostly on the trunk. This is classically precipitated by streptococcal infection.
- *Palmoplantar pustulosis* may be a variant of psoriasis but is thought by some to be a separate condition. It produces sterile pustules with hyperkeratosis on the palms and soles. Pain from resulting fissures may be debilitating. In contrast to the usual distribution, *flexural (or inverse) psoriasis* is sometimes seen. Here, the typical scale is often lost and moist plaques, often with a central fissure in the skin crease itself, are seen (Fig. 18.20).

Topical treatment mostly consists of vitamin D analogues, tar products, salicylic acid and at certain sites steroids, alongside an emollient. Phototherapy is also used, and systemic immunosuppressants, retinoids and biological agents (including monoclonal antibodies and tumour necrosis factor inhibitors) are helpful in severe disease.

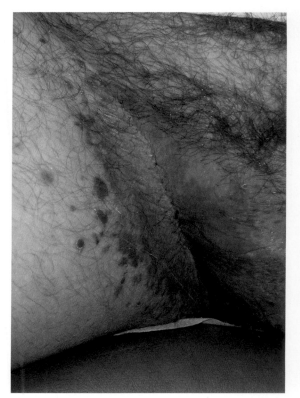

Figure 18.20 Flexural psoriasis.

> **CLINICAL PEARL**
>
> When faced with a widespread rash comprised of erythematous scaly plaques, it may be difficult to differentiate eczema from psoriasis. Remember that eczema is characteristically itchy whereas this is unusual in psoriasis.
>
> With the exception of the discoid pattern, eczematous plaques are ill-defined (Fig. 18.9, p. 310) whereas psoriatic plaques are well demarcated (Fig. 18.19).

Acne vulgaris

Acne is a disorder of the pilosebaceous unit, caused by a triad of excessive sebum production, comedone formation and *Propionibacterium acnes* all contributing to inflammation (Fig. 18.21). It is extremely common in the teenage years, but frequently affects people older than this. The clinical hallmark of the condition is the comedone, which may be open (blackhead) or closed (whitehead). The inflammatory lesions of acne comprise macules, papules, pustules, nodules and cysts (nodules are solid and cysts contain pus – in practice they can usually be lumped together as nodulocystic lesions). Scarring can result, especially from larger lesions in susceptible individuals. The face is usually affected, but lesions are common on the trunk.

As with many skin problems, some patients will experience major psychological problems, usually from the inflammatory lesions but sometimes also from the resultant scarring. Treatment aims to prevent scarring. If scarring is occurring, a more aggressive approach is warranted. Options include topical benzoyl peroxide, retinoids or antibiotics; oral therapy is with long courses of antibiotics (usually 3 months or more) or the oral retinoid

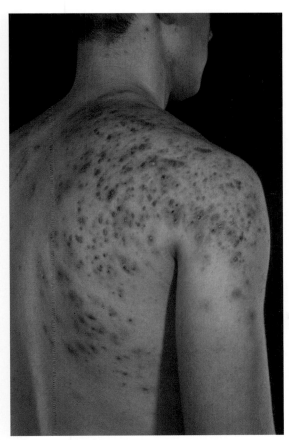

Figure 18.21 Severe nodulocystic acne with extensive scarring.

isotretinoin; some women benefit from taking an oral contraceptive containing an antiandrogen (usually ethinylestradiol/cyproterone acetate). Often a combination approach is used.

Rosacea

Rosacea shares many of the features of acne vulgaris, but lacks comedones. Scarring is very unusual. It tends to come on in the third to fifth decade and usually affects the central face. A variant that affects the area around the mouth is known as perioral dermatitis. Rosacea can produce erythema with numerous telangiectasia, a papulopustular eruption or a combination of the two. Some patients get worse with flushing, which may be precipitated by alcohol, spicy food or stress. If chronic, sebaceous hyperplasia may develop, leading to enlargement of the nose

known as rhinophyma. Up to 15 per cent of individuals with rosacea have associated eye problems, including blepharitis, conjunctivitis and keratitis.

Management involves avoidance of exacerbating factors, topical metronidazole or azelaic acid, oral tetracyclines and occasionally oral isotretinoin.

Lichen planus

Classical lichen planus presents with intensely pruritic violaceous, flat-topped papules, which coalesce into plaques (Fig. 18.3, p. 309). Fine white scaling known as Wickham's striae is visible on the surface. Lesions on the oral mucosa, which are often asymptomatic but may cause discomfort, are common. The sites most often affected are around the wrists and ankles, but the eruption can be widespread. The cause is unknown, but occasionally, there is an infective trigger such as hepatitis C virus. Most cases respond to topical steroids, but systemic treatment is sometimes required.

Urticaria

Urticaria is characterized by the development of red dermal swellings known as weals (Fig. 18.5, p. 309). Scaling is not seen and the lesions are typically very itchy. The lesions result from the release of histamine from mast cells. An important clue to the diagnosis is that individual lesions come and go within 24 hours, although new lesions may be appearing at other sites. Another associated feature is dermographism: a firm scratch of the skin with an orange stick will produce a linear weal within a few minutes. Urticaria is common, estimated to affect up to 20 per cent of the population at some point in their lives.

- Urticaria is labelled *acute* if present for less than 6 weeks. Episodes may be precipitated by infection, including non-specific viral infection, or allergy to foods or drugs. The eruption settles once the patient is clear of infection or avoids the causative substance.
- Rarely, contact urticaria is seen, where the eruption signals allergy to a specific substance that has been in contact with the skin, such as latex. In this case the substance must be avoided, as repeated attacks can become more severe.
- Chronic urticaria may last for years. The vast majority of cases are idiopathic and allergy tests are not indicated.

In some individuals, there are specific triggers for the rash, including pressure, sunlight, cold, exercise or emotion. Certain drugs such as aspirin, nonsteroidal anti-inflammatories and codeine promote histamine release (pharmacologically rather than through hypersensitivity); such triggers should be avoided where possible. Most urticaria can be controlled with antihistamines, though high doses may be required.

Some patients with urticaria also develop angioedema, where swelling of the face, tongue or other sites occurs. Attacks of angioedema may last for 2 or more days and respond less well to treatment.

Though distressing, urticaria and angioedema are rarely serious. However, both may be seen as part of anaphylaxis. Other features of this life-threatening medical emergency are shown in Box 18.5. First-line treatment for this is intramuscular adrenaline (epinephrine). Intravenous antihistamines and steroids are also used, but are no substitute for adrenaline.

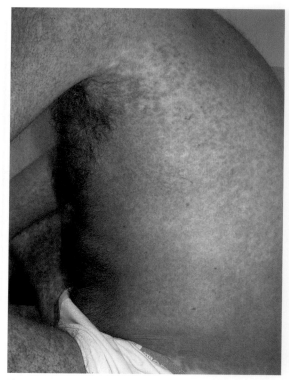

Figure 18.22 A widespread maculopapular drug eruption.

BOX 18.5 FEATURES OF ANAPHYLAXIS

- Onset within minutes of exposure to allergen.
- Urticaria.
- Swelling of lips, tongue and larynx, with potential to threaten airway.
- Bronchospasm causing wheeze and hypoxia.
- Circulatory collapse leading to shock.
- Death if not treated.

Other exanthemata

The term *exanthem* is used to describe an eruption resulting from a reaction to infection or drugs. There are several types.

The prototypical exanthem is the maculopapular rash (Fig. 18.22). In children, this is usually a sign of viral infection. In adults, it tends to reflect a drug allergy. The rash starts on the trunk and then spreads to involve the limbs. It is usually pruritic. If the trigger is removed, the eruption takes around 2 weeks to settle. Desquamation often occurs at around this stage. In the case of drug allergy, the onset is typically 1–2 weeks after the start of the offending drug. The rash can begin even after the drug has been stopped. In previously sensitized individuals who are re-exposed, the eruption recurs within 24 hours.

The 'usual suspects' most often to blame for drug eruptions are shown in Box 18.6, though it is important to bear in mind that virtually any drug can be responsible. Occasionally, other organs can be involved in drug hypersensitivity reactions – if the patient is unwell, a blood screen should be checked (including blood count, urea and creatinine, and liver tests). The main treatment is to stop the culprit agent. Topical steroids, emollients and antihistamines may help with itching. Multiorgan reactions may benefit from systemic steroids.

BOX 18.6 THE 'USUAL SUSPECTS' FOR DRUG ERUPTIONS

- Anticonvulsants – especially carbamazepine, phenytoin and phenobarbital, which may all cross-react
- Sulphonamides such as trimethoprim
- Penicillins and other antibiotics
- Non-steroidal anti-inflammatory drugs
- Allopurinol

Stevens–Johnson syndrome and toxic epidermal necrolysis (TEN)

Stevens–Johnson syndrome (SJS) and toxic epidermal necrolysis (TEN) are thought to be two ends of a spectrum of the same condition. They are usually attributable to drug hypersensitivity, though a precipitant is not always identified. The latent period following initiation of the drug tends to be longer than seen with a classical maculopapular drug eruption. The disease is termed:

- SJS when 10 per cent or less of the body surface area epidermis detaches
- TEN when greater than 30 per cent detachment occurs.

Anything in between is designated SJS/TEN overlap.

Following a prodrome of fever, an erythematous eruption develops. Macules, papules, or plaques may be seen. Some or all of the affected areas become vesicular or bullous, followed by sloughing off of the dead epidermis. This leads to potentially widespread denudation of skin. Mucosal sites, typically two or more, are also affected with blisters or erosions. Haemorrhagic crusts are often seen on the lips. The affected skin is typically painful rather than itchy. Patients appear unwell at presentation. Extensive skin loss leads to impaired thermoregulation, dehydration with potential for hypovolaemic shock, electrolyte derangement and susceptibility to superadded infection. The risk of death relates to the extent of epidermal loss and can exceed 30 per cent.

Key management steps are cessation of all non-essential drugs, emollients, stabilization of fluid status and electrolytes, maintenance of adequate nutrition and ophthalmological review if any eye involvement. Patients are best managed on a specialist burns unit. Supportive treatment and stopping the causative drug are the most important interventions. There is limited evidence that intravenous immunoglobulins may help in TEN.

> **CLINICAL PEARL**
>
> A widespread 'drug rash' that is very painful should ring alarm bells. Look for mucosal involvement and blistering as you may be dealing with toxic epidermal necrolysis.

Erythema multiforme

Erythema multiforme is an acute, self-limiting mucocutaneous disorder characterized by target lesions – annular plaques with at least three different colours within them, commonest on the extremities (Fig. 18.23). They may blister centrally and tend to be sore rather than itchy. Mucosal involvement usually affects the mouth, where ulceration can be severe, but other sites may also be involved. The commonest precipitating factor is herpes simplex infection. Some patients with recurrent viral disease also have recurrent erythema multiforme. Other precipitants include *Mycoplasma pneumoniae* infection and less commonly drugs. A cause is not always apparent. The eruption will settle without treatment after around 10–14 days. However, mucosal disease often requires intervention, as pain from oral ulcers can make eating unbearable; conjunctival involvement can lead to permanent damage to the eye without appropriate care.

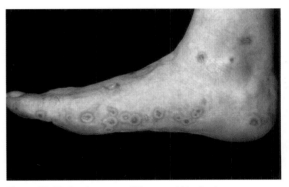

Figure 18.23 Erythema multiforme of the feet.

Erythema nodosum

Erythema nodosum is the most common form of panniculitis (inflammation in the fat). It presents with tender, erythematous, subcutaneous nodules, which feel firm. It usually affects only the lower legs (Fig. 18.24). The overlying skin looks normal except for the colour. There are a variety of triggers, including drugs (especially sulphonamides and the contraceptive pill), infections such as Group A *Streptococcus* and tuberculosis, inflammatory bowel disease and sarcoidosis. In some cases, no underlying cause is found. The condition usually settles with non-steroidal anti-inflammatories or sometimes systemic corticosteroids.

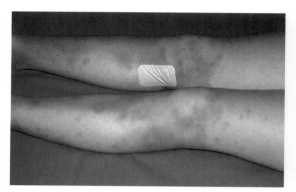

Figure 18.24 Erythema nodosum.

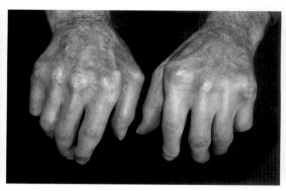

Figure 18.25 Sclerodactyly.

Connective tissue disease and the skin

Purpuric rash

Macular purpura may result from pressure, trauma or suction. They are more likely in the context of anticoagulation or platelet dysfunction (including aspirin therapy), or if the skin is very atrophic such as in elderly people or after long-term steroid use.

Palpable purpura implies a vasculitic process. Lesions are commoner in dependent areas, due to gravitational pressure effects forcing the extravasation of red blood cells through damaged vessel walls. If the process is florid, bullae or ulceration can result (Fig. 18.8, p. 310). Here, the lesions show purpuric changes around the edge. A biopsy may be required to confirm the diagnosis in this situation. Causes of a vasculitic rash are listed in Box 18.7. The history and clinical condition of the patient may be enough to exclude some possibilities, but patients must be screened for other organ disease with a panel of bloods including autoantibodies, and blood pressure and urinalysis to check early for renal involvement. Treatment is of the underlying condition. If there is a causative drug involved, this must be stopped.

BOX 18.7 CAUSES OF A VASCULITIC RASH

- Meningococcal sepsis
- Viral infection (especially hepatitis C)
- Post-streptococcal infection (Henoch–Schönlein purpura)
- Drug-induced vasculitis
- Connective tissue disease
- Idiopathic cutaneous vasculitis

Scleroderma

Systemic sclerosis or CREST syndrome (Calcinosis, Raynaud's phenomenon, oEsophageal involvement, Sclerodactyly (Fig. 18.25) and Telangiectasia) may present initially in the skin. *Localized* scleroderma is known as morphoea; this usually presents with well-defined induration of the affected area, often with an active edge. As the condition evolves, the skin becomes atrophic with prominence of blood vessels. Topical steroids may suffice to treat it; other options are phototherapy or systemic immunosuppression.

Lupus

The best known sign of systemic lupus erythematosus (SLE) in the skin is the macular erythema of the butterfly rash across the face. Photosensitivity is also typical (Fig. 18.26). Acute lupus of the skin can cause a widespread, but often non-specific eruption, sometimes even mimicking toxic epidermal necrolysis. There are certain subtypes of cutaneous lupus.

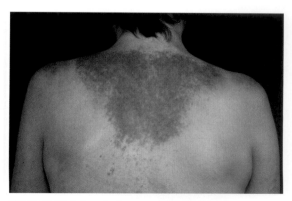

Figure 18.26 Subacute lupus erythematosus.

Whereas these often represent disease confined to the skin, they may present as part of SLE. Subacute lupus presents with annular or polycyclic plaques with peripheral scaling. Chronic cutaneous (discoid) lupus gives rise to scaly, red plaques with follicular plugging, most common on the face and scalp, where scarring alopecia results. Lesions clear to leave marked hypo- and hyperpigmentation which may be very disfiguring.

Dermatomyositis

Characteristic cutaneous features of dermatomyositis include the heliotrope rash around the eyes, Gottron's papules over the knuckles and nailfold inflammation (Fig. 18.27). Ask about symptoms of proximal muscle weakness, such as difficulty climbing stairs or getting up from an armchair. Check creatine kinase levels, but remember that some patients have no detectable muscle disease.

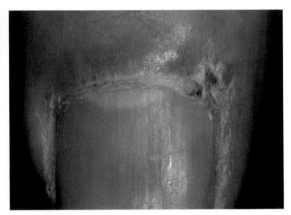

Figure 18.27 Nail fold telangiectasia in dermatomyositis.

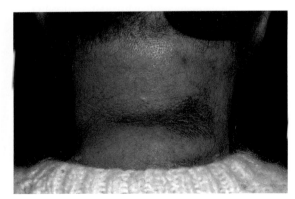

Figure 18.28 Acanthosis nigricans.

Endocrine disease and the skin

Various skin problems arise in patients with diabetes mellitus. Bacterial and fungal infections are more common, due to impaired immunity. Vascular disease and neuropathy lead to ulceration on the feet, which can sometimes be very deep and there may be underlying osteomyelitis. Granuloma annulare (Fig. 18.12, p. 311) and necrobiosis lipoidica have also been associated with diabetes, though many cases are seen in non-diabetic patients. The former produces smooth papules in an annular configuration, often coalescing into a ring. The latter usually occurs over the shins giving rise to yellow-brown discoloration, with marked atrophy and prominent telangiectasia. There is often an annular appearance, with a red or brown border. Acanthosis nigricans, velvety thickening of the flexural skin (Fig. 18.28), is seen with insulin resistance, with or without frank diabetes. It is more common in acromegaly. It can also be associated with internal malignancy, especially gastric cancer. Diabetic bullae are also occasionally seen and diabetic dermopathy produces hyperpigmented, atrophic plaques on the legs. The aetiology of these is unknown.

Other endocrine disorders can also lead to changes in the skin, such as thyroid disease (pre-tibial myxoedema, acropachy), Addison's disease (hyperpigmentation of skin creases and buccal mucosa) and Cushing's syndrome (acne and plethora).

Other internal disease

Sarcoidosis often presents in the skin. It is known as a great mimic and signs can be very variable. It is not uncommon to see the subtype lupus pernio in the examination setting. This is characterized by well-defined purplish infiltration of the skin and is most common on the ear lobes and nose (ask about respiratory symptoms). Mouth ulcers occur in lupus, Crohn's disease and coeliac disease. Crohn's disease can also affect genital and perianal skin. Coeliac disease may be associated with the itchy vesicles of dermatitis herpetiformis.

Internal cancer may induce various cutaneous changes. Skin metastasis can present as a smooth or ulcerated nodule or plaque. As stated above, acanthosis nigricans can indicate malignancy. Pemphigoid (subepidermal split giving a thick blister roof and tense bullae) and pemphigus (intra-epidermal split producing a friable blister roof and usually evidenced by erosions and severe mucosal involvement) may be paraneoplastic, as can dermatomyositis. While there are many other associations, to detail these is outside the scope of this chapter.

Cutaneous infections

Bacterial infections

Most bacterial skin infections are caused by *Staphylococcus aureus* or group A streptococci. There is considerable overlap in the type of problem that each can produce. It is therefore good practice to take a bacterial swab in the case of suspected infection, prior to the use of antibiotics. If antibiotic therapy fails, possible explanations include resistant organisms, poor adherence to treatment, wrong diagnosis or dual diagnosis such as infected eczema (where treatment of both conditions simultaneously may be required).

Cellulitis is infection of the skin and subcutaneous tissues. It is most commonly seen in the leg and presents with swelling, spreading erythema, and warmth (Fig. 18.29). There may be pain and tenderness but this need not be prominent. Some patients will be febrile and a proportion will develop frank sepsis. Risk factors include venous or lymphatic disease, obesity, immunosuppression and any break in the skin. Most cellulitis is caused by *Staphylococcus aureus* or group A streptococci. The latter is responsible for a variant known as erysipelas, which can produce a well-demarcated beefy red plaque on the face. Cellulitis requires systemic antibiotics, usually flucloxacillin or a macrolide, either of which cover most of the likely organisms. In hospital-acquired infection, ensure that therapy also targets methicillin-resistant *S. aureus*.

Necrotizing fasciitis also affects the skin and soft tissues. However, this life-threatening synergistic streptococcal/staphylococcal infection progresses rapidly and can be highly destructive through spread into deeper tissues. It is more common in immuno-

> **CLINICAL PEARL**
> If there is no obvious break in the skin to account for cellulitis, check for tinea pedis. Treating this may prevent recurrent cellulitis.

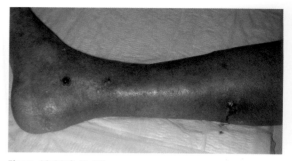

Figure 18.29 Cellulitis.

suppressed individuals. It can present as a rapidly progressive painful cellulitis, usually with associated high fever and severe malaise. It should also be considered where there is fever and intense localized pain, even if there is little to see on the skin. It is a *surgical emergency,* as urgent and aggressive debridement is required to prevent death.

> **IMPORTANT**   *i*
> 'Red flag' findings: necrotizing fasciitis is a surgical emergency, as urgent and aggressive debridement is required to prevent death.

Impetigo is a superficial infection characterized by soreness, erythema and exudate which dries leaving a golden or honey-coloured crust. It can be caused by either staphylococcus or streptococcus; the former can produce a bullous form. It usually affects children. As it is very contagious, siblings may develop it concurrently. Topical antibiotics may be used for localized disease but systemic treatment is indicated if the lesions are more extensive. The crusts should be soaked off with soap and water, as these contain numerous bacteria.

Folliculitis is infection in the hair follicles, usually from *S. aureus* (Fig. 18.6, p. 310). It produces pustules. It may be precipitated by hair plucking, or blockage of the follicles by application of greasy ointments. Antibiotics and antibacterial washes are usually helpful. Nasal carriage of the organism sometimes accounts for recurrent cases.

Viral infections

Various subtypes of human papilloma virus can produce viral warts. These are verrucous hyperkeratotic lesions, common on the fingers and soles, especially in children. Most are self-limiting and clear without treatment within 2 years, but they can be more problematic and numerous in the immunosuppressed. Treatment options for symptomatic lesions include cryotherapy and salicylic acid. Rarely, immunomodulators (e.g. imiquimod) or cytotoxics (5-fluorouracil or bleomycin) are used, but response is variable.

Molluscum contagiosum

Infection with the molluscipox virus gives rise to umbilicated, shiny papules. These are often asymptomatic, but may be itchy. They sometimes become inflamed and sore, especially if traumatized (Fig. 18.30). The condition mostly affects children, especially those with atopy. In adults, the lesions may be mistaken for basal cell carcinoma. Molluscum infection resolves eventually without treatment, usually within 12 months.

Pityriasis rosea

Pityriasis rosea is thought to be due to a virus. The onset of the condition is marked by the appearance of a 'herald patch', a single non-specific erythematous lesion. One to two weeks later, the typical eruption ensues. This is characterized by pink or red plaques with fine scaling, mainly on the trunk, aligned in a so-called Christmas tree pattern along the ribs. They subside after around 6 weeks without treatment.

Herpes simplex virus

Over a third of the world's population experiences recurrent clinical infection by HSV and 80 per cent have antibodies to it. Following primary infection through exposure to respiratory droplets or saliva, the virus becomes latent in the sensory dorsal root, from where it can reactivate due to triggers such as illness, stress or ultraviolet light, causing a 'cold sore'. Be aware that HSV can affect sites other than the lips. Typically, there is a prodrome of pain, paraesthesia or itching, followed by the appearance of a cluster of vesicles. These break down into a 'sore' and then crust over, before healing without scarring. The lesion is usually painful. HSV can affect the eye, causing keratoconjunctivitis, and rarely causes encephalitis. Disease can be much more severe in the immunosuppressed, or in the context of underlying

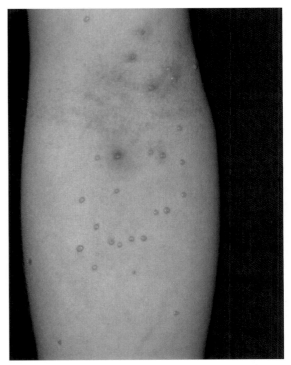

Figure 18.30 Multiple mollusca contagiosa with surrounding eczema.

eczema when it is known as eczema herpeticum (Fig. 18.18, p. 315). Treatment of simple cutaneous disease is with topical or oral antivirals such as aciclovir. Treatment should be instituted at the first indication of a recurrence. Neurological disease requires parenteral therapy.

Varicella zoster virus

Most individuals in the UK contract varicella zoster infection in childhood, leading to primary varicella (chickenpox). The virus is spread via respiratory droplets. The illness begins with fever followed after around 2 days by the typical skin manifestations. The eruption comprises crops of lesions that appear first as erythematous macules. These develop into papules, then vesicles or pustules and finally crust. New crops appear during the illness over 3–5 days – the presence of lesions at different stages is highly characteristic. Itching may be prominent. The condition is usually self-limiting and does not require specific treatment. However, superadded bacterial infection can occur, as well as other complications especially in immunosuppressed individuals. These include encephalitis and pneumonitis, which may be life-threatening. Treatment is with intravenous aciclovir or equivalent antiviral.

Following the initial infection, the virus lies dormant in the dorsal root ganglion. Reactivation leads to the dermatomal rash of herpes zoster (shingles). The first indication is usually pain, which may be severe. A unilateral eruption follows with clusters of vesicles appearing on an erythematous base, rupturing to leave erosions and then crusts. The vesicles may become pustular. Contiguous dermatomes may be affected.

Common complications include superadded bacterial infection and postherpetic neuralgia. Other organs including the central nervous system and heart can also be affected. Herpes zoster arising from the geniculate ganglion of the facial nerve can cause the Ramsay Hunt syndrome. The rash affects the external auditory meatus, pinna or oral mucosa and is associated with some or all of ipsilateral facial palsy, hearing loss and vestibular disturbance. Special care must be taken with shingles affecting the nasociliary nerve – lesions are present on the nasal tip, but the nerve also supplies the eye. Prompt ophthalmological review is required. For uncomplicated cutaneous shingles, treatment is not necessary. However, especially when given early, antivirals may hasten the resolution of symptoms.

Fungal infections

Dermatophytes are a group of fungi that can be acquired from humans, animals or soil. Infection causes 'ringworm', which is referred to clinically as 'tinea', followed by the appropriate body site in Latin. Hence, tinea pedis (foot), manuum (hand), unguium (nail), cruris (groin), capitis (scalp), corporis (elsewhere on the body). The Greek 'onychomycosis' is also used for nail infection.

Ringworm presents with expanding annular plaques, with scaling and tiny pustules at the active edge (Fig. 18.11, p. 310). The lesions may be multiple and are often itchy. Tinea pedis or athlete's foot produces maceration between the toes, sometimes with adjacent scale. Widespread tinea pedis or manuum can give rise to very fine, white scaling in the palmar and plantar skin creases. Nail infection usu-

ally causes thickening and yellow-brown discoloration, which may be indistinguishable from psoriasis. Tinea capitis produces patchy or localized alopecia, inflammation or scaling – the appearances can be quite variable.

If fungal infection is a possibility, send samples for mycological examination. Treatment at most sites is with topical antifungals for localized disease or oral antifungals for more extensive disease. Terbinafine is most effective. Scalp involvement always requires oral treatment and nail disease is also unlikely to respond to topical measures alone.

Pityriasis versicolor (sometimes confusingly referred to as tinea versicolor) refers to a yeast infection. It typically presents in young active adults with hypo- or sometimes hyperpigmented macules or thin plaques. Look closely and fine scaling can be seen at the periphery of the lesions. A skin scraping can confirm the diagnosis. Treatment is with topical ketoconazole and/or oral itraconazole, though patients should be warned that the pigmentary changes take weeks to return to normal and the condition quite commonly recurs.

Infestations

The eggs of head lice are nits, which the louse sticks to the host's hair. Sometimes, lice can be spotted on the scalp. Infestation may be asymptomatic, but severe itching and secondary eczema can occur. Lice are transmitted though close contact with affected individuals so family members and other contacts should be screened. Treatments include insecticides such as malathion, wet combing to remove nits, occlusion with a thick emollient to suffocate the lice or shaving the head to prevent lice which require hairs to which to stick their eggs from reproducing.

Scabies is caused by the mite *Sarcoptes scabiei*. Worldwide, it is estimated that 300 million cases occur annually. Infection is readily transmitted by close contact. Scabies (Fig. 18.31) is one of the causes of an intensely itchy rash. It has a predilection for the web spaces, genitalia (penile papules are typical), flexures and around the nipples. The pathognomonic sign is burrows or tracks – linear crusted lesions of a few millimetres in length, indicating where the mite is burrowing in the skin. The clinical picture is often confused by secondary eczematous

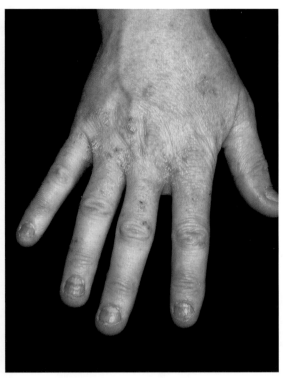

Figure 18.31 Scabies.

changes and excoriations. Lesions can occur all over the body, though scalp involvement is only found in babies and very elderly individuals. Treatment is with scabicides, usually permethrin or malathion. All household and other close contacts must be treated simultaneously, and it is advisable that clothing and bed linen be laundered at the same time.

Benign and malignant lesions

In general, be suspicious if a lesion is rapidly changing. Warning signs in pigmented lesions are: increasing size, darkening colour, irregular pigmentation, multiple colours within the same lesion, and itching or bleeding for no reason. Ask about a history of sun exposure and use of sunbeds (long-term chronic exposure to ultraviolet light is a risk factor for epidermal dysplasia and non-melanoma skin cancer; severe blistering sunburn in childhood is thought to be important in melanoma). Previous personal history and family history are strong risk factors for melanoma. Long-term immunosuppression is another important risk factor for all skin cancers.

Precancerous lesions

Actinic (or solar) keratosis refers to a lesion that displays partial thickness dysplasia of the epidermis. Although this is a histological criterion, most can be diagnosed clinically. Commonest on the face, they present as a mildly erythematous macule or superficial plaque with fine scale. They usually feel rough and dry. Some are hyperkeratotic, but there is no induration of the underlying skin. They may be numerous.

Full thickness epidermal dysplasia is Bowen's disease (also known as intra-epithelial or intra-epidermal carcinoma). Usually there is a well-defined, markedly erythematous plaque, with scaling and/or hyperkeratosis. Lesions are more likely to be single than in the case of actinic keratosis. In men, Bowen's disease is common on the face and to a lesser extent the trunk; in women, the lower leg is the characteristic site.

Treatment options include cryotherapy, topical 5-fluorouracil or curettage and cautery. Formal excision is reserved for lesions suspicious for invasive disease or those where other treatment has failed.

Basal cell carcinoma

Basal cell carcinoma (BCC) is the most commonly occurring type of cancer. There are several subtypes.

- The classical *nodular BCC* presents as a pearly skin coloured nodule, with a rolled edge, central crust or ulceration and surface telangiectasia (Fig. 18.4, p. 309).
- *Superficial BCC*, with a subtle rolled edge, may be a red scaly plaque with no other features.
- *Pigmented BCC* may be varying shades of brown, sometimes dark enough to be mistaken for melanoma.
- *Morphoeic BCC* (also called sclerotic or infiltrative) can be more difficult to spot clinically and often lacks some of the characteristic features. It may not be palpable and can mimic a scar in appearance. Because of the infiltrative growth pattern, morphoeic lesions are often larger than they appear on the skin surface.

Basal cell carcinomas tend to grow very slowly and metastasis is exceptionally rare. However, left untreated, they are very destructive, eating away at normal tissues, hence the common name of 'rodent ulcer'. Treatment is usually surgical excision with a 3–6 mm margin of apparently normal skin; radiotherapy can be a good alternative, depending on the site.

> **CLINICAL PEARL**
>
> Some superficial BCCs are indistinguishable from Bowen's disease and even amelanotic melanoma can present with a red, scaly plaque. Dermatologists often undertake biopsy of such lesions if they are solitary, prior to undertaking treatment.

Squamous cell carcinoma

A typical squamous cell carcinoma (SCC) (Fig. 18.32) manifests as an enlarging red nodule arising on sun-damaged skin. There is often a thick keratin plug centrally. Some present as a plaque with central ulceration. Up to 10 per cent metastasize to local lymph nodes. Particularly high-risk sites for this are the ears and lips. Squamous cell carcinomas can arise in scars or areas of chronic inflammation.

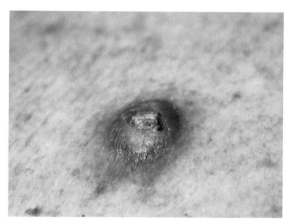

Figure 18.32 Squamous cell carcinoma.

Keratoacanthoma is a benign lesion that mimics SCC. It grows very quickly and may achieve a diameter of over 1 cm in 4–6 weeks. The growth then stops and, after a plateau phase, the lesion regresses spontaneously to leave a small scar. However, because the lesion so closely resembles SCC both clinically and histologically, it is wise to excise it in case it is actu-

ally an aggressive SCC, unless it is definitely already regressing.

> **CLINICAL PEARL**
>
> Beware a leg ulcer that enlarges despite treatment, especially if the edges are raised (Fig. 18.33). Either BCC or SCC can present in this way. Marjolin's ulcer is an SCC arising in a pre-existing ulcer and this too can easily be overlooked. If in doubt, do a biopsy.

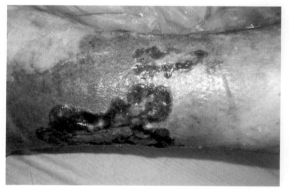

Figure 18.33 A longstanding leg ulcer: elevated, rolled edges aroused suspicion and a biopsy confirmed basal cell carcinoma.

Malignant melanoma

Malignant melanoma is one of the commonest cancers in young adults (Fig. 18.13, p. 311). It is responsible for almost three-quarters of skin cancer deaths, despite only accounting for around 4 per cent of skin cancers. Malignant melanoma can arise *de novo* or from a pre-existing naevus. Most are pigmented, but some are amelanotic. The most important prognostic factor for melanoma is the depth of the tumour when it is excised – Breslow's thickness. As most malignant melanomas undergo a relatively prolonged radial (horizontal) growth phase prior to invading vertically, there is a window of opportunity for early detection and management, while the prognosis remains favourable. The investigation of choice for a suspicious pigmented lesion is *excision* biopsy. Removing only part of the lesion can cause difficulty in interpreting the histology. Factors that should evoke suspicion are summarized above (see ABCDE, p. 311).

> **CLINICAL PEARL**
>
> Eruptive seborrhoeic keratoses (i.e. hundreds that appear suddenly) are thought to be suggestive of internal malignancy. In this context, the phenomenon is known as the sign of Leser–Trélat.

It is common to find moles with certain abnormal features clinically and histologically, but not amounting to malignant melanoma. These are known as dysplastic naevi. Unless very numerous, they are usually excised as they are probably more likely to progress to malignant melanoma than a normal, banal naevus.

Benign melanocytic naevi

The appearances of benign naevi can be quite variable. It is normal for moles to undergo a very gradual evolution as more naevoid cells drop down from epidermis into dermis. The main types are as follows:

- junctional naevi – these are macular and dark brown, and common in younger people
- compound naevi – these are elevated with a warty surface and are usually mid-brown
- intra-dermal naevi – these are smooth papules or nodules and have often lost their pigmentation.

Hairs growing from a mole are not indicative either of a benign lesion or malignant process; however, if the hairs in a mole suddenly stop growing, this may imply destruction of the follicles which could occur in the context of malignant change.

Seborrhoeic keratosis

These lesions are extremely common. Their great variation in appearance frequently leads to diagnostic confusion. They range in colour from pink through skin-coloured to all shades of brown and even virtually black. They are usually elevated from the surrounding skin, but may be macular. They show a fissured or pitted, warty surface which is matt. They are said to look as if they have been 'stuck on'. Most can confidently be diagnosed by dermatologists, but flatter lesions may require a biopsy to exclude actinic keratosis or lentigo maligna. Lesions that mimic malignant melanoma should be excised.

Dermatofibroma

This is another relatively common benign lesion, most often seen on the leg. Most are asymptomatic, but some cause itch. They produce a dermal nodule. The overlying skin may not be discoloured, but there is often hyperpigmentation. The nodule feels firm and if compressed, seems to sink down away from the examiner's fingers, with puckering of the overlying skin. There is a rare, indolently malignant form known as dermatofibrosarcoma protuberans. Warning signs are asymmetry and steady growth.

Pyogenic granuloma

This is a misnomer, being neither pyogenic nor granulomatous. Rather, it comprises blood vessels and granulation tissue. Most are precipitated by minor trauma. They appear as moist, often ulcerated pedunculated nodules (Fig. 18.34). There is often a history of profuse bleeding. Rarely, an amelanotic melanoma or SCC can present similarly. Treatment is usually surgical removal by curettage and cautery.

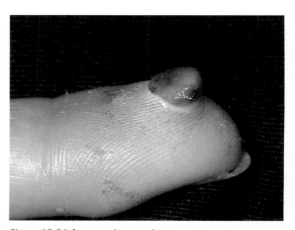

Figure 18.34 A pyogenic granuloma.

THE LAST WORD

Dermatology is not easy! It encompasses over 2000 different conditions. If you're not sure of the diagnosis, give a decent description, come up with a differential diagnosis and speak to a dermatologist.

SUMMARY

History

For rashes, ask about:

- site of onset
- duration
- evolution
- symptoms: itching, soreness, burning
- treatments tried and response
- risk factors (e.g. atopy, family history)
- occupation
- psychosocial impact.

For lesions, ask about:

- site
- duration
- evolution: changes in size, colour
- symptoms: itching, pain, crusting
- treatments tried and response
- previous skin cancer
- risk factors for skin cancer (e.g. outdoor occupation, time abroad, sunbed use, phototherapy, immunosuppression).

Examination

For rashes:

- DCM
  - *Distribution*: what are the affected sites? Is the eruption symmetrical?
  - *Configuration*: what is the pattern (if any) in which individual component parts of the eruption are arranged?
  - *Morphology*: describe the actual features of the component parts of the eruption, e.g. macules, papules, plaques, etc.
- consider typical distributions and examine as necessary (e.g. scalp involvement in psoriasis, penile papules in scabies)
- look for Koebner's phenomenon (e.g. psoriasis, lichen planus, viral warts)
- check for nail disease (e.g. psoriasis, eczema, lichen planus)
- check for mucosal involvement (e.g. drug eruptions, bullous disorders, lichen planus)
- consider underlying medical disease (e.g. examine the abdomen in acanthosis nigricans; chest and abdomen in dermatomyositis; abdomen in pyoderma gangrenosum)

For lesions:

- ABCDE for pigmented lesions
  - Asymmetry
  - Border
  - Colour
  - Diameter
  - Elevation
- remember E for 'everything else'
- solitary or multiple lesions?
- sun exposed site?
- consider the history in conjunction with the examination findings
- examine for lymphadenopathy in squamous cell carcinoma or melanoma.

FURTHER READING

Bolognia JL, Jorizzo JL, Rapini RP (eds). 2003. *Dermatology*. Edinburgh: Mosby.

Burns DA, Breathnach SM, Cox N, Griffiths CE (eds). 2004. *Rook's textbook of dermatology*. Oxford: Blackwell Publishers.

19

THE EYE

Alastair K Denniston and Philip I Murray

INTRODUCTION

It is often assumed that learning how to assess a patient with an ophthalmic problem is all about measuring visual acuity and knowing how to use an ophthalmoscope. Although these are undoubtedly important skills it should be borne in mind that the eye does not exist in isolation and for many patients their 'eye' problems are associated with systemic disease. It is therefore important to consider the ophthalmic assessment in the context of a patient's general history and systemic examination. Figure 19.1 shows external and internal views of the eye illustrating key anatomical structures, and Table 19.1 details the anatomy and function of different eye structures.

HISTORY

Presenting complaint

What's the problem?

Most patients with ophthalmic problems help the practitioner by describing their problem in terms that quickly place it within one of a small number of clinical presentations: uncomfortable/red eye(s), blurred vision, loss of vision, floaters, double vision,

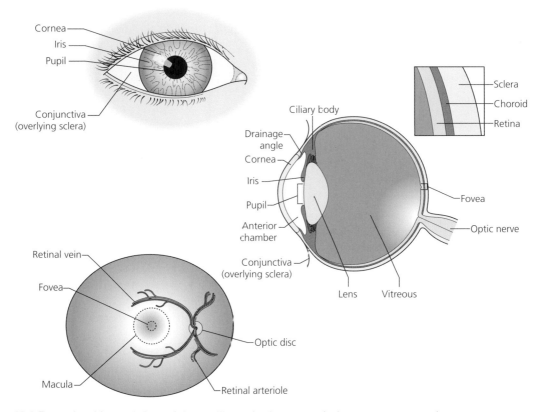

Figure 19.1 External and internal views of the eye illustrating key anatomical structures.

Table 19.1 Parts of the eye

Structure	Anatomy	Function
Conjunctiva	Thin membrane covering most of the anterior surface of the eye, being continuous from the edge of the cornea (the 'limbus') to the edge of the lids; importantly the conjunctiva does not cover the cornea	Mucous membrane; contributes to the tear film
Episclera	A thin connective tissue layer between the conjunctiva and the sclera	Connective tissue
Sclera	A thick white fibrous layer of irregularly arranged collagen fibres forming the posterior five-sixths of the outer coat of the eye	Maintains eye shape and intraocular pressure Barrier to infection Protects against trauma
Cornea	A thick transparent layer of regularly arranged collagen; posteriorly it is continuous with the sclera	The 'window' of the eye: transparency results in excellent light transmission Refraction: the majority of refraction (bending of the light rays) occurs here Barrier to infection Protects against trauma
Aqueous humour	Colourless transparent fluid produced by the ciliary body	Provides oxygen and nutrients to the lens and posterior cornea Maintains the intraocular pressure and shape of the eye
Lens	A transparent biconvex structure of proteins (crystallins); suspended by lens zonules; shape can be altered by the ciliary muscle	Fine focusing Transparency results in excellent light transmission
Uvea	Highly vascular layer comprising iris, ciliary body and choroid; lies deep to the cornea and sclera	Iris: regulates light entry Ciliary body: produces aqueous humour Choroid: provides oxygen and nutrients to the outer retina
Retina	Transparent structure containing multiple neural layers and a photoreceptor layer	Transduction of light into an electrical signal Transparency results in excellent light transmission to the photoreceptor layer
Vitreous humour	Firm transparent gel filling the volume posterior to the lens	Transparent to promote light transmission Protects ocular structures

etc. Subsequent questioning and examination will then pay special attention to those features that are most helpful in narrowing down the diagnosis. We outline these below.

IMPORTANT

One of the commoner ophthalmic emergencies is chemical injury, typically alkaline, from cleaning agents or plaster splashing into the eye(s). This is one time when treatment comes first: irrigate thoroughly before anything else.

Do they know they have a problem?

Some patients may be referred to the hospital eye service after a routine optometrist review (the 'optician eye test'), as the optometrist has a valuable role in screening for asymptomatic disease (especially diabetic retinopathy and glaucoma).

History of presenting complaint

The analysis of most ophthalmic complaints centres on general questions regarding onset, precipitants, associated features (e.g. pain, redness, discharge, photophobia, etc.), duration, relieving factors, recovery and specific questions directed by the presentation. Even after clinical examination further information may be needed to rule in or rule out diagnoses. We consider the main clinical contexts below.

Patient presenting with uncomfortable/red eye(s)

Is there any discomfort?

- Grittiness or foreign body sensation suggests ocular surface problems, such as conjunctivitis.
- Itching is suggestive of allergic conjunctivitis.
- Severe pain (usually 'aching' in nature) suggests serious ocular problems such as acute angle closure glaucoma, or scleritis.
- A completely painless red eye is most commonly seen with a subconjunctival haemorrhage (bleed under the conjunctiva; it is often small, spontaneous and will resolve of its own accord) or episcleritis.

Is there any discharge?

- Discharge suggests ocular surface problems, commonly conjunctivitis.
- Purulent discharge is suggestive of bacterial conjunctivitis.
- Watery discharge is commonly seen in viral or allergic conjunctivitis, or may arise after minor trauma to the cornea (e.g. corneal abrasion).
- Moderately thick 'mucopurulent' discharge may be due to *Chlamydia* infection; consider this especially if the conjunctivitis is unilateral.

Does it affect one or both eyes?

Most ocular surface diseases, such as conjunctivitis or blepharitis (a common chronic inflammation of the eyelids) are bilateral, whereas most serious pathology (usually involving deeper structures) is unilateral:

- *Unilateral causes* include corneal ulcer, acute anterior uveitis, acute angle closure glaucoma and chlamydial conjunctivitis.
- *Bilateral causes* include allergic conjunctivitis, most infective conjunctivitis (note exception of chlamydia, and that at onset, other types of conjunctivitis may be unilateral) and blepharitis.

Is there photophobia (sensitivity to light)?

Photophobia is most commonly seen with acute anterior uveitis, severe inflammation of the cornea (e.g. corneal ulcer – bacterial, viral) or corneal trauma (e.g. abrasion).

Is there any effect on vision?

Any significant reduction of vision suggests serious pathology, such as corneal ulcer, acute angle closure glaucoma, or acute anterior uveitis. Patients with bacterial conjunctivitis sometimes complain of transient blurring but this should clear on blinking.

Table 19.2 summarizes the differential diagnosis of the red eye.

Patient presenting with loss of vision

Did it happen suddenly or gradually?

- *Sudden loss of vision* is commonly due to a vascular event. These may be vessel occlusions giving rise to ischaemia of vision-serving structures such as the retina, optic nerve or brain. Alternatively there may be vessel rupture and consequent bleeding which may either block transmission of light as in traumatic hyphaema (haemorrhage into the anterior chamber) and vitreous haemorrhage, or may distort the retina as in 'wet' age-related macular degeneration (AMD).
- *Gradual loss of vision* is commonly associated with degenerations or depositions. These include cataract, primary open angle glaucoma, 'dry' AMD, macular dystrophies or corneal dystrophies.

Is it painful?

- *Painful blurring of vision* is most commonly associated with diseases at the front of the eye (e.g. keratitis, anterior uveitis) although disease of the orbit, optic neuritis, and giant cell arteritis may also cause painful loss of vision.
- *Painless loss of vision* usually arises from problems in the posterior part of the eye such as cataract, macular and other retinal problems (e.g. AMD, diabetic maculopathy, retinal arterial or retinal venous occlusions), and most optic nerve disease (e.g. primary open angle glaucoma, anterior ischaemic optic neuropathy).

Table 19.2 Differential diagnosis of the red eye

	Discomfort/pain	Photo-phobia	Visual acuity	Redness	Discharge	Other features and associations
Blepharitis	Foreign body sensation	No	Normal	Minimal red eye(s)	Minimal	Crusts on lashes Meibomian cysts Associated with acne rosacea
Bacterial conjunctivitis	Minimal discomfort/gritty sensation	No	Normal	Diffusely red eyes	Purulent discharge	Lashes may be stuck together
Viral conjunctivitis	Minimal discomfort/gritty sensation	No	Normal	Diffusely red eyes	Watery discharge	May have preauricular lymphadenopathy Associated with upper respiratory tract infection
Bacterial keratitis (bacterial corneal ulcer)	Pain	Yes	Reduced	Diffusely red eye	Purulent discharge	White spot (abscess) on cornea Associated with contact lens wear or previous trauma
Viral keratitis (dendritic ulcer)	Pain	Yes	Reduced	Diffusely red eye	Minimal	Classical dendritic staining pattern of herpes simplex virus with fluorescein Reduced corneal sensation Recurrent disease
Marginal keratitis (sterile corneal ulcer)	Moderate discomfort	Yes	Normal	Red eye, may be focal	Minimal	White spots on peripheral cornea which stain with fluorescein Associated with blepharitis and acne rosacea
Acute anterior uveitis (iritis)	Pain	Yes	Reduced	Red eye, especially around limbus	No	May have small, irregular pupil Recurrent disease Associated with HLA-B27 disease
Episcleritis	Nil/mild discomfort	No	Normal	Red eye(s), may be focal or diffuse	No	Recurrent disease Either eye
Scleritis	Severe pain	Not usually	Normal	Deep redness, may be focal or diffuse	No	Associated with autoimmune disease Recurrent disease
Acute angle closure glaucoma	Severe pain	Yes	Reduced (often severely)	Diffusely red eye(s)	No	Nausea/ vomiting Haloes around lights Hazy cornea Semi-dilated pupil Hypermetropia

Is the problem transient or persistent?

- *Transient loss of vision* is commonly due to temporary or subcritical vascular insufficiency (e.g. giant cell arteritis, amaurosis fugax, vertebrobasilar artery insufficiency).
- *Persistent loss of vision* suggests structural changes (e.g. cataract or vitreous haemorrhage) or irreversible damage (e.g. AMD, optic nerve damage).

Does it affect one or both eyes?

- *Unilateral disease* may suggest a local ocular cause.
- *Bilateral disease* may suggest a more widespread or systemic process.

Is the vision blurred, dimmed or distorted?

- *Blurring or dimming* may arise due to pathology anywhere in the visual pathway from cornea to visual cortex; common problems include refractive error, cataract and macular disease.
- *Distortion* is commonly associated with macular pathology.

Where is the problem with their vision?

- *Central blurring of vision* suggests disease of the macula or the optic nerve. In macular disease, patients get a positive scotoma (a blind spot), i.e. they see a 'spot' in the vision where the defect is. In optic nerve disease patients have a negative scotoma, i.e. the defect is not 'seen'.
- *Peripheral field loss* may fall into a number of clear patterns. A superior or inferior hemispheric field loss (i.e. the whole top or bottom half of the vision from one eye) suggests a corresponding inferior or superior vascular event involving retina (e.g. retinal vein occlusion) or optic disc (e.g. a segmental anterior ischaemic optic neuropathy). Peripheral field loss may arise from other retinal disease (e.g. retinitis pigmentosa or retinal detachment), optic nerve disease, compression of the optic chiasm (typically gives a bitemporal hemianopia) or problems in the visual cortex (e.g. strokes, tumours or head trauma resulting in homonymous hemianopic defects).

When does it occur?

Clues may arise from typical precipitants. For example, glare from headlights or bright sunlight is commonly due to certain types of cataract. Episodes of eye pain with 'haloes' occurring in dim light conditions may suggest warning episodes prior to acute angle closure glaucoma.

> **IMPORTANT**
> Sudden visual loss always requires urgent investigation and referral to an ophthalmologist.

Patient presenting with flashes and/or floaters

Are they getting flashes or floaters or both?

- *Flashes and floaters*: most commonly posterior vitreous detachment (the vitreous gel pulling away from the retina), but requires urgent ophthalmic assessment since it may be associated with retinal tear which can lead on to a retinal detachment.
- *Flashes alone*: commonly migraine (may get classic zig-zag lines known as 'fortification spectra' with or without headache), or vitreoretinal problems (impending posterior vitreous detachment causing traction on the retina).
- *Floaters alone*: if floaters have come on gradually consider vitreous degeneration (more common with increasing age and myopia) or uveitis (especially intermediate type); if sudden onset but vision still good consider posterior vitreous detachment (more common with age or myopia); if sudden onset with reduced vision consider vitreous haemorrhage or retinal detachment involving the macula.

> **IMPORTANT**
> Recent-onset flashes and floaters should be presumed to be retinal tear/detachment until proven otherwise – refer urgently to an ophthalmologist.

Patient presenting with double vision

Is the double vision from one eye (monocular) or from both eyes (binocular)?

- If *monocular* (i.e. the double vision is present in the affected eye when the other eye is closed), then it is effectively an optical problem, most commonly cataract.

- If *binocular* (i.e. the double vision is only present when both eyes are open), then the problem is that the two eyes are not correctly aligned. This can be due to a problem anywhere in the neuro-muscular path from brainstem to ocular muscle, but is most commonly due to a palsy of one of the cranial nerves supplying the ocular muscles (i.e. cranial nerves III, IV or VI).

Are the images side by side, vertical or diagonal?

- *Horizontal separation* is usually due to problems with cranial nerve VI, typically a microvascular infarct in a patient with atherosclerotic risk factors. **Note:** This can also result from raised intracranial pressure.
- *Diagonal or vertical separation* may be due to a problem with cranial nerves III and IV.

Is the double vision constant or variable?

Fluctuating double vision may be due to myasthenia gravis, decompensating childhood squint, giant cell arteritis or raised intracranial pressure.

Has the eye/orbit changed in appearance?

- *Proptosis* (i.e. forward protrusion) of the eye due to thyroid eye disease or a tumour can cause slowly progressive double vision.

---

i **IMPORTANT**

Pupil involvement in a cranial nerve III palsy: a third nerve palsy is an ophthalmic emergency since it may arise from a posterior communicating artery aneurysm. In such cases the palsy may be the only warning of impending aneurysmal rupture with subsequent subarachnoid haemorrhage. One helpful feature that warns that a cranial nerve III palsy may be compressive is pupil involvement (i.e. a dilated pupil). This is because the pupil-innervating fibres are on the outside of cranial nerve III, where they are more vulnerable to compression by the expanding aneurysm (or other mass lesion). In contrast, in the more common ischaemic cranial nerve III palsies, the pupil is usually spared as the outer pupillary fibres may get an additional blood supply from the adjacent vasa nervosum.

- *Ptosis* (i.e. drooping lid) and a dilated pupil suggest an ipsilateral cranial nerve III palsy. This is a neuro-ophthalmic emergency since it may represent an aneurysm of the posterior communicating artery.

Has there been recent trauma?

Vertical double vision may occur after trauma causing an orbital floor fracture, or a head injury resulting in a cranial nerve IV palsy.

Table 19.3 summarizes common eye symptoms.

Past ophthalmic history

The background for each presentation is important. Ask about previous surgery/trauma, previous/concurrent eye disease, and refractive error (i.e. what sort of glasses they wear). The differential diagnosis of an acute red eye will be affected by knowing that they had complicated cataract surgery 3 days previously (postoperative endophthalmitis) or that they have a 10-year history of recurrent acute anterior uveitis or even that they wear contact lenses.

Past medical history

Similarly consider the whole patient. Ask generally about any medical problems. In addition, ask specifically about relevant conditions that they may have omitted to mention. The patient with recurrently itchy eyes may not mention that they have eczema or asthma. Similarly, if presenting with a vascular event, ask specifically about diabetes, hypertension and hypercholesterolaemia. Also consider whether the patient's level of disability will affect their ability

Table 19.3 Summary: common symptoms

Symptoms	Source of problem
Pain/redness/photophobia/ discharge	Front of eye
Painless loss of vision	Back of eye (including lens)
Misty vision/glare	Cataract
Distortion of vision/central scotoma	Macula
Flashes and floaters	Vitreous/retina

Note: Some serious eye conditions (notably primary open angle glaucoma) can be asymptomatic.

to take their medication, e.g. not being able to open bottles of eyedrops due to severely arthritic hands.

Family history

This is relevant both to heritable diseases and to infective conditions. Inherited diseases may affect most parts of the eye, and include corneal dystrophies, early-onset cataracts and retinitis pigmentosa. Taking a family and contact history is also important in infectious conditions such as conjunctivitis.

Social history

Ask about smoking and alcohol intake if relevant to the ophthalmic disease (e.g. vascular event or unexplained optic neuropathy respectively). Consider the social context of the patient. Will they remember to instil their drops?

Drugs and allergies

Ask about concurrent medication and any allergies to previous medications (e.g. drops) since these may limit your therapeutic options. In addition to actual allergies consider contraindications (e.g. asthma/chronic obstructive pulmonary disease and β-blocker drops for glaucoma).

EXAMINATION

All medical practitioners should be capable of carrying out an effective basic ophthalmic examination, including testing vision, visual fields and pupil responses, and examining major structures of the eye. This can be achieved with equipment that should be generally available, notably a Snellen visual acuity chart, a pen torch, an ophthalmoscope and basic eye drops (fluorescein and dilating drops such as tropicamide). Where a more detailed examination is indicated, this will be performed by an ophthalmologist using specialized equipment such as the slit-lamp (also known as the bio-microscope).

Visual acuity

Distance vision

This is normally tested using the familiar Snellen chart (Fig. 19.2) that features a series of diminishing high-contrast letters running from a single large

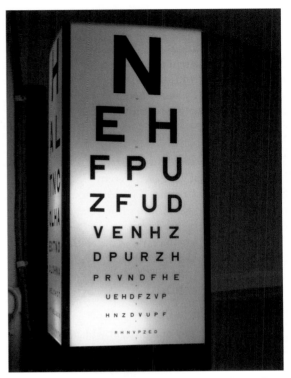

Figure 19.2 The Snellen chart is a familiar tool for testing visual acuity; the standard chart is designed for use at 6 m.

letter at the top to a series of small letters at the bottom. The standard Snellen chart is designed for use at 6 m. Each line is marked with the distance in metres at which a normally sighted person should be able to read that line. Thus a 'normal' person has 6/6 vision, which means they can read the line marked '6' at a distance of 6 m. In contrast somebody with very poor vision may only be able to read top letter of the chart marked '60' (i.e. the letter a normally sighted person could read at 60 m).

- Position the patient 6 m from the illuminated chart, cover the left eye and ask them to read as far down the chart as they can. Record the vision as 6/× where × is the best line read. Repeat the procedure, covering the right eye. If glasses are required for distance (e.g. driving, watching television) then these should be worn.

Pinhole acuity

Use of a pinhole obscures most of the blur caused by refractive error giving a dim but 'in focus' image and therefore gives an indication of the potential vision with correct refraction (e.g. glasses). If the vision is worse than 6/6 in either eye, test acuity (as above) but asking the patient to look through a pinhole for each eye in turn with the other eye obscured (if the vision improves by about two lines then glasses or a new pair of glasses are required).

Near vision

This is usually tested using small books containing paragraphs of text of different sizes (N5 being the 'normal' near vision). The commonest cause of problems with near vision while retaining normal distance vision is presbyopia, i.e. the age-related reduction (usually >40 years) in the ability to accommodate (i.e. focus on near objects).

Pupil examination

Response to light

If light is shone into one pupil it will constrict (the direct response). The pupil of the other eye will also constrict (the consensual response) due to the bilateral nature of the light reflex:

retina → optic nerve → pretectal nucleus → bilateral Edinger-Westphal nuclei → both cranial nerves III → iris sphincter muscle of both eyes.

In the 'swinging flashlight test' light is shone into each eye in turn. Assuming that the electrical signal from both eyes is equal, the pupils should constrict whichever eye the light is being shone in. If the pupil dilates when the light source is transferred from the first to the second eye, the second eye is said to have a 'relative afferent pupillary defect' (RAPD). This is usually due to unilateral or asymmetrical damage to the optic nerve, e.g. glaucomatous optic neuropathy, optic neuritis, anterior ischaemic optic neuropathy or optic atrophy, as well as gross retinal damage, e.g. total retinal detachment.

Ask the patient to look into the distance and shine the pen torch at each eye in turn, observing the pupillary response of both eyes (direct and consensual). Then perform the 'swinging flashlight test', in which the pen torch is directed from one eye to the other in turn (about 1 second gap), and any abnormal dilation is noted.

> **CLINICAL PEARL**
> Testing for an RAPD is probably the most informative pupil test as it can identify optic nerve disease, and is invaluable in those eyes where is it impossible to see the back of the eye.

Colour vision

Colour vision may be reduced when visual acuity is apparently still normal/near normal. This usually indicates optic nerve disease such as optic neuritis.

- Present a bright red target to each eye and ask the patient to say if it appears equally red between each eye; sometimes it helps to ask them to score the intensity of 'redness' out of 10 for each eye (test of red desaturation).
- More detailed analysis requires Ishihara colour plates (See 'Investigations').

Visual fields

Visual field defects which are large and dense can be identified with the confrontational technique. Throughout you should be comparing the patient's visual fields with your own. Therefore it is essential that you position yourself level with them, your hands/pin are equidistant between you and the patient, and that when you ask them to cover one eye, you do likewise: thus if they cover their left, you cover your right.

- Ask the patient, with both eyes open, to look at the bridge of your nose and to note if any part of your face appears to be missing. This should detect any major homonymous defects (i.e. defects affecting the same part of the field from both eyes).
- Ask the patient to cover one eye. Hold up different numbers of fingers in each quadrant and ask patient how many fingers they see. This should detect dense hemianopias or quadrantanopias. Repeat for the other eye.
- To map out any defects in more detail or to detect more subtle defects, a target such as a white hat pin can be used. Again testing each eye in turn, the target should be brought in from the periphery and the patient instructed to say when they first spot it.

- More detailed analysis requires formal perimetry using a machine (see 'Investigations').

Front of the eye

Observation is key. Generally work from outside in, and in particular look for:

- lids: any lumps or inflammation, eyelid turning in (entropion) or turning out (ectropion)
- conjunctiva: any redness (note distribution), discharge, or swelling
- cornea: any loss of clarity or visible white opacities.

Add a drop of fluorescein. This will stain any areas of cornea (or conjunctiva) which have lost epithelium, as seen in a corneal abrasion or bacterial or viral keratitis. The fluorescein-stained area appears green in a blue light (use pen torch or ophthalmoscope with blue filter).

More detailed examination is facilitated by use of a slit-lamp (Fig. 19.3).

Back of the eye

Successful use of the direct ophthalmoscope depends on good preparation and practice. Observe:

- *Red reflex*: loss of the normal healthy orange/red reflection is commonly due to cataract, but may arise due to posterior pathology such as tumours (especially retinoblastoma in children) and inflammation.

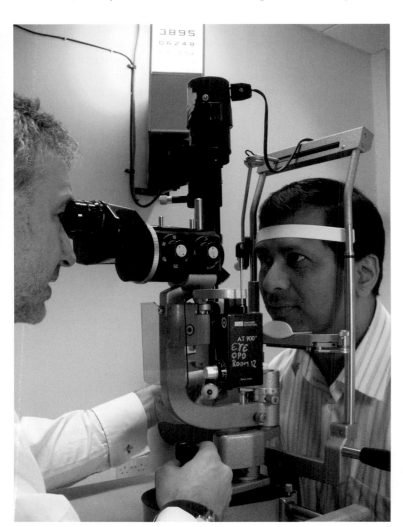

Figure 19.3 The 'slit-lamp' or biomicroscope gives a magnified stereoscopic view of both the anterior and posterior segments of the eye; viewing of the posterior segment requires the addition of a hand-held lens.

In addition in patients who have had cataract surgery the prosthetic intraocular lens may be visible.

- *Optic disc*: note cup:disc ratio, colour and contour.
- *Blood vessels*: check that they of normal calibre, and there are no emboli in the retinal arterioles. Look for irregularities or abnormal new vessels (particularly on the optic disc in proliferative diabetic retinopathy).
- *Peripheral retina*: look for haemorrhages, exudates, microaneurysms, cotton-wool spots, abnormal pigmentation, or detached retina.
- *Macula*: look for any of the above abnormalities involving the macula.

Ophthalmoscopy

Make ophthalmoscopy easier:

- Use a familiar ophthalmoscope, with charged batteries.
- Dim the room lights.
- Where possible, use dilating drops.
- Ask the patient to look slightly up and into the distance at a designated target, and request permission to place a hand on their shoulder to help you get close without collision.
- Your eye should be at the same level as their eye; use your right eye for the patient's right eye and your left eye for their left eye.
- Approach from 15° lateral to their line of gaze; this means that you should be directed straight onto the optic disc.
- Use the red reflex to act as an aiming beam guiding you towards the patient's eye and details should be in focus a few centimetres away from the patient's eye.
- Adjust the lens power of the ophthalmoscope to ensure all details are optimally in focus. If patients neither have a refractive error (nor are wearing contact lenses) the ophthalmoscope will usually be in focus at zero. If either the patient or practitioner usually wears glasses for distance it is likely that the lens power will need adjusting. The strength of lens required can be estimated by adding the refractive error of patient and practitioner (assuming neither is wearing their glasses during the examination).
- Use a systematic approach: note features of the optic disc, the vessels and the peripheral fundus before looking at the macula (lateral to, but on the same level, as the disc; NB it is almost impossible to see the macula through an undilated pupil).

Estimating lens power for ophthalmoscopy

Most ophthalmoscopes include a lens power dial so that you can correct for your own and/or the patient's refractive error. Depending on the model of ophthalmoscope the different lens powers will either be prefixed by a plus (+) or minus (−) or will be black (for plus) and red (for minus).

What you need to know

- *Your own refractive error*: if you are wearing contact lenses or are keeping your glasses on then this will be zero.
- *The patient's refractive error*: ask the patient. They may not know their exact prescription but they often know if they are short-sighted (i.e. myopic) in which case set the dial to a minus lens, or long-sighted (hypermetropic) and so require a plus lens. If they are not sure, first confirm whether they use glasses for distance (television, driving). If they only use glasses for reading you can assume a zero refractive error. If they use glasses for distance, examine the glasses. Hold the glasses at arm's length over some text (as you would a magnifying glass). If they magnify the text they are plus lenses (i.e. the patient is hypermetropic) so dial to the plus/black numbers, whereas if they minify the text (make it smaller) they are minus lenses (i.e. the patient is myopic) so dial to the minus/red numbers. The thicker the lenses the higher the refractive error is likely to be.

CLINICAL PEARL

Setting the dial on the ophthalmoscope: worked examples

EXAMPLE 1 You are short-sighted with a refractive error of −3D *and* the patient is short-sighted with a refractive error of −5D: set the dial on the ophthalmoscope to −8D.

EXAMPLE 2 You are short-sighted with a refractive error of −3D *and* the patient is long-sighted with a refractive error of +5D: set the dial on the ophthalmoscope to +2D.

What you need to do

Add the two refractive errors together and set the lens power dial to this number.

Eye movements

Examination of eye movements is discussed in Chapter 12 as part of the cranial nerve examination.

INVESTIGATIONS

Specialist tests include the following.

Vision and visual function

- *Colour vision* is most commonly tested using the Ishihara plates (Fig. 19.4), a book of coloured numbers that is used to detect red–green colour deficiency – often a sign of optic nerve disease.
- *Visual field testing* can be tested by formal perimetry where the patient stares into a white bowl onto which a bright spot of variable size and intensity is projected. The two main types are Goldmann perimetry and automated perimetry (commonly using the Humphrey machine) (Fig. 19.5). The Goldmann perimeter is manually operated. The operator brings the target (white

spot) in from the periphery, the patient buzzes every time they detect the light, and the operator maps out the points at which the target was spotted. Since a moving target is used this is described as 'kinetic' perimetry. The result looks like a contour map, showing the different levels of visual sensitivity. In automated perimetry the computer directs targets of varying intensity to be projected around the perimeter bowl and again the patient presses a buzzer when they detect them. This is described as 'static' perimetry since the targets do not move. In automated field testing the results are automatically compared to the predicted 'normal' values. Areas of abnormal low sensitivity are highlighted in shades of grey with a corresponding plot giving the actual sensitivity in decibels.

Front of the eye

Intraocular pressure (IOP) testing is part of routine slit-lamp examination for the ophthalmologist. After instillation of an anaesthetic and fluorescein drop, the prism of a Goldmann tonometer (a small piece of equipment attached to the slit-lamp) is brought towards the eye such that the head of the prism just touches the central cornea (Fig. 19.6). Using a blue

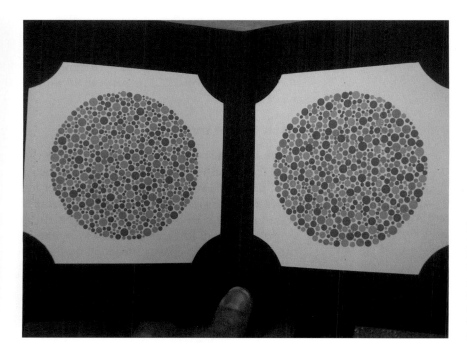

Figure 19.4 Ishihara colour plates comprise a book of coloured numbers that is used to detect problems with red–green discrimination due to either congenital colour blindness or acquired optic nerve damage.

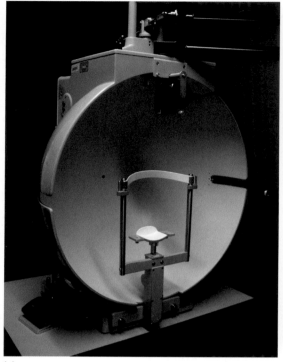

(a)

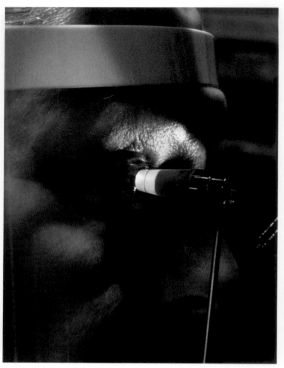

Figure 19.6 The Goldmann applanation tonometer is used with topical anaesthesia and fluorescein to accurately measure the intraocular pressure by a contact method.

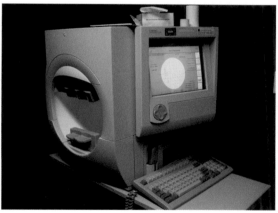

(b)

Figure 19.5 (a) Goldmann Bowl perimeter with which the patient's ability to detect a moving (kinetic) stimulus can be recorded by an observer, and (b) an automated perimeter with which the patient's ability to detect static stimuli is recorded by a computer.

light on the slit-lamp, the operator observes two green semicircles. Adjustment of the tonometer dial changes the pressure that the prism is exerting on the cornea (and thus the corneal deformation) and alters the relative position of the semicircles. Once the correct alignment is achieved (where the two semicircles just overlap) the intraocular pressure can be read off the tonometer dial (1 = 10 mmHg, 2 = 20 mmHg, etc; normal IOP is between 10 mmHg and 21 mmHg).

Back of the eye

Fundus fluorescein angiography is a technique to visualize the retinal vessels. Fluorescein dye is injected into a peripheral vein. Around 15 seconds later the fluorescein dye reaches the retinal circulation. A specialized camera is used that emits blue light at the correct wavelength to excite the fluorescein, and in turn detects the green light emitted from the fluorescein as the molecules return to their resting energy state. Serial photographs are taken to detect the passage of dye through the vessels and any pathological abnormality of the retinal circulation (such as leakage) can be identified.

Optical coherence tomography is a non-contact technique that generates high-resolution cross-sectional images of the retina and optic nerve. By directing a beam of light through the pupil and then measuring the delay and magnitude of the reflected light a detailed cross-sectional map of the retina is built up. It is primarily used for looking at macular problems especially macular oedema.

COMMON OPHTHALMIC DIAGNOSES

Conjunctivitis

Conjunctivitis (inflammation of the conjunctiva) may be due to infection or allergy. Infective causes include bacteria (usually *Staphylococcus* or *Streptococcus*), viruses (usually adenovirus) or *Chlamydia*. For bacterial and viral cases the patient may know that friends or family have recently had a similar problem. Allergic conjunctivitis is usually associated with allergic rhinitis and the patient may have other atopic disease such as asthma or eczema.

Typical presentations

- Infective: bilateral red 'sticky' or 'watering' eyes in any age group.
- Allergic: bilateral itchy eyes with mild redness in younger age group.

Infective conjunctivitis

Symptoms

- Usually bilateral
- Slight discomfort
- Diffusely red
- Sticky/watery eye(s)

Signs

- Diffuse conjunctival redness.
- Normal vision (other than transient blurring which clears on blinking).

Additional sign suggestive of bacterial infection:

- discharge is purulent.

Additional signs suggestive of viral infection:

- discharge is watery

- follicles (visible lumps of lymphoid tissue) on the conjunctival surface of the lids
- enlarged preauricular lymph node
- associated upper respiratory tract infection.

Additional signs suggestive of chlamydial infection:

- chronic unilateral disease.

Investigation

- The specific organism can be confirmed by taking a swab for culture, however most cases are diagnosed clinically and treated empirically with a broad spectrum topical antibiotic.

Treatment

- Bacterial conjunctivitis: frequent topical antibiotics e.g. chloramphenicol.

Allergic conjunctivitis

Symptoms

- Usually bilateral
- Very itchy
- Mild redness
- Watery eye(s)

Signs

- Diffuse conjunctival redness.
- Normal vision (other than transient blurring which clears on blinking).

Investigation

Specific allergens can sometimes be identified e.g. via skin-prick testing.

Treatment

Control with topical antihistamines, mast-cell stabilizers or systemic antihistamine.

Keratitis and corneal ulcer

Keratitis (inflammation of the cornea) may be due to direct infection of the cornea by bacteria or viruses or due to an immune response to bacteria residing the lids (known as 'marginal keratitis'). Bacterial keratitis may be caused by a wide range of Gram-positive and Gram-negative species and is commonly seen in the context of contact lens wear. It requires very frequent topical antibiotics and is an **ophthalmic emergency**, since it may progress to intraocular infection and perforation of the eye. All cases should be referred urgently to an ophthalmologist. Viral keratitis is usually due to herpes simplex virus type 1, and is treated with topical antivirals. In most common types of keratitis there is ulceration, i.e. loss of epithelium with variable deeper corneal involvement according to severity.

Typical presentations

- Bacterial: unilateral red 'sticky' eye with white spot on the cornea which stains with fluorescein.
- Viral: unilateral red watery eye with fine, branching ulcer ('dendritic ulcer') which stains with fluorescein.

Bacterial keratitis

Symptoms

- Unilateral
- Red, sticky eye
- Reduced vision
- Photophobia
- May report contact lens wear or recent trauma to the eye.

Signs

- Conjunctival redness.
- Purulent discharge.
- White spot on cornea with fluorescein staining.
- Occasionally there may be a hypopyon (a visible collection of inflammatory cells in the anterior chamber resulting in a white fluid level) – this indicates a very severe ulcer.

Investigations

The surface of the ulcer should be scraped by an ophthalmologist and the scrapings sent for microscopy and culture to identify the organism.

Treatment

- Patient may require admission.
- Hourly topical antibiotics, e.g. ofloxacin, until resolution.

Viral keratitis

Symptoms

- Unilateral
- Red eye
- Reduced vision

- Photophobia
- May report previous episodes or other herpetic disease (e.g. cold sores).

Signs

- Conjunctival redness
- Fine, branching ulceration which is beautifully highlighted by fluorescein staining
- Reduced corneal sensation in the affected eye.

Investigations

- The presence of virus can be confirmed by taking a swab for viral culture or detection of viral DNA using the polymerase chain reaction; however, most cases are diagnosed clinically and treated empirically.

Treatment

- Aciclovir ointment 5× daily until resolution. Topical steroids must *not* be given as they will make it worse.

Orbital cellulitis

Orbital cellulitis is an ophthalmic emergency in which infection penetrates beneath the orbital septum (post-septal), often from the adjacent air sinuses, and spreads back through the orbit damaging vital structures. It is both a sight-threatening and potentially a life-threatening condition (superficial infection of the skin around the eye is called periorbital or preseptal cellulitis).

Symptoms

- Frontal headache
- Fever
- Double vision
- Loss of vision

Signs

- Pyrexia
- Lid swelling and proptosis
- Limited ocular movements
- Reduced visual acuity

Investigations

Computed tomography (CT) of the orbit can confirm the extent of infection and involvement of sinuses. The organism may be identified from blood cultures and microscopy/culture of material gained during surgical drainage.

Treatment

Patients should be admitted for high-dose intravenous antibiotics, and may require surgical drainage of the involved area.

Acute anterior uveitis (iritis)

Acute anterior uveitis (inflammation of the iris; also known as iritis) is thought to be an autoimmune disease, and is commonly associated with ankylosing spondylitis, and other HLA-B27-related conditions. Recurrent episodes may cause glaucoma and cataract.

Typical presentation

Young adult with unilateral painful photophobic red eye but clear cornea.

Symptoms

- Unilateral
- Red eye
- Reduced vision
- Eye pain
- Photophobia
- May report previous episodes or associated systemic disease.

Signs

- Conjunctival redness (especially around the limbus).
- Small, irregular pupil due to adhesions between the iris and anterior lens capsule (posterior synechiae).
- Clumps of inflammatory cells ('keratic precipitates') may be seen stuck to the posterior surface of the cornea.
- Cloudy anterior chamber – this may be difficult to detect unless there is sufficient inflammation to cause a hypopyon (visible layer of inflammatory cells in the anterior chamber).

Investigations

Investigations are only indicated if the patient has symptoms suggestive of an associated disease such as ankylosing spondylitis.

Treatment

Acute anterior uveitis requires urgent treatment with topical corticosteroid and dilating drops.

Cataract

Although some degree of cataract (loss of transparency of the lens) is almost universal in those >65 years of age, it is only a problem when it is restricting the patient's activity. It is most commonly due to ageing, but it may be associated with ocular disease (e.g. uveitis), systemic disease (e.g. diabetes), drugs (e.g. systemic corticosteroids) or it may be inherited. It is the commonest cause of treatable blindness worldwide.

Typical presentation

Elderly patient with painless, gradually worsening vision without distortion.

Symptoms

- Gradual blurred/cloudy vision.
- Glare – not very common in the typical 'nuclear' pattern of cataract but seen where there are spoke-like opacities around the edge of the lens (known as 'cortical') or an opaque plate at the back of the lens ('posterior subcapsular').

Signs

- Grey/white pupil (viewed with pen-torch).
- Reduced red reflex (viewed with direct ophthalmoscope) – usually diffusely reduced, but spoke-like opacities may be seen if a cortical cataract is present.

Investigations

The diagnosis is clinically evident, but if the cataract is severe enough to warrant surgery an ophthalmologist will carry out biometric investigations (measurement of corneal curvature and axial length of the eye) to determine the power of prosthetic lens to insert.

Treatment

The cataract is removed surgically (phaecoemulsification). This involves removal of part of the anterior lens capsule (capsulorrhexis), ultrasonic removal of the lens nucleus, aspiration of peripheral (cortical) lens matter and insertion of a prosthetic intraocular lens; usually performed under local anaesthesia. One in every 1000 eyes may get severe postoperative infection (endophthalmitis).

Glaucoma

Glaucoma describes a group of eye conditions characterized by a progressive optic neuropathy and visual field loss, in which the intraocular pressure is sufficiently raised to impair normal optic nerve function. Glaucoma may present insidiously or acutely. In the more common primary open angle glaucoma, there is an asymptomatic sustained elevation in intraocular pressure which may cause gradual unnoticed loss of visual field over years, and is a significant cause of blindness worldwide.

IMPORTANT
Acute angle closure glaucoma is an ophthalmic emergency in which closure of the drainage angle causes a sudden symptomatic elevation of intraocular pressure which may rapidly damage the optic nerve.

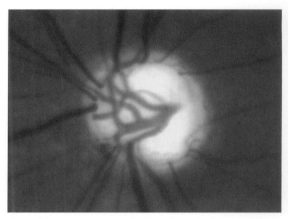

Figure 19.7 Disc photograph of a left optic disc with severe glaucomatous 'cupping' which is recorded in terms of its vertical cup:disc ratio. Cupping arises due to extensive loss of neural tissue, leaving only a thin remnant of healthy tissue around the edge of the disc.

- Raised intraocular pressure >21mmHg (detected on tonometry by optometrist or ophthalmologist).
- Visual field loss – detected by perimetry.
- The drainage angle is open i.e. no obvious obstruction to aqueous outflow (detected on gonioscopy by ophthalmologist).

Investigations

Detailed visual field testing by perimetry may demonstrate a pattern of field loss typical of glaucoma (arcuate scotoma) and will enable disease progression to be monitored.

Typical presentations

- Primary open angle glaucoma – referred by optometrist with elevated intraocular pressure after a routine 'eye-test'.
- Acute angle closure glaucoma – red, hard, severely painful eye(s) with a fixed semi-dilated pupil in a long-sighted patient.

Primary open angle glaucoma

Symptoms

Primary open angle glaucoma is asymptomatic until sufficiently advanced for field loss to be noticeable to the patient.

Signs

- Abnormal optic disc cupping – it is normal to have a small to moderate 'cup' (central white area where the blood vessels run into and out of the eye) to the optic disc, but a vertical cup:disc (C:D) ratio >0.5 or any documented increase in C:D ratio is suggestive of glaucomatous damage (Fig. 19.7).

Treatment

Intraocular pressure is controlled with a range of drops including prostaglandin agonists, β-blockers, carbonic anhydrase inhibitors and α_2-agonists. In resistant cases, laser or surgical treatment (trabeculectomy) is required.

Acute angle closure glaucoma

Symptoms

- Often unilateral
- Red eye(s)
- Reduced vision
- Haloes around lights
- Severe eye pain
- Nausea and vomiting.

Signs

- Conjunctival redness
- Cloudy cornea
- Mid-dilated, fixed pupil
- Drainage angle is closed (detected on gonioscopy by ophthalmologist) thereby preventing aqueous exiting the eye.

Treatment

Acute angle closure glaucoma is treated with topical and systemic drugs to lower the pressure, followed by a laser procedure to make a hole in the iris of both eyes. This acts as a bypass for fluid from the posterior chamber to get to the anterior chamber of the eye and prevents future episodes of angle closure.

Age-related macular degeneration

Age-related macular degeneration is the commonest cause of blindness in the older population (>65 years) in the Western world. Since it is primarily the macula (Fig. 19.8) that is affected, patients retain their peripheral vision and with it a variable level of independence. There are two forms: 'dry' AMD accounts for 90 per cent of cases and the more dramatic 'wet' (also known as neovascular) AMD accounts for 10 per cent.

Typical presentation

- Dry AMD – elderly patient with gradual loss of central vision usually in both eyes, often with distortion.

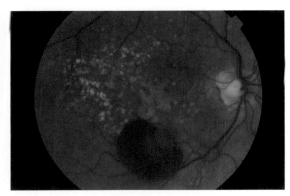

Figure 19.8 Right fundus photograph of a patient with age-related macular degeneration (AMD). This patient has characteristic changes of both dry AMD (yellow drusen and pale atrophic areas) and wet AMD (central scar and inferior haemorrhage).

- Wet AMD – elderly patient with sudden deterioration of central vision in one eye (but may also have features of/been diagnosed with dry AMD). The other eye may be involved later.

Dry AMD

Symptoms

- Bilateral.
- Gradual loss of central vision (central scotoma).
- Often starts with distortion.

Signs

- Yellowish spots around the macula (known as soft drusen).
- Atrophy of the macula.

Treatment

Treatments for dry AMD do not alter the course of the disease but revolve around optimizing the patient's remaining vision, such as using magnifiers.

Wet (neovascular) AMD

Symptoms

- Sudden deterioration of central vision (central scotoma).
- There is often distortion.

Signs

- Elevation, fluid or bleeding around the macula – indicates the presence of a choroidal neovascular membrane.
- With time the membrane scars over, known as a 'disciform scar'.
- Although major loss of vision may have only occurred in one eye, there is almost always evidence of predisposing dry AMD in both eyes.

Investigations

Diagnosis of a choroidal neovascular membrane and monitoring of disease/response to treatment is done with either optical coherence tomography or fundus fluorescein angiography.

Treatment

Treatments for wet AMD seek to reverse the neovascular process by blocking angiogenic factors (anti-VEGF agents – usually given by injection into the vitreous) or photodynamic therapy.

Diabetic retinopathy

Diabetes is the commonest cause of blindness in the younger population (<65 years) in the Western world. Diabetic retinopathy is a microvascular disease of the retinal circulation. In both type 1 and type 2 diabetes glycaemic control and blood pressure should be optimized to reduce progression. Progression of retinopathy to the proliferative stage is most commonly seen in type 1 diabetes, whereas maculopathy is more commonly a feature of type 2 diabetes.

> **CLINICAL PEARL**
> Regular screening by dilated funduscopy/fundal photography is an essential part of diabetic care. If there is no retinopathy or background retinopathy only, then the patient should continue to be screened annually; if there are preproliferative changes or maculopathy they should be referred to an ophthalmologist; if there are proliferative changes they should be referred to an ophthalmologist urgently.

Typical presentation

Asymptomatic patient referred by optometrist or general practitioner with worsening retinal signs.

Symptoms

- Bilateral.
- Usually asymptomatic until either maculopathy or vitreous haemorrhage.
- Gradual loss of vision – suggests diabetic maculopathy (especially if distortion) or cataract.
- Sudden loss of vision – most commonly vitreous haemorrhage secondary to proliferative diabetic retinopathy.

Signs

- Background diabetic retinopathy: microaneurysms, haemorrhages, exudates (usually termed 'hard exudates') (Fig. 19.9).
- Preproliferative retinopathy: cotton-wool spots (signs of ischaemia), venous beading, looping of vessels (Fig. 19.10).
- Proliferative: fine new vessels on disc or elsewhere; may be associated with vitreous haemorrhage,

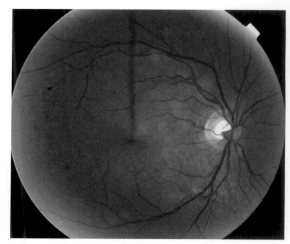

Figure 19.9 Right fundus photograph of a patient with background diabetic retinopathy. Note microaneurysms (red 'dots') and scattered blot haemorrhages (larger red 'spots').

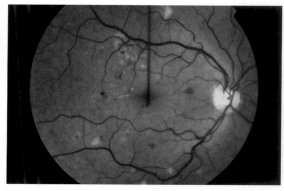

Figure 19.10 Right fundus photograph of a patient with preproliferative diabetic retinopathy. Note widespread cotton wool spots (white fuzzy spots), and more widespread/larger blot haemorrhages.

fibrosis and retinal detachment (and subsequent blindness if untreated) (Fig. 19.11).
- Maculopathy: oedema, exudates, microaneurysms and haemorrhages at the macula (Fig. 19.12).

Investigations

- Optical coherence tomography is useful for diagnosing macular oedema.
- Fundus fluorescein angiography is useful for diagnosing macular oedema, macular ischaemia and new vessels.

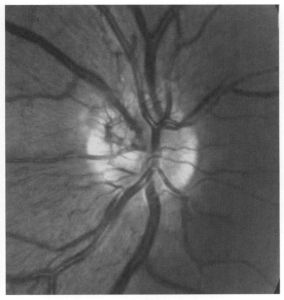

Figure 19.11 Right fundus photograph of a patient with proliferative diabetic retinopathy. Note fronds of fine new vessels in the superior half of the optic disc.

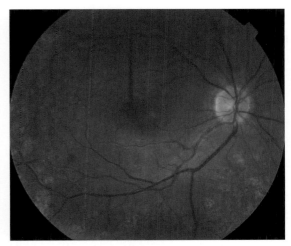

Figure 19.13 Right fundus photograph of a patient who has previously had proliferative diabetic retinopathy which has been successfully treated with pan-retinal photocoagulation and improvement of their glycaemic control. Note peripheral laser scars (pigmented areas) and that signs of severe disease (such as new vessels or cotton wool spots) have resolved.

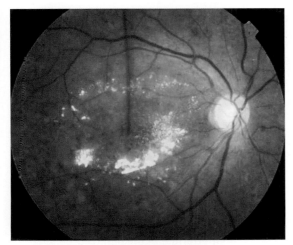

Figure 19.12 Right fundus photograph of a patient with diabetic maculopathy. Note exudates (yellow circinate or ring of exudates) around the macula.

Treatment

The first priority is to prevent retinopathy progressing by controlling risk factors. Proliferative retinopathy requires widespread laser treatment (panretinal photocoagulation, Fig. 19.13). Maculopathy is treated by a combination of laser, corticosteroids and anti-VEGF treatments.

Anterior ischaemic optic neuropathy (AION)

Ischaemia of the anterior part of the optic nerve (i.e. the optic disc) arises from occlusion of the short posterior ciliary arteries. It presents as sudden loss of vision in older patients. It is an emergency since it may be due to life-threatening giant cell arteritis, although it is more commonly due to atherosclerosis.

Typical presentation

Middle-aged/elderly person presenting with sudden painless loss of vision in one eye.

Symptoms

- Unilateral (usually)
- Sudden painless loss of vision

Additional symptoms may point to the underlying cause.

- Features of giant cell arteritis include temporal pain/tenderness, jaw claudication, limb girdle stiffness, night sweats, and weight loss.

- In the absence of the above features atherosclerosis is the more likely diagnosis and would be further supported by the presence of known risk factors (smoking, hypertension, hypercholesterolaemia, diabetes) or other atherosclerotic complications (e.g. strokes, angina/myocardial infarcts, etc).

Signs

- Severe reduction in visual acuity e.g. perception of light.
- Relative afferent pupillary defect.
- Swollen optic disc.
- Disc swelling may be segmental (usually superior) in which case there will be a corresponding inverted visual field defect (i.e. inferior if superior disc swelling).
- Other features of the disc which may be present are pallor and/or surrounding flame haemorrhages.
- If arteritic, fellow eye may become involved in 70 per cent (unusual for fellow eye to be involved if non-arteritic).

Investigations

Giant cell arteritis must be excluded by performing urgent tests for erythrocyte sedimentation rate and C-reactive protein; raised levels of these inflammatory markers support the diagnosis of giant cell arteritis. The gold standard of diagnosis is a superficial temporal artery biopsy.

Treatment

Urgent treatment with high-dose corticosteroids is required.

Retinal vascular occlusions

Occlusion of retinal vessels according to which part of the circulation is affected, i.e. either venous or arterial. They are further classified according to whether the blockage is in a central vessel or in a branch vessel. 'Branch' occlusions may only cause a local field defect whereas 'central' occlusions usually lead to profound drop in visual acuity. Most venous and arterial occlusions are associated with atherosclerotic risk factors, although arterial occlusions may also be caused by giant cell arteritis.

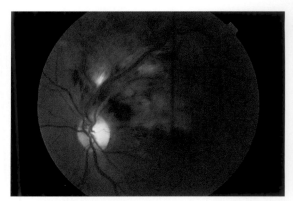

Figure 19.14 Left fundus photograph of a patient with branch retinal vein occlusion. Note extensive haemorrhages and cotton wool spots along the superotemporal arcade.

Central retinal vein occlusion (CRVO) and branch retinal vein occlusion (BRVO)

Symptoms

- Sudden loss of vision (CRVO; or BRVO affecting the macula, Fig. 19.14).
- Asymptomatic or symptomatic field defect (BRVO).

Signs

- CRVO: swollen disc, engorged retinal veins, widespread haemorrhages.
- BRVO: similar changes confined to one sector of the retina.

Treatment

Treatment ranges from observation to laser treatment, anti-VEGF therapies and corticosteroids.

Central retinal artery occlusion (CRAO) and branch retinal arteriole occlusion (BRAO)

Symptoms

- Sudden severe loss of vision (CRAO).
- Asymptomatic or symptomatic field defect (BRAO).

Signs

- CRAO: afferent pupillary defect, pale retina with cherry red spot at the macula, segmentation ('cattle-trucking') of blood in the vessels.

- BRAO: embolus may be visible in a branch arteriole, with pallor of the distal retina.

Treatment

If CRAO is seen within 8–12 hours an ophthalmologist may attempt medical or surgical treatment to lower the pressure in the eye to try to dislodge the embolus and restore the circulation. In all cases consider and exclude the underlying possibility of giant cell arteritis (see above).

Retinal detachment

Retinal detachment is the separation of the neurosensory retina (i.e. the neuronal/photoreceptor layer) from the retinal pigment epithelium. It is a fairly common ophthalmic emergency with an incidence of 1 in 10 000/year.

It usually arises as a result of posterior vitreous detachment – a normal ageing process in which the shrinking vitreous humour detaches from the surrounding neurosensory retina. In most individuals this occurs without a problem other than noticing a few new floaters. In some people, however, especially those who are myopic (short-sighted) or with certain retinal abnormalities the detaching vitreous tears a hole in the retina allowing influx of fluid between the neurosensory layer and the retinal pigment epithelium.

Symptoms

- Unilateral
- Flashes
- Floaters: tadpoles, cobwebs
- Field loss: inverted i.e. superior field loss with inferior detachment
- Reduced vision: profound if a 'macular off' detachment i.e. where the detachment has extended to involve the macula.

Signs

- Detached retina appears grey and balloons forward into the vitreous.
- Sometimes there is associated vitreous haemorrhage.

Investigations

Although usually obvious clinically, ultrasound can confirm the diagnosis and is useful where vitreous haemorrhage obscures the view.

Treatment

Retinal detachments require surgical repair that may be external (suturing a piece of plastic on the sclera to push it towards the retina enabling the retina to reattach) or internal (removal of vitreous gel – vitrectomy); retinal tears detected before the retina has detached can be sealed by laser treatment.

Chemical injury

A common ophthalmic emergency where time is critical and irrigation takes priority over anything else. Although both alkalis and acids can cause severe injuries, alkalis penetrate deeper and tend to result in worse injuries.

Symptoms

- Red eye
- Reduced vision
- Eye pain
- Photophobia
- History of chemical contact with eye

Signs

- Conjunctival redness
- Areas of abnormal conjunctival whiteness – this is a sign of a severe injury which causes vessel occlusion
- Epithelial loss (stains with fluorescein)
- Cloudy cornea

Treatment

1. Irrigate copiously with normal saline (or water if normal saline not available) for at least 30 minutes or until neutral pH.
2. Refer urgently to ophthalmologist.
3. Ophthalmologist will consider admission (depends on extent of burn), and treat with topical and oral vitamin C, cycloplegia, topical steroids, antibiotics and stem cell transplantation.

SUMMARY

History

- Common presenting complaints include: uncomfortable/red eyes, loss of vision, flashes and floaters, and double vision.

- For uncomfortable/red eyes, grittiness, itchiness or a foreign body sensation usually indicate ocular surface problems such as conjunctivitis.
- Severe 'aching' eye pain suggests serious eye pathology such as acute angle closure glaucoma or scleritis.
- Photophobia is most commonly seen with acute anterior uveitis or corneal disease (ulcers or trauma).
- Sudden loss of vision is usually due to a vascular event (e.g. retinal vessel occlusions, anterior ischaemic optic neuropathy, 'wet' AMD).
- Gradual loss of vision is common in the ageing population. It is frequently due to cataract (generalized, i.e. affects central and peripheral field), primary open angle glaucoma (peripheral field loss) or 'dry' AMD (central field loss).
- Recent-onset flashes and floaters should be presumed to be retinal tear/detachment.
- Double vision may be monocular (both images from the same eye) or binocular (different images from each eye). Binocular double vision is serious, commonly arising from a cranial nerve III, IV or VI palsy.

Examination

- Vital examination skills include: measuring visual acuity, examining pupil responses to light, assessing visual fields by confrontation, systematic observation of the front of the eye and ophthalmoscopy.
- Measuring visual acuity is usually performed with the Snellen chart being read at 6 m for each eye in turn. If they can read the line marked '6' they have normal '6/6' vision; if they can only read the top letter (marked '60') then they only have 6/60 vision.

- Tests of pupillary responses to light include the direct, the consensual and the swinging flashlight test. The swinging flashlight test is the most sensitive clinical test of optic nerve damage.
- When examining the front of the eye, a drop of fluorescein is very helpful in highlighting areas of epithelial damage (ulcers, trauma).
- Ophthalmoscopy is a vital skill which rewards practice and preparation. Assessment will include quality of the red reflex, features of the optic disc (cup:disc ratio, colour, contour), retinal blood vessels, peripheral retina and finally macula.
- And finally, even if you cannot confirm the diagnosis on examination, the following presentations are sufficiently serious to warrant urgent referral to an ophthalmologist: sudden loss of vision, severe 'aching' eye pain, new-onset flashes and floaters, new-onset binocular diplopia.

FURTHER READING

Denniston AK, Murray PI. 2009. *Oxford handbook of ophthalmology*, 2nd edn. Oxford: Oxford University Press.

Forrester JV, Dick AD, McMenamin PG, Roberts F. 2007. *The eye: basic sciences in practice*, 3rd edn. Edinburgh: Saunders.

Kanski J. 2007. *Clinical ophthalmology: a systematic approach*, 6th edn. Oxford: Butterworth-Heinemann.

20

EAR, NOSE AND THROAT

Declan Costello

EAR

Presenting symptoms

Hearing loss

Hearing loss is the most common symptom relating to the ear. When taking a history, the following features will be important in reaching a diagnosis:

- age – presbyacusis (age-related degeneration of the hair cells of the inner ear) is very common over the age of 65, and is the most common cause of hearing loss
- speed of onset – a hearing loss that occurs over hours or days is more likely to be due to an acute inner ear pathology such as vascular insufficiency or a viral insult. Glue ear may also present in this way
- laterality – are both ears equally affected? Presbyacusis most commonly affects both ears equally, but an inner ear pathology is more likely to be unilateral
- tinnitus is often present with a hearing loss, and if it is bilateral, it is rarely an indicator of any sinister aetiology
- vertigo – if the hearing loss is sudden in onset and is associated with vertigo (an illusion of movement, see below), suspect inner ear pathology.

Dizziness/vertigo

It is useful, and often very difficult, to attempt to get a clear description of their 'dizziness' from the patient. Encourage the patient to give an exact description, such as 'I feel light-headed' or 'I feel the room spinning round'. These descriptors may point to a cause of the dysequilibrium. The following are useful descriptors:

- 'I feel light-headed when I stand up.' This is classic of postural hypotension, and it will be useful to take the patient's blood pressure when lying and standing to check for a postural drop

Table 20.1 Diagnostic clues from the duration of vertigo attacks

Duration of vertigo attacks	Most likely diagnosis
Seconds to minutes	Benign paroxysmal positional vertigo (BPPV)
Hours to days	Ménière's disease
Days to weeks	Acute vestibular insult

- 'I feel the room spinning around.' This is a good description of true rotational vertigo, and often points to inner ear pathology. True vertigo will make the patient feel very nauseous and (s)he may well vomit. In a vertiginous patient, ask:
  - How long do the spells of vertigo last? This may give clues as to the cause of the vertigo (Table 20.1)
  - Is there any change in hearing? Ménière's disease is a triad of symptoms consisting of vertigo attacks accompanied by unilateral hearing loss and tinnitus
  - Are there any triggers to an attack? Benign paroxysmal positional vertigo (BPPV) typically is started by sudden rotation of the head, such as rolling over in bed
- 'I feel generally unsteady.' This may be seen in multifactorial unsteadiness.

Tinnitus

Tinnitus is a subjective sensation of noise in the absence of external auditory stimuli. Tinnitus is usually high-pitched, described variously as hissing, whining, rushing or whirring. There is little in the description of its quality that helps in finding a cause, but it is important to exclude **pulsatile** tinnitus: if the pulsations are in time with the patient's heart beat, consider a vascular cause. This might include carotid stenosis or a glomus tumour.

IMPORTANT

Tinnitus often accompanies hearing loss, and as such is usually bilateral. If the tinnitus is unilateral, it is important to exclude a vestibular schwannoma (also known as an acoustic neuroma), which may cause either a unilateral sensorineural hearing loss or unilateral tinnitus.

Ear discharge

Ear discharge may be due to disease of the external ear canal (otitis externa) or of the middle ear when a perforation is present (*active chronic otitis media*, previously termed *chronic suppurative otitis media* (CSOM)). Certain types of ear surgery may predispose the patient to discharge, so ask about previous ear operations such as mastoidectomy. Bleeding from the ear is seldom sinister, and is more often a reflection of local trauma (such as with cotton buds) or a grossly inflamed and friable ear canal or middle ear.

Ear pain (otalgia)

Otalgia has numerous causes. In the majority of cases, the pathology will be related to the ear itself, but it is important to remember that referred pain can cause ear symptoms. Pain from the temporomandibular joint typically gives discomfort around the ear during eating, and is mimicked by palpating the joint.

Pain may also be referred from the

- oral cavity via the trigeminal nerve (cranial nerve V)
- pharynx via the glossopharyngeal nerve (cranial nerve IX)
- larynx or hypopharynx via the vagus nerve (cranial nerve X).

IMPORTANT

Constant, dull, unremitting, unilateral ear pain, particularly in a smoker, should alert the clinician to the possibility of a malignancy of the upper aerodigestive tract, a complex of organs that make up the upper respiratory and upper digestive tract, comprising lips and mouth tissues, tongue, nose, throat, vocal cords and portions of the oesophagus and trachea.

Rest of the history

- A family history is important to note: otosclerosis, which is an unusual cause of hearing loss, may be passed down the maternal side of the family.
- An occupational history is important, noting noise exposure as a possible cause of hearing loss. Ask the patient what (if any) ear protection was worn when exposed to any occupational or recreational noise.
- Maintaining balance is only in part under the control of the inner ear: achievement of balance is also reliant on peripheral sensation, eyesight and proprioception. Question patients with dizziness about diabetes (peripheral neuropathy may cause poor peripheral sensation), about joint disease, and about their visual acuity.
- A detailed otological history is essential: previous ear surgery may predispose to ear discharge and any current or previous ear discharge should be noted. A past history of numerous ear infections in childhood may lead to hearing loss in adult life if ossicular damage has occurred.
- Take a drug history – certain drugs such as gentamicin are ototoxic and their use should be asked about.

Examination

Otoscopic examination

Examine the external ear for evidence of erythema or scars, paying particular attention to the postaural sulcus where scars may be hidden. Then examine the ear with an otoscope (auriscope). Hold the otoscope like a pen, in the right hand to examine the right ear and the left hand to examine the left ear (Fig. 20.1). Gently rest the little finger of the hand on the patient's cheek to avoid sudden movements. With the free hand, pull the pinna up and backwards to straighten out the ear canal.

Be methodical when examining with an otoscope: make careful note of the ear canal, and all the quadrants of the tympanic membrane (Fig. 20.2). It is often possible to see some of the ossicles through the drum; this is normal. If wax is present, this may be removed by microsuction or syringing. Infected debris should only be cleared with suction under an operating microscope.

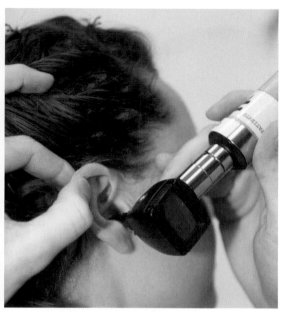

Figure 20.1 Demonstration of use of an otoscope (auriscope).

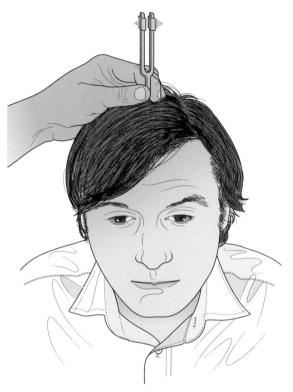

Figure 20.3 Weber's tuning fork test.

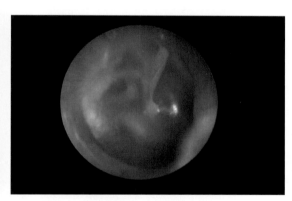

Figure 20.2 Normal tympanic membrane.

 IMPORTANT

If unilateral glue ear (otitis media with effusion) is found, examine the postnasal space to exclude a tumour obstructing the eustachian tube orifice.

Tuning fork tests

Tuning fork tests are useful in clinical practice to help to discern whether a patient has a conductive or sensorineural hearing loss. In **Weber's test** (Fig. 20.3), place the base of a ringing tuning fork on the centre of the patient's head. If the patient's hearing is symmetrical, they will hear the sound equally from both ears. If the patient has a unilateral sensorineural hearing loss, the patient will locate the sound to the *contralateral* ear. If the patient has a unilateral conductive hearing loss, the patient will locate the sound to the *ipsilateral* ear.

In **Rinne's test** (Fig. 20.4), hold the tines of a ringing tuning fork in front of the ear, then place the base of the tuning fork on the mastoid process. If the patient says that the air conduction is louder than the bone conduction, Rinne's test is said to be *positive*. This is normal. To avoid this slightly confusing nomenclature, in practice it is easier to document 'air conduction > bone conduction'.

Balance testing

Tests in a patient presenting with vertigo should include a complete examination of all the cranial nerves, as well as tests of the cerebellar system.

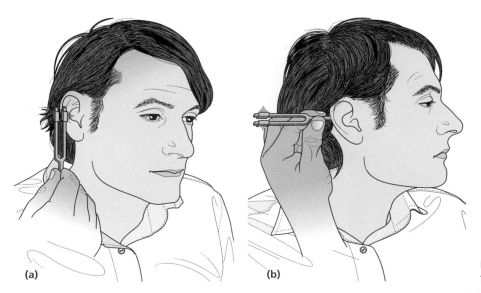

(a)   (b)

Figure 20.4 Rinne's tuning fork test.

Examination of the cranial nerves is covered in Chapter 12. Specific tests of balance should include:

- **Romberg's test**: ask the patient to stand, with the feet together, with their eyes closed. If the patient sways to one side or the other, it is said to be positive. It is a relatively non-specific test, and may be positive in inner ear pathology or in other causes of dizziness.
- **Dix–Hallpike test** (Fig. 20.5): this is a specific test for BPPV. This test requires a good deal of cooperation from the patient. Sit the patient on a couch. Turn the head 45° to the right and then lie the patient briskly down on the couch, allowing the neck to extend so that the head is 30° below the horizontal. Tell the patient to keep their eyes open, and observe the eyes closely for nystagmus. Rotatory nystagmus, accompanied by a subjective sensation of vertigo, is pathognomonic of BPPV.

Facial nerve assessment

Examination of the ear should include an assessment of facial nerve function. Weakness of the facial nerve is graded by the House–Brackmann scale (Table 20.2).

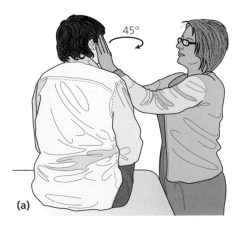

45°

(a)

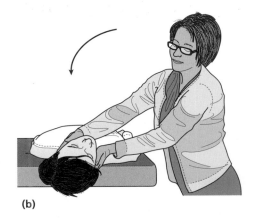

(b)

Figure 20.5 Dix–Hallpike test for benign paroxysmal positional vertigo.

Table 20.2 House–Brackmann scale

I	Normal
II	Normal tone and symmetry at rest; slight weakness on close inspection; good to moderate movement of forehead; complete eye closure with minimum effort; slight asymmetry of mouth with movement
III	Normal tone and symmetry at rest; obvious but not disfiguring facial asymmetry; synkinesis may be noticeable but not severe ± hemifacial spasm or contracture; slight to moderate forehead motion; **complete eye closure with effort**; slight weakness of mouth with maximum effort
IV	Normal tone and symmetry at rest; asymmetry is disfiguring or results in obvious facial weakness; no perceptible forehead movement; **incomplete eye closure**; asymmetrical motion of mouth with maximum effort
V	Asymmetrical facial appearance at rest; slight, barely noticeable movement; no forehead movement; incomplete eye closure; slight movement of mouth with effort
VI	No facial function perceptible

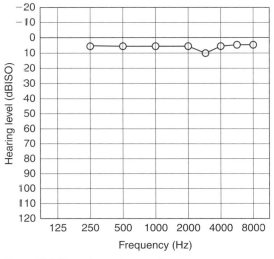
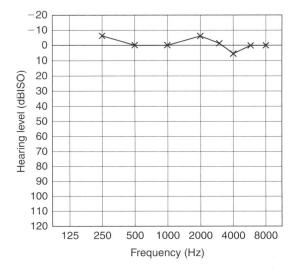

Figure 20.6 Normal pure tone audiogram.

Investigations

- A *pure tone audiogram* (Fig. 20.6) is mandatory to complete the examination of the ear. This will distinguish between conductive and sensorineural hearing loss and may give further valuable information about the potential cause of the hearing loss. An audiogram is also required in any patient with vertigo, as conditions such as Ménière's disease may present with hearing loss.
- *Tympanometry* tests the compliance of the tympanic membrane. A peaked tympanogram (type A, Fig. 20.7) is normal and demonstrates normal movement of the tympanic membrane when air pressure is applied to it. A flat tympanogram (type B), when accompanied by a normal canal volume, indicates that the tympanic membrane's movement is limited, often as a result of 'glue' (otitis media with effusion (OME)) in the middle ear. A tympanogram is performed in seconds and can be helpful in confirming the diagnosis of glue ear.
- If a unilateral sensorineural hearing loss is found, or if the patient complains of unilateral tinnitus, a vestibular schwannoma (acoustic neuroma) should be suspected. *Magnetic resonance imaging* (MRI) of the internal auditory meatuses (IAMs) will confirm or refute the presence of a tumour in the cerebellopontine angle.

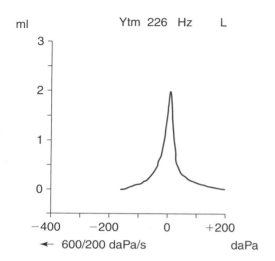

EARCANAL VOLUME: 1.4

	daPa	ml
TYMP 1:	10	2.0
GRADIENT:	35	daPa
REFLEX:	I 1000 Hz	YES

Figure 20.7 Normal tympanogram ('peaked').

- If mastoid or middle ear disease such as cholesteatoma is suspected, *fine-cut computed tomography* (CT) of the temporal bones will guide the clinician as to the extent of the disease and the degree of bone erosion in crucial areas such as the facial nerve and the semicircular canals.

> **SMALL PRINT**
> More specialized tests of hearing may be performed, but are seldom required. Speech audiometry, for example, is useful if a patient's hearing loss is suspected of being non-organic.

Common diagnoses

Glue ear

The most common cause of hearing loss in children is glue ear. This presents with speech problems, poor attention at school and behavioural problems. Teachers or parents may volunteer a hearing loss. Examination shows a dull tympanic membrane, sometimes with evidence of bubbles under the drum (Fig. 20.8). The audiogram will show a con-

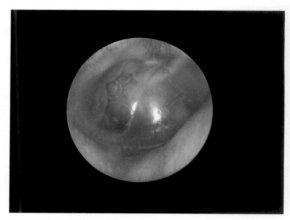

Figure 20.8 Glue ear with bubbles visible under the tympanic membrane.

ductive hearing loss and tympanometry will show flat traces (type B).

Presbyacusis

This is the most common type of hearing loss in adults, and is common over the age of 65. Apart from a confirmatory pure tone audiogram, no specific tests are required.

Benign paroxysmal positional vertigo

This is a common cause of vertigo. The patient will complain of vertigo when moving the head suddenly. The vertigo lasts seconds or a minute and then fades. There is no change in the hearing. A Dix–Hallpike test is diagnostic (see Fig. 20.5, p. 354), and Epley's manoeuvre can rapidly and easily cure this condition.

Ménière's disease

This is a condition characterized by a triad of attacks of tinnitus, vertigo, and worsening sensorineural hearing loss. Many patients also complain of a sensation of aural 'fullness' during attacks. The attacks last hours or days. Between attacks, the patients have no vertigo, but may have underlying progressive sensorineural hearing loss.

Vestibular insult

An acute vestibular event, such as a viral or vascular problem, will present with vertigo that lasts days

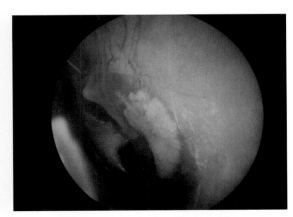

Figure 20.9 Tympanic membrane with perforation and plaque of tympanosclerosis.

or weeks. This is often labelled as 'labyrinthitis', but might equally be called 'vestibular neuronitis' or 'acute vestibular insult'. Rather than the affected ear improving, the brain will adapt to the abnormal information from the affected ear, and compensation will occur over a matter of weeks or months.

Ear discharge

In the presence of ear discharge, it is often difficult to make a diagnosis, but the short-term use of antibiotic drops may settle the discharge enough to allow better inspection of the tympanic membrane. Try to distinguish between disease with an intact tympanic membrane (i.e. otitis externa) and disease with a perforation (i.e. active chronic otitis media, perhaps with cholesteatoma) (Fig. 20.9).

Acute facial nerve palsy

Sudden-onset unilateral facial weakness is a common ENT emergency and must be treated promptly. The history should document ear symptoms (discharge, hearing loss), history of ear surgery, lumps in the head and neck and associated symptoms of pain or dysaesthesia. The list of differential diagnoses is extensive, but the most common are:

- Ramsay Hunt syndrome (herpes zoster oticus) – characterized by pain and vesicles around the ear, this condition should respond promptly to antivirals and steroids

- parotid masses – facial palsy in the presence of a parotid mass is virtually pathognomonic of malignancy
- infection – facial nerve palsy may occur in the presence of acute otitis media. In these circumstances, emergency ENT treatment should be sought
- Bell's palsy – having excluded all other causes of facial palsy, Bell's palsy may be diagnosed. It is a facial palsy of unknown aetiology and is thought to be due to a virally induced immune response. Treatment is with steroids and aciclovir.

Acute sensorineural hearing loss

Patients will occasionally present with a short duration unilateral hearing loss. It is important to establish whether this hearing loss is sensorineural or conductive in nature, and the tuning fork tests outlined above should achieve this.

> **IMPORTANT**
>
> A genuine acute sensorineural hearing loss is an ENT emergency and should be referred immediately to the ENT team.

NOSE

Presenting symptoms

Nasal obstruction

The commonest feature of nasal pathology is nasal obstruction. Ascertain whether one side or both are affected, and when the symptoms occur: a constant nasal obstruction that affects just one nostril, for example, is more likely to be due to deviation of the nasal septum, whereas bilateral obstruction that is worse at night may represent an allergy to house dust mite.

Nasal obstruction may be seasonal, so ask if the symptoms are worse in the hayfever season, as this is suggestive of allergic rhinitis.

Facial pain

This is the one of the cardinal symptoms of sinusitis. In acute sinusitis, it classically occurs in conjunction with nasal obstruction, malaise and foul rhinorrhoea. Facial 'fullness' (sometimes interpreted by patients as pain) may suggest chronic sinusitis, as with nasal polyps. In the absence of any other symptoms of sinusitis, consider other causes (such as dental pain and atypical facial pain).

Facial fullness

A sensation of 'being bunged up' or of facial fullness is rather non-specific, and may be seen in any nasal pathology. Try to distinguish between actual pain and fullness.

Rhinorrhoea

Discharge from the nose may be clear (suggesting coryza rhinitis) or foul (suggesting infective rhinosinusitis) or constant and water-like (suggesting a cerebrospinal fluid (CSF) leak). Bleeding from the nose is usually from Little's area on the anterior part of the nasal septum. However, chronic bloody discharge from the nose, especially if unilateral, suggests more sinister pathology. In this case, a tumour should be ruled out.

> **IMPORTANT**
> Exclude a tumour in patients presenting with a chronic bloody nasal discharge, especially if unilateral.

Hyposmia/anosmia

The sense of smell may be diminished (hyposmia) or absent (anosmia). These are classically seen in nasal polyposis. There may also be an unpleasant smell perceived by the patient (cachosmia), suggestive of infective rhinosinusitis.

Postnasal drip

Patients frequently complain of a sensation of discharge that drips down the back of their throat. Some patients will call this 'catarrh'. In combination with nasal obstruction, this may be due to chronic sinusitis.

Other symptoms

Sneezing commonly accompanies allergic rhinitis, particularly in the hayfever season. Whistling from the nose suggests a septal perforation, which should be visible on anterior rhinoscopy (see below).

Rest of the history

Question any patient with nasal symptoms about previous nasal surgery or trauma. A history of atopy or asthma may suggest an allergic rhinitis or polyposis, as may a positive family history for these conditions. Aspirin sensitivity, in conjunction with asthma and nasal polyposis, is known as Samter's triad.

Examination

Examination of the nose should start with an inspection of the external nose to assess for scars and obvious cosmetic deformity. A discussion of the detailed cosmetic assessment is beyond the scope of this chapter, but it should be possible quickly to assess for nasal bone deviation, columella retraction (the columella is the vertical soft tissue column in between the nostrils that helps provide support to the nasal tip) or supra-tip depression ('saddle nose').

Start by gently pushing up the tip of the nasal septum. If the caudal portion of the septal cartilage is dislocated, pushing up the tip of the nose will cause the cartilage to prolapse into that nostril. This is often accompanied by a deflection of the cartilage to the opposite side further back on the septum.

> **CLINICAL PEARL**
> It is useful (particularly in children) to hold a metal spatula below the nostrils to assess for 'fogging' of the metal. This indicates reasonable nasal airflow.

Proceed to examination with the Thudichum speculum (Fig. 20.10). Examine the nasal septum and the lateral nasal wall, including the inferior turbinate. The middle turbinate is usually also visible with a Thudichum speculum. If a Thudichum speculum is not available, an auriscope may be used.

Full examination of the nose is completed with examination of the internal nose with an endoscope (either a Hopkins' rod rigid endoscope (Fig. 20.11) or a flexible fibreoptic endoscope). Topical anaesthesia (most often lidocaine and phenylephrine) may be used before endoscopy, but is often not required.

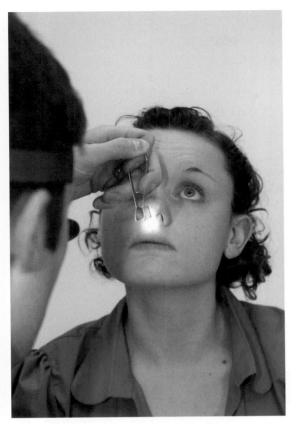

Figure 20.10 Nasal examination with Thudichum speculum.

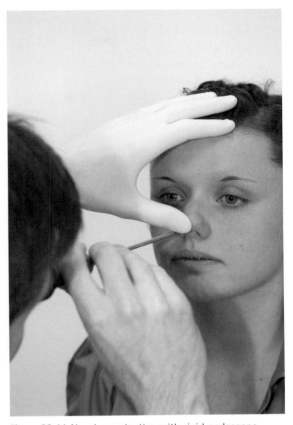

Figure 20.11 Nasal examination with rigid endoscope.

Manoeuvre the endoscope to examine the superior, middle and inferior meatus (below their respective turbinates) as well as examining the postnasal space.

Examine the mouth for evidence of postnasal drip: this will be seen as a trail of mucus or pus on the posterior wall of the oropharynx.

Investigations

Plain X-rays

There is no longer any role for plain X-rays in assessment of the nose or paranasal sinuses. Fracture of the nasal bones is a clinical diagnosis not requiring radiological confirmation, and plain X-rays of the sinuses give very little useful information.

Computed tomography

Computed tomography is now the accepted imaging modality for the paranasal sinuses (Fig. 20.12). It

gives excellent bony definition, and shows soft tissue thickening very clearly.

> **CLINICAL PEARL**
>
> Any patient undergoing cosmetic surgery should have high-quality photographs taken. This will serve as a template for the operation and will be used to monitor postoperative progress.

Allergy testing

In a patient with suspected allergic rhinitis, allergy tests may be useful so the patient can be given advice about allergen avoidance measures. Many ENT departments undertake skin-prick testing: a small volume of a set of known allergens is injected into the dermis and any 'weal and flare' reaction is taken as a positive response to that allergen. Blood tests

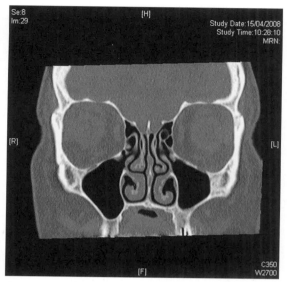

Figure 20.12 Normal CT scan of paranasal sinuses (coronal section).

may also be used: the RAST (radioallergosorbent test) detects specific circulating IgE antibodies.

Other rhinological tests

The University of Pennsylvania Smell Identification Test (UPSIT) may be used to measure olfaction objectively. It is particularly valuable in identifying patients who are feigning anosmia.

> **SMALL PRINT**
>
> Objective tests of nasal airflow (such as acoustic rhinometry, peak expiratory nasal flow and rhinomanometry) are largely of academic interest, and not widely used in clinical practice.

Common diagnoses

Some of the more common nasal pathologies are summarized in Table 20.3.

Deviation of the nasal septum

Nasal septal deflection is often not obvious on external inspection of the nose. However, with a headlight and a Thudichum speculum, the diagnosis is easily made. Deviation of the nasal septum is usually post-traumatic, but the trauma may have occurred in childhood, so may not be remembered by the patient.

Rhinitis

The presence of an oedematous nasal mucosa, along with copious secretions, denotes rhinitis.

Nasal polyps

Nasal polyps are usually visible just with a headlight and a nasal speculum (Fig. 20.13). The inferior turbinate is often mistaken for a polyp, but the pale grey

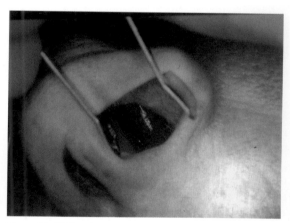

Figure 20.13 Nasal polyp.

Table 20.3 Common nasal pathologies

Disease	Nasal obstruction	Rhinorrhoea	Sense of smell	Facial symptoms
Deviated nasal septum	Constant, unilateral	No	Normal	No
Rhinitis	Intermittent, bilateral	Clear	Normal, possibly hyposmia	None, possibly fullness
Acute sinusitis	Constant, bilateral	Offensive, mucopurulent	Hyposmia/anosmia	Pain and fullness
Sinonasal polyposis	Constant, bilateral	Constant, thick	Anosmia	Fullness
Tumour	Constant, unilateral	Mucopurulent, bloody, unilateral	Normal	Fullness and pain

colour of a polyp is quite different from the pink hue of a turbinate.

Acute bacterial sinusitis

Acute sinusitis presents with nasal obstruction, facial pain (and often redness) and offensive nasal discharge. The patient will have general malaise, and may have a previous history of nasal problems. Examination will show a swollen nasal mucosa with pus in the nasal cavity. The vast majority of cases of sinusitis are self-limiting, or require just oral antibiotics and nasal decongestants. But infection can traverse the very thin lamina papyracea (between the ethmoid sinuses and the orbit, see Fig. 20.12) to cause orbital cellulitis, or a subperiosteal abscess. Proptosis will occur, and the eyelid will become swollen. This is an ENT emergency, and surgery is required within hours to save the eye.

THROAT

Presenting symptoms

Globus sensation

Patients frequently present with an unpleasant sensation of a 'feeling of something in the throat', sometimes abbreviated to FOSIT. As an isolated symptom, this is very unlikely to represent any sinister pathology, but it is important to take the complaint seriously and exclude malignancy. Ask the patient if they have had any difficulty swallowing (dysphagia), voice change or weight loss.

Dysphagia

Patients with dysphagia are usually reasonably accurate in identifying the level of obstruction. Ask them to point on their neck to the location they believe to be the problem.

Pain

Constant, unremitting pain, particularly if it is interfering with sleep, is a sinister symptom, and should be investigated urgently. Because of their shared neural pathways, ear pain may be referred from the oral cavity (including floor of mouth or tongue), nasopharynx, oropharynx, hypopharynx or larynx (Fig. 20.14).

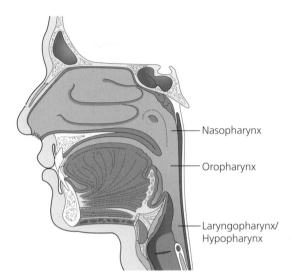

Figure 20.14 Subdivisions of the pharynx.

Recurrent infections

Recurrent tonsillitis is probably the most common reason for referral to the ENT clinic. Episodes of pain on swallowing (odynophagia), accompanied by fever, malaise, and exudate on the tonsils constitute tonsillitis. More than four to five episodes in a year merits a referral to the ENT department for consideration for a tonsillectomy. A peritonsillar abscess (*quinsy*) arises as a complication of acute tonsillitis. Aspiration of the abscess is easy to perform and rapidly resolves the patient's symptoms.

Hoarseness

It is important to ask if the symptoms are constant or fluctuating: a voice that is occasionally hoarse is less likely to have a sinister cause than one which is constantly hoarse. Laryngeal tumours may cause dysphagia, so ask about difficulty swallowing and weight loss. Again, ask about throat and ear pain, mindful of referred otalgia from the pharynx and larynx.

Snoring

Snoring can be enormously disruptive to domestic life, and can cause genuine relationship problems. Ask the patient if they snore every night. Do they snore in every position, or just when sleeping on their back? Ask about alcohol consumption late at night. Smoking causes chronic irritation and can exacerbate snoring. Patients who are overweight are significantly more likely to snore, and should be encouraged to lose weight.

It is important to try to exclude obstructive sleep apnoea. Ask the patient's partner if they witness episodes of apnoea: they are very characteristic and very alarming to the partner. The Epworth Sleepiness Score is a patient questionnaire that assesses for daytime somnolence. If the score is elevated (over 10), suspect sleep apnoea and perform a sleep study.

Dry mouth

Most often, a patient with dryness of the oral cavity will simply require advice on oral hygiene and hydration. Occasionally, however, the symptoms persist, and Sjögren's disease should be suspected. This diagnosis is confirmed by taking biopsies of the minor salivary glands, which show histological evidence of periductal fibrosis and lymphocytic infiltration.

Rest of the history

Many of the salient features of the history are covered above, but to summarize, enquire about:

- hoarseness
- dysphagia
- weight loss
- ear pain
- throat pain
- haemoptysis.

CLINICAL PEARL

The combination of **smoking** and **alcohol** is a potent carcinogen for head and neck cancers, and a detailed history should be noted.

Laryngopharyngeal reflux, in which gastric contents reflux into the larynx and pharynx, is increasingly recognized as a causative factor in ENT disease. Ask about heartburn, an acidic taste in the mouth, and chronic cough. Reflux is characteristically worse at night, so ask about diurnal variation of symptoms.

An occupational history is important: for example, professional voice users, such as singers, clergy, barristers and call centre workers, rely heavily on

their voices and their patterns of voice usage may be inappropriate.

Examination

Good illumination is mandatory for a thorough examination of the mouth. A head torch is useful, but some clinicians prefer to use a head mirror and light. It is helpful to use two metallic tongue depressors when doing this (Fig. 20.15); in this way, the mouth can be systematically inspected, including the difficult retromolar trigone area, sometimes ominously labelled 'coffin corner' for its occult malignancy (Fig. 20.16). The parotid duct orifice should be seen expressing normal saliva, adjacent to the second upper molar tooth. Examine the tonsils for asymmetry (which may point to malignancy).

Thoroughly and systematically examine the neck, making note of any masses, and ascertain

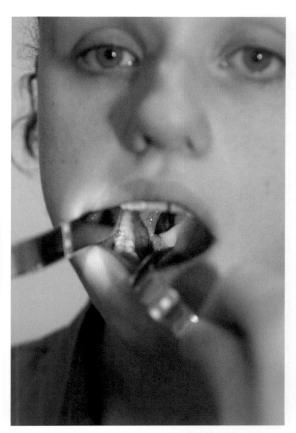

Figure 20.15 Examination of the mouth with two tongue depressors.

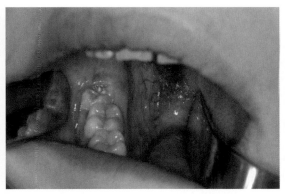

Figure 20.16 Examination of the retromolar trigone – a site of potential 'silent' malignancy.

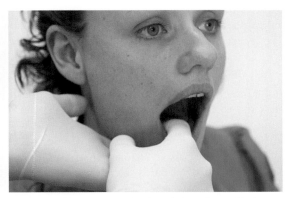

Figure 20.17 Bimanual palpation of the submandibular gland.

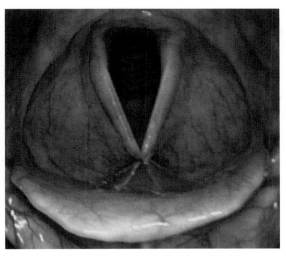

Figure 20.18 Normal larynx, viewed with a 70° rigid endoscope.

- tongue base and valleculae (with the tongue protruded)
- vocal cords (Fig. 20.18) and vocal cord movements – ask the patient to say 'ee-ee-ee'
- false cords
- pyriform fossae – asking the patient to 'puff out your cheeks' will often open the pyriform fossae.

Investigations

Contrast swallow

In a patient with dysphagia, a barium (or Gastrografin) swallow can be useful, but the postcricoid region (the area of the pharynx immediately above the oesophagus) is notoriously difficult to evaluate radiographically; furthermore, it cannot be seen on flexible nasendoscopy. If there is a high index of suspicion of postcricoid malignancy, it may be necessary to undertake an examination under anaesthesia (see 'General anaesthetic panendoscopy and biopsies', below).

Videofluoroscopy

Patients with suspected poor coordination of swallowing, as often occurs after a stroke, are best evaluated with videofluoroscopy. The patient is asked to swallow radio-opaque substances of different consistencies: water, yoghurt, bread, etc. X-ray video images of the patient swallowing are captured and

which level of the neck they occur in (see **Neck**, below).

The submandibular gland can be bimanually palpated (Fig. 20.17), and stones in the submandibular duct are sometimes identified in this way. The tongue, tongue base and tonsils may also be bimanually palpated, but this inevitably provokes a gag reflex, so should be performed at the end of the examination.

Examination of the whole of the upper aerodigestive tract is required, and this is best achieved with a fibreoptic flexible nasendoscope. Local anaesthetic may be used, but is often not required. Be systematic when examining with a nasendoscope so as not to miss pathology. A suggested routine is as follows:

- nasal cavity
- postnasal space
- palate movement

recorded. In this way, it is possible to establish if any solids or liquids are aspirated, or if any residue remains in the valleculae or pyriform fossae.

Fibreoptic endoscopic evaluation of swallowing

This technique gives similar information to video-fluoroscopy: in patients who will tolerate endoscopy, they are given substances of varying textures to swallow. The substances have blue dye added to them so that, when the patient swallows, it is possible to see if there is residue in the valleculae or pyriform fossae, or whether laryngeal penetration occurs.

MRI/CT scanning

Both MRI and CT have their place in imaging the head and neck: MRI may give better soft tissue resolution, but CT is very useful in assessing for cartilage erosion in laryngeal cancer. Check local practices before ordering cross-sectional imaging.

General anaesthetic panendoscopy and biopsies

A tissue diagnosis from the upper aerodigestive tract almost always requires general anaesthesia: it is simply not feasible to biopsy the pharynx or larynx while the patient is awake. The postcricoid region of the hypopharynx is area is not clearly seen even during oesophago-gastro-duodenoscopy (OGD); it is only under general anaesthesia that a clear view is obtained. Panendoscopy consists of laryngoscopy, pharyngoscopy, oesophagoscopy and bronchoscopy.

Chest X-ray

A vocal cord paralysis may result from intrathoracic malignancy due to compression of the recurrent laryngeal nerve. This is particularly true on the left side, where the nerve takes a longer course and is therefore more at risk of damage. A chest X-ray (or CT scan) will help to exclude chest malignancy.

Common diagnoses

Head and neck cancer

Although it is not the most common head and neck diagnosis, cancer must be excluded as a matter of urgency. The presence of any 'red flag' symptoms should prompt an urgent referral to ENT:

- hoarseness (dysphonia) lasting more than 3 weeks
- unremitting ear or throat pain
- persistent neck lump
- dysphagia
- smoking and/or excessive alcohol consumption.

Globus pharyngeus

Previously given the rather more pejorative name 'globus hystericus', globus pharyngeus is a sensation of a lump in the throat in the absence of any objective evidence of a lump. It is important to allay the patient's fear that they have cancer by performing a complete examination and if necessary arranging investigations. The aetiology of globus is poorly understood, but it is believed that muscle tension plays a part, as does laryngopharyngeal reflux.

Benign vocal cord pathology

Numerous non-malignant disease processes can affect the vocal cords, and any of these may cause dysphonia. These include vocal cord nodules (singer's nodules or screamer's nodules), polyps and cysts. Premalignant dysplastic changes may also occur. Oedema of the vocal cords (Reinke's oedema, Fig. 20.19) is commonly seen in smokers, but may also occur in hypothyroidism.

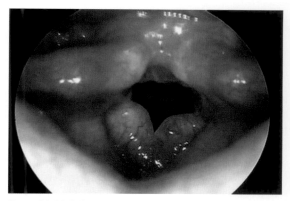

Figure 20.19 Reinke's oedema.

Oral ulceration

Aphthous ulceration may be minor or major. Minor aphthous ulceration is common and may be treated symptomatically with topical anaesthetics. Recurrent debilitating ulceration may be seen with Crohn's disease. If an ulcer persists, it should be biopsied to exclude malignancy.

Pharyngeal pouch (Zenker's diverticulum)

A pharyngeal pouch is a pulsion diverticulum that develops between the muscle fibres of thyropharyngeus and cricopharyngeus. This area is known as Killian's dehiscence. As the pouch enlarges, food and drink can accumulate in the pouch; these may then be regurgitated many hours later. Further expansion of the pouch leads to compression of the upper oesophagus, causing dysphagia and weight loss. A contrast swallow establishes the diagnosis.

NECK

Presenting symptoms

Neck lump

A lump in the neck may represent a metastasis from an underlying head and neck squamous carcinoma, so the history is aimed at excluding this. The history, therefore, consists of questioning about:

- duration of lump
- progression of lump
- dysphagia
- voice change
- haemoptysis
- otalgia
- weight loss
- night sweats
- smoking
- alcohol
- tuberculosis contact and travel history (if tuberculosis is suspected).

Ask about infections of the lump: it is not uncommon, for example, for thyroglossal duct cysts and branchial cysts to become infected and then settle to a smaller size; they still require investigation.

Sinus

A sinus is seen as a pit in the skin. It may discharge or be asymptomatic. Sinuses usually represent an underlying branchial cleft anomaly, but occasionally are seen in malignancy.

Rest of the history

Previous irradiation of the neck predisposes to thyroid malignancy. Radiotherapy was previously used in a surprisingly wide range of benign conditions (including benign goitre), and may not initially be suspected, so direct questioning is required. The patient may require surgery to establish a diagnosis, so establish the status of the patient's general health, to ascertain their fitness for general anaesthesia.

Examination

Groups of lymph nodes may be individually named, but in clinical practice, head and neck surgeons divide the neck into five levels, numbered I–V (Fig. 20.20).

It is important to be specific about the location of a node, as this indicates possible primary sites of malignancy (Fig. 20.21). Nodes in level II, for example, are known to drain the nasopharynx and oropharynx; level III receives drainage from the larynx.

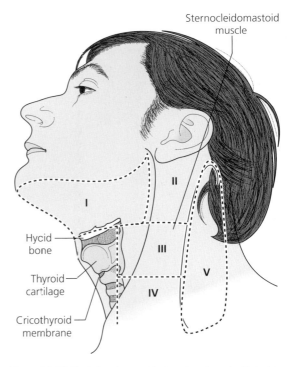

Figure 20.20 Neck levels used in head and neck clinical practice.

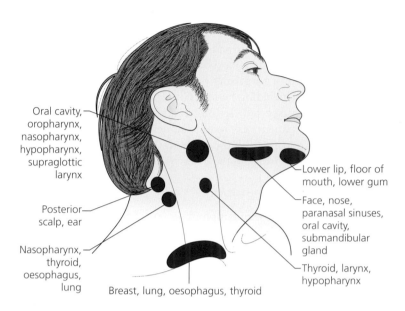

Oral cavity, oropharynx, nasopharynx, hypopharynx, supraglottic larynx

Posterior scalp, ear

Nasopharynx, thyroid, oesophagus, lung

Breast, lung, oesophagus, thyroid

Lower lip, floor of mouth, lower gum

Face, nose, paranasal sinuses, oral cavity, submandibular gland

Thyroid, larynx, hypopharynx

Figure 20.21 Lymphatic drainage sites.

The examination begins with inspection: expose the patient to below the clavicles and examine for scars and obvious masses (Fig. 20.22). If a mass is seen in the region of the thyroid, ask the patient to swallow to assess for upward movement of the mass: with the thyroid bound down by the pretracheal fascia, when the larynx rises, the thyroid moves with it. A midline lump may represent a thyroglossal duct cyst, so ask the patient to protrude their tongue and observe for movement of the lump.

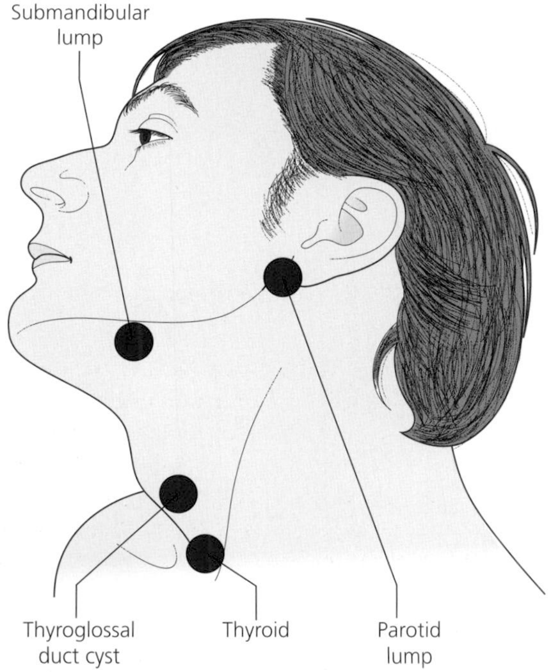

Palpation, performed from behind the patient, should proceed in a methodical manner that does not miss any region of the neck. A suggested order of examination of the neck is:

1. submental
2. submandibular
3. parotid
4. post-auricular
5. levels II, III and IV
6. thyroid (including swallowing again)
7. level V
8. occiput.

By going through a specific routine each time, the examiner will not make omissions. For any lump, describe its:

- site
- size
- shape
- skin changes
- surface (irregular/smooth) and fixity to adjacent structures.

Submandibular lump

Thyroglossal duct cyst

Thyroid

Parotid lump

Figure 20.22 Characteristic locations of neck lumps.

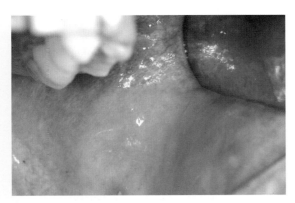

Figure 20.23 Parotid duct orifice.

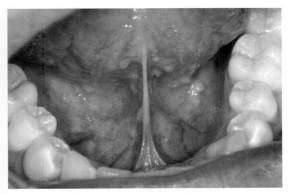

Figure 20.24 Fraenulum of tongue with submandibular duct orifices.

If a parotid lump is found, inspect the parotid duct orifice, inside the cheek adjacent to the second upper molar tooth (Fig. 20.23). Parotid tumours may compromise the facial nerve, so examine this as well.

If a submandibular mass is found, examine the orifice of the submandibular duct, under the tongue and adjacent to the lingual frenulum (Fig. 20.24).

If a cervical lymph node is found, examination now proceeds with trying to identify a primary site of malignancy. It is imperative to examine the oral cavity as well as to perform flexible nasendoscopy to inspect the nasopharynx, oropharynx, hypopharynx and larynx. Squamous carcinoma of the skin may be present as metastasis in the head and neck, so examination should continue with inspection of the scalp, anterior nose and ears.

Document the status of the cranial nerves. Finally, and if appropriate, perform a clinical assessment of the thyroid status: check for tremor, tachy- or brady-cardia, change in skin quality or exophthalmos.

Investigations

Fine needle aspiration cytology

Palpable lumps in the neck should undergo fine needle aspiration (FNA) cytology at the first clinic visit. In experienced hands, this yields good specificity and sensitivity for head and neck malignancy. If initial attempts at FNA yield no result, this should be performed under ultrasound guidance. Many head and neck centres now perform FNA and ultrasound in the head and neck clinic as part of a 'lump in the neck' clinic. The presence of a cytopathologist in the clinic gives an immediate diagnosis, greatly speeding up the diagnostic process.

It is poor practice to excise a neck lymph node when squamous carcinoma is suspected: doing this increases the risk of seeding the tumour to the skin and makes subsequent surgery more challenging. Therefore, FNA is preferred, with excision biopsy used as a last resort. The only exception to this is in suspected lymphoma: in a patient with few risk factors for squamous carcinoma, and who has multiple rubbery nodes characteristic of lymphoma, it is probably reasonable to proceed directly to excision biopsy.

MRI/CT

Cross-sectional imaging will be required. Which investigation to use is really a matter of local preference, as each has its advantages.

General anaesthetic panendoscopy and 'blind' biopsies

If a neck node is found to be malignant and no primary site is obvious on examination or imaging, the patient is said to have an *occult primary*. In this case, it is necessary to take 'blind' biopsies of the most likely primary sites. This entails performing a tonsillectomy and taking biopsies of the postnasal space, tongue base, pyriform fossae and postcricoid region.

Other tests

Positron emission tomography (PET) is increasingly used in occult head and neck malignancy:

the technology relies on 'hot spots' showing areas of increased metabolic activity, such as malignant cells. Thus, if no primary is seen in the clinic or on MRI/CT, a PET scan may show an area of increased metabolism that should be biopsied.

A chest CT scan is mandatory if malignancy is found, to exclude lung metastases or a lung primary as the cause of the neck node.

Common diagnoses

Head and neck cancer

Head and neck cancer is rare, but if caught at an early stage is often curable. Urgent referral is mandatory for any persistent neck lump.

IMPORTANT

Any persistent neck lump mandates urgent referral.

Branchial cyst

Thought to be a cystic degeneration of a lymph node rather than a branchial remnant, branchial cysts present (generally) in young adults. They are smooth, cystic swellings in front of the anterior border of the sternomastoid muscle. Aspiration of the cyst will usually yield characteristic turbid fluid. Microscopy of the fluid may show atypical squamous cells. In older patients, a cystic mass in the neck can, in fact, be a malignancy, so treat any patient over the age of 45 as an urgent case.

Thyroid lumps

These are far more common in women than men and are mostly benign. However, they all require FNA and imaging to confirm this. Most thyroid lumps that initially feel like solitary nodules in fact represent a dominant nodule in a multinodular goitre. Predisposing factors for thyroid malignancy include male gender, a history of previous neck irradiation, previous thyroid cancer and a genetic predisposition.

Parotid masses

The majority of parotid masses are in the superficial lobe, and the majority of these are pleomorphic adenomas. These are slow-growing tumours with a low incidence of malignant degeneration. Perform FNA to confirm the diagnosis, and in most cases a superficial parotidectomy will excise the whole tumour.

Thyroglossal duct cyst

During development, the thyroid gland descends from its initial position at the tongue base to lie in the lower anterior part of the neck. As it descends, the thyroglossal duct is obliterated, but failure of obliteration of the duct can result in formation of a cyst. Hence, a thyroglossal duct cyst occurs in the midline anywhere from the thyroid below to the tongue base above. The radiographic features are characteristic, and surgery involves excision of the cyst and the tract running superiorly. This often necessitates the removal of part of the hyoid bone (Sistrunk's procedure).

Lymphoma

Lymphoma in ENT practice usually presents with enlarged rubbery lymph nodes. The patient may also complain of weight loss, pruritus and drenching night sweats. FNA of the lymph node will usually be non-diagnostic, showing multiple lymphocytes. A diagnosis relies on excision biopsy of an entire node.

Tuberculosis

Tuberculosis may present as a subacute swelling of one or more neck lymph nodes. Enlargement of the nodes occurs over weeks. There are often no skin changes, and it can be clinically very difficult to differentiate from lymphoma or squamous carcinoma. The routine proceeds as before, with history, examination and FNA. If fluid is aspirated on FNA, it should be sent for cytological examination, and also for Ziehl–Nielsen staining and mycobacterial culture. Tuberculous nodes should not be excised, as doing so can lead to a persistently discharging sinus.

Atypical mycobacterium

This condition is most often seen in children, with lymph nodes in the preauricular region most often affected. Over the course of a few weeks, the area becomes swollen and the skin takes on a characteristic purplish hue. The diagnosis is a clinical one, and treatment is with a combination of radical surgery and antibiotics.

Superficial lesions

The skin of the head and neck can be affected by common lesions seen elsewhere. These will not be discussed in detail, but bear in mind that sebaceous cysts, lipomas, basal cell carcinomas, seborrhoeic keratoses, melanomas and many others can be seen. This is particularly true of skin malignancy since the head and neck receive so much sun exposure.

SUMMARY

Ear

- Presenting complaint and associated symptoms:
  - hearing loss
  - tinnitus
  - vertigo
  - ear discharge
  - ear surgery.
- Important related questions:
  - noise exposure
  - family history
  - ear pain.
- Examination:
  - post-auricular inspection – scars; erythema?
  - otoscope – all four quadrants of the tympanic membrane; ear canal
  - tuning fork tests – Weber's and Rinne's
  - facial nerve
  - balance testing.

Nose

- Presenting complaint and associated symptoms:
  - nasal obstruction
  - facial pain
  - rhinorrhoea.
- Important related questions:
  - anosmia/hyposmia
  - nasal surgery.
- Examination:
  - anterior rhinoscopy with Thudichum speculum
  - endoscopy with rigid or flexible endoscope.

Throat

- Presenting complaint and associated symptoms:
  - dysphagia
  - globus sensation
  - pain.
- Important related questions:
  - hoarseness
  - otalgia (ear pain)
  - weight loss
  - haemoptysis
  - alcohol and smoking.
- Examination:
  - oral cavity and oropharynx
  - flexible nasendoscopic examination of nasopharynx, oropharynx, hypopharynx and larynx
  - palpation of the neck.

Neck

- Presenting complaint and associated symptoms:
  - neck lump
  - sinus
- Important related questions:
  - smoking and alcohol
  - dysphagia
  - hoarseness
  - otalgia
  - weight loss.
- Examination
  - thorough examination of all levels (I–V) of the neck
  - examination of oral cavity, oropharynx and flexible nasendoscopic examination of nasopharynx, oropharynx, hypopharynx and larynx.

FURTHER READING

Corbridge RJ, Hellier WPL. 1998. *Essential ENT practice*. London: Hodder Arnold.

Corbridge R, Steventon N. 2006. *Oxford handbook of ENT and head and neck surgery*. Oxford: Oxford University Press.

Ludman H, Bradley PJ (eds). 2007. *ABC of ear, nose and throat*, 5th edn. Oxford: Blackwell Publishing.

21 INFECTIOUS AND TROPICAL DISEASES

Robert N Davidson

THE FEBRILE PATIENT

History

Patients with infection (and inflammatory conditions or, less commonly, malignancy) usually report fever. The fever pattern, often emphasized in older textbooks, is in practice not very helpful. Most people will take antipyretics (paracetamol, aspirin or non-steroidal anti-inflammatory drugs (NSAIDs)) which will change the pattern. Whatever the cause, body temperature generally rises in the evening and falls during the night. The patient thus experiences a sensation of being cold in the afternoon/evening and sweats at night or 30 minutes after taking an antipyretic. Fever is often lower or absent in the morning, or if the patient is on steroids. A sensation of 'feeling hot' or 'feeling cold' is unreliable – healthy individuals often feel these sensations, as may those with menopausal flushing, thyrotoxicosis, stress, panic, or migraine.

The height and duration of fever *are* important. Rigors (chills or shivering, often uncontrollable and lasting for 20–30 minutes) are highly significant, and so is a documented temperature over 37.5°C taken with a reliable oral thermometer. Drenching sweats are also highly significant. Rigors generally indicate *serious bacterial infections* (lobar pneumonia, endocarditis, septicaemia, cholangitis, pyelonephritis, etc.)

Table 21.1 Features that distinguish rigors from a grand mal convulsion

Rigor	Grand mal convulsion
Lasts 20–30 minutes	Lasts 2–3 minutes
Conscious (may be delirious)	Unconscious, later drowsy – will not recall the event
Temperature rises (typically >39°C)	Temperature seldom >37.5°C
No injury	Tongue biting, bruising
No incontinence	May pass urine

or *malaria*. An oral temperature >39°C has the same significance as rigors. Rigors generally do not occur in mild viral infections (e.g. those caused by respiratory viruses, Epstein–Barr virus (EBV), hepatitis), malignancy, connective tissue diseases, tuberculosis and other chronic infections. Table 21.1 lists the features that distinguish rigors from a grand mal convulsion.

Weight loss

Anyone with fever lasting longer than a week should have lost weight – if a patient reports a prolonged fever but no weight loss, the 'fever' usually turns out to be of no consequence.

Travel

The usual incubation periods are:

- malaria – up to 1 year (falciparum malaria usually 0–4 weeks)
- typhoid – up to a month
- dengue – fever up to a week
- tuberculosis – lifelong risk.

Examination of the febrile patient

General

- Has the patient lost weight? Look for prominent cheekbones, caused by wasting of the temporalis and masseter muscles.
- Has the patient's belt been taken in a notch or two? Ask the patient to show you a photograph to compare their facial appearance.
- Is the patient eating well? Look at the food at the bedside: untouched meals indicate ongoing illness; return of appetite is a reliable sign of recovery.

Nails

Leuconychia can represent inflammatory conditions as well as low albumin. The finger nail represents a calendar of the past 3 months – pallor develops from the base. The 'half moon' at the nail base is lost in

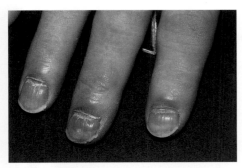

Figure 21.1 Beau's lines. From: Kinirons M, Ellis H (eds), *French's index of differential diagnosis* (14th edition), with permission. © 2005 London: Hodder Arnold.

leuconychia, and looking for the half-moon helps determine if leuconychia is present. A band of brief leuconychia across the nails represents a period of illness or chemotherapy (Beau's line, Fig. 21.1). The toe nails grow more slowly, so the toenail represents the past 6 months. Is there clubbing? If so, consider infective endocarditis, lung cancer and bronchiectasis. Are there splinter haemorrhages? Those caused by infective endocarditis may occur anywhere in the nail, may be any size, and are painless. Are there small, tender infarcts in the palm of the hand (Janeway lesions) or in the finger pulps (Osler's nodes)? These are highly suggestive of infective endocarditis.

Skin and mucosae

- Is the patient sweating?
- Is there pityriasis versicolor? This is a rash of hypopigmented, slightly scaly macules, usually centrally on the chest and upper back. It indicates longstanding sweating – consider tuberculosis or human immunodeficiency virus (HIV) infection.
- Are the conjunctivae pale? Chronic infections usually cause anaemia.
- Is there jaundice? Fever precedes jaundice in hepatitis; fever accompanied by jaundice is a warning sign – consider biliary obstruction with cholangitis, malaria, septicaemia.
- Look in the conjunctivae for small haemorrhages, suggestive of meningococcal septicaemia or infective endocarditis.
- Are there 'cold sores' on the lips? Herpes labialis classically accompanies lobar pneumonia, malaria and HIV infection.

- Is there a definite rash? Petechiae, purpura and ecchymoses often indicate fulminant sepsis.
- Is the skin flushed and erythematous? If so, consider streptococcal and staphylococcal sepsis; consider dengue fever if returned from travelling within the last week.
- Is the erythema blanching?
  - Blanching erythema indicates redness of vasodilated skin capillaries. Blanching erythema is seen in sunburn, in dengue fever and in streptococcal toxic shock syndrome ('scarlet fever') and staphylococcal toxic shock syndrome. Sun-exposed areas of the skin are characteristically worst affected.
  - A non-blanching rash indicates that the red cells causing the rash have extravasated from the capillaries, a form of vasculitis (Fig. 21.2). Sometimes lesions may be partially blanching with a non-blanching purpuric centre.

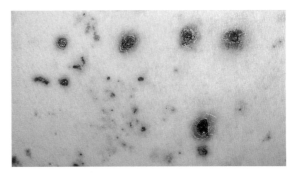

Figure 21.2 Purpuric and necrotic papules in cutaneous vasculitis. From: Marks R, *Roxburgh's common skin diseases* (17th edition), with permission. © 2003 London: Hodder Arnold.

CLINICAL PEARL

Note that in a patient with meningitis or encephalitis cold sores do *not* indicate that herpes simplex is the likely cause of the central nervous system (CNS) infection.

In the mouth

Look for:

- a coated tongue (a non-specific indicator of illness)

- candidiasis inside cheeks and on soft palate (consider HIV, steroids including inhaled steroids)
- leucoplakia on edges of tongue (reliably indicates advanced HIV)
- look for Koplik's spots (on buccal mucosa)
- Kaposi's sarcoma (on hard palate) and other mucosal lesions.

Circulation

Examine for sepsis (see below). Are there heart murmurs? A regurgitant murmur strongly suggests endocarditis.

Respiration

Are there signs of pneumonia? Note: sepsis is often accompanied by hypoxia and tachypnoea (nitric oxide release → vasodilation → intrapulmonary shunting) – a 'false localizing' sign.

Abdomen

Is there an intra-abdominal infection? If there is peritonitis, ask surgeons to advise. Note that sepsis is often accompanied by vomiting or diarrhoea – 'false localizing' signs. Do a rectal examination for:

- pelvic abscess in missed appendicitis
- prostate enlargement – may indicate a urinary tract infection
- a retained tampon – felt on rectal examination as a mass anterior to the rectum; may cause toxic shock syndrome.

Neurological

- Is the patient alert and cooperative? If irritable or stuporose consider CNS infection: meningitis or encephalitis (see below). Other infections should not cause alteration in consciousness unless patient is in septic shock.
- Is there neck stiffness (see below)? Look at the optic fundi for signs of endocarditis (Fig. 21.3), HIV infection and raised intracranial pressure.

Reflection after clinical examination

Once you have finished your clinical assessment of the febrile patient, consider:

- Is there a **site** of infection? Lack of localizing features indicates the infection is primarily in the bloodstream.

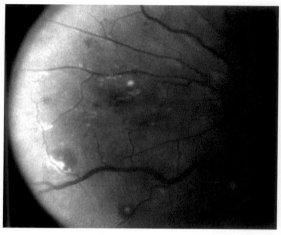

Figure 21.3 Retinal appearances in infective endocarditis. The white spots with haemorrhagic borders (Roth's spots) represent septic emboli. Microscopic haematuria and small lesions on a magnetic resonance image indicate the same phenomena in the kidneys and brain, respectively.

BOX 21.1 TAKING SPECIMENS

- **Blood cultures** must be taken under careful sterile conditions, or contaminants will confuse the picture. Cultures should go into the incubator within an hour or two. For diagnosing endocarditis, typhoid or other bloodstream infections, take three sets from different sites – you need not wait for fever spikes, nor need you wait more than a few minutes between each set.
- A **throat swab** is the best way of growing *Neisseria meningitidis* in meningococcal infection.
- **Urine**: ensure the midstream urine culture is sent to the lab – not discarded once the dipstick has been done.
- **Stool**: if the patient has enteric infection but cannot pass a stool before antibiotics, take a rectal swab instead.
- **HIV tests**: could the patient be immunocompromised? If so, the differential diagnosis is much wider – an HIV test should be offered routinely, and almost all patients will consent. If an ill patient has agreed to an HIV test, do not waste time on pre-test counselling – the result will be back quickly and you can counsel once the result is known.

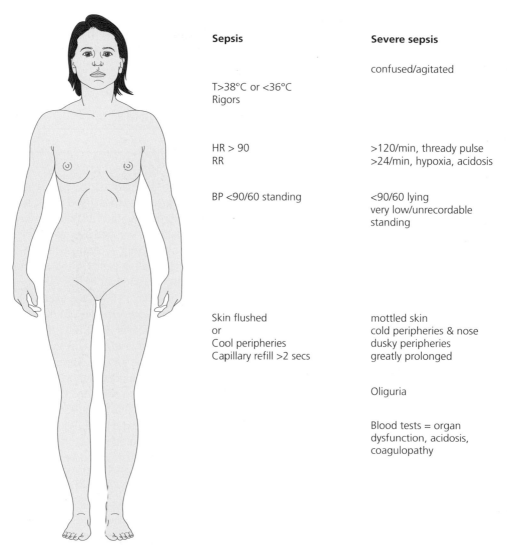

Sepsis

T>38°C or <36°C
Rigors

HR > 90
RR

BP <90/60 standing

Skin flushed
or
Cool peripheries
Capillary refill >2 secs

Severe sepsis

confused/agitated

>120/min, thready pulse
>24/min, hypoxia, acidosis

<90/60 lying
very low/unrecordable
standing

mottled skin
cold peripheries & nose
dusky peripheries
greatly prolonged

Oliguria

Blood tests = organ
dysfunction, acidosis,
coagulopathy

Figure 21.4 The features of sepsis and severe sepsis may be incomplete, so do not be clinically greedy. Take your time to observe the patient. Lying and standing blood pressure is the best single guide to hypovolaemia and early shock. Ask your patient to stand up and walk about the bed, this can reveal the severity of their illness in ways that lying in bed may conceal.

- Does this patient need **urgent treatment** (Fig. 21.4)? If the patient has features of serious infection, take cultures (see Box 21.1) and start treatment based on your clinical diagnosis and the likely infecting organisms. Do not wait for a positive culture, especially if the patient has sepsis or serious infection. Consult local guidelines for choosing antibiotics. Remember, once antibiotics have been started (even if wrongly chosen), further cultures are almost always futile.
- Is this patient part of an outbreak? Do public health authorities need to be notified?
- If you are worried about the patient's condition, admit them to hospital for observation and/or treatment. Reassess the patient regularly, and, in time, the diagnosis is likely to become apparent.

In patients with infection it is essential to distinguish severe from less severe illness. We can infer the likely pathogen, and thus the need for urgent treatment, from the clinical picture.

SEPSIS

Bacterial infections are the most common cause of sepsis, but other serious infections (e.g. falciparum malaria) or inflammatory states (e.g. pancreatitis, pre-eclamptic toxaemia, burns) can cause the same features. Below are listed the indicators of sepsis – the more abnormal the result, the more severe is the patient's condition.

Temperature

- Check if it is above 38 °C or below 36 °C.
- Simple viral infections seldom exceed 39 °C.
- Temperatures (from any cause) are generally higher in the evening than in the early morning.
- As noted above, rigors (uncontrollable shivering) are important indicators of severe bacterial infection or malaria.

Circulatory disturbance

A heart rate greater than 90 beats/min is abnormal, and in severe sepsis a pulse of 140/min is not unusual. While you feel the radial pulse you should assess peripheral perfusion: curl your fingers over the patient's fingers. This detects whether their peripheries are warm and well perfused, or are cold and clammy, or are vasodilated with throbbing digital vessels. In sepsis the radial pulse character may be bounding (especially in patients who have flushed skin and vasodilated peripheries, e.g. staphylococcal or streptococcal sepsis) or thready with cold, clammy peripheries (e.g. Gram-negative shock). Peripheries (fingers, toes, nose) are often markedly cooler than central skin (trunk, forehead) with prolonged capillary refill time (Box 21.2). Fluid resuscitation requires the filling pressure (JVP) to be estimated (see Box 21.3).

Hypotension

Blood pressure (BP) is low in the supine position (systolic BP <90 mmHg) and falls further when the patient is repositioned upright. In septic shock

---

BOX 21.2 CAPILLARY REFILL TIME

Elevate the patient's hand to the level of their heart; firmly press the finger pulp to blanch the skin; count how long the colour takes to return. Less than 2 seconds is normal; if poor peripheral perfusion is present, capillary refill can be greatly prolonged.

BOX 21.3 JUDGING HYDRATION

The cornerstones of treatment of sepsis and septic shock are intravenous fluid resuscitation and antimicrobial therapy. The patient's fluid requirements can be judged against their central venous pressure (CVP). A cannula can be inserted to directly measure the central venous pressure, but this is invasive and carries risk. With careful observation, in many patients the external jugular vein can be used to guide fluid status. Note that the external jugular vein (EJV) is 'unreliable' if it is distended (the EJV may be kinked as it passes through the platysma into the internal jugular). However, if the EJV is not distended, it usually gives very useful information about the CVP.

Method: Prop the patient up at 45°. Place your finger horizontally across the EJV to compress it at the level of the supraclavicular fossa. In a few seconds the EJV should fill and become visibly distended. Then remove your finger – the EJV will empty into the internal jugular. This proves that the CVP was lower than the level of your finger. You can repeat this laying the patient at 30° and at 15°.

BOX 21.4 POSTURAL PULSE AND BP

- In the severely ill patient who cannot stand unaided, prop the patient up with legs hanging down. Keep the BP cuff at the level of the heart.
- In *normal* individuals BP rises slightly on standing.
- In incipient septic shock, the vasodilation and loss of colloid into interstitial spaces means that the circulation is under-filled. A postural drop in BP of >20 mmHg is highly significant. You may also notice the heart rate rising on standing – a rise of >30 beats per minute is highly significant.

sometimes the BP is unrecordable on standing, and the patient may faint when they are helped to stand up (see Box 21.4).

Respiratory disturbance

The first sign is a respiratory rate greater than 20 breaths/min. This is often a combination of two abnormalities: hypoxia caused by intrapulmonary shunts, and lactic acidosis. Observe the character of breathing to give you clues as to the cause of respiratory distress: in hypoxia, the respiratory pattern is normal but rapid. Acidotic breathing has a deep, sighing character (also known as Kussmaul's respiration). If pulmonary oedema or consolidation are present, flaring of the nostrils (alae nasi) is an important sign.

Renal disturbance

- Oliguria is the first sign.
- Catheterize the patient and record the hourly urine output (less than 0.5 mL of urine per kg of body weight per hour = oliguria; less than 5 mL per hour = anuria).

Hepatic dysfunction

See the section on hepatitis below; liver disturbance in sepsis is a form of hepatitis

Confusion

Also called *toxic encephalopathy* or *delirium*, confusion or drowsiness is often present in sepsis. This non-specific feature needs to be distinguished from meningitis and encephalitis (see below), in which the CNS is the site of infection.

> **IMPORTANT**
> Sepsis is always severe when it is accompanied by organ dysfunction. Septic shock is defined as severe sepsis with hypotension despite adequate fluid replacement.

MALARIA

Malaria is the most common and important cause of fever in a returned traveller (or recent immigrant) and should be the first diagnosis considered. Always do a blood film for malaria and/or a rapid diagnostic test (RDT) if malaria is a possibility – that is, within 1 year of travel to an endemic area. Falciparum malaria is potentially fatal, and generally occurs soon (days to weeks) after travel.

> **CLINICAL PEARL**
> Adults and older children from endemic areas (especially West and East Africa) may have low-grade parasitaemia without symptoms (due to partial immunity to malaria). Thus, finding low-grade parasitaemia in these patients does not prove that the fever is caused by malaria – consider additional diagnoses.

Febrile patients with *no malaria parasites visible* on the blood film should not be treated for malaria. It is false to assume that a patient can be ill, even severely ill, with malaria and have no malaria parasites detectable. Blood films or RDTs may need to be repeated daily to be sure they are negative, as parasites are scanty at the start of malaria.

> **IMPORTANT**
> - Remember the essential difference between falciparum malaria and the others. 'Falciparum' means 'bearing a scythe = the Grim Reaper'. Falciparum malaria can be fatal if untreated and is an emergency: hyperparasitaemia, organ failure, cerebral malaria all occur, sometimes unexpectedly.
> - Most malaria from Africa is caused by *Plasmodium falciparum*. Benign malarias (caused by *Plasmodium vivax*, *Plasmodium ovale* and *Plasmodium malariae*) have similar symptoms, but do not kill.
> - If a patient has malaria and shock (low BP) treat for bacterial sepsis as well, as the two conditions may co-exist.

History

Patients generally have evening fevers, so may be afebrile in a morning clinic. Most patients will report rigors (see above). The patterns of tertian (each 48 hours) or quartan (each 72 hours) fever are seen so infrequently as to be clinically almost useless. Beware of the following 'traps':

- some patients with malaria have jaundice, diarrhoea or altered consciousness, and their fever is not prominent
- occasional patients do not volunteer a travel history for various reasons
- patients may have taken some antimalarial treatment – making the parasites scanty without curing the patient.

Examination

Unless malaria has been present for more than 1 week, there are likely to be no abnormal findings. Anaemia and splenomegaly take time to develop. Pallor, splenomegaly and jaundice indicate prolonged or severe malaria. Drowsiness, coma or convulsions could indicate cerebral malaria or hypoglycaemia. Do a rapid glucose test – give 50 mL of 50 per cent dextrose.

Laboratory tests

Most malaria patients will have thrombocytopenia that is not clinically apparent as bleeding is not a feature. The haemoglobin may be low if there is chronic or severe malaria. The white blood cell count (WBC) is usually normal. Raised bilirubin indicates either malarial hepatitis (modestly elevated liver function) or haemolysis. RDTs are very accurate, especially in severe malaria – some will detect falciparum malaria, some detect all forms of malaria. The blood film for malaria (done on a full blood count (FBC) sample) remains the best test, but it is time-consuming and requires skill. Repeat both RDTs *and* blood films daily until the diagnosis is known.

MENINGITIS AND ENCEPHALITIS

Patients with high fever characteristically have a throbbing headache, and may be tremulous – these are non-specific features. However, confusion and decreased level of consciousness indicate there is infection of the CNS itself. The main diagnoses are meningitis and encephalitis.

Meningitis

The patient invariably complains of severe headache which is global and constant, 'the worst headache they have ever had'. If the onset of headache is over 3 hours to 3 days, suspect viral or bacterial meningitis; if more gradual, suspect tuberculous meningitis.

History

The hallmarks of meningitis are:

- headache – severe, global and constant
- photophobia – may resist ophthalmoscopy
- altered consciousness – drowsy and falling asleep unless stimulated
- neck stiffness – on flexion but not rotation
- rash – with bacterial infection.

Examination

General features

Fever is invariably present, highest in the evening, and often with rigors (if bacterial). Patients with meningitis generally have *photophobia* – they avoid the light and may cover their face with a blanket; ophthalmoscopy is sometimes resisted. However, this is a 'soft sign' which is also common in migraine and patients who are irritable for other reasons. There is often *alteration of consciousness* – generally the patient is drowsy or stuporose (falls asleep when not stimulated, falls asleep during the examination). Young patients may be agitated, confused or even aggressive before becoming stuporose – in emergency departments they may be mistaken for patients with drug intoxication or hypoglycaemia. There is frequently evidence of infection outside the CNS, either systemic infection (sepsis, rash) or local infection (otitis media, pharyngitis).

Meningococcal rash

Often with *Neisseria meningitidis* meningitis (and occasionally with other types of bacterial meningitis), there is a characteristic rash:

- scanty blanching macules on the trunk or limbs, usually in mild cases with a longer history

and/or

- non-blanching petechiae, purpura or ecchymoses, typically on the hands or feet, face and conjunctivae – the larger and more numerous the lesions, and the quicker they develop, the more likely it is that septic shock is present or will occur and the worse the prognosis

and/or

- cold, dusky peripheries which resemble frostbite and which become gangrenous (infarcted) if the patient survives – invariably septic shock accompanies these skin appearances.

Sepsis and septic shock (see above) often co-exist with bacterial meningitis – especially when *Neisseria meningitidis* is the cause. Septicaemia multiplies the mortality of meningitis 10-fold and requires aggressive treatment in the intensive care unit.

Testing for neck stiffness

Involuntary neck stiffness ('nuchal rigidity') is a characteristic sign of meningitis, and it is so important that it is essential to examine well for it, and to practise whenever doing a CNS examination so that you know well what is normal.

A useful clue to the absence of neck stiffness may be found during the history taking: if the patient freely nods the head when agreeing with your questions, you can assume the neck is not stiff. Patients with meningitis or subarachnoid haemorrhage characteristically lie still and do not move the head voluntarily. Patients who complain about a stiff neck are often worried about meningitis; patients with meningitis generally complain of a sore *head*, not a sore *neck* – thus neck stiffness is a sign, not a symptom, of meningitis. Neck stiffness (Box 21.5) is not lost if the patient becomes unconscious. If very severe there is arching backward of the spine (opisthotonus) – the patient will be unconscious if this is present. Neck stiffness may be absent in babies.

If you have difficulty making up your mind about neck stiffness, compare flexing with rotating the patient's neck. Meningism leaves rotation relatively unaffected. In mild meningitis, it is only the final part of flexion which is stiff (called 'terminal rigidity').

Kernig's sign

This test detects painful/inflamed nerve roots ('spinal meningitis') and is similar in concept to straight leg raising – it is sensitive in meningitis, but not very

---

BOX 21.5 TESTING FOR NECK STIFFNESS

1. Inform the patient of what you are doing, and reassure them. Remove any pillows so the patient can lie flat in bed.
2. Ask the patient to nod the head so the chin is on the sternum. If a child, you can also ask them to 'kiss their knees'. If the patient can do this, it is unlikely you will find a stiff neck in the next step.
3. Facing the patient, hold the head firmly but gently – put your hands on the mastoid areas behind the ears – slowly rotate the neck all the way from side to side – this will relax the patient, and enable you to compare rotation (which is not stiff in meningitis) to flexion (which is).
4. Slowly flex the head forward – the movement is slow, long and rocking (not a little jog of movement). Repeat this a few times until you are sure – it will be the same every time it is done correctly. If the neck does not flex fully, draw the head still further forwards and watch whether you can lift the patient's shoulders away from the bed.

---

specific. The patient lies supine and the knee and hip on one side are passively flexed to 90°. An attempt is made to passively straighten the knee, until the patient winces and the knee cannot be straightened further. Pain felt in the hamstrings is somewhat suggestive but not specific of meningitis but pain felt in the low back is more specific. Repeat Kernig's test on the other side – the result should be the same. *Brudzinski's sign* is often mentioned but little used – the neck is flexed, and in response to this, the patient actively flexes their hips and knees.

Conditions that mimic meningitis

Meningism is sometimes found in patients with streptococcal sore throats, pneumonia and urinary tract sepsis. The neck is painful and stiff, and with a fever the illness mimics meningitis, but the CSF is normal.

Neck stiffness is also present in subarachnoid haemorrhage. A small subarachnoid haemorrhage is important not to miss ('herald' or 'warning' bleed). The patient is admitted because of headache, and is found to have minimal neck stiffness, temperature normal or up to 38 °C, and blood tests are normal. The patient often settles in hospital overnight, and is thought to have had a 'viral illness with headache'.

BOX 21.6 DECISIONS ABOUT COMPUTED TOMOGRAPHY, LUMBAR PUNCTURE AND TREATMENT IN MENINGITIS

There will be a local policy which you should follow. Useful principles are:

- If septicaemia is present with suspected meningitis, there is no time to lose. Start antibiotics immediately you have taken your blood culture and throat swab.
- In patients who have meningitis without septicaemia, the 20–30-minute delay for lumbar puncture (LP) is acceptable – take specimens to culture blood, throat swab and cerebrospinal fluid (CSF) before the first dose. Usually a computed tomography (CT) scan will add an unacceptable delay, so if CT scan is necessary before LP, start antibiotics first.
- If you are unsure about the presence of neck stiffness, reassess the patient after an hour, when hydration and paracetamol may have improved minor symptoms. If still unsure, reassess again, especially if the patient is clinically relatively well. A patient with mild meningitis is not in mortal danger and can be observed until the diagnosis is clear.

If a patient is admitted because of headache, neuroimaging and LP are an essential part of management.

- Perform a CT scan as early as possible, because a small collection of blood in the CSF may be seen, later it will disperse. See Box 21.6 for more on CT scanning.
- Proceed to LP even if the patient feels better the next day. The CSF might show the subtle changes of xanthochromia, a few red cells, and slightly elevated protein – vital clues which will might enable diagnosis of an aneurysm or arteriovenous malformation before the next (frequently catastrophic) bleed occurs.

CLINICAL PEARL

If a patient has a low or falling level of consciousness, a CT scan must be done before performing a LP. This will help rule out a mass lesion, obstructive hydrocephalus or other contraindication to lumbar puncture. Although the CT cannot tell you the intracranial pressure, it can tell you whether there is abundant CSF in the fourth ventricle and basal cisterns, and help you decide whether LP is safe to perform.

Encephalitis

This is usually viral in origin; the commonest causes are enteroviruses and mumps, but the most serious cause in developed countries is herpes simplex. In tropical environments, arboviruses (Japanese encephalitis, West Nile fever) are common. Rabies is a form of encephalitis that will be considered separately.

History

The hallmarks of encephalitis (see also Box 21.7) are:

- headache – usually severe, continuous, throbbing and getting worse slowly over 1–2 days. Pain is generally felt over the whole head, photophobia is variable
- drowsiness – patient spends increasing periods of time asleep, later becomes unrousable. Confusion or alteration in personality or behaviour may accompany this
- fever – may be low-grade, not usually with rigors
- focal or generalized convulsions may occur (and are a poor prognostic sign in encephalitis).

Examination

- Fever, confusion and drowsiness are characteristic.
- Neck stiffness may be present (= meningo-encephalitis), but if present is not very obvious.
- There are seldom localizing neurological signs.

Laboratory diagnosis

The confirmation of encephalitis is often frustrating: magnetic resonance imaging (MRI) is performed to look for characteristic changes of herpes simplex

BOX 21.7 ENCEPHALITIS – COMMON ERRORS

- One of the common errors is *over-diagnosis*. Encephalitis is unlikely in patients who are behaving oddly, hallucinating, or disorientated, yet perfectly alert and do not have headache or fever. Such patients are far more likely to have psychosis (e.g. schizophrenia) or a toxic confusional state (e.g. hypoglycaemia, recreational drugs).
- Another common error is *under-diagnosis* of meningoencephalitis. Patients, especially young adults, with acute bacterial meningitis often have agitation and confusion for a few hours before they become drowsy. They may wrongly be considered to have psychosis or a toxic confusional state if their headache, neck stiffness and fever are not recognized.
- The key to correct diagnosis is to repeat the examination (including assessing neck stiffness) until the clinical picture is clearer.

virus (HSV) in the temporal lobes. Lumbar puncture may show minor increases in cells and protein and polymerase chain reaction (PCR) can be done to look for viral DNA. However in more than 50 per cent of cases, no aetiological diagnosis can be made, and the patient recovers without treatment or with empirical treatment for HSV.

RABIES AND TETANUS

These are two unusual neurological conditions that are diagnosed by careful observation.

- Rabies can be confirmed by virus isolation, but is invariably fatal.
- Tetanus has no confirmatory tests but, if treated well, the patient should survive.

Rabies

History

The patient or relatives will recall an animal bite in a rabies-endemic area a few weeks earlier. Sometimes the bite was considered insignificant at the time,

though the skin would have been broken. Usually the animal is a dog. Note that a rabid dog is ill, it will behave abnormally and within a few days will have either disappeared or have died.

The only chance of life-saving treatment is immunization given after the bite, but before the symptoms begin. Once symptomatic, a patient with rabies will invariably die. The first symptoms are of itching, pain, or paraesthesia (tingling) at the site of the bite. This is followed by fever, rigors, malaise, weakness, and the symptoms of encephalitis: headache and confusion or drowsiness.

Examination

In 'furious rabies' the characteristic feature is hydrophobia — when the patient is offered a drink of water, or an attempt is made to wash the patient, he or she expresses terror and has an inspiratory muscle spasm (arched, extended back with arms thrown up), with or without laryngeal spasm. Later these spasms become provoked by many stimuli, for example a fan blowing air on the face (aerophobia). It may end in convulsions with cardiorespiratory arrest. Other clinical features include:

- hyperaesthesia
- lucid periods alternating with wild, hallucinating, or aggressive periods
- cranial nerve palsies
- meningism
- involuntary movements
- autonomic nervous system/hypothalamic changes – hypersalivation, lacrimation, fluctuations in BP and temperature, polyuria.

In paralytic (spinal) rabies, there is a flaccid paralysis that ascends from the bitten area, with pain, fasciculation, sensory disturbances, paraplegia and loss of sphincter control.

Tetanus

History

In tetanus the symptoms usually begin 7–10 days after the injury, but this is variable and many patients cannot recall the injury because it was trivial. The first symptom is usually trismus (difficulty in opening the mouth, due to stiffness of the masseters).

Examination

Observe the patient quietly for several minutes and the diagnosis will become apparent.

- As the condition progresses, muscle groups become rigid. These include the muscles of facial expression, producing a characteristic appearance of *risus sardonicus* in which the mouth is fixedly drawn back in a sneer and the eyebrows are raised. In newborn infants with tetanus, there is inability to suckle.
- Stiffness of the chest wall/diaphragm makes breathing difficult. The tone in all the limbs is increased, the back arches backwards and swallowing may become difficult (but not painful – this is not hydrophobia). Later, spasms occur – these are dramatic events lasting 30 seconds to 2 minutes, and are an exaggeration of the underlying rigidity.
- Spasms occur in response to stimuli (touch, sounds, sights, emotions) or spontaneously. They may be mild and brief, or prolonged and very painful: the legs and arms are extended, the back arches (opisthotonus) and the patient cannot swallow or breathe.
- The patient is perfectly conscious throughout. Once the spasm stops, the patient usually gasps a deep breath and may aspirate the saliva from the pharynx. Laryngeal spasms may cause death from anoxia. The importance of recognizing tetanus is to treat the patient – sedate and ventilate the patient for 2 weeks or longer. In severe disease, the autonomic nervous system is involved, giving fever, tachycardia, and an unstable circulation.

INFECTIVE DIARRHOEA

History

The history gives important clues to the diagnosis. Understanding the significance of these symptoms enables you to appreciate what part of the gut is involved, and hence what the cause may be. Does the patient have gastritis (e.g. an ingested *Bacillus cereus* toxin), enteritis (e.g. *Salmonella*), gastroenteritis (e.g. *Rotavirus*), entero-colitis (e.g. *Campylobacter*), dysentery (e.g. *Entamoeba histolytica*), colo-proctitis (e.g. *Shigella*)?

Foregut symptoms

If the patient has epigastric pain, the origin of the pain is the foregut. The foregut starts at the top of the oesophagus and it comprises the stomach and duodenum as far as the ampulla of Vater. Also derived from the foregut are the biliary tree and pancreas, so diseases of these organs also give epigastric pain. Infections of the stomach give vomiting (gastritis) but not diarrhoea, since the stomach is not involved in absorption.

Mid-gut symptoms

If the patient has an infection of the mid-gut, pain is felt centrally (peri-umbilical). The mid-gut structures are the duodenum beyond the ampulla, the remainder of the small bowel, the caecum and appendix, the ascending colon and a third of the transverse colon. Infections of these structures give diarrhoea and central cramping or continuous pain (enteritis). The diarrhoea is watery, there is no mucus (small bowel does not secrete mucus) and no recognizable blood (small bowel enzymes digest any red cells in the lumen).

Hindgut symptoms

If the hindgut is involved, the patient reports lower abdominal pain. Infections of the hindgut (two-thirds of the transverse colon, descending colon, sigmoid and rectum) give crampy lower abdominal pain and diarrhoea (colitis, dysentery). The stools are often very frequent, sometimes being little more than frequent blobs of blood and mucus. An important symptom is *tenesmus*, which indicates that the rectum is inflamed (proctitis). Sensations from the rectum are felt as a strong urge to defecate: the patient cannot pass flatus without sitting on the toilet for fear of incontinence, there is a burning pain in the sacral area and a feeling of incomplete defecation.

Examination

General

Weight loss suggests a chronic condition such as ileocaecal tuberculosis or inflammatory bowel disease. Leuconychia suggests an inflammatory or protein-losing condition. A tachycardia is very significant –

Table 21.2 Signs of dehydration in infants versus adults

Sign	Useful in infants?	Useful in adults?
Dry mouth	✓ (nose breathers)	✗ (often reflects mouth breathing)
Loss of skin turgor	✓ (elastic tissue ++ in skin)	✗ (skin lacks elasticity)
Sunken eyes	✓ (have a fat pad behind eyelids)	✗ (sunken eyes often present, loss of fat pad behind eyelids)
Peripheral perfusion (pulse, capillary refill)	✓	✓
Lying versus standing blood pressure	✗	✓

Table 21.3 Characteristics of the hepatitis viruses

Virus	Incubation period	Route of infection	Chronic disease	Carrier state
HAV	2–6 weeks	Faeco-oral	No	No
HBV	4–26 weeks	Blood contact, sex, neonatal	Common	Common – especially if neonatal infection
HCV	2–26 weeks	Blood contact	Very common	Very common
HEV	2–8 weeks	Faeco-oral	No	No

particularly once the patient is no longer dehydrated – and is a sign of severity, e.g. in ulcerative colitis.

Abdomen

The abdomen is usually flat or even sunken: a distended abdomen is unexpected. If present, look for ascites (suggests tuberculosis) or tympanic distension (suggests toxic megacolon in ulcerative colitis). The site of tenderness should tell you which part of the bowel is inflamed.

Dehydration

This is common in enteritis and gastroenteritis, in which large volumes of fluid are lost. The well-known signs of dehydration which are so useful in infants are of little value in adults (Table 21.2). In adults, hydration is reliably assessed by checking for postural hypotension and peripheral perfusion (see section 'Sepsis' above).

HEPATITIS

- Hepatitis A virus (HAV) infection has become much less frequent since travellers routinely receive the HAV vaccine. This gives almost 100 per cent protection against HAV.

- Hepatitis B (HBV) and hepatitis C (HCV) are both blood-borne viruses, contracted by receiving infected blood products, tattoos, piercings, dental or medical injections, etc. HBV is easily transmitted by sexual intercourse; HCV and HAV are only occasionally transmitted in this way.
- Hepatitis D (delta virus) is a rare infection which may co-infect HBV carriers.
- Hepatitis E (HEV), like HAV, is contracted by ingesting the virus in food or water.

Incubation periods vary according to the dose of virus to which the patient was exposed, the higher the inoculum, the shorter the incubation period (Table 21.3).

History

The history of all types of viral hepatitis is similar.

- Initially, a non-specific viral illness – fever, myalgia, malaise, few or no rigors, loss of appetite, epigastric discomfort and vomiting – is common.
- Travel to an endemic area (or, in the case of HBV and HCV, a high-risk exposure).
- The first specific symptom of hepatitis is, usually, darkening of the urine. Males notice this earlier than females, because they watch their

stream during micturition. Bilirubinuria starts as a dark yellow or orange colour, later becoming darker. Ask the patient to point out something in the room that was the colour of the urine, or offer them alternatives (like honey → Lucozade → beer → black tea) to choose from. The colour is important to distinguish from haematuria (like rosé wine → red wine → frank blood → blood with clots) and haemoglobinuria (like Coca-Cola).

- The patient may notice the sclerae becoming yellow when looking in the mirror. Jaundice is more obvious in the daylight than under artificial light which has a yellow spectrum.
- Once jaundice begins, the viraemic symptoms (fever, myalgia, anorexia) should start to fade and the patient should feel better. The return of appetite is a turning point.
- Even when recovering systemically, the patient may continue to become more jaundiced and develop itching of the skin (cholestatic phase); in this phase, the alanine aminotransferase (ALT)/ aspartate aminotransferase (AST) levels will be falling but the alkaline phosphatase (ALP) and bilirubin levels continue to rise.

IMPORTANT

Warning symptoms in a patient with hepatitis:

- ongoing high fever despite obvious jaundice. Think of: wrong diagnosis – has the patient got malaria, septicaemia or typhoid? Is the patient developing liver necrosis/fulminant hepatitis?
- tachycardia or toxic appearance are further signs for concern.
- drowsiness – is the patient developing encephalopathy/liver failure?

Examination

It is essential to decide whether the liver disease has a chronic or acute-on-chronic component. If there is chronic disease, the prognosis is substantially worse, especially if bleeding from varices occurs. Look for signs of liver disease, including chronic liver disease (cirrhosis) and liver failure (Table 21.4).

Table 21.4 Signs of chronic liver disease and liver failure

Signs of liver disease	Signs of chronic liver disease (cirrhosis)	Signs of liver failure
Jaundice	Leuconychia, clubbing	Encephalopathy
Hepatomegaly	Spider naevi	Bleeding
Splenomegaly	Telangiectasias on cheeks	Hypoglycaemia
	Palmar erythema Thick head of hair Gynaecomastia, testicular atrophy Ascites Ankle oedema Oesophageal varices, caput medusae	

Jaundice

Jaundice is easiest to detect in daylight: the patient is asked to look at their feet and the upper eyelid drawn back to see the sclera normally concealed by the lid. Distinguish the yellow colour of jaundice from the ivory or brownish colour of the exposed sclera in people living in dusty environments. Note that in jaundice, the conjugated bilirubin, which is water soluble, appears in the urine and stains elastic tissues of the sclera (most obvious), soft palate and under the tongue. The opposite is true in carotenaemia, in which the lipid-rich stratum corneum (especially skin of the palms and soles) becomes yellow, but the sclerae are white and the urine colour is normal. Carotenaemia is seen in those consuming a lot of carrots or tomatoes, and is common in African children in the mango season. Note whether the patient has been scratching (clue: the fingernails glisten from being polished against the skin).

Liver examination

Palpate the liver and spleen. Note if the liver is non-tender and firm or even hard suggestive of cirrhosis. A knobbly liver usually indicates malignant deposits. Listen for a bruit over the liver.

Technique

Take the radial pulse to give the timing of the heartbeat; place the diaphragm of your stethoscope just below the right costal margin in the mid-clavicular line and press down with your palm over the stethoscope. A bruit is a humming or whooshing sound heard over the liver. Check that it is not just a heart murmur radiating down from the praecordium. If present, a bruit suggests a primary liver cancer (hepatoma); 50 per cent of hepatomas will have a bruit, or else severe acute alcoholic hepatitis. Listen too for a peritoneal rub. This is rare, and sounds like a soft pleural rub on inspiration. It is sometimes heard over abscesses.

Encephalopathy

It is vital to detect encephalopathy as the sign of liver failure, because transfer to a liver unit will depend on the early detection of the following features.

- **Drowsiness**: at first the patient spends much of the day asleep though is rousable, later rouses with difficulty, then is unrousable.
- **Asterixis** (flapping tremor): this is detected by asking the patient to tense the muscles of upper limbs as follows:
  - ask the patient to extend both arms horizontally
  - then to extend the wrist backwards (to 90° to the arms)
  - then to spread the fingers wide; then to close their eyes and hold that position for 1 minute.

> **CLINICAL PEARL**
>
> A flapping tremor consists of irregular jerking/myoclonic movements of the hands that are not rhythmic nor occurring simultaneously on both sides. During the history-taking, there is often a clue that a flapping tremor will be present because the patient's hands are 'twitchy'. If you take the patient's hand and press it back to extend the wrist, you may often induce the flapping to begin. This persists even when the patient is unconscious.

- **Hepatic fetor**: the patient's breath has a smell like that of stale urine (or the urine in a pet hamster's cage). This is caused by ammonia and ammonia-like substances (methyl mercaptone). Ammonia,

which crosses into the brain causing the encephalopathy, accumulates because the liver fails to synthesize urea.

- **Constructional apraxia**: hepatic encephalopathy seems to affect the non-dominant parietal lobe early, so that the patient cannot properly draw a solid shape.
  - On one side of the patient's notes, draw a five-pointed star (like a sheriff's star).
  - Write 'Dr' underneath it.
  - Ask the patient to copy the star and write 'patient/date' beneath it.

The patient's descent into encephalopathy and emergence from it can be documented in this way (Fig. 21.5).

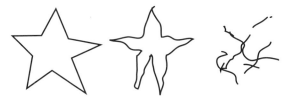

Figure 21.5 Constructional apraxia. The doctor has drawn a solid star (left) in the patient's notes and asked the patient with liver disease to copy it. The patient's attempts show (centre) there is mild constructional apraxia, and (right) severe apraxia later, when the patient developed hepatic encephalopathy. At this stage the patient was sleeping most of the day, had a flapping tremor (asterixis) and had hepatic foetor.

'FLU-LIKE' ILLNESS

General practitioners are generally correct when they say an infection is 'a virus', but the doctor needs to make an accurate assessment to be sure of not missing a serious bacterial infection masquerading as 'flu'. You should know all the features of sepsis intimately (see above), and expect to see none of them in a simple viral respiratory tract infection before diagnosing a 'flu-like illness'.

History

- Influenza is highly infectious, so friends, family, or colleagues should also be affected at the same time – the incubation period is short (1–3 days). If there are no other cases, question the diagnosis.

- The onset of viraemic symptoms is abrupt and often quite severe, with chills, headache, and myalgia. There may be mild rigors on the first day, but these are not sustained.
- As the next few days pass, the fever improves each day, and by day 3 the fever is settling or absent. A fever that continues for more than 3 days is not uncomplicated 'flu, and nor is an illness with rigors after the first day.
- As the viraemia subsides, so the upper respiratory symptoms become prominent. The term 'upper respiratory tract' refers to everything above the trachea: larynx, epiglottis, pharynx, tonsils, middle ears, sinuses. The patient experiences a combination of: rasping sore throat, dry cough, hoarseness, coryza, red eyes, congested sinuses. These persist for a long time (10 days is not unusual) and the patient feels 'miserable' but the fever is no longer prominent.

Examination

Influenza-like illness is very characteristic: the patient has either a viraemic illness with no localizing signs (distinguish this from sepsis by its mildness), or upper respiratory symptoms and signs. The upper respiratory tract infection commonly spreads to give:

- sinusitis – a postnasal drip of muco-pus ± pain in the sinuses
- tracheo-bronchitis – the cough becomes productive of mucus or muco-pus (patients may say, quite accurately, 'The cold has gone to my chest').

These can usually be treated symptomatically with analgesics and decongestants. However, be alert for tachypnoea or signs of hypoxia or consolidation as these suggest secondary bacterial pneumonia. If the tonsils are purulent, or if the picture is of tonsillitis *without* a generalized pharyngitis, then streptococcal tonsillitis is more likely.

CLINICAL PEARL

Be alert for a patient who attends the emergency department late at night for 'flu' – the diagnosis is likely to be more serious! Patients with minor or 'nuisance' illnesses seldom come for help late at night.

GLANDULAR-FEVER-LIKE ILLNESS

Several infections cause a similar picture to 'glandular fever'. The commonest is EBV, with cytomegalovirus (CMV) a close second; HIV seroconversion may look clinically identical, and acute toxoplasmosis similar (except for the lack of sore throat). Glandular fever in the USA is called 'infectious mononucleosis' (or just 'mono').

History

Classically, the patient is an adolescent who has started a close relationship. If an older adult is affected, they have often started a new relationship a few months earlier. Glandular fever is not sexually acquired, but acquired from kissing in most cases, and the history will usually reveal this – once you have won the patient's confidence. EBV and CMV are of relatively low infectivity, so another route of infection, e.g. droplet or aerosol infection is unlikely. The source of infection is perfectly well, but intermittently and asymptomatically excretes EBV or CMV in their saliva. The illness starts with viraemic symptoms of fever (without marked rigors), myalgia, lassitude, and anorexia. A sore throat is characteristic, and the urine often darkens (indicating liver involvement).

Examination

The patient often has a characteristic 'nasal' voice because of enlarged adenoids and with the necrotic tonsils has a characteristic bad breath. The tonsils may be large and covered with a greyish slough – not true pus (in streptococcal sore throats there is often

IMPORTANT   *i*

Be very alert for *any* sign of stridor, or if the tonsils meet in the middle or are threatening to obstruct (a clue is that the patient is unable to swallow their saliva and is drooling or spitting it out). If there are any of these signs of upper airway obstruction, give steroids, intravenous fluids, and call the ENT surgeons urgently – fatal obstruction occasionally occurs in the middle of the night.

pus oozing from the tonsillar crypts). In glandular fever, the soft palate often bears fine petechiae.

Lymph nodes will be enlarged, up to ~2.5 cm diameter, mobile and slightly tender. All regions are involved – not just the tonsillar nodes in the anterior triangle (unlike streptococcal sore throats in which those are usually the only lymph nodes enlarged). The skin may have a macular rash, and if amoxicillin has mistakenly been given for a few days, this rash is very common (80 per cent). This is because most people with EBV glandular fever develop a temporary allergy to amoxicillin. There may be a tinge of jaundice. The abdomen often reveals a soft slightly tender hepatosplenomegaly, each 2–6 cm enlarged.

> ### *i* IMPORTANT
> Be very alert for a painful or tender spleen, or any signs of peritonism. In glandular fever the spleen may rupture spontaneously; it is rare, but tragic. It usually begins as a subcapsular haematoma, with pain and tenderness in the left upper quadrant. A secondary rupture through the capsule then occurs at a later date, and this is often rapidly fatal. If in any doubt about the health of the spleen, get an urgent ultrasound or CT to look for the subcapsular haematoma and ask for an experienced surgeon or physician to check your findings.

In toxoplasmosis, the throat is not inflamed but the rest of the clinical picture may be identical. In HIV seroconversion, the patient may naturally be reluctant at first to tell you of their sexual contact which occurred 2–12 weeks previously, but this is often revealed once you have gained their confidence.

Diagnosis of glandular fever

Basic investigations often hint at the diagnosis:

- a modest elevation of ALT and ALP is invariable in EBV and CMV infection
- the WBC is usually low or normal at the start, but after a week of illness the lymphocyte count starts to rise.

Lymphocytosis may reach levels exceeding 10×10^9/L; microscopy shows these to be characteristic 'glandular fever' cells – hence the name 'infectious mononucleosis'.

TUBERCULOSIS

Tuberculosis mimics many conditions, but has characteristic symptoms and signs.

History

Tuberculosis is much commoner in some population groups than others, so your 'index of suspicion' will be different for a white, UK-born patient (incidence of tuberculosis in this group is well below 5 per 100 000 per year) versus a patient who has immigrated from Somalia within the past 5 years (incidence in this group >500 per 100 000 per year). The patient has usually spent time in a country where tuberculosis is prevalent (though this may have been decades previously), or has been in contact with a known case of pulmonary tuberculosis, or is elderly and has been exposed to tuberculosis in the UK in the era when it was common (before 1950).

Tuberculosis is never an acute illness – typically the symptoms will emerge over weeks.

- **Weight loss:** this is almost always present. It is caused by anorexia, although the patient is eating as much as they feel like, so it is usually the family who report the loss of appetite.
- **Fever:** there are seldom rigors (except miliary tuberculosis, in which the infection is blood-borne). The fever is intermittent, but eventually has a characteristic pattern of feeling colder in the evenings and with sweats at night. Typically, the TB patient will describe waking in the middle of the night or early morning with pyjamas that are soaked with sweat; commonly they have to change pyjamas in the night, or sleep on a towel.

> ### SMALL PRINT
> Night sweats are *characteristic* but not *specific* for tuberculosis – they also occur in other chronic infections and inflammatory diseases.

- **Localizing symptoms:**
  - in ~50 per cent of tuberculosis patients the disease is pulmonary. This gives rise to a cough which persists for weeks; it becomes productive of scanty mucoid or blood-streaked sputum

- in ~25 per cent of tuberculosis patients, the disease is localized to lymph nodes. Commonly, these are in the neck, and the patient may notice them when bathing or looking in the mirror. The lymph nodes enlarge gradually and with little pain or overlying inflammation
- in ~25 per cent of tuberculosis patients, the disease affects almost any other site: if in the pleura there may be little pleuritic pain; if in bone (e.g. spine) there is constant discomfort which does not settle when lying down/resting; if in the abdomen or peritoneum there is gradual discomfort and distension, with diarrhoea being mild or absent.

Examination

General

- The patient is usually thin, but often surprisingly sprightly and seldom spends time lying in bed.
- Uneaten meals and snacks will be evident in the room, indicating anorexia.
- The temperature chart will show up to 39–40 °C, characteristically in the evening (though consuming paracetamol will transform the chart into irregular spikes).
- Leuconychia is common, clubbing absent (unless there is bronchiectasis secondary to severe pulmonary tuberculosis).
- The patient is coughing, but this is seldom hacking or continuous. With pulmonary tuberculosis there is frequently laryngeal involvement, and the patient's voice may have a slightly hoarse or whispering quality.
- Lymph nodes are most frequently found in the neck – generally a few are clustered together, each ~2–4 cm in diameter, mobile and non-tender. Once a tuberculosis lymph node is >3 cm in diameter, the centre should be necrotic when the node is needled; once it is >5 cm in diameter the node should be fluctuant on examination. Note: If nodes >3 cm are solid, the diagnosis of tuberculosis is unlikely.
- A 'cold abscess' may be found anywhere, typically arising from a lymph node or bone.

Cardiac

Tachycardia indicates severe disease and is a 'warning sign'. Check for signs of pericardial effusion with tamponade or constriction: elevated jugular venous pressure, pulsus paradoxus, impalpable apex beat, increased cardiac dullness on percussion and soft heart sounds.

Respiratory

While a cough and tachypnoea may be found, the stethoscope is generally useless in predicting the presence of pulmonary tuberculosis; the chest X-ray is the key to diagnosis (Fig. 21.6). Pleural TB is easily detected clinically, as the effusions are almost always large.

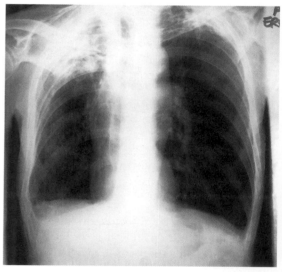

Figure 21.6 Right upper lobe tuberculous infection. From: Kinirons M, Ellis H (eds), *French's index of differential diagnosis* (14th edition), with permission. © 2005 London: Hodder Arnold.

Abdomen

In peritoneal tuberculosis, the abdomen is usually distended with a mixture of peritoneal fluid (shifting dullness) and thickening of intraperitoneal tissues, giving a characteristically 'doughy' feel.

Neurological

Tuberculous meningitis is associated with gradually evolving neck stiffness. Drowsiness, cranial nerve palsies or motor weakness are signs of severity.

Locomotor

- In spinal tuberculosis there will often be tenderness when you percuss over the infected vertebra.
- Method: use fingers first, then the tendon hammer onto your fingers, and finally the side of your fist, work your way down the spine and watch the patient for wincing).
- Deformity (an angulation when you run your hands down the contour of the spine) is a warning sign.
- In spinal tuberculosis, motor weakness, a sensory level or bladder involvement are all extremely serious findings, and may require emergency management (MRI, steroids, surgical referral).
- Tuberculosis affecting a bone or joint outside the spine is usually clinically unimpressive; the lesion is slightly swollen but no acute inflammation is present.

Diagnosis of TB and common pitfalls

TB is confirmed by seeing (down a high-powered microscope, under Ziehl–Neelsen or auramine staining) or culturing *Mycobacterium tuberculosis*.

For the laboratory to report a specimen as *smear positive*, there are >5000 organisms per mL of sample – a situation which commonly occurs *only* in the sputum of patients with *cavities on chest X-ray*. Thus a negative smear result from any other sample is still consistent with tuberculosis: CSF, pus, lymph node aspirate, sputum from a tuberculosis patient without cavities, etc. All of these are usually culture positive, but smear negative.

However, if a patient with cavities on the chest radiograph produces three sputum samples that are of *good quality* (i.e. not saliva) and which are *smear negative*, then tuberculosis can be virtually ruled out in that patient.

Be sure to request tuberculosis culture – it is a slow process (up to 6 weeks for a positive result) and labour-intensive, so routine specimens are not cultured for tuberculosis unless specified.

IMPORTANT
Mycobacterium tuberculosis will not grow once specimens have been preserved – be sure that biopsy specimens are cultured without being put into formalin.

SUMMARY

- The pattern of fever is unimportant, but the duration of fever, the height of the fever and the presence of rigors give crucial clues.
- Weight loss due to loss of appetite is invariable in febrile patients.
- A travel history is essential, especially for malaria.
- Look for signs of infective endocarditis.
- There are important clues in the skin and mucous membranes.
- Be very familiar with the signs of sepsis, and especially severe sepsis.
- Be sure to take all your cultures before starting antibiotics, but do not delay treatment in sepsis.
- Know how to assess hydration: in an adult it is done by assessing the circulation and is not the same as in infants.
- Be sure to examine carefully for a stiff neck (meningism) and, if unsure, repeat your examination until the picture is clearer.
- Headache, fever and drowsiness are the hallmarks of encephalitis – you should be able to distinguish this condition from a toxic confusional state, and distinguish psychosis from both.
- Rabies and tetanus are diagnosed clinically.
- Gastrointestinal infections: there characteristic clues on the history indicating what part of the digestive tract is involved, and hence what pathogen is responsible.
- The examination of the jaundiced patient can easily distinguish acute from chronic liver disease, and detect liver failure.
- Know the features of upper respiratory and pharyngeal infections, so you do not label serious infections as being 'flu-like'.
- Know the features of tuberculosis, and who is likely to be at risk of it.

FURTHER READING

Eddlestone M, Davidson R, Brent A, Wilkinson R (eds). 2008. *The Oxford handbook of tropical medicine*, 3rd edn. Oxford: Oxford University Press.
Peters W, Pasvol G. 2006. *Atlas of tropical medicine and parasitology*, 6th edn. Edinburgh: Mosby.

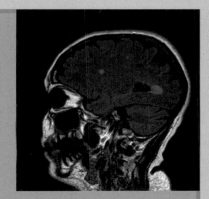

C SPECIAL SITUATIONS

22

ASSESSMENT OF THE NEWBORN, INFANTS AND CHILDREN

Chris Dewhurst and Leena Patel

INTRODUCTION

Paediatric history taking and examination require some basic skills and the need to consider special attributes that differentiate children from adults (Box 22.1). When referring to children use the appropriate term, depending on their age (Table 22.1). Children's ability to understand, communicate, express feelings, cooperate with clinical assessment, make decisions and participate in their healthcare is age dependent, and the role of the parent will vary accordingly. Therefore an individually tailored approach is required.

BOX 22.1 CORE SKILLS IN RELATION TO ACUTE ILLNESS

'Foundation doctors will provide care for children in primary care and in a variety of secondary care settings such as surgery and the emergency department. They must learn to recognize serious illness in infants and children in these settings so that they can seek help promptly. The trajectory of illness is generally different from that in adults, and the signs of critical illness are often subtle or vague in the early stages.'

Foundation Programme Curriculum (2007)

Table 22.1 Terms used to describe children in different age groups, and the characteristics to be aware of during history taking and examination

Term	Characteristics
Neonate: birth to 28 days	Depends on parents for all needs Makes different sounds and cries to indicate pleasure, hunger and pain
Infant: 1 month to 1 year	Depends on parents for all needs Makes eye contact, recognizes parents and smiles Older infants are wary of strangers and anxious if separated from parents Infants >6 months look at faces and listen when spoken to, respond to name and familiar words (e.g. mummy, milk); and respond to simple requests (e.g. 'Give to mummy'; 'More milk?')
Toddler: 1–2 years	Uneasy with strangers and unfamiliar places: clings to parents, shy, sucks thumb, hits, kicks, cries, says 'No!' Understands simple questions (e.g. 'Where is teddy?'), shows objects and body parts by pointing Can express needs (e.g. 'More milk', 'No more', 'No wee wee')
Pre-school: 2–5 years	Understands questions, gives answers that can be understood, and will also ask questions ('What?' and 'Why?') By 4 years of age, clear fluent speech and will talk to strangers Can revert to toddler behaviour in unfamiliar environments or if unwell Can dress and undress, indicate toilet needs Very active and curious, but limited concentration span and easily distracted
School: 5–11 years	Begins to challenge adults Better social skills Develops interests and hobbies Begins to take some responsibilities
Adolescent: 11–18 years	Should be allowed to think for self and make informed choices Likes to assert independence Does not like being referred to as a child Concerned about physical appearance Influenced by peers and social acceptance

Table 22.2 Components of the paediatric history

Presenting problem	Sequence, duration and evolution of symptoms Parent and child's perspective of events Associated symptoms, predisposing factors, background problems Impact on child's life and the family, e.g. school absence and time off work Treatment if any and response Thoughts and feelings about the problem, e.g. self-blame Reason for seeking medical advice and expectations, e.g. parents may simply be seeking reassurance
Medicines and allergies	Treatment, including doses and compliance Allergic reactions (including nature of reaction), other side effects
Pregnancy and birth	Mother's age Pregnancy planned or unplanned During pregnancy: mother's health, medication, smoking, recreational drugs, events, e.g. accident, bleeding, antenatal monitoring and scans Delivery: gestation (born when expected or earlier), labour spontaneous or induced, drugs in labour, prolonged rupture of membranes, mode (vaginal, forceps or Caesarean section) At birth: birth weight, spontaneous breathing or need for resuscitation Initial feeding: breast or bottle, vomiting, poor feeding Neonatal problems: e.g. jaundice, low blood glucose, blue, floppy, admission to baby unit
Immunizations and health promotion	Ascertain immunizations given according to nationally recommended schedule; reasons if not given (e.g. pertussis or measles–mumps–rubella vaccine, Fig. 22.1) Check personal child health record (the 'Red book') Healthy eating and regular exercise Accident prevention Adolescents: safe sex and contraception; advice against smoking, alcohol and drug abuse
Past medical and surgical history	Previous illnesses, hospital admissions, operations Professionals involved in management Common childhood illnesses, e.g. chickenpox, measles
Diet	Feeding in infancy and age at weaning Type and amount of fluid intake, snacks and meals, food variety, eating behaviour
Growth and puberty	Weight, length/height and head circumference measured and plotted on growth charts Check previous measurements, e.g. child health record (the 'Red book') Size compared with peers Puberty in adolescents • Girls: onset of breast development, menarche • Boys: onset of testicular enlargement, genital changes, shaving
Neurodevelopment and school	Age <4 years: gross motor, fine motor, vision, hearing and language, social School-age: school progress and ability compared with peers
Family	Home: lives with parents, foster carer (i.e. 'looked after child') Structure and dynamics: parents married, separated or single; siblings Health: problems similar or relevant to those of the child, e.g. atopic disease; epilepsy; mental illness; family history of type 2 diabetes, high cholesterol, high blood pressure or heart disease for an overweight child; disability in parents or siblings Smoking, alcohol or substance abuse Family tree (Fig. 22.2)
Social	Ethnic, cultural, religious background, beliefs and values Parents' occupation or social benefits Support mechanisms, e.g. family/friends or isolated family Accommodation Pets Transport Travel abroad

HISTORY TAKING FROM CHILDREN AND PARENTS

Taking a history and doing the examination are complementary in the clinical assessment of children, and many aspects are done simultaneously. Thorough examination may not be possible in a young child who is unwilling or not able to cooperate but a comprehensive history (Table 22.2) along with astute observations can provide valuable information about:

- what the child and parents are concerned about
- whether there is anything wrong with the child.

Whenever possible, start by talking to the child. Infants are unable to pinpoint or verbalize but their behaviour conveys how they feel. The information elicited from preschool-age children will be limited but they can point to painful body parts (e.g. 'Show me the sore?'). By 4 years a child can communicate fluently, whereas older children and teenagers should be allowed to relate their own history.

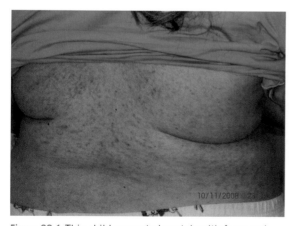

Figure 22.1 This child presented acutely with fever and confluent macular erythematous rash. It started on the face and behind the ears before spreading to the rest of the body. An increased number of cases of measles are due to poor uptake of the measles–mumps–rubella vaccine. Unsubstantiated links with autism in the 1990s resulted in many parents declining the vaccine for their children. Photograph courtesy of Dr Harold Sackey and Dr Julie Ellison, Leighton Hospital, Crewe.

> **CLINICAL PEARL**
> *How babies and young children communicate*: even babies and young children who have not yet developed fluent speech can convey a lot about what is wrong with them:
> - be patient and offer encouragement
> - listen attentively
> - watch facial expressions, gestures and behaviour closely.

Consent

Consent to undertake the clinical assessment should be obtained from the child as well as the parents, and includes:

- introductions and asking the child's name
- explaining the purpose for taking a history and examining, and your role
- asking permission from parents and also the child if they are old enough to understand
- respecting privacy and confidentiality.

Establish rapport

An open and mutually trusting relationship is necessary to elicit the history, unveil the family's anxieties and expectations, and gain cooperation from the child. Attention to what the child sees, hears, perceives and does throughout the consultation contributes to establishing rapport. This includes the following:

- greeting with a warm sincere smile, a welcoming voice and using the child's name creates a powerful first impression
- shake hands with the child – this will make them less apprehensive when you later ask to examine their hands
- ask the child their age – this gives them an opportunity to speak (a child knows this by age 4 years)
- communicate with both the child and parents
- arrange seating in a way that avoids physical barriers, allows good eye contact with the child and maintains a professional distance (Fig. 22.3). Have available a variety of toys
- tailor the tone of your voice, manner and approach according to the age and level of understanding of the child

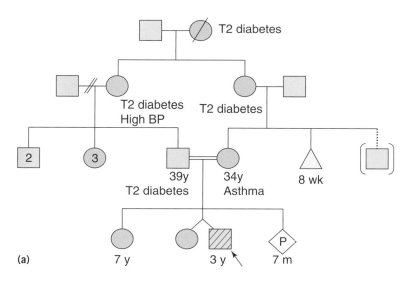

Figure 22.2 Symbols to represent the family tree: (**a**) example of a family tree; (**b**) symbols.

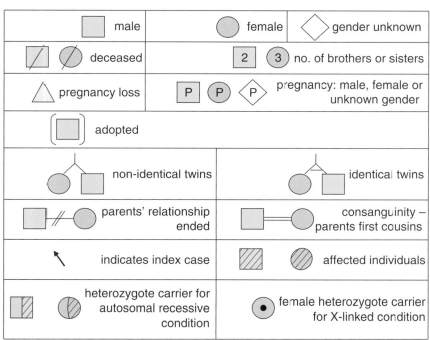

(b)

- listen attentively – maintain eye contact, nod encouragingly, pick up cues from what they say as well as their body language and then explore these with probing open questions
- match and mirror the language, phrases and words used by the child and parents (e.g. 'He's got the runs'; 'She's always got a pot belly'; 'There's a wobble in her eyes') but clarify the meaning
- engage the child by exploring interests, such as favourite toys, pop group, hobbies, the football team they support, television characters and their school activities

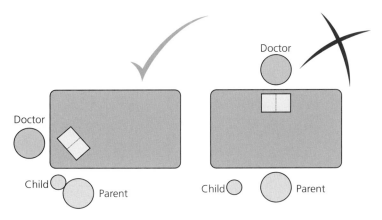

Figure 22.3 Seating arrangements during a paediatric consultation.

- attend to the child's and sibling's needs (e.g. by holding the door open; offering a chair, giving an appropriate toy and allowing to play; pausing if the child needs a feed or the toilet)
- be humble and ask parents what they think about the problem, their concerns and their expectations
- compliment, respect and thank parents and children for what they do and say (e.g. to the parents: 'It's very good that you gave paraceta- mol and you did the right thing in asking for an appointment' or 'You have thought of very

important issues' ; to the child: 'What a clever boy'; 'Good girl. Thank you for letting me feel your tummy').

Procedure to elicit the history

The history should be structured and comprehen- sive but at the same time focused and relevant to the presenting problem (see Table 22.2).

- Explain the context and objective of the clinical assessment.
- Initiate with open questions and explain the reasons for questions. This helps elicit more information.
- Identify cues and explore them with further open questions ('What?' and 'Why?').
- Use closed questions to ascertain specific points.
- Ask parents to describe what happened to the child and their interpretation (e.g. 'Why do you think he has had this cough for so long? What do you think the cause is?'). Although symp- toms in infants and toddlers are frequently vague and non-specific, parents know their child best and are able to recognize when the child is unwell.
- Document symptoms reported by parents verbatim.
- Clarify the meaning of terms used by parents as they may be different from your understanding (e.g. wheezy, diarrhoea, constipation, fits). Ask parents to mimic what they heard or observed

CLINICAL PEARL

Create a safe environment and build rapport: these are essential during history taking and will allow children and parents to reveal their concerns, fears, thoughts and feelings. Avoid:

- stern appearance, white coat and stethoscope round the neck
- interrupting when the child or parent is talking
- judgements about what they tell you
- dismissing or ignoring what they tell you
- too many closed questions
- distractions, e.g. people going in and out of the room, telephone calls
- appearing rushed or preoccupied with something else.

(e.g. the 'wheezy' noise or the movements in the 'fits').

- Explore labels given to them by other professionals (e.g. chest infection, silent reflux, urine infection, allergy to penicillin) and do not unquestioningly accept these.
- Do not be content with vague or general statements and try to obtain precise details (e.g. in treatment history, 'penicillin liquid four times a day for 5 days' instead of merely 'a course of antibiotics'; 'two puffs of a brown inhaler twice a day with a spacer' instead of simply 'an inhaler').
- Enquire about hidden anxieties (in a child with headaches, parents might fear they have a brain tumour) and feelings (e.g. a child with fits: 'This can be a very frightening experience for parents. How did you feel?').

The history thus elicited will provide plenty of clues to possible diagnoses and problems. These help to select aspects of the physical examination that are relevant.

CLINICAL PEARL

Ask 'Why?'. Probe throughout the history, for example if:
- parents think a child can't hear – 'Why do they think that?'
- a child was born by caesarean section – 'Why?'
- a child was admitted to baby unit – 'Why?'
- a child was not given the measles–mumps–rubella vaccine – 'Why?' (see Fig. 22.1, p. 392).

---

i **IMPORTANT**

Pain which must be taken seriously in a child includes:
- morning headaches
- neck pain
- backache
- chest pain worse on coughing or deep breathing
- epigastric pain which occurs at night and disturbs sleep
- joint pain associated with swelling.

PHYSICAL EXAMINATION IN PAEDIATRICS

The importance of observation

The examination should be focused and relevant to the problems identified in the history. Observation is crucial, from the time you first set eyes on the child until the end of the consultation. This means listening and watching simultaneously for the child's:

- size and appearance, including clothes
- posture, movements and gait
- vocalization, speech and body language
- interest in what is around them, what and how they play, and behaviour
- reactions and interaction with parents and others.

Observations need to be compared and interpreted with:

- what the child is like when well (parents are the ones who know their child best)
- what you might expect in an otherwise normal child of comparable age.

IMPORTANT   *i*

The holistic approach: physical examination of a child includes actively listening and observing throughout history taking, examination and discussion of management.

Approach to physical examination

The approach to the physical examination should be age appropriate, gentle and non-threatening.

- Children under 4 years of age can become anxious if separated from parents and placed on an examination couch. Leave them wherever they are (e.g. in the safety of parent's lap, standing or sitting next to parents, or playing with toys) and start by observing them from a distance.
- In a gentle tone, ask the child permission to examine, e.g. 'Please can you show me your hands?' Start with the hands as this allows the child to gain confidence in you.

- Thereafter you can request the child to be positioned comfortably and appropriately for you to do a systemic examination. A young child can be examined sitting and lying on a parent's lap. If examination necessitates positioning the child on a couch, having the parents standing close by and holding the child's hand can be reassuring.
- Defer undressing until after examination of exposed parts as it can be frightening for young children and embarrassing for older ones. Leave any unpleasant examination (e.g. throat, genitalia) until the end. If an adolescent patient requests being examined in the absence of parents, ensure that a chaperone (e.g. a nurse) is present.
- In infants and toddlers, the examination is opportunistic and the sequence followed for adults is frequently not possible. If a child is asleep, start with auscultation rather than palpation as the latter is likely to wake up the child.
- Explain to the child and parents what you are going to do and why.

> **CLINICAL PEARL**
> *The reluctant child*: do not force a child to be examined. A child's apprehension and unwillingness can be recognized from:
> - 'No!' or head shaking
> - crying, hitting, kicking or resisting
> - hiding their face or running away.
>
> In these situations explain the examination, gently persuade, distract with toys, offer a feed or dummy, and/or seek the parent's assistance to help you examine the child.

Specific examination techniques in paediatrics

The components of general and systemic examination in children are the same as adults but in addition there are two unique assessments (presented in detail later in this chapter):

- neurodevelopment
- growth and puberty.

Examination techniques for older children and adolescents are virtually the same as for adults. Some aspects of examination for infants and toddlers are different, and these along with particular attributes in this age group are highlighted below.

> **CLINICAL PEARL**
> Respect the child's dignity and body. Do not start the physical examination by:
> - undressing the child
> - putting your hands on the child
> - asking the child to lie down on the couch.
>
> Start with examining parts that are already exposed. Later explain what parts need to be exposed and why. Children older than 3–4 years age can undress and expose themselves on request. For younger ones, seek the parent's advice and assistance: they will know what their child will allow, will be adept at undressing their child and this is also less threatening for the child.

Respiratory and ENT examination

- Nature of the cough and sputum: with a wet or 'productive' sounding cough, airway mucus tends to be swallowed and then brought up in vomit rather than being expectorated.
- Position of comfort: infants prefer sitting upright or being carried by a parent, with the head resting on the parent's shoulder, when there is airway obstruction.
- Respiratory rate is normally faster in infants and decreases with age (Table 22.3).
- Chest shape: bilateral grooves over the lower part of the chest – Harrison's sulci – result from chronic indrawing of the lower ribs (Fig. 22.4).
- Percussion: use a light tap as the chest is normally more resonant than in older individuals.

Table 22.3 Normal respiratory and heart rates in children

Age group	Respiratory rate/minute	Heart rate/minute
<1 year	30–40	110–160
1–5 years	25–30	95–140
5–12 years	20–25	80–120
>12 years	15–20	60–100

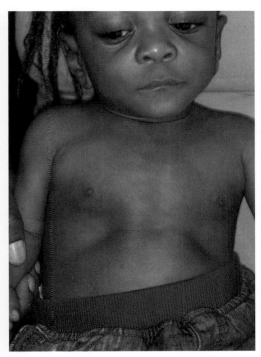

Figure 22.4 Infant with Harrison's sulci: bilateral grooves at the insertion of the diaphragm with flaring of the lower ribs. This is seen in chronic airway obstruction and rickets. In this infant, flaring of the nostrils and pursed lips suggest increased effort to breathe.

> **IMPORTANT**
>
> Respiratory distress can be due to a respiratory or a cardiac problem. Signs include:
> - increased respiratory rate or tachypnoea, i.e. need for increased ventilation
> - pursing lips on expiration to increase pressure and prolong expiration
> - expiratory grunt from exhaling against a partially closed glottis in order to increase end-expiratory pressure
> - nasal flaring, and intercostal, subcostal and sternal recessions owing to increased work of breathing
> - head bobbing from use of sternomastoid as an accessory muscle
> - laboured breathing.

- Auscultation: use the bell of the stethoscope as it is smaller and the rubber does not feel cold. The bell placed on the hand first and gently moved towards the chest is more likely to be accepted by an infant, and if necessary let them grasp your or a parent's finger.
- Breath sounds: in infants these are broncho-vesicular owing to the thin chest.

Cardiovascular examination

- Heart rate is normally faster in infants (Table 22.3).
- Palpate the brachial pulses rather than the radial as they are easier to feel; simultaneously compare with femoral pulses. In the newborn and first few months, palpate the femoral pulses by gently flexing and abducting the hips. Impalpable pulses suggest coarctation of the aorta. Bounding pulses are present in haemodynamically significant patent ductus arteriosus (PDA).
- Measure the blood pressure using an appropriate sized cuff (covering two-thirds of the arm) and interpret from age- and gender-specific normal ranges.
- Breathlessness is indicated by tiredness when feeding and not completing feeds.
- Heart failure is indicated by puffiness of the face (but oedema of the feet is unusual), respiratory distress and liver enlargement.
- Check for dysmorphic features in the face and hands, as a heart defect may be part of a syndrome (e.g. atrioventricular septal defect in Down's syndrome, coarctation of the aorta in Turner's syndrome and pulmonary stenosis in Noonan's syndrome).
- Apex beat is in the fourth left intercostal space in the mid-clavicular line in infants and fourth to fifth intercostal space in older children.
- Heart murmurs in infants can be innocent or associated with congenital heart defects. The timing, quality, location and presence of a thrill help to differentiate them (Table 22.4).
- Percussion is superfluous in children.

Table 22.4 Heart murmurs in infants and children

Systolic murmurs are found in up to 50 per cent in the first week of life and usually arise from: • the changing dynamics of the circulation or • an incompletely closed patent ductus arteriosus (continuous systolic or machinery murmur) or • patent foramen ovale (mid-systolic murmur)	
Check preductal and postductal oxygen saturation in infants with a persistent murmur or if features suggest it is not innocent, and consider referral to a paediatric cardiologist	
Clinical features to differentiate innocent from significant heart murmurs	
Innocent if	**Not innocent if**
Mid-systolic or continuous (venous hum)	Diastolic Pansystolic
Soft, grade 1 or 2	Grade 3–6 associated with a thrill
Musical, vibratory or rumbling	Heard all over the praecordium and/or radiates to axilla, back or neck
Localized to left sternal edge or below clavicles	Other positive findings, e.g. low volume or collapsing pulse, absent femoral pulses, displaced apex beat, abnormal heart sounds, signs of heart failure
Changes with position and respiration	
Transient or only heard when child is unwell	

Examination of the abdomen

- Examine the mouth for thrush or ulcers.
- Once they have learnt to sit and stand, children do not like to lie down to be examined. A reasonable examination can be done with the child reclined on a parent's lap, or sitting or standing (Fig. 22.5).
- Owing to the thin abdominal wall, the normal abdomen can appear protuberant but soft. A tense, distended abdomen arouses suspicion.
- Liver and spleen can normally be felt on gentle palpation up to 2 cm below the costal margin, moving with the diaphragm and abdominal wall during respiration. Normal liver span in mid-clavicular line is about 2.5–3 cm in infants, 4–5 cm by age 5 years and 6–10 cm in adolescents. The spleen enlarges towards the left iliac fossa in infants and across towards the right iliac fossa in older children.
- Kidneys are not normally palpable except in the newborn.
- A distended bladder may be visible in infants and can be palpated.
- Genuine tenderness and guarding from peritoneal irritation are involuntary. Assess during auscultation by applying gentle pressure with the stethoscope.

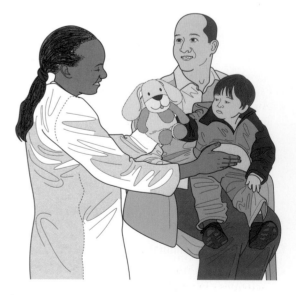

Figure 22.5 Examination of the abdomen in a child reclined on the parent's lap.

Table 22.5 Assessment of cranial nerves in infants and young children

Cranial nerve	Assessment
I	History of recognizing day-to-day smells (e.g. food, sweet flavours, stools)
II	History Observe visual behaviour, squint, nystagmus Check with different-sized objects or toys, and moving objects
III, IV and VI	History Observe for squint, eye movements, eye lids, head tilt Use hand puppets to assess range of movements and distract during funduscopy
V, VII, IX and X	Observe sucking, chewing, swallowing (drooling), crying, smiling and eye closure Listen to speech Gag reflex
VIII	History Observe response to whispers, normal conversation and other noises
XI	Observe head turning
XII	Observe tongue protrusion through imitation

- Expose the nappy area for any perianal excoriation (e.g. lactose intolerance) or rash (e.g. thrush), anal fissures, rectal prolapse (as in cystic fibrosis) and appearance of genitalia. Rectal examination is not routinely done in children.
- Check nappy contents for colour of urine (e.g. dark orange in obstructive jaundice) and appearance of stool (e.g. bulky, greasy and offensive in fat malabsorption).

Nervous system examination

- Observe while taking the history and examine through play as this is most informative.
- Assess cranial nerves from the child's everyday activities (Table 22.5).
- Assess tone, power, movements and coordination from observation of the child's posture (e.g. frog-like in hypotonia (Fig. 22.6), activity (e.g. no anti-gravity movements) and play (e.g. building with 2.5 cm (1 inch) cubes, threading beads, drawing

skills, unusual grasp and handedness). Check tone with passive full range of movements, and shaking of wrists and ankles.
- Use play to assess different muscle groups:
  - offer a toy and hold it up – watch for going on toes and lifting arms to reach for the toy
  - roll a ball or car and ask the child to get it – watch gait, sitting or stooping and getting up, reaching and holding object

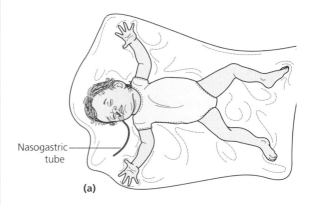

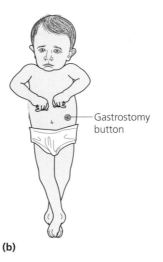

Figure 22.6 (a) Infant with frog-like posture indicating generalized hypotonia. (b) Infant with scissoring of the lower limbs, fisting of the hands, and flexion and pronation of the upper limbs. These are features of spastic quadriplegia. The nasogastric tube in (a) and gastrostomy button in (b) suggest problems with feeding (i.e. sucking and swallowing).

- ask the child to pull paper – small muscles of hand
- ask the child to squeeze your fingers – hand grip
- hold by fingertips – forearm muscles
- lift from under the arms – shoulder adductors
- observe sitting up from lying down – abdominal muscles
- observe getting up from sitting – proximal muscles
- observe crawling up steps – proximal and distal muscles of lower limbs.
- Hand dominance under 1 year is abnormal.
- The plantar response is up-going in infants and before a child is able to walk.

Musculoskeletal examination

- Assess the child's posture (Fig. 22.6), activity and play including gait (e.g. waddle, limp, toe walking), sitting and getting up.
- Look for deformity and asymmetry in limbs (e.g. shortening), chest (e.g. Poland's anomaly), neck (e.g. torticollis) and spine (e.g. scoliosis).

IMPORTANT

Interpreting features from the history and examination: children 'do not read textbooks' when they become unwell and there is a degree of natural variability in the manifestations and course of an illness. Listen to, and respect, what parents tell you. However, be aware of inflicted injuries and fabricated illnesses if there are discrepancies between the history and:

- your examination findings
- your knowledge of normal growth and development, pathological disease processes and natural variations.

ASSESSMENT OF NEURODEVELOPMENT

Child neurodevelopment (frequently referred to as 'development') refers to the neurological, cognitive and psychosocial processes that occur from birth through to the teenage years. A complete paediatric consultation includes a relevant developmental screen to determine if the child's development is age appropriate. A detailed assessment is required when parents or professionals have specific concerns about a developmental problem.

The four main areas of development

Normal development is a continuous integrated process but for the purpose of assessment it is subdivided into four areas:

- gross motor – tone and posture, body-limb movements and locomotion, e.g. sitting, walking
- fine motor and vision – hand skills that are partly dependent on intact visual functioning, e.g. picking up small objects
- hearing, speech and language – these are interrelated and also dependent on cognitive ability, e.g. answering questions such as 'What is your name?'
- social, personal and emotional – including self-help, behaviour and social interaction, e.g. dressing, feeding, listening to a story, playing with others.

For each of these areas, development progresses through predictable stages or milestones (Table 22.6). There is a wide age range at which these milestones are normally reached, and the sequence in achieving them is more important than age.

The developmental assessment

History

The history will help ascertain:

- current level of functioning
- pattern of prior development and any unusual or abnormal development
- potential aetiological factors for developmental delay (Table 22.7).

Parents naturally compare their child's development and abilities with other children in the family or their social environment. If they cannot recall precise details regarding the age at which a particular milestone was reached, referring to common calendar events is helpful, e.g. 'She is really steady on her feet. When did she start walking? Around Christmas?'

Table 22.6 A simplified guide to key developmental milestones

Age	3 months	6 months	9 months	12 months	2 years	3 years	4 years	5 years
Gross motor	Finger play Lifts head+chest	Sits supported	Stands supported Crawls or Creeps	Walks	Runs Climbs, Jumps	Up stairs	Hops Kicks ball	Skips Rides bicycle
Fine motor and vision	Holds rattle Follow 180°	Palmar grasp Reaches for cube	Immature pincer grasp Bangs two cubes	Mature pincer grasp Draws	Two-handedness Draws Stacks 6 cubes	Draws Use 9 cube tower thread beads	Draws man and cross	5 Draws man and cross
Hearing, speech and language	Turns head to sound Chuckles aah, ngah, uh Vowel sounds	Understands voice tones p b m babbles	Responds to name, 'No' mama, dada, bye bye, night night Repetitive sounds	Responds to familiar words: milk, mummy Few words with meaning	Respond to 2 key words 50 words 2–3 word sentence	Name and age Nursery rhyme Who, Why Asks Counts to 3	Responds to simple instructions Speech fluent How, When Ask	Grammar + complex sentences Reads words Count to 20 or more
Social and personal	Recognizes mother and smiles Face expressive Anticipates feeding	Shows likes and dislikes, prefers mother Puts objects in mouth Chews	Looks for familiar people Waves, claps, plays peek-a-boo Holds bottle	Stranger anxiety Hugs doll Simple ball play Drinks from cup	Solitary play Imitates domestic tasks Undresses Uses spoon	Plays with other children Day toilet trained Dresses Washes hands	Pretend play Buttons fully Brushes teeth	Ties shoelaces Uses knife + fork
Warning signs	Abnormal tone Does not fix Does not grasp No smile	Persistence of primitive reflexes Little vocalization Squint	Cannot sit Hand preference No babble Little interest in surroundings	No weight bearing No pincer grasp	No walking Few words Does not point Poor attention	Clumsy Cannot draw straight line Loner	Cannot stack 10 cubes or copy O Unintelligible speech	Cannot copy + Does not know colours or letters

To allow for normal variations, developmental age is defined within 2–3 months in children under age 2 years and within 6 months in children 2–5 years of age. Until age 12 months, allow for prematurity. For a detailed summary of important milestones, refer to the Denver Developmental Screening Test. Line drawings courtesy of Shaili Patel.

Table 22.7 Clues in the history about potential aetiological factors for developmental delay

Prenatal and birth history	Maternal illness (e.g. rubella), medicines (e.g. sodium valproate), smoking, alcohol or recreational drugs in pregnancy Perinatal asphyxia Prematurity and associated complications
Postnatal events	Insult to the brain from injury, infection (meningoencephalitis), hypoglycaemia, kernicterus, tumour Constellation of features suggestive of inborn errors of metabolism or syndrome
Family history including non-immediate family	Familial or genetic conditions, e.g. a boy with learning difficulties may have fragile-X syndrome, with affected males being present on the maternal side
Social history	Environmental or social stimulus, e.g. a child who spends all day in a pram or baby walker will not walk, a child who is rarely spoken to has poor language skills

IMPORTANT

Non-acquisition of a skill significantly outside the normal range serves as a 'warning sign' for a more detailed developmental assessment.

Opportunistic observation

Throughout the consultation observe and pay attention to what the child does – how they play, communicate (see Box 22.2) and interact.

CLINICAL PEARL

A good estimate of a child's level of development can be elicited in an unstructured way during the consultation. If you remain alert and observant, the child will show you their developmental skills. For example, they may walk into the room and say hello when you greet them. Then they might begin playing with a doll, dressing it and combing the hair. Thus, all four key areas of development have been demonstrated without the child being aware of being examined!

Semi-structured examination

- Observe appearance (including head size and dysmorphic features) and obvious neurological abnormality (e.g. nystagmus, floppy posture, limb deformity, involuntary movements) but do not pre-judge development.

- Start the assessment with whatever the child is occupied with and make it playful, e.g. a 2.5-year-old child looking at a book: 'Can you show me what is in the book?'. You would expect the child to name some pictures in the book.
- Then engage the child with a few selected toys and activities (Table 22.6). Each will incorporate several different developmental skills, e.g. the ability of a 4-year-old child to draw a picture of a man on request requires intact hearing, comprehension, cognitive ability to associate a two-dimensional picture with the concept of a man, vision and good fine motor skills.
- Keep instructions simple; do not try to do too much and do not overwhelm the child by cluttering their surroundings with a lot of objects.

BOX 22.2 CAUSES OF DELAYED SPEECH
- Delay in maturation – most common cause and frequently familial.
- Hearing impairment – history of impacted wax, ear infections, meningitis or head injury; tendency to turn up the volume on the television.
- Cognitive and intellectual impairment – learning disability, cannot comprehend.
- Difficulty with articulation – history of cleft lip and palate, nasal regurgitation, can comprehend.
- Environmental from neglect, emotional deprivation and lack of stimulation.
- Social interaction and communication problems – as in autistic spectrum disorder.

- Give the child adequate time and a few attempts to show what they can do.
- Remember to encourage and praise the child.

Observe parents

Findings in the child may prompt examination of parents e.g. a child with hypotonia and delayed gross motor skills whose mother has myotonic dystrophy.

Questions to consider if a child's development is delayed

The answers will provide a plan for further assessment, investigations for potential aetiological causes and direct management.

- Which areas appear to be delayed? All areas (global developmental delay) or restricted to one area (e.g. motor development, Fig. 22.7)?
- What is the magnitude of the delay? Is it within the wide range of normality?
- What is the pattern of abnormal development:
  - development delayed from birth
  - normal progress initially and development delayed after a certain time
  - normal or slow progress with development initially and loss of previously acquired skills, i.e. developmental regression.
- Is there a recognizable pattern to the developmental delay? For example, a child with absent speech, poor eye contact and little social interaction is likely to have autism.
- Has the history and examination revealed any potential aetiological factors (see Table 22.7)?

> **i IMPORTANT**
> Developmental regression means loss of previously acquired physical skills or mental abilities. The causes are:
> - progressive neurodegenerative and metabolic disease, e.g. mucopolysaccharidoses, amino acidurias, organic acidurias
> - uncommon types of epilepsy
> - endocrine: hypothyroidism
> - acute psychotic episode
> - systemic illnesses and psychological disturbances.

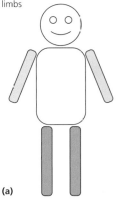

Spastic diplegia – all limbs affected but lower limbs significantly more than upper limbs

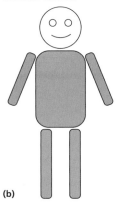

Quadriplegia – upper and lower limbs affected equally trunk also affected

(a)   (b)

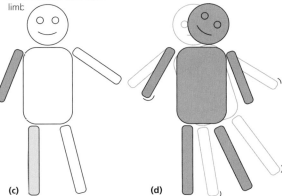

Hemiplegia – unilateral involvement but upper limb more affected than lower limb

Choreo-athetoid – involuntary movements of the whole body

(c)   (d)

Figure 22.7 Patterns of motor deficit in cerebral palsy: (a) spastic diplegia, (b) quadriplegia, (c) hemiplegia and (d) choreo-athetoid cerebral palsy. Cerebral palsy is a disorder of movement and posture. Although non-progressive, its clinical features become increasingly apparent over time as anticipated motor developmental milestones are not achieved.

ASSESSMENT OF GROWTH AND PUBERTY

Assessment of growth

Growth is a dynamic process that occurs throughout childhood and ends after achieving full pubertal

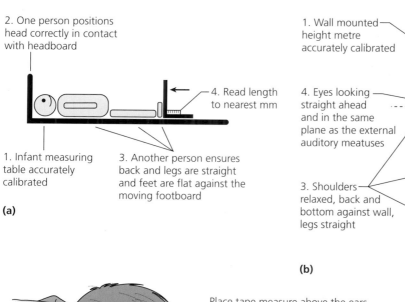

2. One person positions head correctly in contact with headboard

4. Read length to nearest mm

1. Infant measuring table accurately calibrated

3. Another person ensures back and legs are straight and feet are flat against the moving footboard

(a)

1. Wall mounted height metre accurately calibrated

4. Eyes looking straight ahead and in the same plane as the external auditory meatuses

3. Shoulders relaxed, back and bottom against wall, legs straight

7. Read height to the nearest mm

5. Ensure headboard is on top of the head

6. Ask child to breathe in: exert gentle but firm pressure under the mastoid processes as the child breathes out and relaxes

2. No shoes and socks: heels together, flat and against the wall

(b)

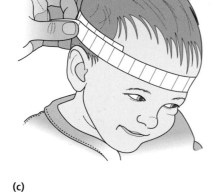

Place tape measure above the ears and midway between the eyebrows and the hairline passing over the occipital prominence at the back of the head

Ensure hair does not interfere with the measurements and remove plaits or braids

If the head is abnormally shaped, place the tape measure over the largest measurable circumference

(c)

Figure 22.8 Techniques for measuring: (**a**) length (if child under 2 years or not able to stand), (**b**) standing height and (**c**) head circumference.

development. Assessment of growth provides a sensitive guide to a child's:

- well-being
- nutritional status
- pubertal development
- disease activity and response to treatment of any underlying illness.

History

- Ask about the child's growth.
- Ask for the parents' height, weight, body mass index (BMI; weight in kg/height in m²) and head circumference if there are concerns about the child's growth.

Measurements (using reliable equipment and correct techniques)

- To measure the weight:
  - use accurately calibrated electronic scales
  - measure with child wearing minimum clothing and infant naked
  - record weight to nearest 100 g.
- Measure the length, height and head circumference (Fig. 22.8):
  - single measurements provide limited information
  - serial measurements show the pattern of growth and growth velocity.
- Calculate the BMI if a child appears overweight or weight is on a higher centile than height.

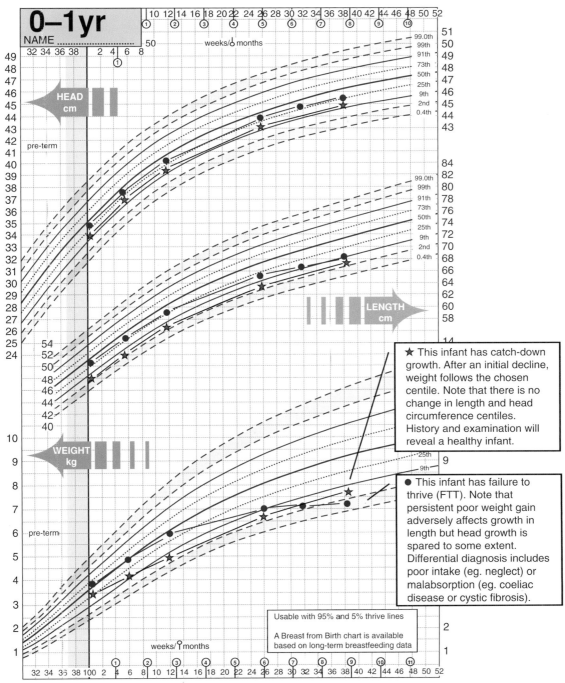

0–1yr

NAME ....

pre-term

HEAD cm

LENGTH cm

WEIGHT kg

pre-term

99.0th
99th
91th
73th
50th
25th
9th
2nd
0.4th

★ This infant has catch-down growth. After an initial decline, weight follows the chosen centile. Note that there is no change in length and head circumference centiles. History and examination will reveal a healthy infant.

● This infant has failure to thrive (FTT). Note that persistent poor weight gain adversely affects growth in length but head growth is spared to some extent. Differential diagnosis includes poor intake (eg. neglect) or malabsorption (eg. coeliac disease or cystic fibrosis).

Usable with 95% and 5% thrive lines

A Breast from Birth chart is available based on long-term breastfeeding data

weeks/♀months

Figure 22.9 Infant growth chart to show (**a**) normal catch-down in weight and (**b**) failure to thrive (or poor weight gain in infancy). Failure to thrive is defined as fall in weight by ≥2 centiles. © Child Growth Foundation. Reproduced with permission; further information www.healthforallchildren.co.uk.

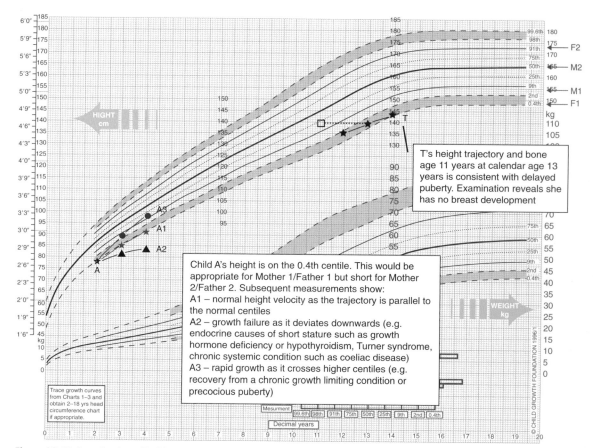

Figure 22.10 Growth chart (0–20 years) to show the importance of plotting measurements, the value of serial height measurements, and interpreting in the context of pubertal status and parents' heights (indicated on the right as M = Mother and F = Father). © Child Growth Foundation. Reproduced with permission; further information www.healthforallchildren.co.uk

- Plot values on standard growth centile charts:
  - centile charts represent the distribution of growth in the normal population but do not account for differences in ethnic backgrounds
  - disease-specific growth charts are available for some conditions, e.g. Down's syndrome, Turner's syndrome, achondroplasia.

Correctly interpret the measurements

- Compare each to normal centiles.
- Examine the relationship between weight, height/length and head circumference centiles (Fig. 22.9).

- Identify overt deviation from the normal pattern of growth and normal variations.
- Assess height in relation to pubertal status (Figs 22.10 and 22.11).
- Consider height, weight, BMI and head circumference in relation to parents (Table 22.8).

Assessment of pubertal development

The physical changes during puberty and the timing of the pubertal growth spurt normally occur in a fixed order (Fig. 22.11). Assessment of pubertal development is indicated when there are concerns about:

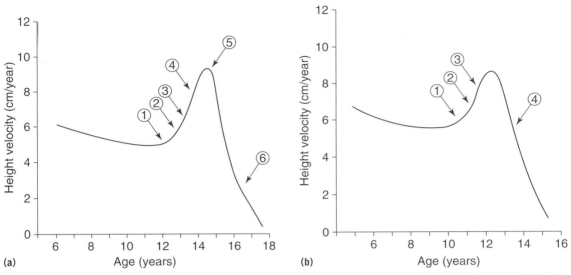

Figure 22.11 The sequence of physical changes during puberty in relation to peak height velocity in (**a**) boys and (**b**) girls. In boys (**a**) the stages are: (1) onset of puberty with testes volume 4 mL; (2) pubic hair develops; (3) growth of penis; (4) axillary hair appears; (5) voice breaks; and (6) facial hair appears and necessitates shaving (when growth slows). Peak height velocity occurs at testes volume 12–15 mL, G4–G5. In girls (**b**) the stages are: (1) onset of puberty with development of breast buds; (2) pubic hair develops; (3) axillary hair appears; and (4) menarche when growth rate slows, usually at breast stage 3–4. Peak height velocity occurs at B2–B3. From: Ryan S, Gregg J, Patel L, *Core paediatrics*, with permission. © 2003 London: Hodder Arnold.

Table 22.8 Determining mid-parental height and target adult height

	For a boy	For a girl
Father's height, cm	Plot height	Plot (height − 14 cm)
Mother's height, cm	Plot (height + 14 cm)	Plot height
Mid-parental height (ht) (MPH), cm	$\dfrac{\text{father's ht + mother's ht + 14}}{2}$	$\dfrac{\text{mother's ht + father's ht − 14}}{2}$
Adult target range, cm	MPH ± 10 cm	MPH ± 8.5 cm

- growth in height – short stature, tall stature or rapid growth, lack of pubertal growth spurt
- the timing of puberty – precocious or late
- genital appearance
- pubic hair development – precocious
- abnormal sequence of physical changes during puberty (Table 22.9).

Ask about **puberty in parents** – time of onset of puberty, growth spurt, menarche, shaving. Assess **growth** including pubertal growth spurt (Fig. 22.11). Examine and assess **pubertal status** using Tanner's stages for changes in breast development, genital development (Fig. 22.12), pubic hair and axillary hair.

NEONATAL HISTORY AND EXAMINATION

Assessment at birth

A brief examination of the newborn is performed immediately after birth to check for:

- successful adaptation to the transition from *in utero* to *ex utero* life and any need for resuscitation – using the Apgar score (Table 22.10)
- gender from appearance of genitalia
- conditions which may require urgent management, e.g. anal atresia, oesophageal atresia (if history of polyhydramnios)

Table 22.9 Onset of puberty

Onset of puberty	Girls	Boys
First sign of normal puberty	Breast bud development (not pubic hair)	Enlargement of testes ≥4 mL (not pubic hair)
Average (range) age for normal children	11 years (8–13)	12 years (9–14)
Age definition for precocious puberty	Before 8 years	Before 9 years
Age definition for delayed or absent puberty	After 13 years	After 14 years

(a) Breast development in girls

B1. Prepubertal: no breast development

B2. Onset of puberty: noticeable elevation of breast bud (uni- or bilateral)

B3. Enlargement of breast and areola with no separation of contours

B4. Areola projects separately from enlarging breast

B5. Areola merges with contour of breast but papilla projects

(b) Testes size and genital development in boys

G1. Prepubertal and testes under 4 mL size

G2. Onset of puberty: testes ≥ 4 mL, scrotum enlargement and reddening of skin

G3. Penis grows in length and breadth

G4. Development of glans. Further enlargement of testes, scrotum and penis

G5. Mature adult appearance. Testes 20-25 mL

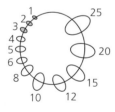 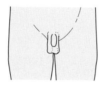 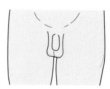 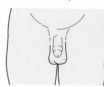 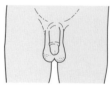

Orchidometer

Figure 22.12 Assessment of pubertal status from (a) breast development in girls and (b) testes size and genital development in boys.

- obvious syndrome, e.g. Down's syndrome
- malformations, e.g. cleft lip, spinal anomalies.

Routine newborn examination – 'the first day check'

All newborns (see Box 22.3 for terms) are routinely examined within the first 24–48 hours. This has three main purposes:

- to identify congenital malformations not evident at birth

- to reassure parents regarding 'normal' variants
- to provide information to parents about health promotion (e.g. sleep positioning to reduce sudden infant death syndrome, immunization schedules) and respond to any questions or concerns the parents may have.

Prenatal history

The newborn has a significant past history: the *in utero* life. Review maternal notes and ask mother about her health, events in pregnancy, labour and

Table 22.10 The Apgar Newborn Score

Sign	0 points	1 point	2 points
A – appearance and colour	Pale	Cyanosed	Pink
P – pulse and heart rate	Absent	<100/min	>100/min
G – grimace and cry	No response	Grimace	Vigorous cry
A – activity and muscle tone (allow for prematurity)	Flaccid	Some flexion of limbs	Active
R – respiratory effort	Absent	Slow, irregular	Good, crying

The Apgar Score was developed by Virginia Apgar, an anaesthetist, as a quick and efficient way to evaluate the effects of maternal anaesthesia on newborn babies. It is now performed 1 minute and 5 minutes after birth, and also after 10 minutes in an unwell baby (score <6) to ascertain adaptation to extrauterine life.

IMPORTANT

The unwell newborn can be difficult to identify as signs are subtle and non-specific. Any of the following must prompt further assessment:

- heart rate less than 100
- tachypnoea (respiratory rate >60 per minute)
- grunting respiration
- cyanosis
- hypotonia
- pallor.

At birth these signs indicate that the neonate may require resuscitation to assist in transition to *ex utero* life. After birth they should prompt a full assessment to exclude serious underlying pathology such as sepsis, cardiac or respiratory failure.

BOX 22.3 DEFINITIONS OF TERMS USED

- Premature: born before 37 weeks' gestation.
- Postmature: born after 42 weeks' gestation.
- Small-for-gestational age: birth weight and/or length >2 standard deviations below the mean for gestational age.

Examination

Examine the baby in the cot in the presence of parents and in a warm, well-lit environment. First stand back and observe the baby's appearance and posture. Look at the face, head and hands. In stages undress the baby fully, and while doing this be opportunistic. Remember to examine the back (Fig. 22.13). Leave

family history (for details, see the section 'The child with dysmorphic features and birth defects', p. 414).

Newborn's health

Ask the mother, and check midwife's records, for:

- method of feeding and how successful this is
- meconium and urine passed within the first 24 hours; urine stream in a male infant
- temperature
- blood glucose if premature, small-for-gestational age or maternal diabetes.

Family history

Ask about:

- genetic abnormalities (e.g. early onset deafness)
- congenital defects (e.g. dislocated hips, congenital heart defect).

CLINICAL PEARL

Be opportunistic when examining a baby. For example:

- if eyes are open, look for the red reflex (Fig. 22.14)
- if the baby cries or yawns, inspect the mouth
- if the baby is quiet, expose the chest and auscultate the heart (Fig. 22.15)
- if the baby sucks your finger, palpate the palate
- if the baby cries, note how lusty
- as the baby is undressed in stages, note how the baby handles (i.e. tone)
- if the baby is upset, you can try to settle them by sitting them up, holding them vertical, gently raising them up and down, softly blowing on their face, letting them grasp parent's finger, letting their parent hold them or offering a finger to suck on. Sometimes, however, only a feed will do!

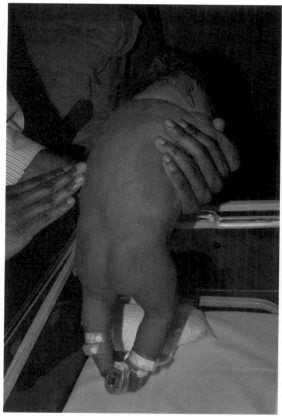

Figure 22.13 Technique for examination of the back in a neonate.

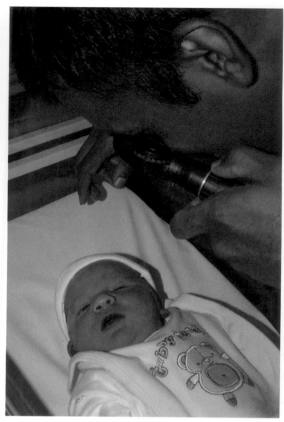

Figure 22.14 Eliciting the red reflex using an ophthalmoscope. This can be difficult in dark-skinned babies. Absence of the red reflex suggests congenital cataract, retinoblastoma or congenital glaucoma.

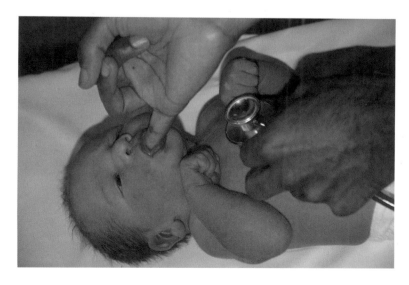

Figure 22.15 Auscultation of the heart while palpating the palate.

examination of the hips until the end as this is the most distressing part for both the baby and the parents. Check weight, measure the head circumference and plot on growth charts at the correct gestational age for the baby.

Specific aspects of the examination and common findings

Head to toe examination

During the examination, identify and differentiate common relatively benign findings from those that require further evaluation (Table 22.11, Fig. 22.16). The following are particularly important:

- red reflex (Fig. 22.14)
- hard and soft palate – look with a pen torch and also feel as the baby sucks on your finger (Fig. 22.15)
- femoral pulses – weak or absent pulses suggest coarctation of the aorta
- hip stability – first see if the skin creases are equal on the inner aspect of the thigh, that the legs are the same length when extended and that you can fully abduct each hip. The absence of any of

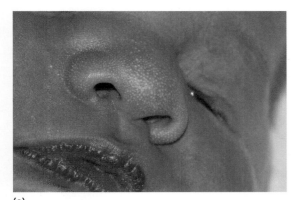

(a)

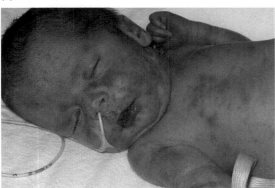

(b)

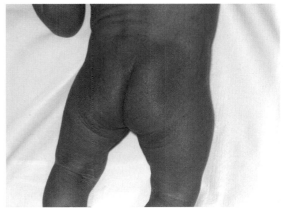

(c)

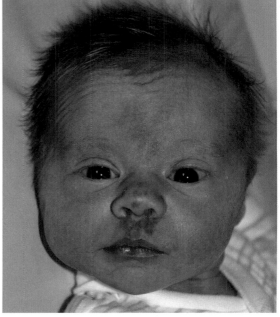

(d)

Figure 22.16 Common benign skin lesions on newborn examination: (**a**) milia – small white papules on the face; (**b**) erythema toxicum – erythematous rash with yellow vesicles which fleet around different sites for up to 2 weeks. Note the nasogastric tube in this preterm infant; (**c**) Mongolian blue spot – discrete blue/grey pigmentation classically, but not exclusively, seen in dark-skinned babies on the lower back/buttocks; (**d**) superficial capillary haemangioma on the face – pink patches over the eyelids, glabella, nose and philtrum that generally fade but tend to persist if on the neck.

Table 22.11 Common and relatively benign versus sinister findings on examination of the newborn

Examination	Findings which if isolated are not usually suggestive of a serious problem	Findings which may need further evaluation
General	Jitters that settle on handling/sucking Bruising to the face – do not confuse with cyanosis	Abnormal movements, tone or posture – opisthotonus, hypotonia or hypertonia Asymmetrical movements Irritability
Colour and skin	Milia (milk spots) (Fig. 22.16a) Erythema toxicum (Fig. 22.16b) Mongolian blue spot (Fig. 22.16c) Superficial capillary haemangiomas (Fig. 22.16d) Cutis marmorata – mottled appearance when exposed Skin tags	Pallor Cyanosis Plethora – polycythaemia Jaundice within the first 24 hours Bullous lesions
Head and face	Caput – diffuse swelling over presenting part of head, chignon – well-circumscribed swelling following ventouse extraction Cephalhaematoma – swelling limited by individual skull bones	Dysmorphic features Facial nerve palsy Deep capillary haemangioma (dark red/purple with overlying skin 'thick') – Sturge–Weber syndrome Midline swellings – meningocoele and encephalocoele Subaponeurotic haemorrhage
Eyes	Subconjunctival haemorrhage Epicanthic folds Transient squint Clear discharge – common due to non-patency of nasolacrimal duct	Absent red reflex Coloboma Purulent or profuse discharge – day 2–5: gonococcal if copious, staphylococcal if less severe; after day 7: chlamydia
Nose	Distorted nasal septum – due to pressure against maternal pelvis during delivery	Choanal atresia – if bilateral, airway patency needs to be established as an emergency
Ears	Preauricular tags – usually of no significance but requires audiological assessment	Low-set ears – trisomies, Turner's syndrome Preauricular pits – can be associated with sinuses and become infected
Mouth and palate	Ebstein's pearls – equivalent to milia on the palate Tongue tie – frenulum attached to anterior of tongue Ranula – mucous retention cyst under the tongue Neonatal teeth – may need removal if interfere with feeding	Cleft lip/palate Poor suck
Neck		Webbing – Turner's or Noonan's syndrome Torticollis – sternomastoid tumour Midline swelling – goitre Lateral swelling – branchial cyst, cystic hygroma
Back and spine	Sacral dimple – ensure you can see the base, and that it is not a sinus	Pits, sinuses, naevi or hair tufts – suggest underlying abnormality such as spina bifida Deformity or asymmetry – hemi-vertebra
Chest	Breast engorgement and/or discharge – due to acute cessation of maternal hormones Prominent xiphisternum	Respiratory distress Stridor – laryngomalacia common and improves when baby held prone; but exclude other causes of upper airway obstruction Abnormal shape – Poland anomaly, thoracic dystrophy

Table 22.11 *Continued*

Examination	Findings which if isolated are not usually suggestive of a serious problem	Findings which may need further evaluation
Umbilicus	Cord – stays attached for up to 10 days Three vessels usually (two arteries and one vein) but may only be two – no evidence of association with renal anomalies	Erythema of surrounding abdominal wall – suggests omphalitis and may require antibiotics
Abdomen	Liver/spleen palpable up to 2 cm below costal margin Diastasi of the recti – visible as a fusiform bulge on crying Vomiting milk – small possets are common Umbilical hernia	Bile-stained vomiting – intestinal obstruction Failure to pass meconium within 48 hours – Hirschsprung's disease, cystic fibrosis or meconium plug Abdominal mass Kidneys – hydronephrosis, cystic changes or tumour Bladder – outlet obstruction, e.g. posterior urethral valves in the male Groin – inguinal hernia
Genitalia and perineum	Unilateral undescended testes occur in 5 per cent at birth Retractile testis – present in scrotum but cremasteric reflex causes retraction Vaginal bleeding/discharge – acute cessation of maternal hormones at birth Pink urine – is usually urate crystals seen in the nappy and has no significance	Imperforate anus – do not be fooled by meconium in the nappy. It may have been passes through a rectovaginal fistula Hypospadias or epispadias – urethral meatus opens onto the dorsal aspect of the penile shaft Ambiguous genitalia (see Fig. 22.22, p. 418) Anterior placed anus – may be normal but can be associated with imperforate anus Bilateral undescended testis – may actually be ambiguous genitalia and will need careful assessment Poor urinary stream – posterior urethral valves
Hands	Single palmar creases – unilateral in 5 per cent and bilateral in 1 per cent of the general population Clinodactyly	Lymphoedema – Turner's syndrome (see Fig. 22.21, p. 417) Syndactyly or polydactyly – isolated or associated with a syndrome (e.g. Apert's)
Feet	Positional deformity – talipes equinovarus or calcaneovalgus	Fixed deformity – ventral aspect of foot does not touch anterior shin
Cardiovascular	Transient, soft systolic murmur – likely to occur during transition to ex-utero circulation owing to turbulent flow through closing ductus arteriosus or foramen ovale	Bradycardia <100/min – neonatal heart block Absent femoral pulses – coarctation of aorta Loud harsh systolic or diastolic murmur

these signs raises concern about developmental dysplasia of the hips. Next perform Barlow's and Ortolani's manoeuvres (Fig. 22.17).

Neurological examination

This is influenced markedly by gestational age. A detailed examination may be required if a neurological abnormality is suspected or if there has been a potential hypoxic insult to the brain. However, simple observation provides valuable clues. The normal term newborn:

- has a flexed posture, with smooth, symmetrical movements of the limbs

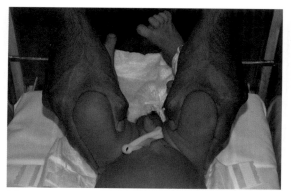

(a)

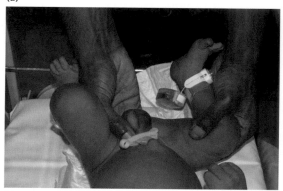

(a)

Figure 22.17 Examination for developmental dysplasia of the hips. (a) With the hip and knee flexed place your middle finger over the greater trochanter and your thumb on the medial aspect of the femur. Push the femur and in turn, the femoral head downward. If dislocatable the femoral head will be pushed posteriorly out of the acetabulum – Barlow's manoeuvre. Note the presence of meconium in the nappy. (b) Now stabilize the pelvis with one hand and with the other abduct the hip and push the femoral head back toward the pelvis. A dislocated hip will slip into the acetabulum with a clunk (not a click!) – Ortolani's manoeuvre.

- may open their eyes intermittently and be quiet or be active and crying
- sucks with strong rhythmic movements, either for a feed or on a finger
- does not slip through your hands like a 'rag doll' when picked up and held under the arms – if they do, it indicates hypotonia and requires further assessment
- demonstrates primitive reflexes, reflecting brainstem activity (Fig. 22.18).

THE CHILD WITH DYSMORPHIC FEATURES AND BIRTH DEFECTS

One in 40 babies is born with a birth defect and 3 per cent of these are major (Box 22.4). The diagnosis is obvious in some (e.g. Down's syndrome

BOX 22.4 CLASSIFICATION OF BIRTH DEFECTS
- **Deformities** – these occur when external mechanical factors alter normal development (e.g. talipes or torticollis due to alterations in amniotic fluid or intrauterine space).
- **Disruptions** – these are destruction of normally developed structures by external factors (e.g. limb amputation defects from amniotic bands).
- **Malformations** – these are defects that arise from the intrinsically abnormal development of body structures (e.g. heart defects, neural tube defects).

Birth defects can be:
- **minor** (i.e. cosmetic, e.g. clinodactyly) or **major** if normal function is affected (e.g. absent thumb).
- **isolated** or **multiple** (e.g. syndactyly can be isolated or associated with other defects in Apert's syndrome).

Multiple defects can occur as a sequence, association or syndrome:
- **sequence** – in this, the first defect directly leads to a series of malformations (e.g. cleft lip–palate sequence).
- **association** – two or more major defects that do not occur by chance (e.g. VACTERL – Vertebral, Anal, Cardiac, Tracheo-oesophageal, Ear, Renal, Limb defects; CHARGE – Coloboma, Heart, Choanal atresia, Retarded growth and development, Genital, Ear defects).
- **syndrome** – minor (e.g. single transverse palmar crease) and major defects (e.g. cardiac) with a recognized pattern of occurrence and a common cause (e.g. Down's syndrome, Turner's syndrome).

(a) Rooting reflex	(b) Palmer and plantar grasp	(c) Placing and stepping reflexes	(d) Asymmetric tonic neck reflex	(e) Moro reflex
Stroke the cheek near the angle of the mouth. The baby will open his mouth and turn towards your finger.	Gently press your finger in the palm of the baby's hand or the ball of the foot. Fingers or toes grasp onto the examining finger.	Hold the baby erect and draw the dorsum of the foot along the under edge of a table top. Flexion followed by extension of the legs occurs.	With the baby lying down turn his head to one side (and then the other). He will adopt a 'fencing' posture, i.e. limbs on the face side will be extended and opposite side will be flexed.	With the baby lying down raise his head with your hand under the occiput. Abruptly move your hand toward the bed, and catch the head as it drops down. This results in symmetrical abduction and extension of the arms followed by flexion and adduction.

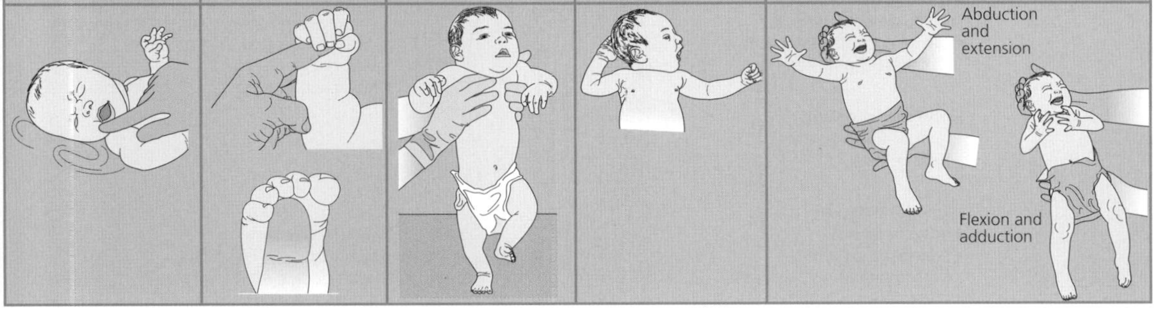

Figure 22.18 Primitive reflexes in the newborn. (**a**) rooting reflex; (**b**) palmar and plantar grasp; (**c**) placing and stepping reflexes; (**d**) asymmetrical tonic neck reflex (ATNR); (**e**) Moro reflex. Persistence of these reflexes beyond 4–6 months is abnormal, suggests that cortical inhibition of the brainstem has not occurred and progress with normal development is hindered.

or oculocutaneous albinism) but others require the expertise of a geneticist. A correct diagnosis is important to:

- check for known medical associations (e.g. cardiac abnormalities in Down's syndrome or Turner's syndrome)
- inform the family about the likely prognosis and child's future health
- offer appropriate management (e.g. developmental physiotherapy programme for Down's syndrome, growth hormone treatment for Turner's syndrome)
- inform parents about the nature of the condition and recurrence in future pregnancies.

Prenatal and birth history

A detailed prenatal and birth history will provide clues about the aetiology (Fig. 22.19).

Family history

Ask about:

- consanguinity – increased risk for autosomal recessive defects
- pregnancy loss or early childhood deaths.

Examination

- Check birth weight, length and head size for intrauterine growth retardation, overgrowth, micro- or macrocephaly.
- Perform a thorough head-to-toe examination. Follow the same approach as for the routine neonatal examination, paying particular attention to the face (Fig. 22.20), hands (Fig. 22.21), heart and genitalia (Fig. 22.22).
- Identify any unusual or dysmorphic features and defects.

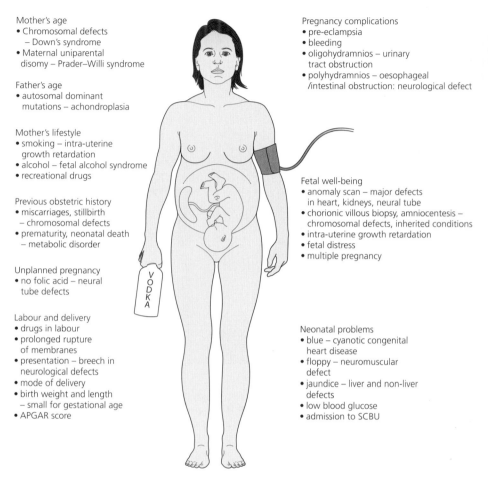

Mother's age
- Chromosomal defects
  – Down's syndrome
- Maternal uniparental
  disomy – Prader–Willi syndrome

Father's age
- autosomal dominant
  mutations – achondroplasia

Mother's lifestyle
- smoking – intra-uterine
  growth retardation
- alcohol – fetal alcohol syndrome
- recreational drugs

Previous obstetric history
- miscarriages, stillbirth
  – chromosomal defects
- prematurity, neonatal death
  – metabolic disorder

Unplanned pregnancy
- no folic acid – neural
  tube defects

Labour and delivery
- drugs in labour
- prolonged rupture
  of membranes
- presentation – breech in
  neurological defects
- mode of delivery
- birth weight and length
  – small for gestational age
- APGAR score

Pregnancy complications
- pre-eclampsia
- bleeding
- oligohydramnios – urinary
  tract obstruction
- polyhydramnios – oesophageal
  /intestinal obstruction: neurological defect

Fetal well-being
- anomaly scan – major defects
  in heart, kidneys, neural tube
- chorionic villous biopsy, amniocentesis –
  chromosomal defects, inherited conditions
- intra-uterine growth retardation
- fetal distress
- multiple pregnancy

Neonatal problems
- blue – cyanotic congenital
  heart disease
- floppy – neuromuscular
  defect
- jaundice – liver and non-liver
  defects
- low blood glucose
- admission to SCBU

Figure 22.19 Taking the prenatal and birth history for a child with birth defects.

- Check parents for familial characteristics (e.g. single transverse palmar crease, large head size, facial features).

Genitalia

Ambiguity in the genitalia is defined as external genitalia that are neither entirely female nor entirely male in appearance (Fig. 22.22). It includes clitoromegaly or micropenis, varying degrees of fusion of the labioscrotal folds and abnormal position of the urethral orifice. The parents' immediate question about whether their baby is a boy or a girl cannot be answered without careful evaluation by a team of specialists. A calm and sensitive manner is essential. Check:

- the male genitalia – penile length (measured with wooden tongue depressor held perpendicular to symphysis pubis), position of urethral orifice, size of scrotum and presence of testes
- the female genitalia – clitoris is normally prominent in preterm babies but not otherwise visible without separating labia majora.

INVESTIGATIONS

Other than the national neonatal screening tests, there are no *routine* investigations in paediatric medicine. Investigations should only be done if:

- serious underlying pathology is considered in the diagnosis (e.g. jaundice in the first 24 hours after birth) or differential diagnosis

or

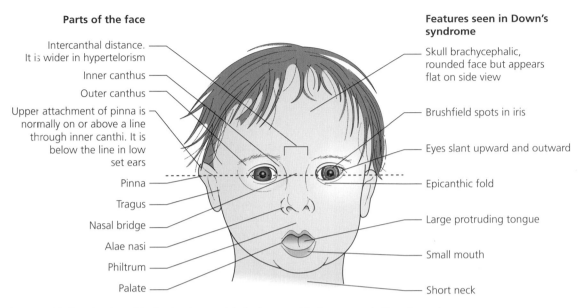

Parts of the face

Intercanthal distance. It is wider in hypertelorism

Inner canthus

Outer canthus

Upper attachment of pinna is normally on or above a line through inner canthi. It is below the line in low set ears

Pinna

Tragus

Nasal bridge

Alae nasi

Philtrum

Palate

Features seen in Down's syndrome

Skull brachycephalic, rounded face but appears flat on side view

Brushfield spots in iris

Eyes slant upward and outward

Epicanthic fold

Large protruding tongue

Small mouth

Short neck

Figure 22.20 Examination of facies for dysmorphic features and features seen in Down's syndrome.

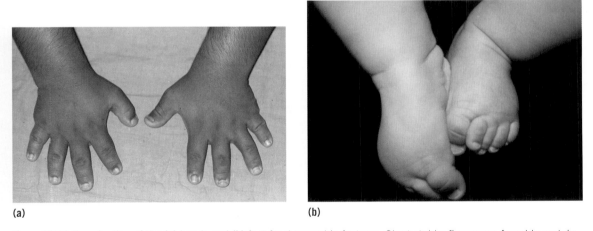

(a)   (b)

Figure 22.21 Examination of the (a) hands and (b) feet for dysmorphic features. Short stubby fingers are found in certain skeletal dysplasias and Albright's hereditary osteodystrophy. Puffy feet in a newborn or infant are seen in Turner's syndrome. Adapted from: Ryan S, Gregg J, Patel L, *Core paediatrics*, with permission. © 2003 London: Hodder Arnold.

- results of the test will alter management (e.g. increasing yellow pigmentation in a baby with jaundice when investigation will inform about the need for phototherapy).

The plan for investigations must be informed by findings from history and examination. Results need to be interpreted using age- and gender-appropriate reference ranges for children.

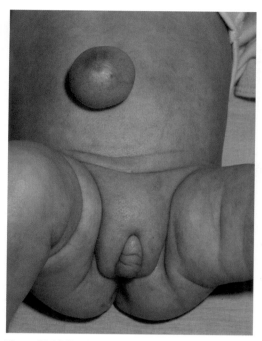

Figure 22.22 Newborn with ambiguous genitalia. This requires detailed assessment for possible disorders of sex development (DSD) – the group of anomalies affecting the sex chromosomes, gonads, internal genitalia (i.e. reproductive organs) and external genitalia. The umbilical hernia is an incidental finding and parents simply need reassurance that it will resolve spontaneously. Photograph courtesy of Dr Nandhini Prakash, Pennine Acute Hospitals, Oldham.

 IMPORTANT

All newborn babies have a heel prick blood sample taken in the first week of life to screen for:

- phenylketonuria
- congenital hypothyroidism
- cystic fibrosis
- sickle cell disease
- medium chain acyl-CoA dehydrogenase deficiency.

These are serious diseases which are amenable to early treatment.

COMMON OR SERIOUS PAEDIATRIC PRESENTATIONS AND DIAGNOSES

Acute febrile illness

Assessing an acutely febrile child is akin to detective work.

- Identify the focus: the most likely suspects are nose, throat, ear, chest and urinary tract.
- Determine the likely pathogen: viral infections are more common than bacterial but the latter are more serious.

History

This frequently offers clues to the focus of infection but can be non-specific (fever, vomiting and poor appetite) in infants under 3 months of age and in certain infections such as septicaemia and urinary tract infections.

IMPORTANT   *i*

Duration, severity and progress of symptoms can help differentiate relatively uncomplicated viral from more serious bacterial infections.

Examination

The tympanic membranes and tonsils *must* be visualized to exclude acute otitis media and tonsillitis, respectively. Chest signs can be subtle in lower respiratory tract infection (pneumonia) but the presence of increased respiratory rate with increased work of breathing raises suspicion. The signs of meningitis in infants and toddlers are different from those in older children and adults (Table 22.12).

Explore predisposing pathology and complications, e.g. for vesicoureteric reflux and renal scarring from urinary tract infection.

Investigations

- Check urine if symptoms are non-specific and the focus is not identified from examination.

Table 22.12 Comparison of signs of meningeal irritation in infants and toddlers and older children

Infants and toddlers	Older children
Shrill high-pitched cry	Severe headache
Neck stiffness unusual. If present, observed as arched neck and back	Neck stiffness – unable to touch chest with chin, kiss knees or look up
Kernig's sign unreliable	Kernig's sign, Brudzinski's sign
Irritability and drowsiness	Prefers to be left alone in a dark (photophobia), quiet room (phonophobia)
Resents being handled	
Bulging anterior fontanelle	

- In infants under age 3 months, have a low threshold for performing an infection screen and treating with antibiotics.

i **IMPORTANT**

Acute infections with no obvious focus:

- urinary tract infection
- septicaemia
- meningitis
- appendicitis
- osteomyelitis
- septic arthritis
- psoas abscess
- malaria.

Febrile convulsions

One in 20 children between 6 months and 5 years of age will have a febrile convulsion.

History and examination

- Fit occurs when the child has a high fever.
- Fit usually lasts less than 5 minutes, is generalized and the child recovers full consciousness within an hour.
- Rigors can also occur with high temperature but differ because:
  - the child can communicate and does *not* lose consciousness
  - limb movements are usually less rhythmic, less pronounced and at a faster rate than in a seizure.
- Parents often say that they thought their child was going to die.

- Ask about family history of febrile convulsions.
- Determine the underlying cause for the fever (see above) – exclude serious underlying pathology such as meningitis.

The seriously unwell infant

Young children, and especially infants, can become unwell rapidly from:

- shock, e.g. septicaemia (Fig. 22.23), intussusception
- severe dehydration, e.g. severe gastroenteritis
- respiratory failure, e.g. severe asthma, epiglottitis
- heart failure, e.g. large left to right shunts
- status epilepticus, e.g. encephalopathy
- meningitis or encephalitis.

Correctly identifying the seriously unwell child can be difficult. It is often described as an art rather than a science. Experienced paediatricians can identify these seriously unwell children from initial

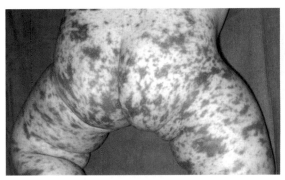

Figure 22.23 Confluent purpuric rash of meningococcal septicaemia in a seriously unwell infant. From: Ryan S, Gregg J, Patel L, *Core paediatrics*, with permission. © 2003 London: Hodder Arnold.

Table 22.13 Clues to a seriously ill infant

Symptoms	Signs
High fever but cold hands and feet	General: • cold extremities, mottled skin and prolonged capillary refill • confluent purpuric rash (Fig. 22.23)
Difficulty breathing, rapid breathing, noisy breathing with grunting, stridor or wheeze	
Blue or pale and lethargic or tired	
Stridor, drooling of saliva and unable to swallow	Respiratory: • tachypnoea, recessions, grunting
Refusal to feed	
Persistent vomiting	Cardiovascular: • cyanosis, pallor, tachycardia or bradycardia, gallop rhythm, hypotension or hypertension
Profuse diarrhoea and lethargic	
Irritability, unusually drowsy or difficult to arouse	Neurological: • bulging fontanelle, photophobia, meningism • apathetic demeanour or altered conscious level • floppiness, paucity of movements • abnormal posture, arching of back • altered pupil size and reactivity
Persistent high-pitched cry	
Prolonged convulsion	
Child 'not himself' and behaviour exceptionally different from normal, e.g. quiet and prefers to sleep when the child would normally be vocalizing and active	

observations of their general demeanour and behaviour. However, there are many clues which can assist the novice (Table 22.13).

Wheezing and asthma

'Wheeze' is often used by parents and children to describe any type of noisy breathing, e.g. inspiratory upper respiratory rattles in a coryzal child or stridor (Table 22.14). Ask parents to imitate the noise to clarify. Young children, up to the age of 5 years, may wheeze if they are coryzal; this is termed 'viral-induced wheeze'. These children may continue to wheeze through childhood and develop asthma. If asthma (see also Box 22.5) is suspected, check for:

- potential triggers for acute attacks – cigarette smoke, animal dander, coryza, exercise, excitement, dust, hot or cold weather, night-time
- the effect of asthma on the child's life – the three S: sleep, sport and school
- family history of atopy (asthma, eczema, hayfever)
- peak flow readings in children older than 6–7 years
- excluding other chronic conditions such as cystic fibrosis.

BOX 22.5 'NON-ASTHMA' FEATURES
- Chronic productive cough with yellow or green mucus
- Poor weight gain
- Frequent offensive stools
- Clubbing
- Localized wheeze with or without crackles
- Poor response to bronchodilator (i.e. irreversible airway obstruction).

IMPORTANT   *i*
Beware of the unwell child with asthma who does not have a wheeze on auscultation – 'the silent chest'. This occurs when there is not enough air moving in and out of the lungs to generate the wheeze sound. It indicates severe airway obstruction.

Vomiting in infants

Common causes of vomiting in infants include:

- gastro-oesophageal reflux
- gastroenteritis

Table 22.14 Features of upper versus lower airway obstruction in children

Extrathoracic or upper airway obstruction	Intrathoracic or lower airway obstruction
Stridor during inspiration	Wheeze predominantly on expiration
Suprasternal and lower sternal retraction. Causes: • viral laryngotracheobronchitis • epiglottitis	Intercostal and subcostal recession. Causes: • asthma • bronchiolitis • cystic fibrosis

- pyloric stenosis
- urinary tract infections.

Serious causes include:

- meningitis
- intestinal obstruction
- congenital adrenal hyperplasia
- metabolic disorder.

Acute vomiting with or without diarrhoea

This is usually viral (e.g. norovirus or winter vomiting viruses; rotavirus gastroenteritis) and self-limiting but can be due to other pathogens. Check for:

- degree of dehydration – from depression of anterior fontanelle and other clinical features as in adults
- complications – a history of blood in the stool, pallor and child appearing unwell are warning signs of serious complications:
  - haemolytic uraemic syndrome – other features are oliguria/anuria and/or petechiae/purpura
  - intussusception – typically occurs in children aged between 3 and 12 months. Vomiting is bile stained. Spasms of pain when the child screams and looks pale alternate with periods when the child is exceptionally quiet and still.

Abdominal pain

Medical and surgical causes of abdominal pain are summarized in Table 22.15.

Recurrent non-specific abdominal pain occurs in around 10 per cent of children over 5 years of age. The pain is typically periumbilical, sharp, colicky and does not wake the child at night. It is not associated with eating, activity, bowel habits or somatic symptoms. Thorough history and examination are

Table 22.15 Medical and surgical causes of abdominal pain

	Acute abdominal pain	Recurrent abdominal pain
Medical	Urinary tract infections Mesenteric adenitis Diabetic ketoacidosis Lower lobe pneumonia	Constipation Inflammatory bowel disease Peptic ulcer disease Non-specific (non-organic)
Surgical	Appendicitis Intestinal obstruction	Malrotation

essential to identify the minority of children who have an underlying organic cause for their pain.

Autistic spectrum disorder

Children with autistic spectrum disorder find any changes in their routine, such as a visit to see a doctor, especially unsettling. Clues from the history and observation include:

- history of an unrecognized or recognized syndrome
- family history – autistic spectrum disorder in a sibling
- restricted interest – child does not:
  - engage in 'pretend' or imaginative play, e.g. make a cup of tea with a toy tea set
  - point to objects of interest in the room or a book e.g. if asked, 'Where is the teddy?', or look at objects pointed out to them by someone else, e.g. if told, 'Look, there's a train.'
- unusual behaviour – repetitive and stereotyped movements and activities e.g.
  - rocking, head banging
  - play with same toy or watch the same DVD
  - twirl a string or wash hands repeatedly.

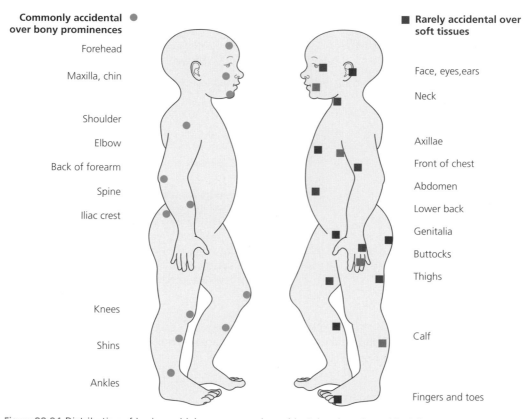

Commonly accidental ●
over bony prominences

Forehead

Maxilla, chin

Shoulder

Elbow

Back of forearm

Spine

Iliac crest

Knees

Shins

Ankles

■ **Rarely accidental over**
soft tissues

Face, eyes, ears

Neck

Axillae

Front of chest

Abdomen

Lower back

Genitalia

Buttocks

Thighs

Calf

Fingers and toes

Figure 22.24 Distribution of bruises which are commonly accidental and rarely accidental.

- Social interaction – 'in a world of their own':
  - prolonged solitary play
  - no awareness of children or people around them.
- Communication abnormal or inappropriate:
  - poor non-verbal skills – eye contact, facial expressions, gestures
  - delayed speech

- speech repetitive, and abnormal in tone and rhythm.

Bruises

Accidental bruises are common in normally active children. They predominantly occur over bony prominences, and the pattern and distribution will be consistent with the child's age, lifestyle and activity (Fig. 22.24). When a child presents with unexplained or unusual bruises, consider two possibilities:

- bleeding disorder such as idiopathic thrombocytopenic purpura, haemophilia or leukaemia – ask about a history of:
  - easy bruising
  - frequent nose bleeds, prolonged bleeding after teeth extraction
  - family history of easy bruising or unusual bleeding
- Non-accidental or inflicted injury, i.e. physical abuse (Fig. 22.25).

> ℹ️ **IMPORTANT**
>
> Attention deficit hyperactivity disorder is an inherited neurobehavioural problem. Features include difficulties at school and at home. The child appears disruptive, disobedient and anti-social owing to:
> - hyperactivity
> - impulsive behaviour
> - difficulty paying attention.

History
- Changing history
- Injury unexplained – incidental discovery
- Explanation not consistent with:
    - place and pattern of bruises
    - age and development of child
- Inappropriate action by carer:
    - delay in seeking medical attention
    - refuse assessment or management
    - unprovoked aggression
- Other features of abuse, e.g. neglect
- Behaviour problems or specific worries about child
- Previous injuries but managed at different hospitals
- Family and social history
    - other children
    - domestic violence
    - known to Social Services
- No medical cause of bruising

Listen to the child
Observe interactions between child and parents

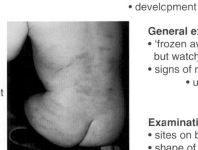

Assess growth and development
- weight, height, head circumference
- development

General examination
- 'frozen awareness' – expressionless but watchful appearance
- signs of neglect or emotional abuse
    - unkempt clothes, hair, body

Examination for bruises
- sites on body (Figure 22.24)
- shape of bruises/pattern
- different colours

Examination for other injuries
- mouth: gums, teeth, frenulum
- head, eyes, fundi, abdomen
- genitalia
- bite marks, pinch marks
- burns/scalds, cigarette burns
- joints and bones

Record of bruises and injuries
- use a body chart
- obtain consent and arrange photographs

Figure 22.25 Clinical assessment in a child with unexplained bruises and suspected non-accidental injury. Adapted from: Ryan S, Gregg J, Patel L, *Core paediatrics*, with permission. © 2003 London: Hodder Arnold.

SUMMARY

General points:

- each child is unique and clinical assessment requires an individually tailored approach
- a neonate brings legacies from the critical period of growth and development *in utero* as well as the potentially hazardous process of being born
- problems of prematurity and congenital anomalies are major causes of morbidity in childhood and account for 60 per cent of deaths under age 15 years
- infants and children are more vulnerable and respond differently to certain illnesses (e.g. acute infections) owing to the time taken for body systems and physiological processes such as the immune system to mature
- growth in size, physical changes of puberty, and neuro-behavioural, cognitive and social development occur during childhood and adolescence.

The basic skills in the clinical assessment of children are to:

- take a history from parents or other carers as well as from the child if the child is able to communicate
- assess the child's growth and development
- examine the child using an age-appropriate approach
- determine whether the child is seriously ill
- identify the problems or diagnoses, predisposing/influencing factors and any complications.

These skills require:

- a holistic approach
- basic generic knowledge about physiology, normal variations and disease processes
- specific understanding about normal growth and development through childhood
- the ability to communicate with children and parents
- an understanding about how to assess children at different ages
- common sense.

IMPORTANT

Forms of child abuse include:

- physical abuse
- emotional abuse
- neglect
- sexual abuse
- fabricated illness (Munchhausen's syndrome by proxy).

FURTHER READING

Arthritis Research Campaign. DVD: Paediatric Gait, Arms, Legs, Spine (pGALS). Available at: www.arc.org.uk/arthinfo/emedia.asp#pGALS.

Foster HE, Jandial S. 2008. pGALS – A screening examination of the musculoskeletal system in school-aged children. Arthritis Research Campaign, *Reports on the Rheumatic Diseases Series 5: Hands on.* No. 15. Available at www.arc.org.uk/arthinfo/medpubs/6535/6535.asp (accessed 23 November 2009).

Goldbloom RB. 2002. *Pediatric clinical skills.* Philadelphia: WB Saunders

Ryan S, Gregg J, Patel L. 2003. *Core paediatrics. A problem-solving approach.* London: Hodder Arnold.

UK Department of Health. 2009. *Spotting the sick child.* Available at: https://www.spottingthesickchild.com

23 THE ACUTELY ILL PATIENT

Hina Pattani and Bob Winter

INTRODUCTION

Patients in hospital may become acutely ill at any time. This is more likely in certain groups of patients, for example emergency admissions, after surgical or radiological intervention and after discharge from critical care. There is often a delay in recognizing and appropriately managing acutely ill patients. This is likely to result in increased length of hospital stay, mortality and morbidity.

Abnormal physiology is often seen in patients on hospital wards; however, observations are frequently incomplete or not acted on. Early warning or 'track and trigger' scores allocate points to observations (such as pulse and blood pressure) that are outside the normal range. This weighted score can then be used to highlight such patients and trigger early assessment and treatment.

Acutely ill patients require prompt assessment with simultaneous treatment. A systematic approach to this ensures that all immediately life-threatening problems are recognized and the correct treatment is started promptly. In order to achieve this, the classical approach to assessment of the stable patient must be modified (Table 23.1).

On the topic of the recognition and management of acutely ill patients, the Foundation Programme Curriculum (2007; see also Box 23.1) states that the following core competencies and skills should be acquired by foundation doctors:

- promptly assesses the acutely ill or collapsed patient
- identifies and responds to acutely abnormal physiology
- where appropriate, delivers a fluid challenge safely to an acutely ill patient
- reassesses ill patients appropriately after starting treatment
- requests senior or more experienced help when appropriate
- undertakes a secondary survey to establish differential diagnosis
- obtains an arterial blood gas sample safely, interprets results correctly
- manages patients with impaired consciousness, including convulsions
- uses common analgesic drugs safely and effectively
- understands and applies the principles of managing a patient following self-harm
- understands and applies the principles of managing a patient with an acute confusional state or psychosis

Table 23.1 Patient assessment

Stable patient	Acutely ill patient
Full history ↓	Immediate assessment and management (A B C D E)
Systematic examination ↓	
Investigations ↓	History and systematic examination with a review of charts and investigations ↓
Differential diagnosis ↓	
Management plan	Diagnosis and further targeted investigations ↓
	Management plan with planned reviews of response

BOX 23.1 CORE SKILLS IN RELATION TO ACUTE ILLNESS

'On completing the two years of foundation training, all foundation doctors should be competent and feel confident in the early management of emergency patients and of those with acute problems on a background of chronic disease. They will be expected to show how individual competencies can be combined to provide appropriate and timely care within the clinical settings of primary and secondary care.' The Foundation Programme Curriculum (2007) www.foundationprogramme.nhs.uk

- ensures safe continuing care of patients on handover between shifts, on-call staff or with 'hospital at night' team by meticulous attention to detail and reflection on performance
- considers appropriateness of interventions according to patients' wishes, severity of illness and chronic or co-morbid diseases.

> **IMPORTANT** i
>
> Acutely ill patients require prompt assessment using a systematic approach to ensure that all immediately life-threatening problems are recognized and the correct treatment is initiated promptly.

IMMEDIATE ASSESSMENT AND MANAGEMENT

The most widely used system for assessment and treatment of acutely ill patients is the A B C D E system (Table 23.2). The rationale for this system is that conditions causing airway compromise are likely to kill more quickly than those causing breathing dysfunction and in turn those causing circulatory problems. Therefore the most life-threatening problems are both identified and treated in order of priority. Many of these assessments and treatments can be carried out simultaneously if more than one person is attending to the patient.

Table 23.2 Immediate assessment and management

A	Airway assessment and treatment if needed
B	Breathing assessment and treatment if needed
C	Circulation assessment and treatment if needed
D	Disability of the central nervous system
E	Exposure to allow full examination

The A B C D E approach is a clinical approach, and a system of:

- LOOK
- LISTEN
- FEEL
- TREAT

can be adopted for each of the components.

Airway

The first step when assessing the airway is to talk to the patient. A patient who is able to respond in an appropriate way not only has a patent airway but also has adequate oxygenation, ventilation and cerebral perfusion to be able to respond appropriately.

Look

- Central cyanosis – purplish tinge of skin and mucus membranes due to the presence of deoxygenated haemoglobin close to the surface of the skin. This occurs when oxygen saturations are below 88 per cent.
- See-saw respiration – paradoxical movement of the chest and abdomen with respiratory effort. On inspiration the chest is drawn in and the abdomen expands and the opposite occurs on expiration.
- Use of accessory muscles of respiration – the patient may brace the shoulder girdle by resting forwards on outstretched arms.
- Tracheal tug – downward tug of the trachea that is manifest by downward movement of the thyroid cartilage.
- Altered level of consciousness – this can be the cause of airway compromise but can also result from airway obstruction.
- Foreign bodies, blood or vomit – open the mouth to ensure it is clear.

Listen

- Grunting – this is an instinctive mechanism to keep the alveoli open and is caused by exhalation against a partially closed glottis.
- Snoring – this is due to partial collapse or swelling of the soft tissues of the upper airway.
- Hoarseness – raspy or harsh sounding voice caused by upper airway inflammation or lesions on the vocal cords.
- Stridor – high-pitched *inspiratory* stridor is caused by airway obstruction at the level of the vocal cords. Lower-pitch stridor that occurs mainly on *expiration* is most commonly associated with tracheal obstruction.

Feel

- Air flow with inspiration and expiration.

Treat

If there are signs and symptoms of airway compromise then the steps should be taken to immediately open and secure it (Box 23.2). Initially basic manoeuvres can be used such as chin lift, jaw thrust and suction to remove secretions. An oropharyngeal or nasopharyngeal airway can be used to aid this process (Fig. 23.1). If these simple methods are not successful then a definitive airway in the form of an endotracheal tube is indicated. As soon as the airway is patent, administer high-flow oxygen.

BOX 23.2 CAUSES OF AIRWAY OBSTRUCTION
- Central nervous system depression
- Blood
- Vomit
- Foreign body
- Trauma to the face or neck
- Epiglottis
- Pharyngeal swelling
- Laryngospasm
- Bronchospasm
- Secretions

Breathing

The respiratory rate is a very early and sensitive sign of acute illness. A respiratory rate of fewer than 12 or greater than 30 breaths per minute or the inability to speak in full sentences are signs of impending respiratory failure (Box 23.3).

BOX 23.3 CAUSES OF BREATHING COMPROMISE
- Reduced respiratory drive:
  - central nervous system depression.
- Reduced respiratory effort:
  - spinal cord lesion
  - muscle weakness
  - nerve damage
  - restrictive chest wall abnormalities
  - pain.
- Lung disorders:
  - pneumothorax
  - haemothorax
  - infection
  - aspiration
  - exacerbation of chronic obstructive pulmonary disease
  - asthma
  - pulmonary embolism
  - lung contusion
  - acute respiratory distress syndrome
  - pulmonary oedema.

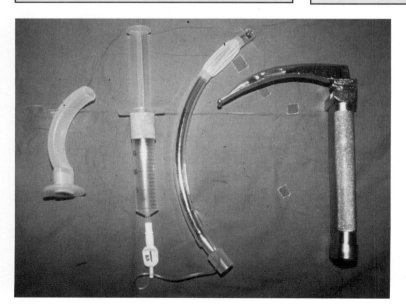

Figure 23.1 Airway adjuncts – an oropharyngeal airway is shown on the left, and an endotracheal tube (and laryngoscope) are shown on the right.

Look

- Look for central cyanosis.
- Look for use of accessory muscles of respiration.
- Depth and equality of respiration – look for rapid shallow respirations. Asymmetrical movements of the chest wall on either side give an indication of pathology on one or the other side.
- Sweating – this may be a sign of the exertion required to maintain the increased respiratory effort.
- Raised jugular venous pressure – this is an indirect measure of central venous pressure. The internal jugular vein connects to the right atrium without any intervening valves and therefore acts as a column for blood in the right atrium. A tension pneumothorax can cause a raised jugular venous pressure.
- Patency of any chest drains – any chest drains *in situ* should be examined to check that they are still in place: this may mean removing wound dressings. Ensure that the drain is not clamped. The drain should be swinging, a sign that it is in the pleural cavity.
- Look for see-saw respiration.
- Inspired oxygen concentration and oxygen saturations – note the inspired oxygen concentration and the delivery device. It is important to remember that the oxygen saturation *does not* give any indication of the partial pressure of carbon dioxide.

Listen

- Noisy breathing – this may be an indication of airway compromise.
- Audible wheeze – this is wheeze that can be heard without the aid of a stethoscope.
- Coughing – this may indicate that the patient is trying to clear secretions. It is important to examine any sputum that is being cleared as it may give a clue to the diagnosis, for example purulent secretions may indicate pneumonia.
- Ability of the patient to talk in full and comprehensible sentences – this indicates that the patient has adequate oxygenation, ventilation and cerebral perfusion to be able to respond appropriately.
- Percussion note:
    - dull – check for a pleural effusion or pneumonia

    - normal – suggests healthy lungs
    - hyper-resonant – check for pneumothorax or emphysema.
- Auscultate for breath sounds – these can be absent or present, normal or abnormal:
    - crackles – popping sounds that originate within the airways. They sound similar to the sound produced by rubbing your hair between your fingers
    - wheeze – musical sounds that are most commonly heard at the end of inspiration or in early expiration.

Feel

- Position of the trachea – this is an indication of the position of the upper mediastinum. The trachea may be central or deviated to the right or to the left. If the trachea is deviated to one side then it is either being pushed or pulled towards that side. A tension pneumothorax (Fig. 23.2) or a massive pleural effusion will push the trachea over to the opposite side. Collapse of one or multiple lobes will pull the trachea over to the affected side (Fig. 23.3).
- Equality of chest wall movement – it is often easier to feel for this with hands on either side of the chest rather than by inspection alone. Reduced motion suggests pathology.
- Presence of surgical emphysema or crepitus – surgical emphysema occurs when air enters the

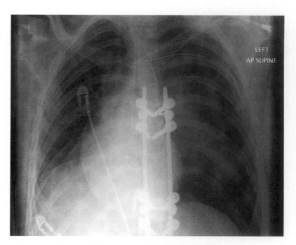

Figure 23.2 Chest X-ray showing a left-sided tension pneumothorax.

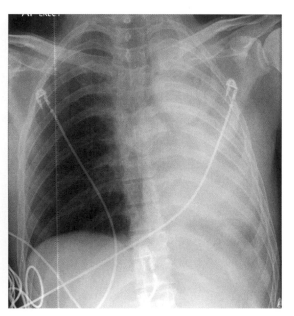

Figure 23.3 Chest X-ray showing left lung collapse.

soft tissues and feels like crackling under the surface of the skin when gentle pressure is applied.
- Tactile vocal fremitus – this is increased over areas of consolidation and decreased or absent over areas of effusion or collapse.

Treat

All acutely ill patients should be given high flow oxygen initially. Other simple manoeuvres such as sitting the patient up may be beneficial. The cause of respiratory compromise then has to be determined before specific treatments can be administered.

Circulation

Look for signs of shock (Box 23.4), defined as 'a state where there is acute circulatory failure with inadequate tissue perfusion causing cellular hypoxia'. In both medical and surgical patients who are acutely ill hypovolaemia must be considered as the primary cause of shock. Unless another cause is obvious a fluid challenge should be administered.

Look

- Look at the colour of the fingers and toes – they may be blue, pink or mottled indicating peripheral vasoconstriction.

BOX 23.4 CLASSIFICATION OF SHOCK
- Hypovolaemic shock:
  - haemorrhage
  - gastrointestinal fluid loss
  - trauma
  - infection
  - burns
  - renal loss
  - iatrogenic.
- Cardiogenic shock:
  - myocardial infarction or ischaemia
  - acute arrhythmia
  - acute cardiomyopathy
  - acute valvular lesions
  - myocardial contusion.
- Obstructive shock:
  - cardiac tamponade
  - tension pneumothorax
  - pulmonary embolism.
- Neurogenic shock.
- Anaphylaxis.
- Septic shock (Fig. 23.4).

- Reduced peripheral perfusion – look for collapsed or under-filled veins, which indicate hypovolaemia. Shocked patients may have a normal blood pressure.
- Haemorrhage – this may be external from either wounds or drains or it may be concealed within the chest, abdomen, pelvis or soft tissues.

Listen

Heart sounds (Table 23.3).

Feel

- Limb temperature – the skin may be cool if the patient has peripheral vasoconstriction or warm if the patient has peripheral vasodilation.

Table 23.3 Abnormal heart sounds and their meaning

Heart sound	Interpretation
Gallop rhythm	May indicate heart failure
Quite heart sounds	May indicate cardiac tamponade
New murmur	May occur after a myocardial infarction or may be a sign of endocarditis

GUIDELINES FOR MANAGEMENT OF SEVERE SEPSIS AND SEPTIC SHOC

Surviving Sepsis Campaign This is a summary of the Surviving Sepsis Campaign *International Guidelines for Management of Severe Sepsis and Septic Shock: 2008*, condensed from *Dellinger RP, Levy MM, Carlet JM, et al: Surviving Sepsis Campaign: International guidelines for management of severe sepsis and septic shock. Intensive Care Medicine (2008) 34:17- 0.*

This version does not contain the rationale or appendices contained in the primary publication. The SSC guidelines do not cover every aspect of managing critically ill patients, and their application should be supplemented by generic best practice and specific treatment as required. Please refer to the guidelines for additional information at www.survivingsepsis.org

Strength of recommendation and quality of evidence have been assessed using the GRADE criteria, presented in brackets after each guideline.
For added clarity:
◆ Indicates a strong recommendation or "we recommend"
◇ Indicates a weak recommendation or "we suggest"

This pocket uide is distributed by the ESICM

January 2008

SSC Guideline have been endor ed by
American Association of Critical-Care Nurses
American College of Chest Physicians
American College of Emergency Physicians
Canadian Critical Care Society
European Society of Clinical Microbiology and Infectious Diseases
European Society of Intensive Care Medicine
European Respiratory Society
International Sepsis Forum
Japanese Association for Acute Medicine
Japanese Society of Intensive Care Medicine
Society of Critical Care Medicine
Society of Hospital Medicine
Surgical Infection Society
World Federation of Societies of Intensive and Critical Care Medicine.
Participation and endorsement by erman Sepsis Society and Latin American Sepsis Institute.

Initial resuscitation (first 6 hours)

◆ Begin resuscitation immediately in patients with hypotension or elevated serum lactate >4mmol/l; do not delay pending ICU admission. (1C)
◆ Resuscitation goals: (1C)
• Central venous pressure (CVP) 8–12 mm Hg*
• Mean arterial pressure ≥ 65 mm Hg
• Urine output ≥ 0.5 mL.kg⁻¹.hr⁻¹
• Central venous (superior vena cava) oxygen saturation ≥ 70%, or mixed venous ≥ 65%
◇ If venous O₂ saturation target not achieved: (2C)
• consider further fluid
• transfuse packed red blood cells if required to haematocrit of ≥ 0% and/or
• dobutamine infusion max 20 μg.kg⁻¹.min⁻¹
* A higher target CVP of 12-15 mmHg is recommended in the presence of mechanical ventilation or pre-existing decreased ventricular compliance.

Diagnosis

◆ Obtain appropriate cultures before starting antibiotics provided this does not significantly delay antimicrobial administration. (1C)
• Obtain two or more blood cultures (BCs)
• One or more BCs should be percutaneous
• One BC from each vascular access device in place >48 hours
• Culture other sites as clinically indicated
◆ Perform imaging studies promptly in order to c onfirm and sample any source of infection; if safe to do so. (1C)

Antibiotic therapy

◆ Begin intravenous antibiot ics as early as possible, and always within the first hour of recognising severe sepsis (1D) and sep-tic shock. (1B)
◆ Broad-spectrum: one or more agents active against likely bacte-rial/fungal pathogens and with good penetration into presumed source. (1B)
◆ Reassess antimicrobial regim en daily to optimise efficacy, prevent resistance, avoid toxicity & minimise costs. (1C)

◆ Epinephrine, phenylephrine or vasopressin should not be administered as the initial vasopressor in septic shock. (2C)
• Vasopressin 0.0 units/min maybe subsequently added to norepineph-rine with anticipation of an effect equivalent to norepinephrine alone.
◆ Use epinephrine as the first alternative agent in septic shock when blood pressure is poorly responsive to norepinephrine or dopamine. (2B)
◆ Do not use low-dose dopamine for renal protection. (1A)
◆ In patients requiring vasopressors, insert an arterial catheter as soon as practical. (1D)

notropic therapy

◆ Use dobutamine in patients with myocardial dysfunction as supported by elevated cardiac filling pressures and low cardiac output. (1C)
◆ Do not increase cardiac index to predetermined su pranormal levels. (1B)

Steroids

◇ Consider intravenous hydrocortisone for adult septic shock when hypotension remains poorly responsive to adequate fluid resuscitation and vasopressors. (2C)
◇ ACTH stimulation test is not recommended to identify the subset of adults with septic shock who should receive hydro cortisone. (2B)
◇ Hydrocortisone is preferred to dexamethasone. (2B)
◇ Fludrocortisone (50 µg orally once a day) may be included if an alternative to hydrocortisone is being used which lacks significant mineralocorticoid activity. Fludrocortisone is optional if hydrocortisone is used. (2C)
◇ Steroid therapy may be weaned once vasopressors are no longer required. (2D)
◆ Hydrocortisone dose should be < 00mg/day. (1A)
◆ Do not use corticosteroids to treat sepsis in the absence of shock unless the patient's endocrine or corticosteroid history warrants it. (1D)

◇ Non invasive ventilation may be considered in the minority of ALI/ARDS patients with mild-moderate hypoxemic respiratory failure. The patients need to be haemodynamically stable, com-fortable, easily arousable, able to protect/clear their airway and expected to recover rapidly. (2B)
◆ Use a weaning protocol and a spontaneous breathing trial (SBT) regularly to evaluate the potential for discontinuing mechanical ventilation. (1A)
• SBT options include a low level of pressure support with continuous positive
    airway pressure 5 cm H₂O or a T-piece.
• Before the SBT, patients should:
    – be arousable
    – be haemodynamically stable without vasopressors
    – have no new potentially serious conditions
    – have low ventilatory and end-expiratory pressure requirement
    – require FiO₂ levels that can be safely delivered with a face mask or nasal cannula
◆ Do not use a pulmonary artery catheter for the routine monitor-ing of patients with ALI/ARDS. (1A)
◆ Use a conservative fluid strategy for patients with established ALI who do not have evidence of tissue hypoperfusion. (1C)

Sedation, analgesia, and neuromuscular blockade in sepsis

◆ Use sedation protocols with a sedation goal for critically ill mechanically ventilated patients. (1B)
◆ Use either intermittent bolus sedation or continuous infusion sedation to predetermined end points (sedation scales), with daily interruption/ lightening to produce awakening. Re-titrate if necessary. (1B)
◆ Avoid neuromuscular blockers where possible. Monitor depth of block with train of four when using continuous infusions. (1B)

Glucose control

◆ Use IV insulin to control hyperglycaemia in patients with severe sepsis following stabilisation in the ICU. (1B)
• Aim to keep blood glucose <8. mmol/L (150 mg/dl) using a

◇ Consider combination therapy in Pseudomonas infections. (2D)

◇ Consider combination empiric therapy in neutropenic patients. (2D)

◇ Combination therapy no more than ˜5 days and de-e scalation following susceptibilities. (2D)

◇ Duration of therapy typically limited to 7˜10 days; longer if response slow, undrainable foci of infection, or immunologic deficiencies. (1D)

♦ Stop antimicrobial therapy if cause is found to be non-infectious. (1D)

Source identification and control

♦ A specific anatomic site of infection should be established as rapidly as possible (1C) and within the first 6 hours of presentation. (1D)

♦ Formally evaluate patient for a focus of infection amenable to source control measures (eg: abscess drainage, tissue debridement). (1C)

♦ Implement source control measures as soon as possible following successful initial resuscitation. (1C)

◇ Exception: infected pancreatic necrosis, where surgical intervention best delayed. (2B)

♦ Choose source control measure with maximum efficacy and minimal physiologic upset. (1D)

♦ Remove intravascular access devices if potentially infected. (1C)

Fluid therapy

♦ Fluid-resuscitate using crystalloids or colloids. (1B)

♦ Target a CVP of ≥8mmHg (≥12mmHg if mechanically ventilated). (1C)

♦ Use a fluid challenge technique while associated with a haemodynamic improvement. (1D)

♦ Give fluid challenges of 1000 ml of crystalloids or ˜00–500 ml of colloids over ˜0 minutes. More rapid and larger volumes may be required in sepsis-induced tissue hypoperfusion. (1D)

♦ Rate of fluid administration should be reduced if cardiac filling pressures increase without concurrent haemodynamic improvement. (1D)

Vasopressors

♦ Maintain MAP ≥65mmHg. (1C)

♦ Norepinephrine or dopamine centrally administered are the initial vasopressors of choice. (1C)

Recombinant human activated protein C (rhAP C)

◇ Consider rhAPC in adult patients with sepsis-induced organ dysfunction with clinical assessment of high risk of death (typically APACHE II >25 or multiple organ failure) if there are no contraindications. (2B: 2C for post-operative patients)

♦ Adult patients with severe sepsis and low risk of death (eg: APACHE II <20 or one organ failure) should not receive rhAPC. (1A)

Blood product administration

♦ Give red blood cells when haemoglobin decreases to <7.0 g/dl (<70 g/L) to target a haemoglobin of 7.0 – 9.0 g/dl in adults. (1B) A higher haemoglobin level may be required in special circumstances (eg: myocardial ischaemia, severe hypoxaemia, acute haemorrhage, cyanotic heart disease or lactic acidosis)

♦ Do not use erythropoietin to treat sepsis-related anaemia. Erythropoietin may be used for other accepted reasons. (1B)

◇ Do not use fresh frozen plasma to correct laboratory clotting abnormalities unless there is bleeding or planned invasive procedures. (2D)

◇ Do not use antithrombin therapy. (1B)

◇ Administer platelets when: (2D)
- counts are <5000/mm˜ (5 X 109/L) regardless of bleeding.
- counts are 5000 to ˜0,000/mm˜ (5– 0 X 109/L) and there is significant bleeding risk.
- Higher platelet counts ≥50,000/mm˜ (50 X 109/L) are typically required for surgery or invasive procedures.

Mechanical ventilation of sepsis-induced acute lung injury (AL)/ARDS

♦ Target a tidal volume of 6ml/kg (predicted) body weight in patients with ALI/ARDS. (1B)

♦ Target an initial upper limit plateau pressure ≤ ˜0cmH2O. Consider chest wall compliance when assessing plateau pressure. (1C)

♦ Allow PaCO2 to increase above normal, if needed to minimise plateau pressures and tidal volumes. (1C)

♦ Positive end expiratory pressure (PEEP) should be set to avoid extensive lung collapse at end expiration. (1C)

◇ Consider using the prone position for ARDS patients requiring potentially injurious levels of FiO2 or plateau pressure, provided they are not put at risk from positional changes. (2C)

♦ Maintain mechanically ventilated patients in a semi-recumbent position unless contraindicated. (1B)
  ◇ Suggested target elevation ˜0 – 45 degrees. (2C)

validated protocol for insulin dose adjustment. (2C)

♦ Provide a glucose calorie source and monitor blood glucose values every 1-2 hours (4 hours when stable) in patients receiving intravenous insulin. (1C)

◇ Interpret with caution low glucose levels obtained with point of care testing, as these techniques may overestimate arterial blood or plasma glucose values. (1B)

Renal replacement

◇ Intermittent haemodialysis and continuous veno-venous haemofiltration (CVVH) are considered equivalent. (2B)

◇ CVVH offers easier management in haemodynamically unstable patients. (2D)

Bicarbonate therapy

♦ Do not use bicarbonate therapy for the purpose of improving haemo dynamics or reducing vasopressor requirements when treating hypo perfusion-induced lactic acidaemia with pH ≥ 7.15. (1B)

Deep vein thrombosis (DVT) prophylaxis

♦ Use either low-dose unfractionated heparin (UFH) or low-molecular weight heparin (LMWH), unless contraindicated. (1A)

♦ Use a mechanical prophylactic device, such as compression stockings or an intermittent compression device, when heparin is contra indicated. (1A)

◇ Use a combination of pharmacologic and mechanical therapy for patients who are at very high risk for DVT. (2C)

◇ In patients at very high risk LMWH should be used rather than UFH. (2C)

Stress ulcer prophylaxis

♦ Provide stress ulcer prophylaxis using H2 blocker (1A) or proton pump inhibitor. (1B) Benefits of prevention of upper GI b leed must be weighed against the potential for development of ventilator-acquired pneumonia.

Consideration for limitation of support

♦ Discuss advance care planning with patients and families. Describe likely outcomes and set realistic expectations. (1D)

Prepared on behalf of the SSC by Dr Jeremy Willson & Professor Julian Bion

Figure 23.4 Guidelines for management of severe sepsis and septic shock. From: Wilson J, Bion J, 2008: *Guidelines for management of severe sepsis and septic shock* poster. Mount Prospect, Illinois: Society of Critical Care Medicine. Reproduced with permission of the publisher. Copyright 2008. Society of Critical Care Medicine.

- Measure the capillary refill time – hold the fingertip at the level of the heart and apply cutaneous pressure for 5 seconds in order to cause blanching of the skin. On releasing the pressure, time how long it takes the skin to return to the colour of the surrounding tissues. A normal capillary refill time is less than 2 seconds. A prolonged capillary refill time indicates poor peripheral perfusion.
- Peripheral and central pulses – assess for volume, equality and rhythm.

Treat

All patients with shock need to have two large bore peripheral cannulas inserted. Draw blood at the same time. Administer a fluid challenge of 20 mL/kg of crystalloid. The cause of cardiovascular compromise then has to be determined before specific treatments can be administered.

Disability

Rapidly assess the central nervous system using the AVPU scale (Box 23.5). This is easier to remember than the Glasgow Coma Scale (Table 23.4). If the Glasgow Coma Scale is used then the various components should be recorded separately.

Examine the pupils, looking for size, symmetry and response to light. Obtain a blood glucose as this is a relatively common and easily reversible cause for reduced consciousness in hospital patients (Box 23.6).

Exposure

Expose the patient to allow full examination. Care must be taken to maintain dignity and prevent hypothermia.

BOX 23.5 AVPU SCALE

- A – alert and orientated
- V – vocalizing
- P – responsive only to pain
- U – unresponsive

BOX 23.6 CAUSES OF REDUCED CONSCIOUS LEVEL

- Primary brain injury
- Hypoxia
- Hypercapnia
- Reduced cerebral perfusion
- Sedatives or opiates
- Hypoglycaemia
- Uraemia
- Hypothyroidism

Table 23.4 Glasgow Coma Scale

Response	Score
Best motor response	1 – no response to pain 2 – extensor posturing to pain 3 – abnormal flexion to pain 4 – withdrawal to pain 5 – localizing to pain 6 – obeys commands
Best verbal response	1 – none 2 – incomprehensible sounds 3 – inappropriate speech 4 – confused conversation 5 – orientated
Best eye response	1 – no eye opening 2 – eye opening in response to pain 3 – eye opening in response to speech 4 – spontaneous eye opening

SUMMARY

Immediate assessment and management of the acutely ill patient is best undertaken using the A B C D E approach:

- A – Airway
- B – Breathing
- C – Circulation
- D – Disability (of the central nervous system)
- E – Exposure (to allow full examination).

FURTHER READING

Advanced trauma life support student course manual, 8th edn. Can be purchased from the American College of Surgeons. Available at: www.facs.org (accessed 16 November 2009).

Dellinger RP, Levy MM, Carlet JM, *et al.* 2008. Surviving Sepsis Campaign: International guidelines for management of severe sepsis and septic shock. *Critical Care Medicine* **36**:296–327.

National Institute for Health and Clinical Excellence. 2007. *Acutely ill patients in hospital – recognition of and response to acute illness in adults in hospital.* Available at www.nice.org.uk/CG50 (accessed 16 November 2009).

Resuscitation guidelines. 2005. Published by the Resuscitation Council (UK). Available at www.resus.org.uk/pages/guide.htm (accessed 16 November 2009).

The Foundation Programme Curriculum. 2007. Available at www.foundationprogramme.nhs.uk (accessed 16 November 2009).

THE PATIENT WITH IMPAIRED CONSCIOUSNESS

Hina Pattani and Bob Winter

INTRODUCTION

Impairment of consciousness can occur from either local (i.e. cranial) or generalized causes (Table 24.1). Many critically ill patients will have impaired consciousness as part of their presentation. The initial assessment and management of the patient with impaired consciousness is the same as that of any acutely unwell patient and focuses on the A B C D E system (see Chapter 23).

Table 24.1 Common causes of impaired consciousness

Cranial causes	Generalized causes
Encephalitis	Alcohol
Epilepsy	Diabetic ketoacidosis
Head injury	Drugs
Meningitis	Hypoglycaemia
Subarachnoid haemorrhage	Hypoxia
	Sepsis

i IMPORTANT

A patient with impaired consciousness is at risk of airway compromise, aspiration of gastric contents and ventilatory or circulatory embarrassment.

CLINICAL HISTORY

The clinical history can be extremely valuable in patients with impaired consciousness; however, often there is initially very little clinical history available. In many patients, the cause of impaired consciousness is obvious from the history, for example a period of impaired consciousness following a witnessed convulsion may be post-ictal and investigation and management should be focused on the cause of the seizure.

Problems may arise in the patient who has been found with a reduced level of consciousness. Important information such as the presence of a suicide note or stigmata of drug or alcohol use should not be overlooked. Head injury as a cause for unconsciousness is usually obvious; however, in the elderly or alcoholic patient, there may be little history of trauma and you should have a low threshold for investigations such as computed tomography (CT). Head injury is often associated with spinal cord injury, therefore if head trauma is suspected, precautions should be taken to reduce the likelihood of worsening a spinal injury.

PHYSICAL EXAMINATION

The immediate assessment and management of the patient with impaired consciousness should follow the A B C D E system (as described in Chapter 23). This systematic approach ensures that all immediately life-threatening problems are recognized and the correct treatment is started immediately. Be constantly alert to 'clues' that indicate the reason for the patient's reduced conscious level (Fig. 24.1). Specific areas that require a more detailed examination are outlined below.

Airway

Reduction in conscious level is a symptom/sign rather than a diagnosis in its own right and management should be aimed at the underlying cause while protecting basic functions threatened by the clinical condition of the patient.

Securing the airway with a definitive airway such as an endotracheal tube should be considered carefully and early. This may require expert assistance. Management of the patient with severe depression of consciousness will often require intubation and ventilation in a critical care area unless the cause is

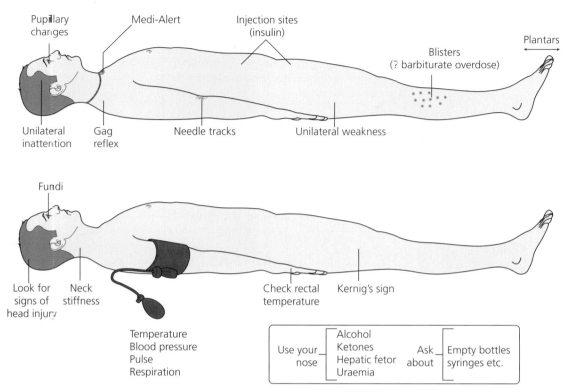

Figure 24.1 What to look for in the patient with impaired consciousness. From: Gray D, Toghill P (eds), *An introduction to the symptoms and signs of clinical medicine*, with permission. © 2001 London: Hodder Arnold.

rapidly amenable to therapy (such as hypoglycaemia). Even in overdose where there is an antagonist, such as opiates or benzodiazepines, it is often safer and easier to ventilate the patient rather than reverse the drug effects other than for diagnostic reasons.

Breathing

Examination of the respiratory system should include an assessment of depth and rate of breathing which may indicate causes in other systems such as the air hunger of diabetic ketoacidosis or the shallow slow respiration pattern of opiate intoxication. Assessment of breathing should also include measures to augment it if inadequate. As a rule all comatose patients should receive oxygen in the first instance. Assessment of arterial blood gases is useful as it is important to recall that adequate oxygen saturation does not equate to adequate ventilation, especially in the context of oxygen supplementation.

Circulation

Hypertension in the context of coma may be the result of Cushing's response to raised intracranial pressure or vasospasm following subarachnoid haemorrhage, and should not be specifically treated in the first instance. Rather, urgent measures to reduce intracranial pressure such as mannitol 0.25–0.5 g/kg and consideration of anaesthesia and sedation for immediate CT scan should take precedence. If a CT scan indicates that hypertensive encephalopathy is the likely diagnosis rather than secondary hypertension, then rapid reduction of blood pressure is indicated.

Hypotension is more often a marker of systemic disease such as sepsis than a cause for impairment of consciousness in its own right. The discovery of a low blood pressure should prompt efforts to restore it and simultaneous efforts to elucidate the cause. The depression of diastolic blood pressure associated with the vasodilation of sepsis contrasts with the elevated or maintained diastolic blood pressure produced by the vasoconstriction of hypovolaemic or cardiogenic shock.

Disability

Examination of the nervous system should include a formal assessment and documentation of the level of consciousness. The Glasgow Coma Scale (Table 23.4, p. 432) is the most recognized method of doing this and ideally the individual elements rather than just the total should be recorded.

SMALL PRINT

When the Glasgow Coma Scale was first described in 1974, it was scored out of a total of 14 points. Soon afterwards, a Modified Glasgow Coma Scale was proposed with a total score of 15 points (adding the Motor category of 'abnormal flexion to pain'). The modified scale is now the more widely used, although some centres still use the original 14-point scale.

Assessment of the pupils including size, reactivity and symmetry may give important clues.

- The post-ictal pupils of either opiate intoxication or brainstem stroke are associated with either slow shallow respiration or rapid shallow respiration, respectively.
- Bilateral dilated reactive pupils are often associated with drugs such as tricyclic antidepressants in overdose whereas dilated fixed pupils are more commonly associated with brainstem damage or barbiturate overdose.
- A unilateral dilated pupil may herald impending uncal herniation and brainstem coning but may also be seen with a complete cranial nerve III palsy in posterior communicating artery aneurysm.

Lack of corneal reflex is usually associated with deep coma or drug overdose. Lateralized motor signs are most commonly associated with structural brain damage such as that following intracerebral haemorrhage, although hypoglycaemia or migraine may also produce lateralized signs. Generalized abnormal movement such as myoclonus suggests a metabolic or hypoxic cause for coma.

Exposure

An examination of temperature may reveal a generalized disturbance as a cause for impairment of consciousness.

- Both elevation and reduction of body temperature may be associated with impairment of consciousness.
- Low temperature may of itself cause coma but may also be associated with other conditions and exposure to low environmental temperature.
- Fever is more often a marker of infection which may be localized to the central nervous system such as meningitis or encephalitis or in another system such as respiratory where systemic infection and hypoxia may co-exist.

If an elevated temperature is found then examination of the skin may reveal the purpuric rash of meningococcaemia. The skin may also show tracks from intravenous drug use or icterus associated with liver disease.

INVESTIGATIONS

Any patient with reduced consciousness and either focal signs, a history of trauma or meningism should be urgently investigated with CT. In the patient with meningism and fever, blood cultures and intravenous antibiotics should also be instituted immediately.

In the absence of these signs the likelihood is that the reduction in conscious level is being produced by a generalized cause, i.e. metabolic or toxic, and investigations should be focused on eliminating these. Key investigations include:

- full blood count
- urea and electrolytes
- calcium
- liver function tests
- thyroid function tests
- cortisol
- toxicology screen (including paracetamol and salicylate levels).

Electroencephalogram is occasionally required to eliminate rare cases of non-convulsive status epilepticus.

SUMMARY

- Impairment of consciousness can occur from either local (i.e. cranial) or generalized causes.
- The initial assessment and management of the patient with impaired consciousness is the same as that of any acutely unwell patient and focuses on the A B C D E system.
- Management of the patient with severe depression of consciousness will often require intubation and ventilation in a critical care area, unless the cause is rapidly amenable to therapy.
- As a rule all comatose patients should receive oxygen in the first instance. Adequate oxygen saturation does not equate to adequate ventilation, especially in the context of oxygen supplementation.
- Hypertension in the context of coma may be the result of Cushing's response to raised intracranial pressure or vasospasm – urgently reduce intracranial pressure and arrange immediate CT. If this indicates hypertensive encephalopathy rather than secondary hypertension, then rapid reduction of blood pressure is indicated.
- The Glasgow Coma Scale is the most recognized method of formally assessing and documenting the level of consciousness.
- Lateralized motor signs are most commonly associated with structural brain damage.
- Pupil signs are informative:
  - pin-point pupils suggest opiate intoxication (associated with slow shallow respiration) or brainstem stroke (associated with rapid shallow respiration)
  - bilateral dilated *reactive* pupils are often associated with drugs such as tricyclic antidepressants in overdose
  - bilateral dilated *fixed* pupils are more commonly associated with brainstem damage or barbiturate overdose
  - unilateral dilated pupil may herald impending uncal herniation and brainstem coning or complete cranial nerve III palsy in posterior communicating artery aneurysms
  - lack of corneal reflex is usually associated with deep coma or drug overdose.
- Reduced consciousness with focal signs, a history of trauma or meningism should be urgently investigated with CT.

FURTHER READING

Teasdale G, Jennett B. 1974. Assessment of coma and impaired consciousness. A practical scale. *Lancet* **304**: 81–84.

25 THE OLDER PATIENT

Rowan H Harwood

INTRODUCTION

Are older people different from younger adults?

Assessing problems with individual systems in older people is done the same way as for younger people: the history taking and examination is fundamentally the same.

The majority of older people are basically healthy, free from severe disability and mental illness, and 'feel' little different from a younger person in their attitudes and responses to illness. Cancer is no less threatening, incontinence no less humiliating, and bereavement no less devastating than it would be for you or me. Older people are not 'them' – a race apart; they are 'us', just older, or 'us' in the future.

However, older people vary one from another more than younger people do. This holds at all levels: enzyme activity, cellular and organ function, gross physical function. Some run marathons, some can't walk. Older people get ill more frequently. They have had longer exposure to environmental and physiological determinants of disease (smoking, diet, exercise, trauma, cholesterol, blood pressure), and longer for genetic determinants to manifest.

Health problems themselves vary. There may be:

- a mixture of multiple acute and chronic illnesses
- medical, psychological and social dimensions
- multiple stakeholders, including relatives, carers, and services (such as care homes) as well as the patient.

This means that doctors must be flexible in how they approach older people. Some are dealt with fairly simply and no differently from younger adults. Others are complex, difficult to assess, and frustrating to manage (Box 25.1). Ailments may be curable or incurable. Chronic illness may be stable or progressive. Acute illness may be but a temporary episode in a much longer 'illness career'. Problems

---

> **BOX 25.1** HOW MEDICINE IN OLDER PEOPLE IS DIFFERENT
> - Non-specific or atypical presentations
> - Multiple pathologies
> - Rapid loss of function
> - Increased propensity to complications of both disease and its treatment
> - Need for explicit rehabilitation
> - Importance of assessing the environment
>
> From: Evans JG. 1990. How are the elderly different? In: Kane RL, Evans JG, MacFadyen D. *Improving the health of older people: a world view*. Oxford: OUP, 50–68, by permission of Oxford University Press.

---

with function ('disability') and social situation are frequent enough to make them worth asking about routinely.

The notion of frailty can be helpful. Frailty implies a combination of limitation in function and propensity to deterioration. Frail patients are the core business of geriatric medicine. Unfortunately, frail older patients often put doctors (and medical students) in the wrong frame of mind, with numerous pejorative terms in common use. More positively, it can be useful to ask 'What can medicine contribute to helping this person's problems?' Your history taking and examination are not an end in themselves, but a prelude to action, so when taking a history you have to know how you might intervene, and what information is needed to support action. Interventions may aim for:

- prevention (of diseases or complications)
- cure (of diseases or complications)
- prolonging life
- relieving symptoms
- maximizing function
- giving information
- supporting families and carers.

The mechanisms for achieving these include:

- risk assessment
- diagnosis
- drug treatment
- surgical treatment
- remedial therapies (speech and language therapy, physiotherapy, occupational therapy, rehabilitation nursing)
- nutritional therapies
- psychotherapies, counselling, advising
- teaching
- supporting decision making and advanced planning.

None of these is unique to geriatric medicine, and they apply equally to a sick child or younger adult with disabling chronic disease. To borrow a line from Professor Archie Young: 'Geriatric medicine is general medicine … done obsessively'. In fact, the practice of geriatric medicine presupposes expertise in all of general internal medicine and more: psychiatry, ophthalmology, rheumatology, urology, health psychology, sociology, ethics and law.

Effective care for older people will almost always involve other people than doctors alone: nurses, therapists, social workers. The team (often a 'virtual team' with flexible membership and no direct line management) works best when members know both their own contribution, and what others can do. There will be multiple assessments, which will often overlap. Share information: therapists will know things doctors also need to know.

The doctor should be clear what his or her contribution is (because they often forget). They must get the medicine right, with an unusual thoroughness and comprehensiveness, attention to disability and planning for the future, and knowledge of interventions from the level of pathology to the environment. The starting point is diagnosis. Problems must be explained in biomedical terms. Only then can thinking about therapy and prognosis begin. In hospital, an experienced practitioner will also start to build discharge options very early on, managing expectations and keeping possibilities open, as well as proactively involving and informing the patient and carers.

INFORMATION GATHERING

History taking from complex older patients takes time. A 'typically complex' older patient will take an hour or more to clerk and 15 minutes to review on a post-take ward round.

'History taking' is perhaps too narrow a term. There is a more prolonged process of 'information gathering' that extends over several days or even weeks. An initial assessment in an emergency department or medical admissions unit is unlikely to be complete, and may need revisiting and revising, involving:

- third party history taking (e.g. to establish a diagnosis or to collect basic information in cognitive impairment, or to assess loss of consciousness)
- observation, both for change or fluctuation (e.g. alertness and cognition in delirium)
- assessment of function (which will probably involve nurses and therapists).

Presenting symptoms

An older person may present with any 'typical' medical symptom, such as weight loss, pain, breathlessness, or disturbance of consciousness, and these should be investigated and managed as for anyone else. In addition, there are four classical 'non-specific' presentations of disease, the so-called 'geriatric giants'. Non-specific means that they can be caused by many different pathologies. These are:

- immobility
- falls
- confusion
- incontinence.

Add to this the even more non-specific 'not coping'. Emphasizing non-specificity can be overdone, however. Most presenting symptoms in medicine are non-specific. Breathlessness, for example, may have cardiac, respiratory, metabolic and psychogenic causes, and weight loss may be malignant, gastrointestinal, metabolic or psychiatric.

The non-specificity of the 'headline' presenting complaint is often easily unravelled by simple questioning and probing for more 'typical' symptoms.

signs of heart failure, no more than half of patients actually need it (ankle swelling may also be caused by dependency, immobility, hypoalbuminaemia, venous or lymphatic obstruction).

stay. If not, consider a trial of stopping it.

Ask if withdrawal of a drug has been considered, in particular antidepressants, antipsychotics, analgesics, corticosteroids and hypnotics. In dementia, people may go through 'psychotic' or agitated phases, sometimes associated with relocations or life events, and 3 or 6 months later medication can be withdrawn. If not, dose minimization may be possible (e.g. can furosemide be reduced to a lower than prescribed dose in stable heart failure?).

Distinguish between preventive drugs, e.g. vascular (antithrombotics, cholesterol and blood pressure lowering), anti-osteoporotic (calcium and vitamin D, bisphosphonates and other anti-resorbatives) and those controlling active current problems, e.g. antiarrhythmics, analgesics, antianginals, heart failure, diabetic, and antiepileptic drugs, bronchodilators. If a preventive drug is causing problems, stop it. The odds on it doing good are usually too slim to justify side effects.

Ask about medicines management and compliance. Who supervises? Are compliance aids used (dosette box, blister pack, family supervision)?

Ask about past allergies and adverse effects. Specify the exact problem if possible. Calls to GPs and reviews of case notes may be needed to clarify. Many adverse effects get called 'allergies' – few actually are, but you will still need to know about them. If an expected drug is missing (e.g. a statin in vascular disease, angiotensin-converting enzyme (ACE) inhibitor in heart failure) search the case notes and phone the GP to find out if there is a reason.

Social and functional history: activities of daily living

Social history is often brushed over in younger adults – perhaps limited to marital status, occupation and smoking and alcohol consumption histories. For many older people it is key to understanding their problems and planning discharge.

- Who, if anyone, does the patient live with?
- And in what sort of accommodation (house with stairs, ground floor flat, care home)?
- Is there help from family, or paid carers?
- Ask about the health of an elderly spouse or co-resident.

Function tells us several things. It provides a baseline against which we can consider changes in health. A problem with function (a *disability*), such as walking or safety awareness, may have been the presenting problem. Quantifying function tells us about disease severity. Function is the 'final common pathway' for the effects of many different diseases or combinations of diseases. Problems with walking may be due to pain, weakness, breathlessness, falling, blindness, dementia, depression or fear. We may have to start with the disability and work 'backwards' to identify the signs and symptoms (*impairments*) that are associated with it, and from that work out the underlying diagnoses. Function will give you insight into cognition, confidence, physical ability and available support networks. Usually it is problems with function that make discharge difficult, so assessing function is part of discharge planning.

What someone does day to day depends both on their capacity to do tasks, and the physical and social environment in which they do them. It also depends on the use of aids and appliances. In assessing function you must also assess the environment and levels of help available and used.

The range of activities that might be considered is wide. At a minimum, ask about mobility, continence and behaviour. An otherwise fit older person might be asked about driving, shopping, cooking and money management. Stair climbing, walking outdoors, walking indoors, dressing, getting to the toilet, wheelchair use and bed to chair transfers can all be considered. If problems are identified ask how they are overcome (Who gets your food? How do you get to the toilet?). Falls and incontinence and other lower urinary tract symptoms (LUTS) are common so ask specifically about these. Incontinence and LUTS may not be volunteered – develop a form of words that is not open to offence, but do not be embarrassed yourself.

'How do you occupy your time?' can be a revealing question. Many people do little more than watch television.

Discharge anticipation

'Discharge planning begins on day 1' is a slogan that may not be applicable in many complex cases. The answer to questions about discharge destinations will often be 'It depends'. Do not suggest that care home placement is necessary before a full assessment and decision-making process has been undertaken.

Make life as easy as possible for your colleagues by recording basic aspects of social and functional history, and sources of support, as early as possible, especially if you have a relative present at first clerking who may not be available later. If strong opinions about the future are expressed early on ('She's not coming home'), record them, but do try to keep all options open as long as possible.

Discharge home with support is not always possible, but is usually preferable, and quicker, than care home placement. Moreover, it may be that despite severe disability and dependency, someone already well supported at home can be discharged quickly after resolution of a minor crisis, when you would have anticipated a long and difficult admission, but only if you know the support arrangements that are in place.

Sometimes you need to identify quickly that terminal care is appropriate, and plan accordingly.

Third party and cognitive history

Most older people are able to give a full account of themselves and their symptoms. Technically it is a breach of confidentiality to involve anyone else without their permission – if the person has capacity, it is courteous to ask at least, although in many cases the consent will be implicit, and need not be explicit. However, if someone cannot give an account of themselves, best practice, best interests, and, in the UK the law, require that others be consulted.

This is usually required in cases of cognitive impairment, aphasia or other communication difficulties. It is also useful in cases of non-specific 'not coping', loss of consciousness and falls (30 per cent of people experiencing syncope have no recall of losing consciousness; epilepsy is a diagnosis made primarily on third party history; the deathly pallor of cardiovascular syncope or pre-syncope can be a helpful diagnostic pointer).

Think of it as 'clerking the relatives'. Re-take the history. Identify and characterize prior activities of daily living, as in the functional history. Also find out about cognition, especially time course of deterioration, severity and impact on behaviour (Box 25.3). Ideally do this without the patient present (by telephone if necessary). Carers may wish to ensure that you fully understand what they are experiencing, especially where there is fluctuation, and this may include information upsetting to the patient.

BOX 25.3 COGNITIVE HISTORY

- What led the patient to present to medical attention?
- Duration, fluctuation or progression of symptoms. When did you first notice a problem? When was he or she last normal? How were things last Christmas? Last summer?
- Ask about:
  - forgetfulness, repetitiveness, misplacing or losing things (and any consequent accusations of theft)
  - safety concerns, leaving the gas on, burning out pans, getting lost, leaving the front door open, dealing with strangers
  - reasoning and judgement
  - change in personality and behaviour
  - night-time disturbance, sleep reversal
  - daytime occupation
  - management of complex or mentally taxing tasks – bills, shopping, cooking, driving
  - loss of hygiene and house sense (living in squalor)
  - continence
  - falls
  - availability of outside help, family or statutory services
  - insight.

Early forgetfulness, lapses in judgement, or personality changes, may not be recognized as such, or may be ignored, suppressed or compensated for (by family members taking on more mentally difficult tasks). You have to probe: Who does the bills? The shopping? What does he or she do to occupy their time? Inability to do mentally taxing tasks may only be apparent when a daughter goes on holiday, or a spouse becomes ill or dies.

Impairment of recent memory is often dismissed by patients and families as part of normal ageing. In fact there is no clear distinction between 'normal' and 'abnormal'; measurements of cognitive function lie on a continuum. Problems in multiple cognitive domains, which are progressive and interfere with social function, without an alternative explanation, are required to diagnose dementia.

It is important to identify fluctuation. Sudden onset (or abrupt change in prior dementia) along with fluctuation in cognition and attention are the defining features of delirium, and also occur in dementia with Lewy bodies.

Others may also have useful information. Consider phoning the family doctor, or social care providers (home care, or wardens of assisted living facilities). The drug history is important, especially recent changes, and will often not be reliably given by the patient.

Check whether mental state or physical function were recorded during a previous hospital admission.

Mental state examination

Examining the mental state is a basic competency, but one with which most physicians are unfamiliar and uncomfortable. Many resort to a fairly uncritical use of screening tools such as the Abbreviated Mental Test score or Geriatric Depression Scale, without realizing that interpretation of these requires follow up with a formal mental state examination.

Examination is a combination of observation and questioning (Box 25.4). This may be difficult if the patient is suspicious or uncooperative. The objective is to identify and characterize cognitive function, depression, anxiety, psychosis or other psychiatric diagnoses.

Speech

Assess language, syntax (are sentences put together properly?) and content. Remember aphasia: misinterpreting aphasia for confusion is so common that you should specifically test for it (understanding motor commands, fluency in spontaneous conversation or picture description, naming, sequences such as counting, answering yes/no questions).

Mood

Strictly 'mood' is a person's inner feelings, and the 'affect' is how the individual appears to the outside world. People with depression usually complain of feeling sad or miserable, but not always. Look for persistent negative ideas – blame, being a burden, not deserving other people's efforts, or lack of motivation. It can be difficult to separate understandable reactions to difficult life circumstances (like being disabled or

---

BOX 25.4 SUMMARY OF MENTAL STATE EXAMINATION

- Appearance – grooming, dress, distress
- Behaviour – agitation, apathy, cooperation, eye contact
- Cognition
  - Alertness and attention
  - Orientation (person, place, time)
  - Concentration
  - Memory – registration and short-term recall
  - Intellect
  - Logical and abstract thought and decision making
- Speech – aphasia, syntax, content
- Mood, objective and subjective
- Thoughts, including delusions
- Hallucinations
- Insight

---

ill) from depressive thoughts. Severe depression is pervasive (all aspects of thinking) and persistent (2 or 3 weeks minimum). Other conditions are more variable or distractible. Most useful is to find out if the person can experience any enjoyment at all. Inability to cheer up in normally rewarding situations (*anhedonia*) is a reliable sign of depression. If someone is depressed ask about thoughts of self-harm or suicide. This is easier than might be first thought ('Do you ever think that life isn't worth living? Or that you would rather be dead? Have you ever thought about harming yourself? Have you ever actually thought about taking your own life?').

Ask about sleep, tiredness on waking, appetite, weight loss and diurnal variation (mornings worse). However, many physical symptoms in depression can reasonably be put down to poor physical health, and in older people (or anyone with physical ill health), psychological symptoms are a better guide. Some people with depression may also have periods of elation, inappropriate happiness or a sense of importance or grandeur – hypo-mania or mania, part of bipolar affective disorder.

Anxiety is a state of apprehension, fearfulness or premonition. It is commonly associated with depression. The key feature of severe anxiety is of autonomic arousal – palpitation, tremor, sweating, dry mouth, abdominal discomfort, and also restlessness, choking or breathlessness and irritability. Anxiety can be subdivided into three syndromes: *panic disorder*, *generalized anxiety* and *phobia* (fear in response to a particular trigger, such as confined spaces or spiders). Both anxiety and depression can be part of delirium. In fact, among general hospital inpatients, depressive symptoms are more likely to represent delirium than they are to represent major affective disorder.

Abnormal beliefs

Delusions are firmly held false beliefs, not amenable to rational argument. They may occur in dementia, delirium, depression or delusional disorder. In dementia they can be the direct result of poor memory: if you cannot remember where you put something, either someone moved it, or there must have been burglars. Other delusions may result from imagining that you are much younger than you really are. Delusions in delirium are more irrational, lack structure or system, may be inconsistent, and fleeting (short lasting).

Depressive delusions are usually obvious, but may be somatized (appear as physical symptoms) or hypochondriacal (delusion of illness). In 'delusional disorder', paranoid (persecutory) delusions may occur, with accusations against neighbours, landlords, public services or utilities. It may also involve delusions of infestation or bodily abnormalities (and so present to physicians).

Abnormal perceptions

Hallucinations are abnormal perceptions (hearing or seeing things that are not there). Auditory hallucinations are most commonly seen in functional psychoses (schizophrenia or severe depression). Visual hallucinations occur in delirium and dementia with Lewy bodies (DLB). In DLB, they are typically formed and animated (moving), and may involve seeing strangers in one's home. (See also the section 'Abnormal experiences/perceptual disorders' in Chapter 13.)

Using standardized scales

Some people advocate checking cognition (using the 10-point Abbreviated Mental Test score, AMT, or 30-point Mini-Mental State Examination, MMSE) and depression (using the Geriatric Depression Scale or Hospital Anxiety and Depression Scale) in all older inpatients. This is not bad advice but is not strictly necessary. The AMT is very crude and sufficient only in admissions units and non-specialist settings. The MMSE is much more sophisticated, but is also only a screening test, and still requires proper history taking and diagnosis. Experienced practitioners will often pick up clues that there are cognitive or other mental health problems, but are still sometimes caught out. Nurses, occupational therapists and physiotherapists may also spot problems, for example, in day-to-day behaviour, remembering what is said in therapy sessions, or when doing more complex tasks such as kitchen assessments. It may not be until a speech therapist or translator is available that someone with apparent aphasia is found to have underlying cognitive impairment as well.

> **CLINICAL PEARL**
> - You cannot diagnose dementia or depression using a standardized scale alone. You need to take a history, and establish interference with social function, as well.
> - Besides dementia, low scores can be caused by delirium, aphasia, deafness, visual impairment, prolonged hospital stays, low intellect and not speaking English.
> - A previous MMSE score recorded in the notes can be very useful during subsequent admissions if things have changed.
> - Many 'depressive' symptoms are caused by physical illness and high scores on depression scales must be interpreted with care. They are also common in delirium.

PHYSICAL EXAMINATION

The ritual for examining each system is no different from that used in any other adult. At least once during a hospital admission someone should do a full physical examination. Some parts of the examination are often neglected and these are discussed below.

Measure postural blood pressure

Blood pressure varies with circumstances. Drugs or autonomic failure make postural hypotension quite common (25 per cent over 65 years). When investigating dizziness or falls, measure blood pressure after 5 minutes lying, then after 1–2 minutes standing (using an automated sphygmomanometer, remembering that the machine takes about 15 seconds to make a reading). Record if the patient was dizzy on standing.

Musculoskeletal system

Joint disease is very common in older people (50 per cent of 80 year olds have knee arthritis), and may contribute to immobility, falls, dizziness and pain. Look at the shoulders and hands if symptoms dictate. Look at the knees, and the bulk of quadriceps muscles. Record if the knees can be fully extended (they should go into a few degrees of hyperextension), and the extent of any fixed flexion deformity. Test flexion/extension and internal/external rotation of the hips. If painful, think about the shortened externally rotated leg in hip fracture. Remember that an apparently painful hip, with a normal X-ray, may be due to a pelvic fracture. Neck arthritis may be associated with dizziness on standing when the neck is extended (due to disordered proprioception, not vertebrobasilar ischaemia).

Feet

Look for ulcers, deformities, and neglected nails (onychogryphosis).

Neurological examination

There is so much that can potentially be done in this area, that doing it all is both time consuming and beyond the stamina of an ill patient. Problems such as arthritis may make it difficult to interpret. You may have to resort to skilled observation alone if the patient is uncooperative. The key is to ask yourself 'What you are examining for?'

The nervous system is actually many systems: consciousness, vision, brainstem, hearing, balance, speech, pyramidal motor, extra-pyramidal motor, coordination, sensory and autonomic. Your first aim is to use your knowledge of neuroanatomy to determine where the lesion is. Where you look will be determined by the nature of the problem and the symptoms revealed in the history.

- If you are investigating falls, you will want to examine vision, vestibular and pyramidal function, coordination, feet tactile sensation and proprioception.
- If you expect the examination to be normal (in the absence of specific neurological symptoms) you can define a minimum examination, which should reassure you that a structural brain lesion is unlikely. It takes perhaps 5 minutes to perform, and comprises: gross acuity, visual fields, eye, face, palate and tongue movements, speech, arm tone, pronator drift, shoulder abduction, first dorsal interosseous (index finger abduction), finger-nose coordination, dysdiadochokinesis, hand and feet sensation, standing balance/Romberg's test and gait.
- If cooperation is lacking, look. You can detect spatial inattention and visual field loss, facial asymmetry, speech and swallow problems, abnormal limb movements, symmetry of limb movement and coordination, ability to stand from sitting, gait, maybe limb tone, and hand grip, possibly via a hand shake.

Today, access to computed tomography (CT) or magnetic resonance imaging (MRI) is generally easy, but remember that in the absence of red-flag symptoms (focal onset epilepsy or raised intracranial pressure – headache, drowsiness) a competently performed, normal neurological examination almost rules out significant structural brain pathology.

Dentition

Problems with the dentition can explain dysarthria and swallowing difficulties, as well as being an endocarditis risk. If there are dentures do everything possible to prevent them being lost in hospital.

Vision

Distinguish between uni-ocular loss (anterior to the optic chiasm – broadly ophthalmology, apart from amaurosis fugax) and homonymous loss (posterior to it – broadly neurology). Sudden vision loss is an emergency that requires immediate explanation (do funduscopy, and/or refer to an eye emergency department). In any visual loss ensure that an adequate explanation has been reached. Refer on to ophthalmology if this is not clear.

Pressure areas

New sores on specialist wards are rare, but some may be 'imported', from surgical wards and nursing homes. Sacrum, greater trochanters and heels are vulnerable. Specifically look for them, know the warning signs (non-blanching erythema or blisters), and how to grade a pressure sore (1= erythema, 2 = skin break, 3 = subcutaneous tissue, 4 = muscle cavity). Assess dead tissue or slough, and look for cellulitis.

Continence assessment

The commonest diagnoses will be detrusor instability and incomplete bladder emptying. A post void bladder ultrasound scan and urine dipstick test provide the 'quick wins', but more involved assessment may include a neurological examination of the legs, inspection of the vulva for atrophy or prolapse and a rectal examination for the prostate and constipation.

Functional assessment

In someone who is fairly well you can assess sit-to-stand and bed transfers and gait yourself. Anything more difficult is associated with risk, both to the patient (falling) and to you (back injury). Your hospital will have a manual handling policy. Nurses usually have good judgement about what someone can do, but you may require formal physiotherapy and occupational therapy assessments. Do not try to supervise a difficult transfer (e.g. to get someone on a bed) if you are not confident or have not been trained. The golden rule is, if in doubt, use the safest possible transfer, using a hoist if necessary.

INVESTIGATIONS

Some doctors claim that older people are over-investigated, others say that ageist discrimination denies older people access to the best modern investigation technology. In fact, it is not a matter of investigate more or investigate less, it is: investigate with a clear purpose.

Investigation is important in older people since diagnosis is more difficult due to non-specific and atypical presentation, multiple pathologies and uncertain information if history taking is compromised by cognitive impairment or communication difficulties. This can mean that older people need more, not less, access to high-tech tests.

However, some tests are unpleasant, and most carry a cost, if only in terms of time, travel to hospital and inconvenience. For the frail, cognitively impaired or bewildered, this can become a major trial, so tests for defensive or academic reasons cannot be justified. It is not quite true to say that a test is only justified if it is going to change management. Tests provide information, and information has value. It may or may not lead to therapeutic intervention. A test result can tell you to stop investigating further (for example a scan showing widespread cancer). Clinical judgement is important. If there is doubt, discuss with the patient and family and use the principles of decision making (benefits, burdens, autonomy, justice) to decide.

The practicality of tests must also be discussed. Retaining barium in the colon may be impossible and CT colonography or colonoscopy preferable. All bowel investigations are impossible without fully evacuating the bowel, which itself may require hospital admission. A plain abdominal X-ray is a good way to assess faecal loading (but radiologists may frown on this as an indication).

Blood tests 'come cheap'. Make sure there is a recent blood count, renal, liver and thyroid function tests, and calcium. Patients with anaemia and neurological and psychiatric symptoms also need vitamin B_{12} and folate tests. C-reactive protein (CRP) level is a useful screen for sepsis but (like temperature and the white cell count) is not 100 per cent sensitive (there can be false negatives).

Dipstick urinalysis is useful when negative, it virtually excludes urinary infection. Urinalysis positive for nitrites and leucocyte esterase still needs culture to confirm infection, but remember that 30 per cent of elderly women, and anyone with a urethral catheter, have asymptomatic bacteriuria, so the test must be interpreted in the light of symptoms. If someone is non-specifically unwell and there is no other explanation, treating the 'urinary tract infection' is unavoidable.

CLINICAL PEARL

Do not repeat tests unnecessarily. B$_{12}$ and thyroid function will not change over 6 months or so. Do not measure vitamin D in someone on supplements.

PROBLEM LISTS

A problem list is a way of assembling complex, disparate, information, to give you an overview of where work needs doing. It is more a working tool than a formal document.

You may use a problem list as part of the 'history of the presenting complaint', especially where there are a lot of different symptoms. In subacute settings (e.g. medical or rehabilitation ward or intermediate care) where more information has emerged from tests and assessments, and as issues develop over time, the problem list becomes a reassessment of 'where we have got to'. You may also use it at a ward round or weekly review. It is a way of making sure that things do not get overlooked.

Problems can be symptoms or impairments (e.g. breathlessness, weakness, spasticity, pain), diagnoses, disabilities (mobility, continence, behaviours), social or environmental issues, abnormal test results, risks or predispositions.

DECISION MAKING

Although not strictly history taking, gathering information to inform decision making is an increasingly important part of clinical practice. To make decisions you need to set out benefits and burdens of a proposed intervention, test or course of management, consider what the patient wants (autonomy) and respect justice (working within available resources and avoiding discrimination).

Where the patient lacks capacity, seek the existence of an advanced decision for the refusal of treatment (living will), or the holder of a health and welfare Lasting Power of Attorney (LPA). If there is none, legally you then need to involve the patient in deciding and ascertain their current wishes (even if they do not fully understand what they are saying), find out their previously expressed wishes (from an informant) and seek the views of family members. In the UK, if someone has no family or friends you must involve an Independent Mental Capacity Advocate for any serious decision.

These issues form part of the broad spectrum of information gathering that may be added to history taking at admission or done separately later. Information may be needed rapidly to help decision making in emergency situations (e.g. resuscitation and aggressive medical intervention versus terminal care).

COMMON DIAGNOSES

Immobility

Immobility describes an 'activity limitation' or 'disability'. It is often the end result of multiple pathologies and other factors, such as volition and environment, although a single cause may be identified (Table 25.1).

A common crisis is when someone has 'gone off their legs' due to an acute or acute on chronic illness. Immobility is one of the 'geriatric giants', the non-specific presentations of acute disease. It also results from chronic illness, including musculoskeletal, neurological, cardio-respiratory and dementia.

An important additional feature is the role of 'deconditioning': the loss of muscular strength and stamina, and cardio-respiratory fitness, following a period of illness, immobility or under-activity (possibly over months or years). Fortunately this is reversible with sustained and progressive exercise, and, along with restoration of confidence, probably accounts for a large part of what is achieved in general geriatric rehabilitation.

The medical role is to assess and identify causes, intervene to reverse treatable causes, palliate outstanding symptoms, and initiate rehabilitation to improve motor function, and other functional abilities.

Gross mobility can be quantified at a series of levels, from sitting balance, to transfers, through indoor

Table 25.1 Causes of immobility

System	Problem	Investigation
Musculoskeletal	Arthritis, especially knees, hips, back Covert fractures (pelvis, hip, tibial plateau) Limb loss Foot deformities (toenails, ulcers, hallux valgus) Myopathy	Mainly clinical. X-ray may help X-ray Clinical Clinical Vitamin D status, thyroid function, creatine kinase, ESR
Neurological	Hemiparesis (usually stroke) Paraparesis (including spinal cord compression or ischaemia, cervical myelopathy) Parkinson's disease Peripheral neuropathy	Clinical, CT/MRI brain MRI spine, B_{12} Clinical Nerve conduction studies, glucose, B_{12}, ESR, autoantibodies
Vision	Blindness Hemianopia and inattention	Clinical Clinical, CT brain
Cardiovascular	Heart failure (breathlessness, oedema) Chest pain Postural hypotension Intermittent claudication	Clinical, chest X-ray, ECG, echocardiography Clinical, ECG, chest X-ray, angiography Clinical Clinical, duplex ultrasound, angiography
Respiratory	Breathlessness (chronic obstructive pulmonary disease, pulmonary embolism, fibrosis, effusion, pneumonia, cancer)	Chest X-ray, spirometry, blood gases, CT thorax
Skin	Leg or foot ulcers Oedema (dependency, heart failure, hypoalbuminaemia, venous or lymphatic obstruction)	Clinical Clinical, albumin, as for heart failure
Psychological	Anxiety, loss of confidence Depression with psychomotor retardation Dementia (apraxia, executive failure)	Clinical Clinical Clinical

CT, computed tomography; ECG, electrocardiography; ESR, erythrocyte sedimentation rate; MRI, magnetic resonance imaging.

mobility, stairs, outdoor mobility and crossing roads or rough ground. Further qualification can be in terms of:

- human help (number of persons, hands on, or supervision)
- aids required (wheelchair, pulpit frame, gutter frame, wheeled Zimmer frame, three-wheeled delta frame, crutches, sticks)
- degree of difficulty experienced
- distance or speed achieved.

A report may, for example, describe someone as being able to walk 10 m with a Zimmer frame and the supervision of one person.

Assessment will identify symptoms and signs contributing to the problem, which must then be explained by diagnoses. This requires history taking and thorough examination of the neurological and musculoskeletal systems, heart and chest. Reports from nurses and therapists can help. When mobility declines suddenly, consider an acute medical illness (infection, metabolic disturbance, new stroke, drug side effect).

Immobility may not always be 'curable' but at a minimum do not miss a treatable cause. Consider if part, at least, of a progressive decline might be due to deconditioning, which is eminently reversible. After an acute illness, the ambition should always be a return to pre-morbid mobility.

Falls

Falls, and fear of falling, are common, and limiting. A third of older people fall each year. Falls are inevitable if activity and mobility are encouraged – a complete absence of falls suggests inactivity or restraint.

To assess someone who has fallen or who is at risk of falls, you must understand the balance system. Four mechanisms detect postural instability:

- vision
- the vestibular system
- proprioception in the neck and legs
- tactile sensation in the feet.

The motor and musculoskeletal systems provide the effector mechanism for adjusting to disturbances. Balance is not just static (e.g. standing still), however, and posture must be maintained during walking, climbing stairs and other activities. Anticipation, sequencing, planning and judgement are also required. Abnormalities of any of these increase the tendency to fall.

Falls can be classified in several different ways.

- By main cause (about a third each):
  - acute illness – falling is a non-specific presentation of any illness in an older person, so be on the lookout for an acute illness, such as pneumonia, drug adverse effect, arrhythmia, stroke, gastrointestinal bleed, metabolic or electrolyte disturbance
  - chronic illness – in particular neurological disease, especially Parkinson's disease and stroke, but also including dementia, arthritis, visual problems
  - environmental – accidents, tripping, lighting.
- Predisposition and precipitation:
  - anyone can fall – what varies is chance that any given activity, trauma or insult will result in failure to maintain balance, and the likelihood of a resulting injury
  - a long list of risk factors has been described – including previous falls, chronic neurological disease, lower limb arthritis and proximal muscle weakness, abnormal gait, history of heart disease, postural hypotension, taking four or more prescription drugs (especially sedative, neuroleptic, and antidepressant medication), poor vision and foot problems. The more risk factors the greater the chance of falling, so interventions tend to be multi-factorial, to remove or reduce as many risk factors as possible
  - the precipitant may or may not be obvious – a single adequate explanation (syncope, acute stroke, heart attack, pulmonary embolus, trauma, tripping, misjudgement) should be sought, but will often be uncertain.
- Syncopal or non-syncopal, or association with dizziness:
  - syncope (loss of consciousness) has particular diagnostic implications that must be recognized (head trauma, cardiovascular, epileptic, hypoglycaemic – Table 25.2)
  - syncope is often associated with amnesia for the event (in 30 per cent)
  - dizziness may give diagnostic clues – there are three main types:
    - presyncope – 'light headedness, as if about to faint', blurred or darkened vision, possibly tinnitus. Generally implies a cardiovascular cause
    - vertigo – a spinning sensation. Implies vestibular or brainstem dysfunction
    - dysequilibrium – the perception of unsteadiness, more non-specific, but may be neurological or musculoskeletal in origin. A brief (few seconds) dysequilibrium occurs when the (arthritic) neck is extended during standing.

Falls assessment

- Most helpful is the 'predisposition and precipitant model':
  - First explain the fall – what happened and why did it happen?
  - Then identify what risk factors make this individual prone to fall.
- If there is syncope, an unexplained fall, or memory impairment you need a history from a witness.
- What were the circumstances of the fall?
  - What was the patient doing?
  - Was there a clear and sufficient cause (tripping, being pushed, falling out of bed, standing without habitually required supervision)?
- Was there any warning?
  - Did the patient complain of feeling dizzy?

Table 25.2 Causes of presyncope and syncope

Factor	Comment	Investigation
Head trauma	Usually obvious, look for lacerations, beware cervical spine injury	CT brain if suspected intracranial bleeding (drowsy, features of raised intracranial pressure, focal neurology)
Epilepsy	Generalized seizures. Get a description from a witness. Ask about ictal and post-ictal features.	CT brain, glucose, electrolytes, electroencephalogram
Intracranial bleeding	Primary or subarachnoid haemorrhage. Highly unlikely to be transient unless it precipitates a seizure	CT brain ± angiography
Hypoglycaemia	Loss of consciousness only if severe, unless it precipitates a seizure	Glucometer
Vasovagal syncope	3Ps – provocation, posture, prodrome	Clinical diagnosis
Postural hypotension	Usually due to drugs, also autonomic neuropathy, or age related autonomic dysfunction	Lying and standing blood pressure, or head up tilt test; autonomic function tests
Carotid sinus hypersensitivity	Cardioinhibitory and vasodepressor types	Head up tilt-table test
Other provoked syncopes	Micturition, defecation, cough	Clinical diagnosis
Bradyarrhythmias	Heart block, Stokes–Adams attacks, sick sinus syndrome	ECG, 24-hour ECG
Tachyarrhythmias	Sustained or paroxysmal, atrial fibrillation, supraventricular tachycardia, ventricular tachycardia	ECG, 24-hour ECG
Severe aortic stenosis	Typically exertional syncope (but uncommon)	Echocardiography
Acute myocardial infarction	Temporary or permanent myocardial damage and pump failure; provoked transient arrhythmia; vasovagal secondary to pain	ECG, cardiac markers (e.g. troponins)

CT, computed tomography; ECG, electrocardiography.

- Was there time to sit down, or did they fall to the ground?
- What did they look like? Cardiovascular causes often cause a 'deathly pallor'. Generalized epilepsy causes transient respiratory arrest, and the patient may go blue. Convulsion, tongue biting or incontinence may be evident.
- Were there associated symptoms such as chest pain, or breathlessness? Or ear symptoms such as (new) deafness, pain, tinnitus or discharge?
- Did anyone take the pulse?
- Has this happened before?
  - If so, how often?
  - Are there obvious precipitants?
- Take a drug history.
  - Is there anything recently started?
  - Is acute or chronic alcohol excess involved?

- Assess general function, including transfers, walking, stairs, outdoor mobility, dressing and bladder function (hurrying to the toilet can lead to lapses of judgement; nocturia is another occasion of risk).
- Examination during a syncopal episode is invaluable, especially pulse, blood pressure (ECG rhythm strip if available), respiratory rate or neurological signs (tone, plantar responses).
- Between attacks a thorough cardiovascular, neurological, musculoskeletal and ear examination is required:
  - check postural blood pressure. Examine for heart murmurs, suggesting aortic stenosis or other structural abnormalities such as hypertrophic cardiomyopathy. Get an echocardiogram if suspicious

- test visual acuity (separately in each eye) and examine for cataracts. Are the spectacles up to date?
- test visual fields, and for visual inattention. Examine for parkinsonism (cogwheel rigidity, best felt at the wrist), bradykinesia (touch the thumb on each finger in turn) and tremor. Examine for pyramidal (upper motor neurone) lesions – weakness, increased tone and reflexes, upgoing plantar responses. Pronator drift is a sensitive test for subtle weakness. Also test proximal muscle power (shoulder abduction, hip flexion), and for lower limb sensation loss (pin prick, vibration, proprioception)
- test cerebellar function (finger–nose ataxia, dysdiadochokinesia)
- examine the neck for cervical spondylosis, hips and knees for arthritis (unsteadiness either due to mechanical instability or 'nociceptive inhibition', giving sudden loss of supporting muscle tone around an acutely painful joint). Examine the feet for overgrown toenails (onychogryphosis), corns and calluses, ulcers and other deformities
- check hearing, examine the tympanic membranes, and do Romberg's test.

CLINICAL PEARL

- Transient ischaemic attack (TIA) does not cause syncope or presyncope.
- Isolated vertigo (with no other associated neurological features) is usually due to vestibular dysfunction.
- Hyperventilation can cause dizziness (symptoms are reproduced by hyperventilating).
- Vasovagal syncope always occurs standing up; there is a clear precipitant (pain, fear, smell) and some presyncopal warning symptoms before the loss of consciousness.

Tests

Choice of tests will be guided by prior assessment:

- If on insulin or sulphonylurea drugs (e.g. gliclazide) always test the blood sugar by glucometer (finger prick test).

- If syncopal or presyncopal, postural blood pressure, electrocardiogram (ECG), echocardiography and 24-hour ECG can be useful. Other autonomic function tests may be useful to make the diagnosis of autonomic neuropathy. The diagnostic yield of echocardiography and 24-hour ECG is low, and these tests should not be used indiscriminately in the absence of appropriate findings from the history or clinical examination.
  - A 24-hour ECG recording can be difficult to interpret. It will often show multiple ventricular or supraventricular ectopic beats (often of no significance), and even runs of such beats (of no particular diagnostic value). Paroxysmal atrial fibrillation requires that the rhythm be sustained for some minutes at least. There may be bradycardia, particularly at night, which is only of importance if associated with second or third degree heart block, or is clearly symptomatic. Pauses less than 3 seconds are usually not significant. There may be false negatives – if there are no symptoms during the 24-hour period, it is unlikely that a diagnostic rhythm will be captured. If the clinical features are sufficiently suspicious, you can go on to 48- or 72-hour recordings, cardiomemo (a device which records during symptoms only), or an implantable loop recorder.
  - 70° head up tilt testing is useful to investigate otherwise unexplained syncope, looking to diagnose carotid sinus syndrome. However, this is lengthy (45–60 minutes), labour intensive to perform, and may give false positive results.
- CT or MRI is only required when specifically indicated. Fits require neuroimaging. Bony injury resulting from falls will require appropriate imaging.

Falls prevention programmes commonly employ environmental assessment and modification, usually by an occupational therapist, to reduce hazards, optimize equipment and appliances, and review lighting.

Incontinence and lower urinary tract symptoms

There are three caveats on urinary incontinence:

- As a non-specific presentation, new incontinence can be caused by any acute illness, as likely as not outside the urinary tract. You only know if the incontinence is new by asking about what went before. This type of incontinence gets better with the underlying illness.

- Not all incontinence is caused by urinary tract infection – but a urine dipstick screen, and culture if positive, is mandatory. Over-diagnosing urinary tract infection causes other things to be missed.
- Beware 'functional incontinence' – wetting caused not because the bladder is abnormal but because of immobility, communication difficulties or inability to find a toilet (especially after stroke or for a demented person in a strange hospital ward).

The majority of longer-term bladder problems among older people are caused by detrusor instability (overactive bladder), followed by incomplete bladder emptying (retention). Urgency and nocturia can be almost as troublesome as incontinence itself. Urologists have a saying that 'the bladder is an unreliable witness', meaning that it is difficult to make accurate diagnoses from symptoms alone.

> **IMPORTANT**
> Remember that urethral catheters are always a last resort. If someone is admitted with one, find out why it is there, and if there is no good reason (i.e. retention) suggest a trial without.

The cardinal feature of an overactive bladder is urinary urgency (inability to postpone the desire to void). Urgency may be brought on by trigger factors: the 'key in the door phenomenon', bumpy rides, the sound of running water. Other symptoms include urinary frequency and nocturia. Many cases represent primary detrusor instability, but other causes include any neurological disease (e.g. stroke, dementia, multiple sclerosis), prostatic hyperplasia, bladder infections, cancers and stones, and oestrogen deficiency. Fast filling also provokes unstable bladder contractions, in part responsible for the havoc caused by loop diuretics.

Examination has a limited role, apart from excluding neurological disease, and feeling for an enlarged bladder and prostate gland per rectum (but even then this is a poor guide). Older women may

be examined for atrophic urethritis, but essentially all older women are oestrogen deficient. The gold standard for diagnosis is cystometry, which is invasive and unpleasant, but may be useful if an enlarged prostate is responsible. A frequency volume diary over 3 days gives a lot of information, including functional bladder capacity (normal is 350–600 mL), which is likely to be low (150–250 mL) in detrusor instability, frequency (less than seven times by day and once at night is normal) and the day/night split of urine production.

Some people with incontinence, especially in dementia, will not be cured, and a routine of prompted voiding (say every 2 hours), along with adequate containment is the best that can be achieved. However, in assessment, do not miss quick wins such as infection, the effects of drugs or retention.

Nocturia is a big issue for older people, resulting in disturbed sleep and falls. There are many 'medical causes' that must be identified, including:

- diabetes
- heart failure, especially with leg oedema
- hypercalcaemia
- alcohol or tea drunk in the evening
- lithium drugs.

Many cases of nocturia are due to age-related nocturnal polyuria – a loss of diurnal production of antidiuretic hormone and renal insensitivity to it. A day/night split with more than a third produced at night is diagnostic (in younger adults urine production halves during sleep).

Incomplete emptying is easier to assess nowadays with the use of portable ultrasound scanners. They must be used post void. Anything less than 100 mL is normal, and although symptoms are unlikely with anything less than 300 mL residual, any residual over 100 mL precludes the use of anticholinergic bladder-stabilizing drugs. Causes include anticholinergic drugs, prostatic enlargement, faecal impaction, spinal cord disease and detrusor failure. Check renal function and prostate specific antigen, and do a rectal exam (or abdominal X-ray) to assess for faecal loading (as well as examining the prostate).

You can ask about 'obstructive' urinary symptoms including poor stream, hesitancy (slowness to get started), intermittency (stop–start flow) and terminal dribbling. A urine flow rate (the urology clinic will have a machine), cystoscopy or cystometry make the diagnosis formally.

Faecal incontinence may be due to diarrhoea, in which case investigate it in its own right. Describe stool type if possible using the Bristol Stool Scale. Do not miss cases caused by drugs or laxatives. Otherwise it can be due to constipation with overflow (the rectum produces mucus, which gets stained with faeces and passed as 'spurious diarrhoea'), or more commonly, a disinhibited 'neurogenic' colon (equivalent to the unstable bladder), caused by neurological disease (Box 25.5). This is a diagnosis of exclusion. Apart from a 'bowel regimen' (constipate with loperamide and electively evacuate with an enema – unpleasant and disliked by patients unless it is the only way to remain at home), trying to predict bowel movements and containment are all that can be done. A diary may help to identify patterns.

BOX 25.5 CAUSES OF FAECAL INCONTINENCE
- Constipation with overflow incontinence
- Disinhibited 'neurogenic' colon
- Diarrhoea
- Laxatives or other drugs
- Diminished level of consciousness or unawareness
- Immobility
- Anorectal sphincter damage

Confusion

Confusion is a vague term. It needs to be specified more precisely, in terms of behaviours and observations, and mimics such as aphasia excluded. The key distinction to make is between:

- *delirium* – abrupt onset, caused by drug or physical illness, and usually reversible

and

- *dementia* – insidious onset, long term, progressive.

But bear in mind that dementia is the strongest risk factor for delirium, and about half of cases of delirium seen in hospital will be on the background of dementia. Both have impairment of cognition –

memory, orientation, intellect, judgement. You can screen for this using the AMT or MMSE.

To distinguish between *delirium* and *dementia*, you need:

- a cognitive history from an informant
- an assessment of:
    - attention – can the patient stay on the subject and maintain a coherent stream of thought?
    - conscious level – drowsy or over-vigilant?
    - fluctuation – seen in delirium.

In delirium, there may be agitation, although apathetic hypo-active and depressive forms are equally common. Hallucinations and delusions may occur (but so may they in dementia with Lewy bodies). The presence of a physical illness may be obvious, but you may need to look hard (and in some cases no physical illness is found to explain a convincing delirium).

Dementia involves progressive impairment across several cognitive domains which is socially disabling. This is diagnosed primarily by history, but requires cognitive testing and investigation for rare 'reversible' causes and co-morbidities (brain imaging, vitamin B_{12}, folate, thyroid, liver and renal function).

SMALL PRINT
Diagnosis of subtypes (Alzheimer's, vascular, Lewy body and fronto-temporal) can be done by applying research diagnostic criteria, but is difficult, and primarily done by specialists.

Stroke

Stroke is a syndrome, a collection of signs and symptoms. It is a sudden onset (or rapidly progressive over 24 hours) focal neurological deficit of presumed vascular origin. A newer, pathologically based definition is 'focal brain injury caused by sudden interruption of blood flow'. Transient ischaemic attack is a stroke that gets better quickly, usually within the hour, and by definition within 24 hours. The importance of TIA (and other minor stroke) lies in its propensity to recur (8 per cent in a week, 17 per cent in 3 months), requiring rapid investigation and institution of secondary prevention.

The clinical manifestation of stroke depends on the site of the injury and can include: hemiparesis, hemisensory loss or hemi-neglect, visual field loss, speech and swallowing disorders, cranial nerve palsies, incoordination and cognitive impairment.

The first diagnostic task is to exclude mimics (including hypoglycaemia, fits, migraines, tumours, intercurrent illness and old stroke). The next task is to distinguish infarction from haemorrhage, which requires early brain imaging (preferably immediately, certainly within 24 hours). This has assumed a new urgency with the availability of thrombolytic therapy for use within 4.5 hours of onset for infarcts.

Stroke syndrome still requires an explanation – although in up to half of fully investigated cases no convincing cause is found. Defining stroke subtypes (e.g. using the Oxford classification system – total anterior circulation (TACS), partial anterior circulation (PACS), lacunar and posterior circulation) can help define both cause and prognosis.

- TACS is due to an occlusion of the middle cerebral artery, and so damages cortical and subcortical structures, including hemiparesis, visual field loss and higher cortical function (and often drowsiness).
- PACS is due to occlusion of a branch of the middle cerebral artery, so is often embolic (from the heart or a carotid plaque).
- Lacunar strokes (pure motor or sensory hemi-symptoms) involve small end arteries to the internal capsule – typical in hypertension, diabetes and smoking.
- Posterior circulation strokes involve the occipital cortex (isolated hemianopia), cerebellum (isolated cerebellar syndrome) or brainstem (sometimes damaging cranial nerve nuclei with contralateral hemiparesis).

Investigation requires assessing cardiac rhythm and ischaemic damage (ECG), carotid or vertebrobasilar arteries (duplex ultrasound or MR/CT angiography), and risk factors. In younger patients with no obvious cause, a bubble contrast or transoesphageal echocardiography study can identify patent foramen ovale and atrial septal aneurysms. Catches include endocarditis (clinical signs, temperature, inflammatory markers, blood cultures, echocardiography), and arteritis (specifically temporal arteritis – ask about headache and check ESR).

Intracerebral bleeds may need investigation with MR or CT angiography (for aneurysms, or vascular malformations), or interval rescanning (for tumours or vascular malformations), although in older people many deep bleeds are put down to hypertension, while superficial (lobar) bleeds are attributed to amyloid angiopathy.

> **IMPORTANT**
> Watch for patients on anticoagulants. Anyone on warfarin with new neurological signs or a persisting headache needs an immediate CT head scan; if there is bleeding reverse the anticoagulation immediately.

Hip fracture

A hip fracture results from an interplay of three things:

- trauma, usually a fall (1 per cent of hip fractures are spontaneous)
- sufficient impact (and 'correct' geometry) to break the bone
- bone that is weak enough to break, usually due to osteoporosis, but sometimes due to metastases.

Its incidence increases exponentially with age. A third of victims are dead within a year of a hip fracture. Co-morbidity and acute medical complications are very common, and are associated with mortality. Assessment should include:

- identifying why the patient fell, and whether intervention is required to prevent further falls
- identifying and optimizing co-morbidities, and rationalizing medications
- assessment of osteoporosis – it is safe to assume that all older people with a hip fracture are osteoporotic. Seek a secondary cause (steroid drugs or Cushing's syndrome, postmenopausal women, hypogonadism in men, thyrotoxicosis, smoking, alcoholism, myeloma, hyperparathyroidism), check vitamin D status, and consider treatment options.

Polymyalgia rheumatica

One of a small number of pure disorders of ageing, polymyalgia rheumatica (PMR) is almost unheard of under the age of 50. It presents with pain and stiffness around the shoulders or hips and buttocks, worse in the morning, and sometimes quite disabling. It may be undiagnosed for months as it is ascribed to arthritis, age or other co-morbidity. Once thought of, the diagnosis is confirmed by a greatly raised ESR, and a rapid response (within 48 hours) to high dose prednisolone (30 mg a day – but remember that rheumatoid arthritis may also rapidly respond to steroids). Thirty per cent also have temporal arteritis, where the urgency is greater, lest optic ischaemia or stroke occur. Ask about headache (possibly unilateral) and palpate the temporal arteries. Arrange for temporal artery biopsy if there is doubt.

Osteoarthritis

This is the commonest disabling condition in Western populations, and is seem in the majority of very elderly people, but is often ignored by their hospital doctors. Arthritis contributes to immobility, falls, depression and deconditioning. Examine the joints, exclude inflammatory arthropathies, assess function and consider therapy options, starting with analgesia (paracetamol and work upwards) and joint stabilizing muscle strengthening. Involve a physiotherapist and occupational therapist. Assess for aids and appliances, and consider arthroplasty.

SUMMARY

- Older people may present with non-specific or atypical symptoms, have multiple pathologies, lose abilities fast, be prone to complications, need explicit rehabilitation and require consideration of their environment.
- The first medical goal in assessing an older person is to explain (all) their problems in terms of diagnoses. This needs patience, commitment, thoroughness and time.
- Information gathering is a longer-term process than mere history taking. History may need to be reviewed or expanded, examination may have to be spread over more than one session, and combined with observations from nurses and therapists.
- There are many practical problems to history taking – become skilled in methods to make life easier for yourself and your aphasic, cognitively impaired, deaf, or non-English speaking patients.
- For many patients third party history (or histories) may be required, especially where there is cognitive impairment, aphasia, syncope or unexplained falls.
- Drug history is crucial and may need some effort to obtain.
- Full social and functional histories are required, in particular living arrangements, accommodation type and help available or used. Function is summarized in mobility, continence and behaviour, but a very wide range of activities should be considered, tailored to the individual being assessed.
- Learn how to examine the mental state.
- Neglected aspects of physical examination include postural blood pressure, joints, vision, and nervous system.
- Use investigations with discretion, but difficulties and complexities in diagnosis makes access to high-tech tests more rather than less necessary for older people.
- Doctors must support multi-professional working, both taking account of others' assessments and observations, but also providing help in terms of diagnostic explanation and assessment of problems or complications identified by nurses or therapists.
- Use problem lists to catalogue multiple problems and map areas of uncertainty.
- Immobility, falls, confusion and incontinence are all syndromes or disabilities that require explanation, diagnosis and assessment of where intervention might help.

FURTHER READING

Cottrell S, Davies A. 2006. *Stroke talk: a communication resource for hospital care*. London: Connect Press.

Department for Constitutional Affairs. 2007. *Mental Capacity Act 2005 Code of Practice*. London: The Stationery Office. Available at: www.dca. gov.uk/legal-policy/mental-capacity/mca-cp.pdf (accessed 19 November 2009).

Evans JG. 1990. How are the elderly different? In: Kane RL, Evans JG, MacFadyen D (eds). *Improving the health of older people: a world view*. Oxford: Oxford University Press, pp. 50–68.

Parr S, Pound C, Byng S, *et al*. 2004. *The stroke and aphasia handbook*. London: Connect Press.

26 DEATH AND THE DYING PATIENT

David Gray

INTRODUCTION

Modern medical care and procedures often extend the life expectancy of people with serious illness, delaying the point at which death seems imminent. At this point, the aim is to provide palliative care, which often requires a multidisciplinary approach to meet the needs of the patient and family.

Once it has been agreed that death cannot be avoided, and that all possible reversible causes have been considered and excluded:

- document this in the notes and, if in hospital, complete a *Do Not Attempt Resuscitation* (DNAR) form (following discussion with the patient and, where appropriate, their family)
- agree the goals of care with the patient, their family and the staff providing care
- plan a 'Last days of life' care pathway (see below)
- carry out an initial assessment, recording mental state and conscious state, current symptoms, hydration state, urinary and faecal continence, degree of pain
- make available medication to control pain, agitation, nausea and vomiting – whether for use by syringe driver, subcutaneous injection or orally
- discontinue unnecessary, non-essential treatment such as antibiotics, oxygen and intravenous fluids
- discontinue unnecessary nursing observations (temperature, pulse, blood pressure)
- avoid further blood tests
- deactivate implantable cardioverter defibrillator (ICD) if fitted – further 'shocks' are distressing and inappropriate.

It is important to talk with the patient and, with the patient's consent, with their family and close friends, to establish any preferences they have regarding care in the final stages of life; this ensures that the wishes of the dying are known and guides the most appropriate care.

> **CLINICAL PEARL**
>
> Agreement that an illness is 'terminal' should not be taken to mean that treatment should *not* be given – controlling symptoms of pain, nausea or anxiety remains a priority.

LAST DAYS OF LIFE CARE PATHWAY

- Carry out an assessment of the patient's needs: this includes their conscious level, mental state, pain control and ability to swallow.
- Assess present and future comfort measures: you may need to deal with constipation, diarrhoea, continence, oral hygiene.
- Consider appropriate means of pain control – a palliative care team will be happy to advise on oral medication, subcutaneous injection and intravenous infusion via a syringe driver. If two doses of a drug prescribed on an *as required basis* are needed, prescribe a *regular* dose
- Prescribe medication on a *prn* basis for pain, agitation, respiratory secretions, nausea and vomiting, dyspnoea.
- Review and discontinue all unnecessary medical and nursing interventions: including nursing observations, blood tests, antibiotics, intravenous fluids and medication, oxygen therapy, implantable cardioverter defibrillator.
- Complete a *Do Not Attempt Resuscitation* form.
- Assess the patient's and family's spiritual needs.
- Record the family's preference regarding notification of deterioration or death – this avoids the 'midnight phone call'.
- Provide the family with information on visiting times, car parking and hospital facilities.
- Inform the patient's general practitioner.
- Record the multidisciplinary team's care plan and goals prominently in notes.

- If the patient dies in hospital:
  - ensure the GP is informed as soon as possible
  - agree the procedure regarding 'laying out', taking into account religious, cultural and spiritual requirements
  - update the patient's details on the hospital computer system and make sure all departments cancel any outstanding appointments
  - pack the patient's property for collection by the family
  - provide the relatives with the Department for Work and Pensions booklet 'What to do after a death in England and Wales'. This can be reviewed at: www.jobcentreplus.gov.uk/JCP/stellent/groups/jcp/documents/website-content/dev_016117.pdf.

Medication

As taking medication may involve a lot of effort for a patient, try to keep the number of drugs to a minimum. In the absence of nausea and vomiting, difficulty in swallowing or coma, oral medication is usually preferred to parenteral.

You will need to be aware of the therapeutic interventions, pharmacological and non-pharmacological, for common symptoms due either to the underlying disease process or its treatment; if possible, try to establish the cause of the symptom before starting treatment. Please refer to the palliative care section of the British National Formulary for advice. Common symptoms include:

- pain
- headache
- nausea and vomiting
- intractable hiccup
- constipation
- breathlessness
- anxiety and distress
- 'death rattle'
- agitation and delirium.

TALKING TO THE PATIENT

It may seem obvious, but the patient needs to know that medical care can no longer influence the out-come and death is inevitable. Reassure the patient that treatment can still be given to control symptoms such as pain or nausea. Remember that each person has unique needs and wishes. Knowing that death cannot be postponed allows family relationships to be mended and may bring a sense of peace; involve members of the clergy if appropriate.

The emotional rollercoaster

Faced with the prospect of dying, some may 'clutch at straws' and unrealistically seek any form of treatment, usually unconventional, that might prolong life, however briefly and regardless of the potential for side effects. This is part of a well-recognized emotional process of grieving (the 'Kübler-Ross model'):

- *denial*, acting normally without accepting the inevitability of death, is often temporary and is a natural response to fear and uncertainty. This may be followed by
- *anger* ('Why me?'), followed by
- *bargaining*, and then
- *depression* once realization sets in. Finally,
- *acceptance* of the inevitability.

Frank discussion with family, friends and carers helps some to progress rapidly through these stages, though the sequence of stages may emerge in a slightly different order. Expect an emotional rollercoaster in other patients. Eventually, almost all will achieve a sense of peace that will be influenced by family support, philosophy of life and religious belief.

Staying in control

How much a patient wants to stay in control of the terminal stages of disease varies. Some wish to 'surrender' total responsibility for their care, others to retain control, even to the point of planning a funeral in great detail. Being honest is the best policy – explain that the team is still concerned about maintaining dignity and quality of life as much as possible. Give individuals a chance to express their needs and be prepared to discuss organ donation if this is appropriate.

DIFFICULT QUESTIONS

Questions the patient may ask

How long have I got?

This is hard to answer. The doctor cannot know when any individual will die – any statement is just an estimate based on everything known about the site of any cancer, its natural history, how far (and how fast) it may have spread, co-morbid factors and duration of illness. Overestimating how much time is left may raise false hopes while underestimating may destroy hope altogether. The shortest and longest a person is likely to live is more realistic.

What symptoms can I expect and what can be done to control them?

Common symptoms are pain, breathlessness, bedsores, fatigue, incontinence, poor appetite, depression, anxiety, confusion, disability and stress. These symptoms can be controlled.

Can I make my wishes known in advance of a crisis?

A 'living will' is a written statement (an *advanced decision*) or a verbal statement (an *advanced statement*) of a person's wishes relevant to a later stage when the individual is no longer able to make decisions. Only the former is legally binding, though the latter should be taken into account when deciding what is in an individual's best interests. The legal support for this process was enacted in the Mental Capacity Act 2005, enforced in late 2007. It is binding on those providing care if capacity to make decisions is lost.

If the patient has made a will, this may include an individual's preferences for treatment or care, or an advanced decision to refuse treatment. If this includes life-saving treatment, strict rules need to be adhered to:

- the decision must be in writing
- it must be signed and witnessed
- it must include a written statement that the advance decision applies to treatment *even if life is at risk*.

A *Lasting Power of Attorney* (LPA) can record an advanced statement, giving another person or persons the power to make decisions on their behalf if the individual cannot do so.

The care plan may involve decisions regarding interventions such as providing a feeding tube, resuscitation or ventilation. A useful information sheet is available from www.ageconcern.org.uk/AgeConcern/is5.asp. Different rules apply in Scotland (www.ageconcernscotland.org.uk) and Northern Ireland (www.ageconcernni.org).

Can I still become an organ donor?

This is a decision that needs to be made well in advance of death and with the full knowledge of the family. Generally, those dying of a chronic disease can donate skin, bone and corneas. Donation of organs is more likely to be considered when death occurs suddenly. A standard organ donation card should be completed.

A patient may express a desire to donate his or her body to medical science. According to the Human Tissue Authority, with the patient's consent the donated body can be used for:

- anatomical examination – for teaching the structure and function of the human body to students or healthcare professionals
- research – for scientific studies which improve the understanding of the human body
- education and training – usually for those learning surgical techniques, as opposed to anatomical examination.

Patients can find further details regarding body and tissue donation at www.hta.gov.uk/donations.cfm.

Questions caregivers may ask

How can we get the best care?

There are several options, depending on the degree of help and the amount of support needed. Emotional and social support for a dying person and family members may be provided:

- at home – some prefer to spend their last days at home. If so, arrange for all necessary treatment for comfort to be available on arrival. Also make sure all are aware of the individual's preferences regarding further medical intervention

- in a nursing home – supervision by medical and nursing staff allows regular assessment and dispensing of drugs in a timely and appropriate manner
- in a hospice – where the emphasis is to promote quality of life and ensure a dignified and comfortable death
- respite care – temporary care either in the home, nursing home or hospice intended to give carers a rest from the fulltime responsibility of providing care, and time to themselves to sort out their own affairs. Voluntary organizations such as Macmillan Cancer Relief (www.macmillan.org.uk) or Marie Curie Cancer Care (www.mariecurie.org.uk) can provide support for patients and respite care for the family.

Will the family be able to cope if we wish to take a loved one home?

Each family is different – a large extended close family can provide just about everything that is needed whereas other families will need a lot of assistance. Some families cope very well, but others may need to be advised that coping with problems arising with pain and discomfort, breathing, bodily functions, unsteadiness and mood changes (especially depression) and their own grief may be unrealistic and hospice care may be more appropriate. Spend time to discuss day-to-day issues and how doctors, nurses, carers and Macmillan nurses can provide emotional comfort and support during the last days of life.

Will we know when the time has come?

Patients may experience a change in symptoms when close to death, such as drowsiness and unresponsiveness, increasing confusion, becoming withdrawn, loss of control of bodily functions, difficulty with breathing, and increasing pain. Explain that when death does occur, there will be no respiratory effort or pulse, the pupils become dilated, the jaw relaxes, there is no response to being spoken to and bowel and bladder sphincters relax and release their contents.

What should we do when death occurs?

If the person has expressed a desire not to be resuscitated, advise the family not to dial '999' but to let immediate family members and friends (and hospice personnel if they have been involved) know. Contact the person's local doctor so that death can be officially confirmed and a death certificate issued. Call the undertaker who will arrange to remove the body.

It is a criminal offence not to register a death with the Registrar of Births, Deaths and Marriages within 5 days (a further 9 days is permissible if the registrar is aware that a death certificate has been issued); the registrar will want to know the deceased person's date and place of death; full name (including maiden name) and address; place and date of birth; occupation (if a married woman or widowed, husband's occupation); if still married, date of birth of husband/wife; and whether in receipt of pension or social security benefits.

For useful advice see:

- Citizens Advice Bureau, Advice Guide, Family – in England, What to do after a death (www.adviceguide.org.uk/index/family_parent/family/what_to_do_after_a_death.htm)
- Department for Work and Pensions booklet 'What to do after a death in England and Wales (www.jobcentreplus.gov.uk/JCP/stellent/groups/jcp/documents/websitecontent/mdev_016117.pdf).

PREPARING THE FAMILY FOR DEATH OF A LOVED ONE

Observing a loved one's gradual physical and mental decline towards death may be very distressing, especially in the last hours with the onset of confusion, fading of consciousness, skin mottling and, finally, as pharyngeal secretions accumulate, the 'death rattle'. These moments can have a lasting effect on those family members and caregivers present. Even so, seeing the body after death is important – it helps avoid denying that an individual has died and is at peace.

Disbelief, anger, depression, loneliness and disorientation, followed by yearning for a loved one are all part of the grieving process. It rarely involves getting over the death of a loved one, more coming to terms with loss and getting on with life. Disseminating the news to the more distant family members, friends and work colleagues often helps, as does planning for and attending the funeral.

DIAGNOSIS AND CONFIRMATION OF DEATH

Helpful guidelines on the diagnosis and confirmation of death are contained within the Academy of Medical Royal Colleges (AoMRC) publication *A code of practice for the diagnosis and confirmation of death* (2008). This important document covers both the diagnosis of brainstem death and the confirmation of death following cardiorespiratory arrest.

> *Death entails the irreversible loss of those essential characteristics which are necessary to the existence of a living human person and, thus, the definition of death should be regarded as the irreversible loss of the capacity for consciousness, combined with irreversible loss of the capacity to breathe.*
>
> *A code of practice for the diagnosis and confirmation of death* (AoMRC, 2008)

Death following cardiorespiratory arrest

Following cardiorespiratory arrest, the confirmation of death requires recognition of the irreversible cessation of:

- cardiac activity
- respiratory activity
- neurological (pupillary) activity.

The AoMRC code of practice advises that the point of death after a cardiorespiratory arrest is identified by the following conditions:

- simultaneous and irreversible onset of apnoea and unconsciousness in the absence of the circulation
- full and extensive attempts at reversal of any contributing cause to the cardiorespiratory arrest have been made (Box 26.1).

In addition, one of the following criteria must be fulfilled:

- the individual meets the criteria for not attempting cardiopulmonary resuscitation
- attempts at cardiopulmonary resuscitation have failed

BOX 26.1 POTENTIALLY REVERSIBLE CONTRIBUTING CAUSES OF CARDIORESPIRATORY ARREST

- Hypothermia
- Hypoxia
- Hypokalaemia and hyperkalaemia (and other metabolic causes)
- Hypovolaemia
- Toxic/therapeutic (e.g. narcotics, tranquillizers)
- Tension pneumothorax
- Tamponade (cardiac)
- Thrombosis (coronary/pulmonary)

- treatment aimed at sustaining life has been withdrawn because:
  - it has been decided to be of no further benefit to the patient and not in their best interest to continue *and/or:*
  - it is in respect of the patient's wishes via an advance decision to refuse treatment.

Under these circumstances, the person responsible for confirming death should observe the patient for at least 5 minutes while noting the:

- absence of a central pulse on palpation
- absence of heart sounds on auscultation
- absence of respiratory movements and breath sounds on auscultation.

If there is any return of spontaneous cardiorespiratory activity during this period of observation, a further 5 minutes of observation is required (commencing at the next onset of cardiorespiratory arrest). After 5 minutes of cardiorespiratory arrest has been observed, the next step is to confirm:

- fixed, dilated pupils (pupils unresponsive to light)
- absence of corneal reflexes
- absence of motor response to painful stimulus (supraorbital pressure).

These observations should be recorded in the case notes, with the date and time of death being the point at which these criteria were met.

Brainstem death

For a comatose patient who has a heartbeat but is apnoeic (and therefore supported by a ventilator),

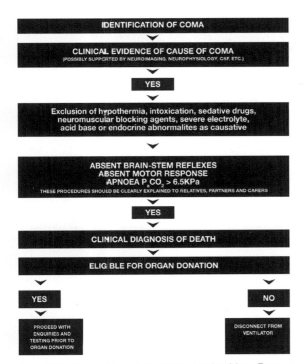

Figure 26.1 Diagnostic and management algorithm. From: Academy of Medical Royal Colleges (2008) *A code of practice for the diagnosis and confirmation of death.*

death can by diagnosed (in the UK) by confirming the irreversible cessation of brainstem function. From a legal standpoint, the UK does not have a statutory definition of death, but the courts have adopted the criteria for brainstem death as part of the law. The situation is different in the USA, where 'whole brain death', rather than death of the brainstem alone, is the diagnostic criterion (www.bioethics.gov/reports/death/index.html).

Figure 26.1 outlines the key steps in establishing a diagnosis of brainstem death. Brainstem testing should only be undertaken if there is irreversible brain damage, of known aetiology, and potentially reversible causes of coma have been excluded:

- depressant drugs
- primary hypothermia
- potentially reversible circulatory, metabolic and endocrine disturbances
- potentially reversible causes of apnoea (e.g. neuromuscular blocking agents).

The diagnosis of death following irreversible cessation of brainstem function is confirmed by the following criteria:

- pupils fixed and unresponsive to sharp changes in light
- absent corneal reflex
- absent oculo-vestibular reflexes (Fig. 26.2)
- absent motor responses within the cranial nerve distribution despite adequate stimulation of any somatic area
- absent cough reflex response to bronchial stimulation (by a suction catheter placed down the trachea to the carina), or absent gag response (to stimulation of the posterior pharynx with a spatula)
- apnoea test (absence of a spontaneous respiratory response to hypercarbia ($PaCO_2$ >6.5 kPa) over a 5-minute period). The apnoea test should be performed last, and only if all the preceding tests have shown absent brainstem reflexes.

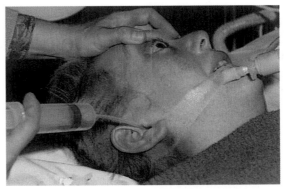

Figure 26.2 Testing vestibulo-ocular reflexes by injecting ice-cold water into the external auditory canal. From: Ogilvie C, Evans CC (eds), *Chamberlain's symptoms and signs in clinical medicine* (12th edition), with permission. © 1997 London: Hodder Arnold.

The brainstem tests should be undertaken by two medical practitioners, acting together, who have been registered for over 5 years, who are competent in performing and interpreting brainstem tests, and at least one of whom is a consultant. There must be no clinical conflicts of interest and the medical practitioners should not be members of the transplant team. It is common for one doctor to perform the tests while the other observes and then (if the first set

Diagnosis is to be made by two doctors who have been registered for more than five years and are competent in the procedure. At least one should be a consultant. Testing should be undertaken by the doctors together and must always be performed completely and successfully on two occasions in total.

Patient Name: **Unit No:**

Pre-conditions

Are you satisfied that the patient suffers from a condition that has led to irreversible brain damage?

Specify the condition:

Dr A: **Dr B:**

Time of onset of unresponsive coma:

Dr A: **Dr B:**

Are you satisfied that potentially reversible causes for the patient's condition have been adequately excluded, in particular:

	DR A:	DR B:
DEPRESSANT DRUGS		
NEUROMUSCULAR BLOCKING DRUGS		
HYPOTHERMIA		
METABOLIC OR ENDOCRINE DISTURBANCES		

TESTS FOR ABSENCE OF BRAIN-STEM FUNCTION	1ST SET OF TESTS	2ND SET OF TESTS	1ST SET OF TESTS	2ND SET OF TESTS
DO THE PUPILS REACT TO LIGHT?				
ARE THERE CORNEAL REFLEXES?				
IS THERE EYE MOVEMENT ON CALORIC TESTING?				
ARE THERE MOTOR RESPONSES IN THE CRANIAL NERVE DISTRIBUTION IN RESPONSE TO STIMULATION OF FACE, LIMBS OR TRUNK?				
IS THE GAG REFLEX PRESENT?				
IS THERE A COUGH REFLEX?				
HAVE THE RECOMMENDATIONS CONCERNING TESTING FOR APNOEA BEEN FOLLOWED?				
WERE THERE ANY RESPIRATORY MOVEMENTS SEEN?				

Date and time of first set of tests:

Date and time of second set of tests:

Dr A Signature: **Dr B Signature:**

Status: **Status:`**

Figure 26.3 Procedure for the diagnosis and confirmation of cessation of brainstem function by neurological testing of brainstem reflexes. From: Academy of Medical Royal Colleges (2008) *A code of practice for the diagnosis and confirmation of death.*

of tests shows no evidence of brainstem activity) for the doctors to swap roles for a repeat set of tests after a period of time has elapsed. The findings should be documented using a pro forma such as the one shown in Figure 26.3.

SUMMARY

The dying patient:

- at some point, the focus of medical treatment switches from active intervention to palliative care. Death is inevitable
- document this in the notes and plan a 'Last days of life' care pathway
- carry out an initial assessment and agree among caring staff the goals of care
- discontinue unnecessary treatment, avoid further blood tests, stop temperature, pulse, blood pressure checks and deactivate ICD if fitted
- even though an illness is 'terminal', treatment should still be available to control common symptoms, especially pain, agitation, nausea and vomiting
- establish the patient's wishes and any preferences regarding care in the final stages of life.

Following cardiorespiratory arrest, death is confirmed by:

- absence of a central pulse on palpation
- absence of heart sounds on auscultation
- absence of respiratory movements and breath sounds on auscultation
- fixed, dilated pupils (pupils unresponsive to light)
- absence of corneal reflexes
- absence of motor response to painful stimulus (supra-orbital pressure).

Brainstem death – irreversible cessation of brainstem function is confirmed by the following criteria:

- pupils fixed and unresponsive to sharp changes in light
- absent corneal reflex
- absent oculo-vestibular reflexes
- absent motor responses within the cranial nerve distribution despite adequate stimulation of any somatic area
- absent cough reflex or gag response
- apnoea test (absence of a spontaneous respiratory response to hypercarbia).

FURTHER READING

Academy of Medical Royal Colleges. 2008. *A code of practice for the diagnosis and confirmation of death*. Available at: www.aomrc.org.uk/aomrc/admin/reports/docs/DofD-final.pdf (accessed 1 November 2009).

Ellershaw J, Wilkinson S, Saunders C. 2003. *Care of the dying: a pathway to excellence*. Oxford: Oxford University Press.

Firth S. 2001. *Wider horizons: care of the dying in a multicultural society*. London: National Council for Hospice and Specialist Palliative Care Services.

Liverpool Care Pathway (LCP) for the dying patient. Available at www.liv.ac.uk/mcpcil/liverpool-care-pathway/index.htm (accessed 1 November 2009).

National End of Life Care Programme. Available at www.endoflifecareforadults.nhs.uk/eolc/ (accessed 1 November 2009).

FURTHER READING

CLINICAL EXAMINATION AND DIAGNOSIS

Douglas G, Nicol F, Robertson C. 2009. *Macleod's clinical examination*, 12th edn. Edinburgh: Churchill Livingstone.

Epstein O, Perkin GD, Cookson J, *et al.* 2008. *Clinical examination*, 4th edn. London: Mosby.

Huw Llewelyn H, Ang HA, Lewis KE, Al Abdullah A. 2009. *Oxford handbook of clinical diagnosis.* Oxford: Oxford University Press.

Talley NJ, O'Connor S. 2005. *Clinical examination: a systematic guide to physical diagnosis*, 5th edn. Edinburgh: Churchill Livingstone.

Thomas J, Monaghan T. 2007. *Oxford handbook of clinical examination and practical skills.* Oxford: Oxford University Press.

GENERAL MEDICINE

Boon NA, Colledge NR, Walker BR, Hunter JAA. 2006. *Davidson's principles and practice of medicine*, 20th edn. Edinburgh: Churchill Livingstone.

Kumar P, Clark M. 2009. *Kumar and Clark clinical medicine*, 7th edn. London: WB Saunders.

Longmore M, Wilkinson I, Turmezei T, Cheung CK. 2007. *Oxford handbook of clinical medicine*, 7th edn. Oxford: Oxford University Press.

Index